Short Textbook of
Orthopedics
for Undergraduate Students

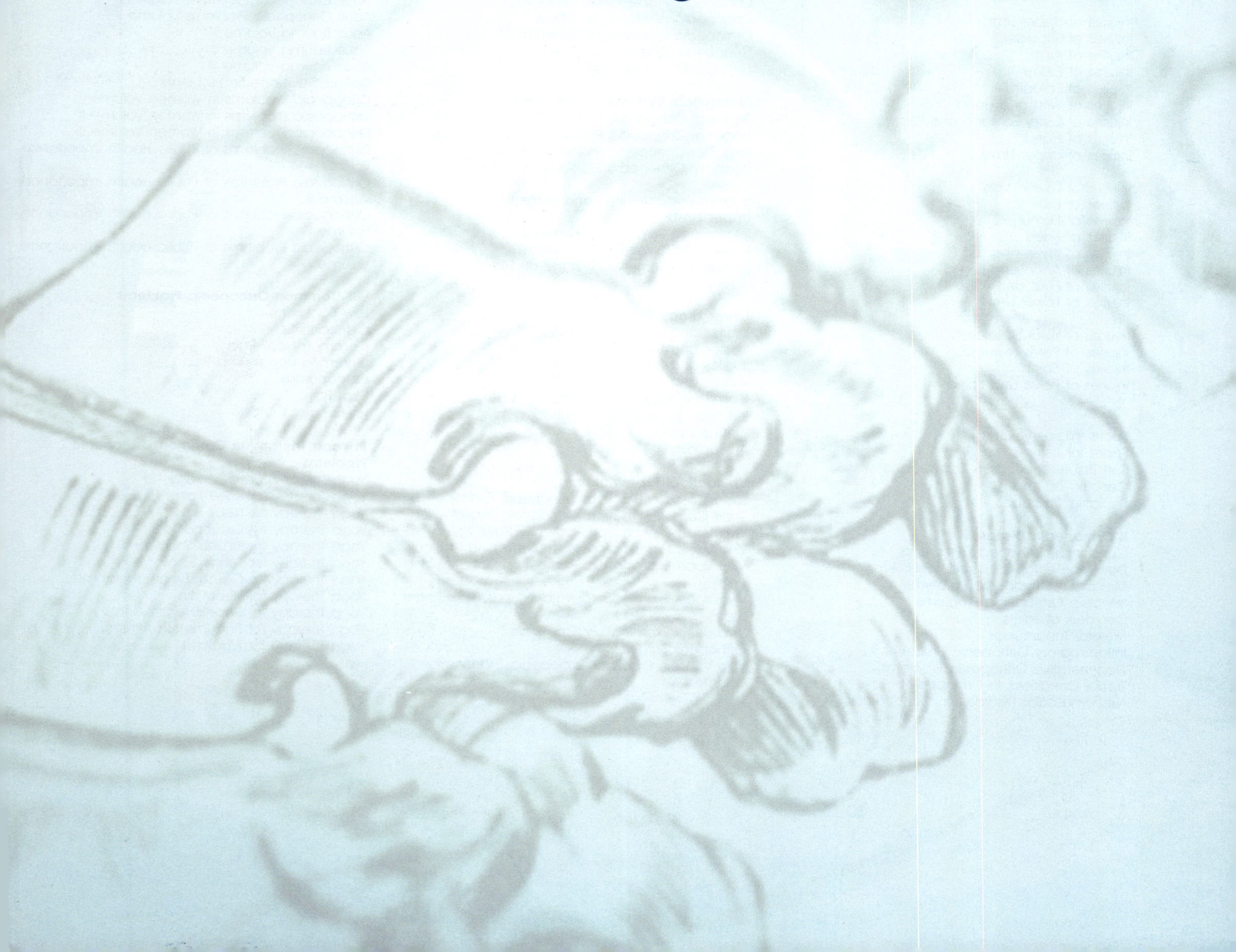

Dr John Ebnezar

Guinness World Record Holder
in writing the maximum number of books (8)
in one year

—An outstanding performance

Other CBS Book by the Same Author

• Common Orthopedic Problems

103 titles

I Orthopedic Trauma
General Fractures
General Principles of Fractures and Dislocations
Fracture Treatment Methods
Fractures and their Complications
Atypical Fractures

Injuries of Upper Limb
Injuries of Shoulder
Injuries of Arm
injuries of Elbow
Injuries of Forearm
Injuries of Wrist and Hand
Injuries of Distal Forearm and Wrist
Injuries of Hand
Injuries of Upper Limb

Injuries of Lower Limb
Injuries of Hip
Injuries of Femur
Injuries of Knee
Injuries of Knee and Leg
Injuries of Ankle and Leg
Injuries of Foot and Ankle
Injuries of Lower Limb

Injuries of Axial Skeleton
Injuries of Pelvis and Hip
Injuries of Spine
Injuries of Pelvis and Spine

Sports Injuries Volume I
Sports Injuries Volume II
Soft Tissue Problems in Orthopedics
Geriatric Trauma
Pediatric Trauma

II Orthopedic Disease
Congenital Orthopedic Problems
Developmental Orthopedic Problems
Metabolic Orthopedic Problems
Infective Orthopedic Problems
Disorders of Joints
Skeletal Tuberculosis
Inflammatory Orthopedic Problems
Degenerative Orthopedic Problems
Tumor Conditions in Orthopedics
Neuromuscular Disorders in Orthopedics

III Specific Orthopedic Problems
Orthopedic Problems of Spine
Orthopedic Problems of Neck
Orthopedic Problems of Hip
Orthopedic Problems of Knee
Orthopedic Problems of Foot
Orthopedic Problems of Shoulder
Orthopedic Problems of Elbow
Orthopedic Problems of Forearm
Orthopedic Problems of Wrist
Orthopedic Problems of Hand

IV Regional Orthopedic Problems
Regional Orthopedic Problems of Upper Limb
Regional Orthopedic Problems of Lower Limb
Regional Orthopedic Problems of Spine
Regional Orthopedic Problems of Hand

V Orthopedic Injuries and Surgeries
Upper Limb
Injuries and Surgeries of Humerus
Injuries and Surgeries of Forearm
Injuries and Surgeries of Hand and Wrist

Lower Limb
Injuries and Surgeries of Hip
Injuries and Surgeries of Femur
Injuries and Surgeries of Tibia
Injuries and Surgeries of Foot and Ankle
Common Surgeries of Spine
Interlocking Surgeries in Orthopedics
Arthroscopy
Arthroplasty

VI Practical Examination
Long Cases in Practical Orthopedic Examination
Short Cases in Practical Orthopedic Examination
Viva Voce Examination: Typical X-Rays
Viva Voce Examination: Instruments and Implants
Viva Voce Examination: Prosthetics, Orthotics and
Traction
Viva Voce Examination: Ward Rounds, Specimen
Slides and Spotters
Viva Voca Examination: Common
OrthopedicSurgeries
Viva Voce in Practical Orthopedic Examination
Volume I

Viva Voce in Practical Orthopedic Examination
Volume II

VII Orthopedic Problems of Different Ages
Pediatric Orthopedic Problems
Adult Orthopedic Problems Volume I
Adult Orthopedic Problems Volume II
Adult Trauma Volume I
Adult Trauma Volume II
Adult Trauma Volume III
Geriatric Orthopedic Problems
Orthopedic Problems in Women Volume I
Orthopedic Problems in Women Volume II
Orthopedic Problems in Women Volume III
Orthopedic Problems of Public Health Importance
Volume I
Orthopedic Problems of Public Health Importance
Volume II
Orthopedic Problems of Public Health Importance
Volume III
Orthopedic Problems of Public Health Importance
Volume IV

VIII Common Orthopedic Problems
Low Backache
Osteoarthritis
Common Neck Pain
Common Upper Limb Pain
Osteoporosis
Foot Pain
Rheumatoid Arthritis

IX Yoga Therapy in Common Orthopedic
Problems
Yoga Therapy for Low Backache
Yoga Therapy for Knee Pain
Yoga Therapy for Neck Pain
Yoga Therapy for Osteoporosis
Yoga Therapy for Frozen Shoulder
Yoga Therapy for Tennis Elbow
Yoga Therapy for Carpal Tunnel Syndrome
Yoga Therapy for Heel Pain
Yoga Therapy for Repetitive Stress Injury
Yoga Therapy for Rheumatoid Arthritis
Yoga Therapy for Fractures

Short Textbook of
Orthopedics
for Undergraduate Students

John Ebnezar

MBBS, D'Ortho, MD (Ortho-Hons), DNB (Ortho), MNAMS (Ortho), Honorary Doctorate in Medicine (Ortho)
PhD (Yoga), Sports Medicine (Australia), IOA-INOR Fellow (United Kingdom)
Padma Shri Awardee (2016) • Dr BC Roy National Awardee
Author of over 200 books in orthopedics
Consulting orthopedic surgeon, sports specialist, spine surgeon and wholistic orthopedic expert
Geriatric orthopedic surgeon
Former Vice President, Indian Orthopedic Association
Founder President, Geriatric Orthopedic Society of India
Founder Director, Geriatric Orthopedic Association of India
Founder President, Orthopedic Authors' Association, and All India Medical Author's Association
President, Neuro-Spinal Surgeons Association of India (Karnataka)
Chairman, Karnataka Orthopedic Academy®
President, Bangalore WHOlistic Academy
President, Vaidya Kala Ranga, Bangalore
Medical Superintendant, CV Raman General Hospital, Indiranagar, Bangalore
CEO, Parimala Health Care Services (An ISO 9001:2008 Hospital), Bangalore
Chief Orthopedic and Spine Surgeon, Dr John's Orthopedic Center, Bangalore
Chairman, Ebnezar Medical Institute
Editor in Chief, *Journal of the Geriatric Orthopedic Association of India*
Editor, *Journal of Yoga and Physiotherapy*
Guinness World Record Achiever in Book Writing (2010)
2nd World Record in Book Writing—103 Books (2012)
Email: *johnebnezar@gmail.com* Website: *www.johnebnezar.com*

Rakesh John
MBBS, MS (PGI), DNB, MRCS (England), Dip. SICOT, MNAMS
Completed Senior Residency from PGIMER, Chandigarh

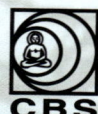

CBS Publishers & Distributors Pvt Ltd

New Delhi • Bengaluru • Chennai • Kochi • Kolkata • Mumbai
Hyderabad • Jharkhand • Nagpur • Patna • Pune • Uttarakhand

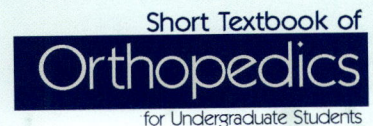

Short Textbook of
Orthopedics
for Undergraduate Students

ISBN: 978-93-86478-69-6

First Edition: 2018

Published by Satish Kumar Jain and Produced by Varun Jain for
CBS Publishers & Distributors Pvt Ltd
4819/XI Prahlad Street, 24 Ansari Road, Daryaganj, New Delhi 110 002, India.
Ph: 23289259, 23266861, 23266867   Fax: 011-23243014   Website: www.cbspd.com
e-mail: delhi@cbspd.com; cbspubs@airtelmail.in.

Corporate Office: 204 FIE, Industrial Area, Patparganj, Delhi 110 092, India
Ph: 4934 4934   Fax: 4934 4935   e-mail: publishing@cbspd.com; publicity@cbspd.com

Branches

- **Bengaluru:** Seema House 2975, 17th Cross, K.R. Road,
  Banasankari 2nd Stage, Bengaluru 560 070, Karnataka, India
  Ph: +91-80-26771678/79   Fax: +91-80-26771680   e-mail: bangalore@cbspd.com
- **Chennai:** 7, Subbaraya Street, Shenoy Nagar, Chennai 600 030, Tamil Nadu, India
  Ph: +91-44-26260666, 26208620   Fax: +91-44-42032115   e-mail: chennai@cbspd.com
- **Kochi:** Ashana House, No. 39/1904, AM Thomas Road, Valanjambalam, Ernakulam 682 016, Kochi, Kerala, India
  Ph: +91-484-4059061-65   Fax: +91-484-4059065   e-mail: kochi@cbspd.com
- **Kolkata:** No. 6/B, Ground Floor, Rameswar Shaw Road, Kolkata-700014 (West Bengal), India
  Ph: +91-33-2289-1126, 2289-1127, 2289-1128   e-mail: kolkata@cbspd.com
- **Mumbai:** 83-C, Dr E Moses Road, Worli, Mumbai-400018, Maharashtra, India
  Ph: +91-22-24902340/41   Fax: +91-22-24902342   e-mail: mumbai@cbspd.com

Representatives

- **Hyderabad** 0-9885175004
- **Jharkand** 0-9811541605
- **Nagpur** 0-9021734563
- **Patna** 0-9334159340
- **Pune** 0-9623451994
- **Uttarakhand** 0-9716462459

Printed at: Magic International Pvt. Ltd, Greater Noida, UP, India

to

my mother
(Late) Sampath Kumari
who taught me that life is more than self
and there is more joy in giving and sharing
than taking

my family
who are an epitome of love,
sacrifice, encouragement and inspiration

all my teachers
who made me what I am today

and

all my students
past and present

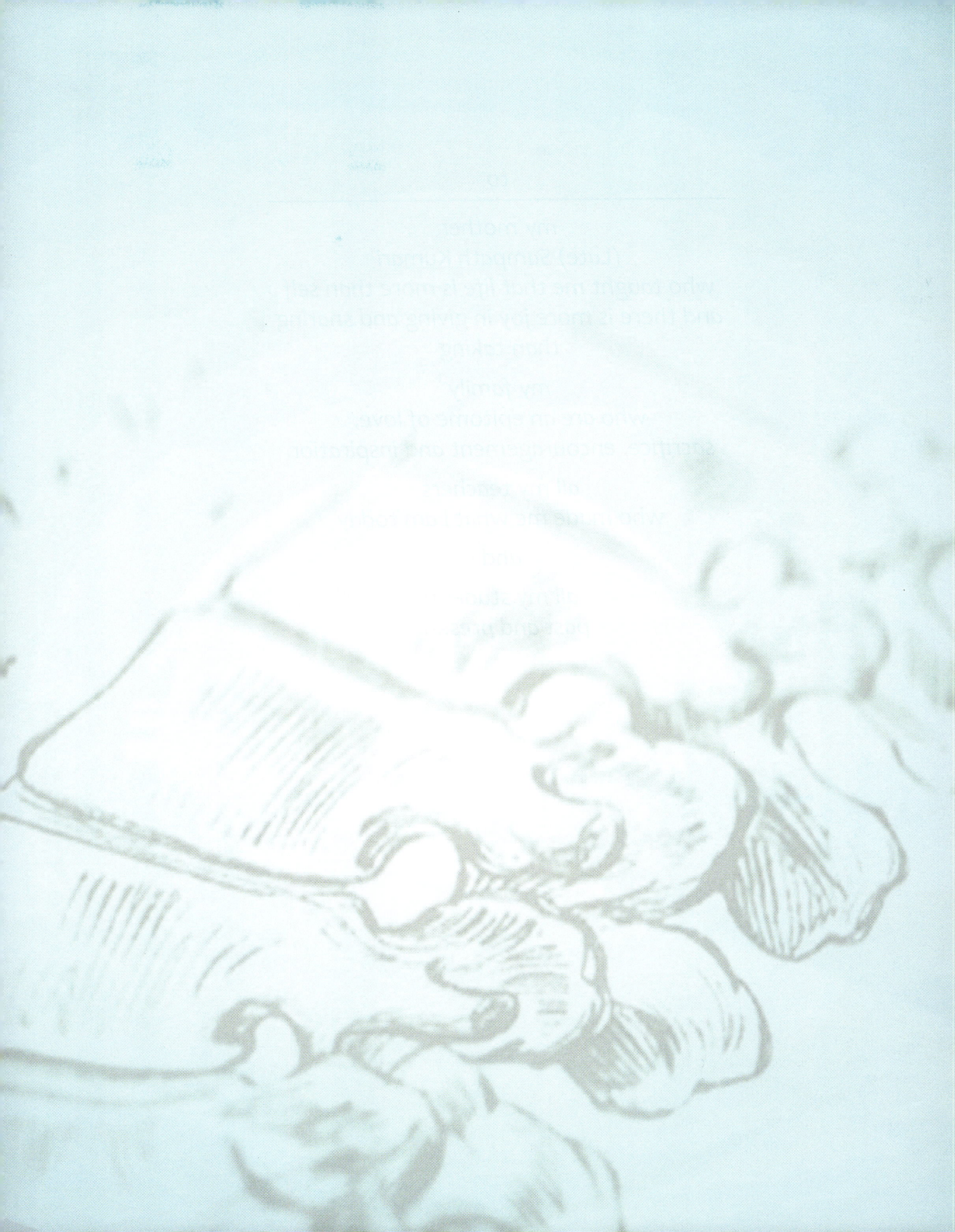

Preface

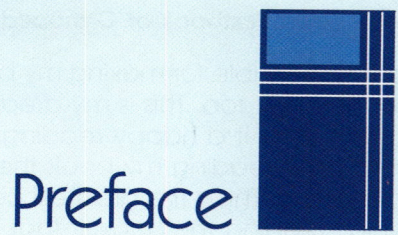

When my *Textbook of Orthopedics* hit the market 21 years back it was an instant hit with the students. Students liked the format of the book immensely and the innovations and certain special features which were hitherto unknown in the field of medical book writing made it very appealing to the students. But slowly I realized that though the book was universally liked, undergraduate students were slowly distancing themselves away from the book due to the contents which they felt was more for them and were reading other smaller books. Meanwhile I noticed another trend, that though I had written the book keeping undergraduates in mind, the book had gained acceptance among the unexpected postgraduate students of orthopedics. This was totally unexpected but the book had gained more acceptances with them. The undergraduate students felt that the matter in my book was more for them and they found it difficult to read as they were already burdened with the major clinical subjects in the final year.

Wherever I went, be it medical colleges or conferences or CMEs, undergraduate students used to flock to me and express their anguish that though they liked my book immensely they were forced to read other books as the book was slightly beyond them. They urged me to bring a smaller version of the book so that they could read my book. This set me thinking. Then some of the teaching colleagues in various medical colleges across the country also urged me to bring a smaller book for undergraduates and upgrade the present book to the postgraduate level as they were already reading my book and was possessed almost by every postgraduate student.

Respecting their feelings, sentiments and requirements I decided to bring out a book exclusively for the undergraduate medical students. Then I was faced with another dilemma, some of the existing books for UG students were too short and condensed and very elementary. I was in a fix whether to emulate them or keep the book short but yet give adequate and necessary information. After dilly-dallying for long and after confabulating with students and teachers, I chose the middle path of not condensing the book too much or giving too much information. So this book is now in your hands. Believe me it has taken enormous effort on my part and also on the part of the publishers to make this a unique book which will be cherished by the medical students.

Highlights

- The text is printed in 4-color and has a very attractive design
- The text has been divided into 12 sections.
- The chapters are short and crisp for easy reading.
- Language is kept simple and lucid.
- Good color diagrams.
- Includes a number of good clinical photographs
- Good classical X-rays have been incorporated wherever necessary
- Breaking away from the conventional practice, lots of original, innovative and thought-provoking diagrams have been introduced, which hopefully the students will like.

My earlier books have been widely appreciated for columns like quick facts, vital facts, flow charts, points to ponder, mnemonics, etc. and many students have told me that they read these just before the examinations. These columns give them the gist of the entire chapters in a jiffy and it is a great boon to them. Hence I have retained them in this book. Copying is the best complement and I now see so many new books coming out in the market in orthopedics are copying this method of mine thereby stamping their approval of my beliefs and thoughts. To make these features more attractive, I have added many new exciting sub-columns. Section on Clinical Examination Methods in Orthopedics is being given at the end of the chapter.

I welcome the students and the teachers to give me their valuable feedback, criticisms constructive suggestions. This will help me to come out with a better revised edition in the future. I thank all those who

are responsible for making my books successful and hope that the same kind of patronage will be extended to this book too. This is my dream book and hope it strikes the right chord with the undergraduate students and makes it a happy reading and great learning experience. Lots of students have written to me saying that after reading my book they have fallen in love with orthopedics and would love to take it up as their profession. This is the greatest compliment I have received from my students. Hope, my students benefit and enjoy reading this book. If that happens my effort has been worth it.

John Ebnezar

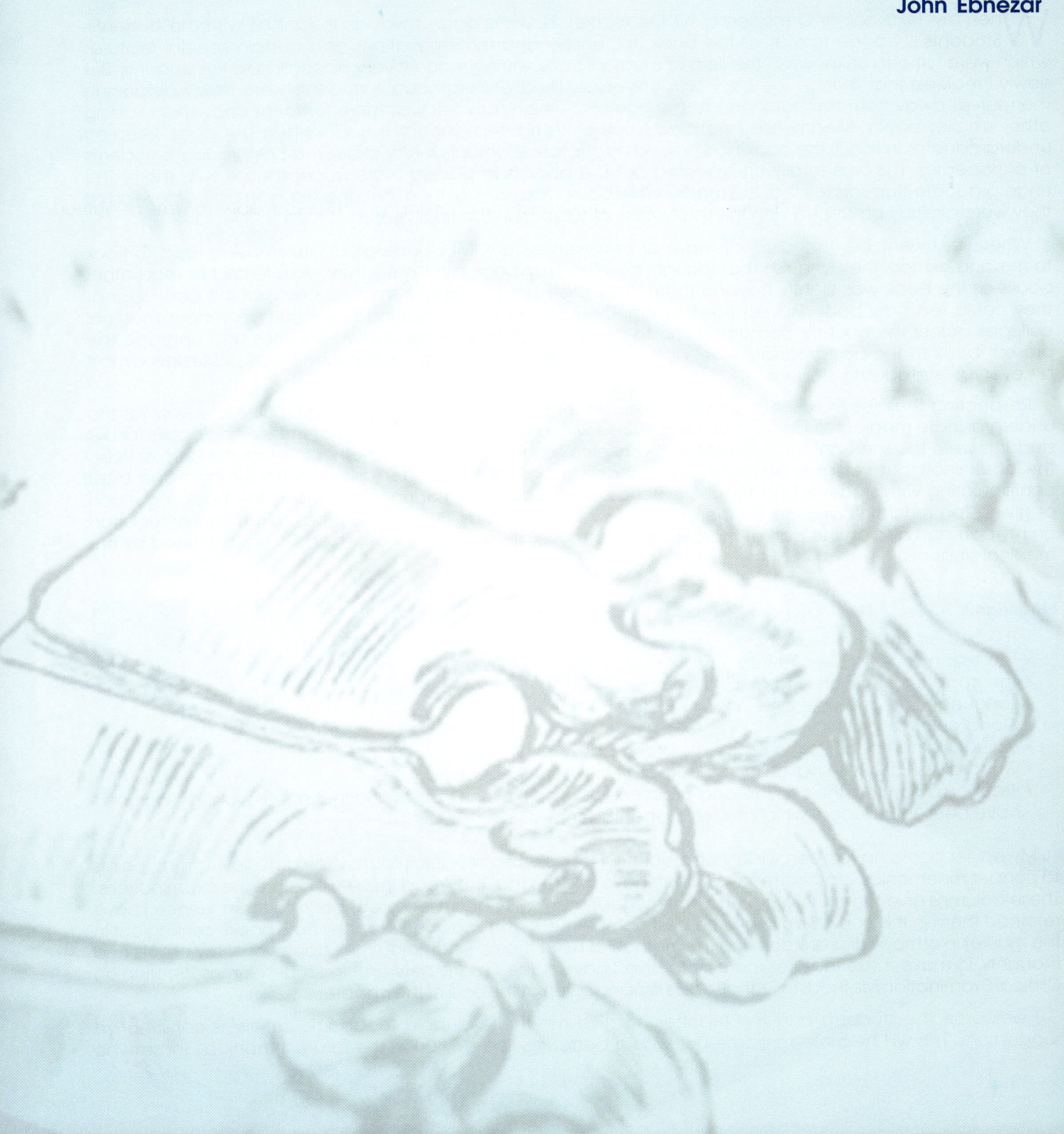

Acknowledgments

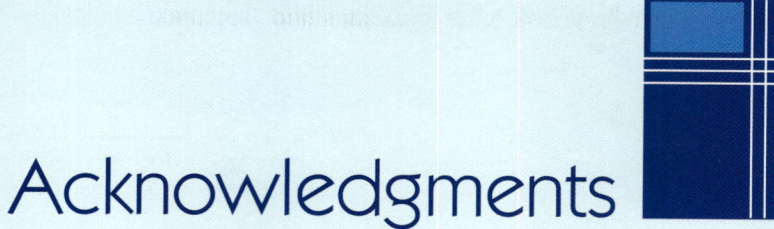

I sincerely thank all the members of my family for their unstinted and unflappable love, warmth, encouragement and support.

I thank all my teachers who shaped my personality and career right from primary school to my postgraduation in orthopedics at JN Medical College, Belgaum. I thank all the colleagues at Bangalore Medical College for their cooperation and support when I first wrote the book in 1996.

I thank Mr Satish K Jain, Managing Director, CBSPD, for bringing out this book. He has been very supportive and cooperative and took extra interest and went out of his way to bring out a book of international standards. My special thanks to my dear disciplinarian friend Mr YN Arjuna who showed special interest in bringing out this book. He is extremely dedicated and hardworking and is responsible for the beautiful format of the book which believe me was a Herculean task. I also thank Mrs Ritu Chawla for the tremendous amount of hard work put in by her in the preparation of this book. I thank the entire team of CBS PD comprising DTP operators, graphic designers, proofreaders, artists, printers and supporting technical staff, who have worked hard behind the scenes to bring out this book.

My special thanks to Dr Yogitha, the chief Ayurvedic and Yoga professional of my center, and all the staff of my hospital who have helped me in bringing out this book.

It is the teachers and students who need a big thumbs up for patronizing and supporting my book. Finally, I thank the Supreme God for the life he gave me and blessing me immensely in all spheres of life so that I could leave a legacy of my own when I quit this beautiful world created by him.

John Ebnezar

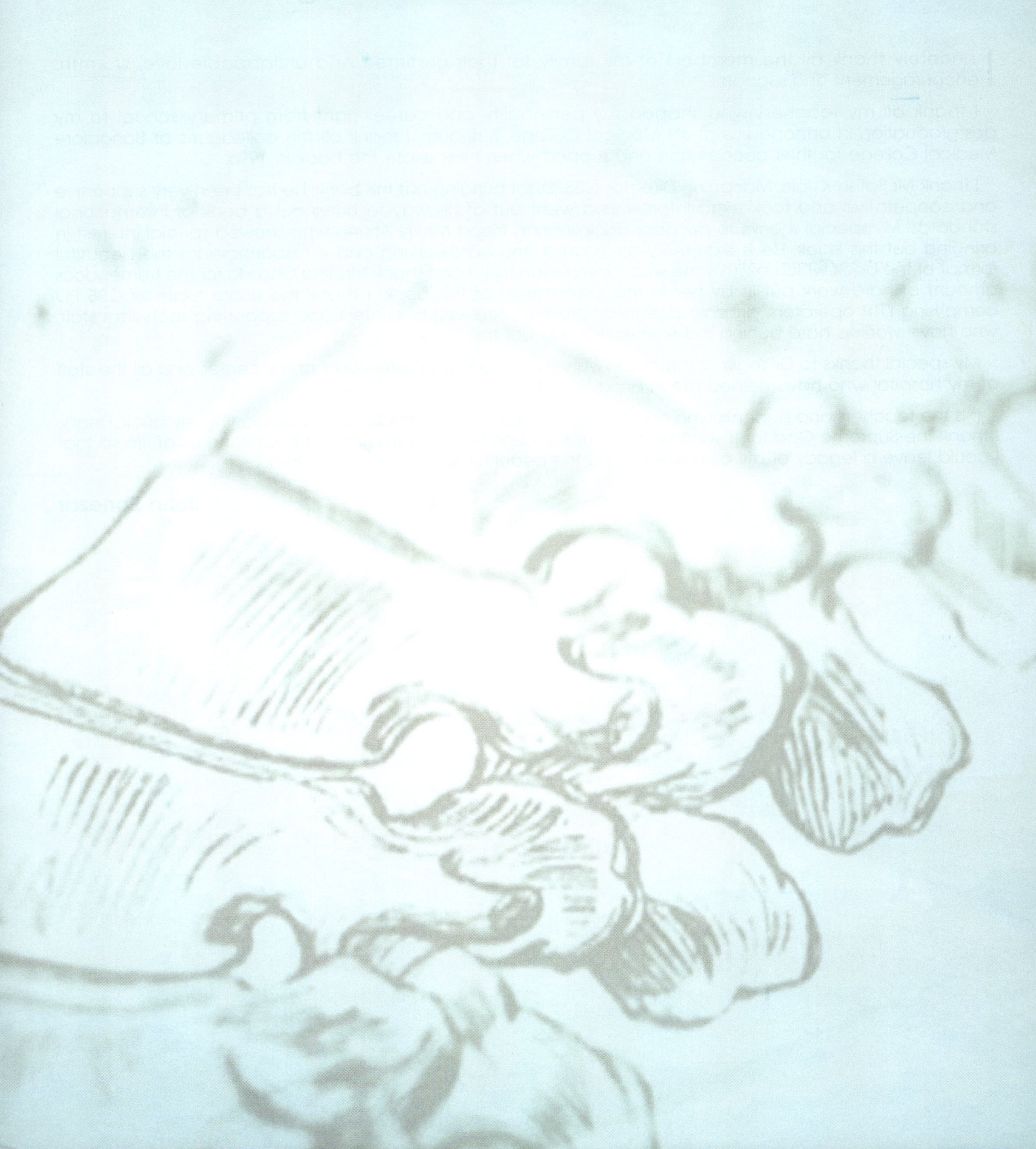

Contents

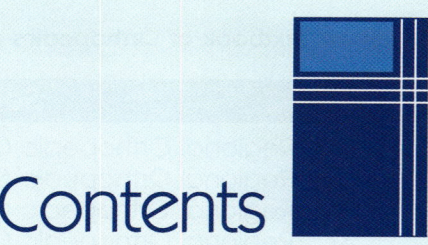

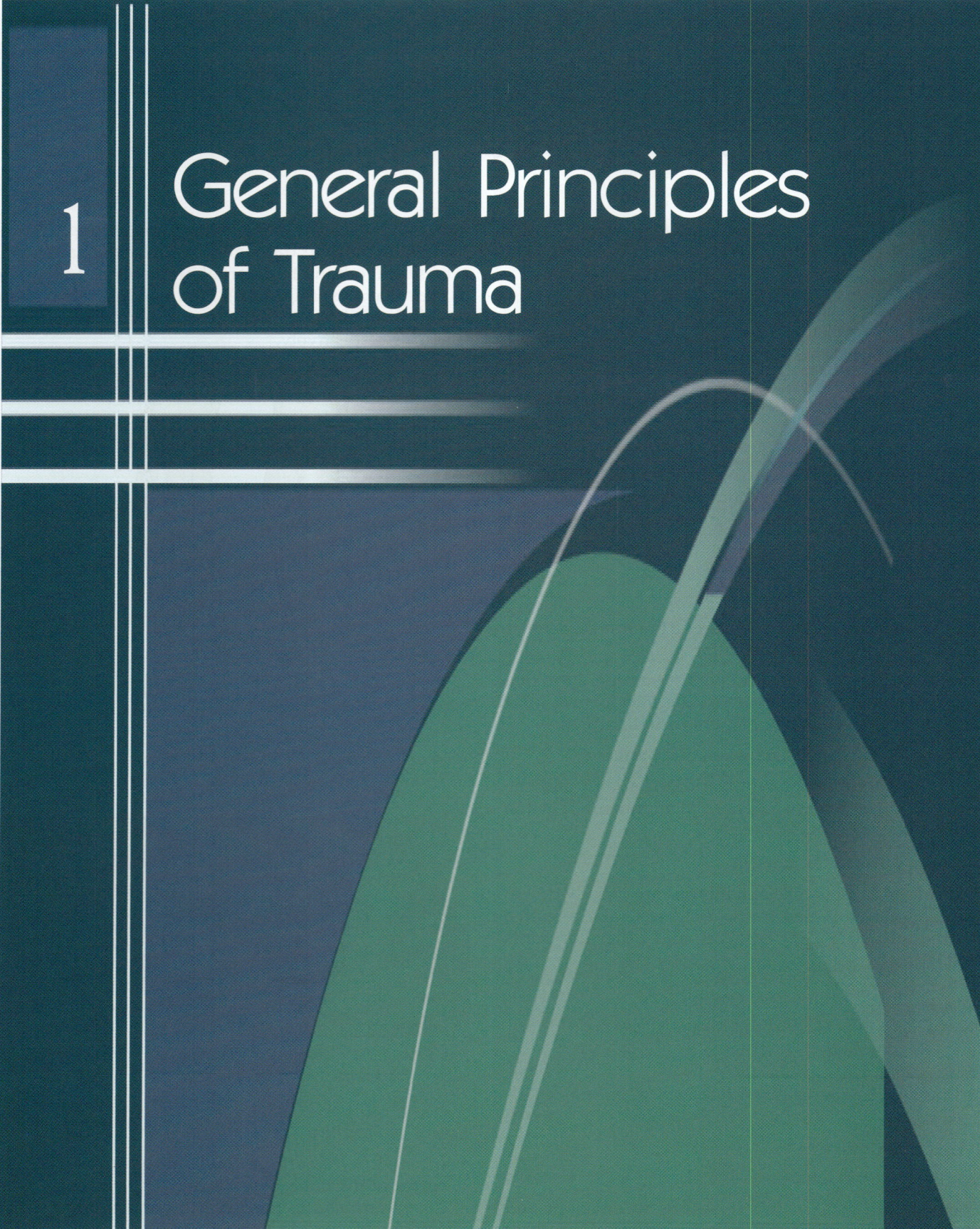

1 General Principles of Trauma

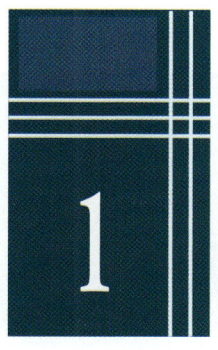

Fracture Basics

Before dealing with the fractures per se, let us familiarize ourselves with the various spectra of musculoskeletal injuries. Simple fractures could be either incomplete or complete and could be undisplaced or displaced.

DEFINITION

Fracture is a break in the surface of a bone, either across its cortex or through its articular surface.

Dislocation is a complete and persistent separation of a joint in which at least part of the supporting joint capsule and some of its ligaments are disrupted.

Subluxation is partial separation of a joint.

Sprain is a temporary subluxation of a joint and the articular surfaces return to normal alignment. It is due to ligament tear.

Strain is a tear in the muscle.

Mechanism: Musculoskeletal injuries are usually due to trauma following road traffic accidents, falls, assaults, sports, industrial, agricultural, and other accidents (see Fig. 6.1).

Remember
Forces required to cause damage to a bone could be:
- Large and sudden (e.g. RTA)
- Repetitive (e.g. stress fracture)
- Trivial (e.g. pathological fractures).

Types of Fracture
Simple or compound

The bone can break within its soft tissue envelope and may not communicate to the exterior (*simple* or *closed*

fractures) (Fig. 1.1A) or it may even rip through its soft tissues or may be damaged by the external forces, exposing the bone to external atmosphere (*compound* or *open fractures*) (Fig. 1.1B). Figures 1.2A and B show the clinical photograph of a simple and compound fractures respectively.

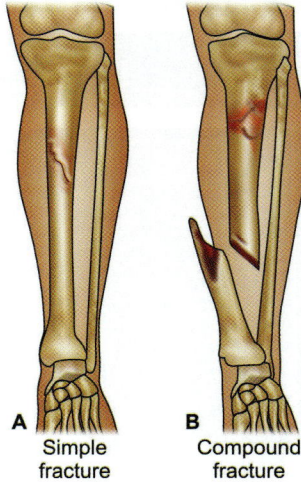

Figs 1.1A and B

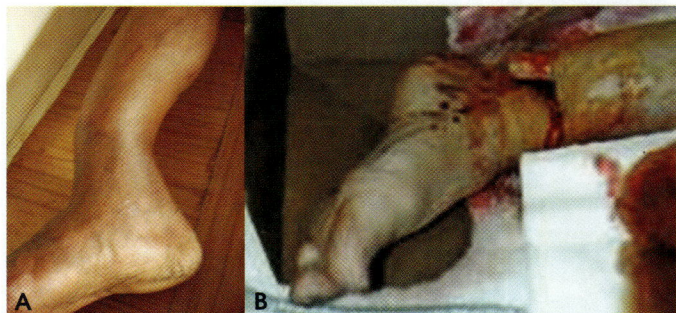

Figs 1.2A and B: Clinical photograph showing simple fracture (left) and compound fracture of the tibia (right)

Extent of Fracture

- *Incomplete fracture*: Involves only one surface or cortex of the bone.
- *Complete fracture*: Involves the entire bone which could be *displaced* or undisplaced.

Displacement of Fractures

Usually a complete fracture is displaced due to various factors, depending on the direction of force, mode of injury, pull of the muscles, etc. A fracture may show any of the following displacements or angulations (Figs 1.3A to D):
- Anterior angulations or displacement
- Posterior angulations or displacement
- Varus or medial angulations or displacement
- Valgus or lateral angulations or displacement
- Shortening
- Translational

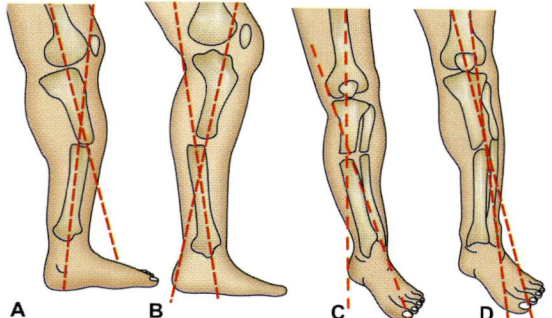

Figs 1.3A to D: Different angulations in fractures: (A) anterior, (B) posterior, (C) medial, (D) lateral

Note: Deformities following fractures are due to displacements of the bone fragments.

Causes

- Muscle forces
- Gravity
- Obliquity of the fracture line
- Improper handling of the fracture.

Classification of Fractures (Orthopedic Trauma Association)

- *Linear fracture:* These could be *transverse, oblique or spiral.* Any fracture, which forms an angle less than 30° with the horizontal line, is called *transverse* (Fig. 1.4A). Angle equal to or more than 30° is termed as *oblique.* The oblique fracture could be long oblique or short oblique (Fig. 1.4B).
- *Spiral fracture:* This could be long spiral or short spiral (Fig. 1.4C).
- *Intraarticular fracture:* In this type, fracture line extends into the joint.
- *Comminuted fracture:* The fracture fragments are more than two in number. They are further classified into comminution less than 50% and comminution more than 50%. *Butterfly-shaped fractures* are also included in this group (Fig. 1.4D).
- *Segmental fracture:* A fracture can break into segments and each segment could be in two levels, three

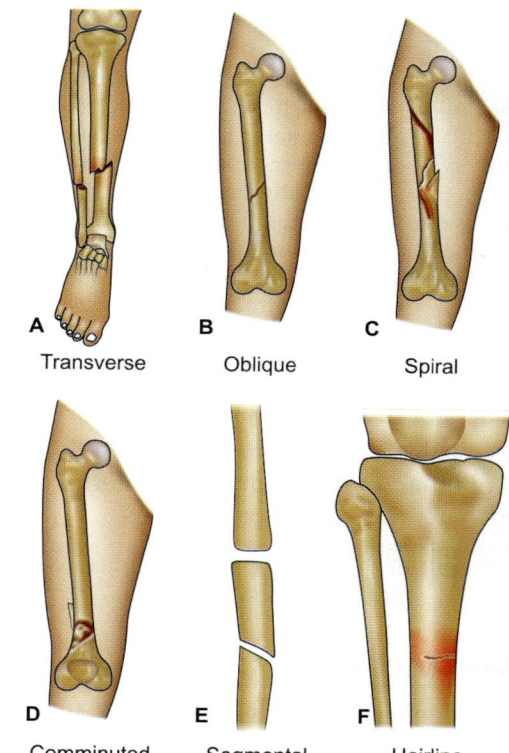

Figs 1.4A to F: Types of fractures based on fracture patterns

levels, and a longitudinal split or comminuted (Fig. 1.4E).

- *Avulsion fracture:* This occurs due to the pull of the tendon or muscles at the point of its insertion, e.g. mallet finger (Fig. 3.2B).

- *Bone loss:* This could be less than 50% or more than 50% bone loss or a complete loss of bone (see Fig. 6.3).

HISTORY

Orthopedic injuries encompass a wide range of problems starting from bone and joint injuries, strains, sprains and damage to associated neurovascular structures.

The value of a systematic clinical approach to unravel the myth and mysteries of orthotrauma cannot be less emphasized. Time-honored and time-tested clinical formulae applied so successfully in the diagnosis of various system disorders can be applied for ortho-trauma also which consists of the following.

Contrary to popular beliefs, a proper history gives vital clues and goes a long way in arriving at a proper diagnosis.

Age: Certain fractures have predilections for certain age groups. Hence, the practice of first enquiring about the age of the patient is a step in the right direction (Table 1.1).

Table 1.1: Age vs fractures and dislocations

Age	Types of fractures and dislocations
• Birth	Brachial plexus injury, fracture, clavicle, humerus fracture, etc.
• Early childhood	Supracondylar fracture of humerus, epiphyseal injuries.
• Late childhood	Posterior dislocations of elbow. Slipped capital epiphysis. Monteggia's fracture.
• Adult	Fracture of long bones, hip and shoulder dislocations.
• Elderly	Colles' fracture, neck femur fracture.

Sex Colles' fracture is more common in females and supracondylar fracture humerus, posterior dislocations of elbow are more common in males.

Note: In spite of age predilections, any fracture can be seen in any age group as an aberration.

MECHANISM OF INJURY

Musculoskeletal injuries are usually due to trauma because of road accidents, fall from height, crime, etc. However, the forces, which break, could be direct or indirect and this depends on the mode of injury. This could be different in different age groups as in table 1.2.

Table 1.2: Common modes of injury in different age groups

Age	Common modes of injury	Examples
Children	Fall with outstretched hands usually while on play or from a height	Fracture clavicle and dislocation of any upper limb bones
Adults	Fall from height	Upper limb injuries, spine injuries, etc.
	Diving injuries	Cervical spine injuries.
	RTA	Any combination of injuries. • Whiplash injury. • Dashboard injuries like patella fracture, posterior hip dislocation, etc.
	Sports injuries	Ankle and shoulder, elbow and knee joint injuries.
	Assaults	Long bone fractures (e.g. nightstick fracture of ulna).
Elderly	Trivial fall	Colles' fracture or neck femur fracture, etc.

Note: High-velocity trauma due to RTA can produce any combination of bone and joint injuries.

Clinical Presentations

Presenting Complaints

A patient with limb injuries may complain the following:
- *Pain:* This is very subjective symptom and is invariably the first and the most important complaint. It may be mild, moderate, severe and may be due to tearing of periosteum (which contains the nerve endings), soft tissue injury, nerve injury, etc.
- *Swelling*: It is due to soft tissue injury, medullary, bleeding and reactionary hemorrhage. Swelling is usually more in fractures and less in dislocations.
- *Deformity:* Patients with displaced fractures and dislocations usually present with some deformity.
- *Inability* to use the affected part is another frequent complaint.

Clinical Signs

Having made a note of the history and presenting complaints, effort is now directed towards eliciting the signs, some of which are general and some are injury specific.
- *Tenderness*: This is an important clinical sign in bone and joint injuries and is usually seen after trauma. Importance of tenderness, methods of elicitation and grading is mentioned below in the box.

Remember

Tenderness may be the only evidence of fracture in:
- Crack fracture
- Hairline fracture
- Stress fracture
- Fatique fracture
- Torus fracture
- Pathological fracture

Method of eliciting: By proceeding from normal area to the affected part for better patient compliance.

Grading
- Grade I: Just a suspect
- Grade II: Patient winces on pressure
- Grade III: Patient winces and withdraws
- Grade IV: Patient will not allow to touch

This grading of tenderness is superior to the conventional mild, moderate and severe grading.

- *Swelling*: The swelling is examined for shape, size, consistency, tenderness, fluctuation, etc. The swelling is classified as mild, moderate and severe based upon the size and extent.
- *Deformity*: This is usually seen in displaced fractures and dislocations. Undisplaced fractures, mild strains and sprains usually show no deformities. Some of the deformities are very characteristic and specific and help in making a spot diagnosis (Figs 1.5A to D).
- Table 1.3 shows classical deformities in orthopedic trauma.

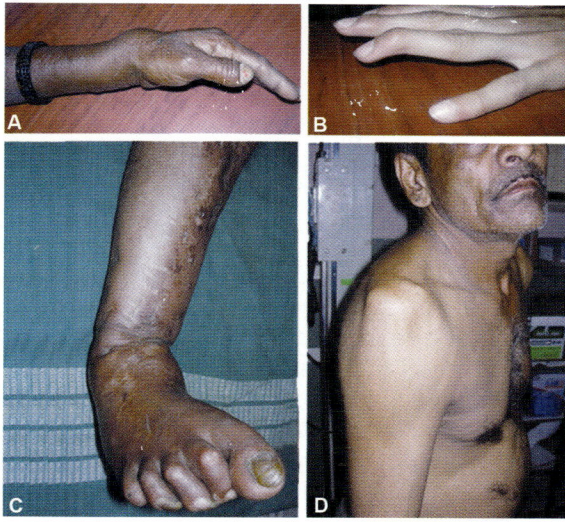

Figs 1.5A to D: (A) Dinner fork deformity, (B) Mallet finger, (C) Lower end of tibia, (D) Anterior dislocation of shoulder

Remember

"D" in fracture
- Deformity is seen often in displaced fractures.
- Displacement could be anterior, posterior, medial or lateral.
- Distal fragment is the reference point to suggest the type of displacement.
- Dislocation of joints usually presents as a deformity.

Table 1.3: Classical deformities in orthopedics	
Classical deformities	*Possible diagnosis*
Upper limbs	
Wry neck	Cervical spine injuries
Drooping of shoulder	Clavicle fracture
Flat shoulder	Anterior dislocation of shoulder
S-shaped deformity	Supracondylar fracture of humerus
Dinner fork deformity	Colles' fracture
Boutonnière deformity of finger	Rupture of central extensor slip
Mallet finger	Rupture of distal end of index extensor
Jersey finger	Rupture of distal end of flexor digitorum profundus of index finger
Lower limbs	
Flexion, adduction and internal rotation	Posterior dislocation of hip.
Flexion, abduction and external rotation of lower limb	Anterior dislocation of hip.
Incomplete external rotation of lower limbs	Fracture neck femur (intracapsular)
Complete external rotation of lower limbs	Trochanteric fractures, shaft femur, leg bones fractures.
S-shaped ankle	Ankle dislocations.

- *Abnormal mobility*: Normally movements occur only at the joints and not in between. When such movements are noticed, it is a sign of a fracture (Fig. 1.6).
- *Loss of transmitted movements*: When one end of the limb is rotated, it is transmitted automatically to the other end. Due to break in the continuity, the movement is not transmitted. This is due to displaced fracture.
- *Crepitus*: This is an abnormal grating sensation produced by the friction between two ragged surfaces of the fracture fragments. It is elicitable only in displaced fractures and should be elicited very gently to avoid hurting the patient.
- *Shortening of the limb:* Shortening of various degrees is common in bone and joint injuries (see Fig. 8.25).

Note: Crepitus, abnormal mobility, deformity and loss of transmitted movements cannot be elicited in undisplaced fractures, stress fractures, impacted fractures, etc.

About Crepitus

It is defined as an abnormal grating sensation either felt or heard. It could be:
- Fine, e.g. osteoarthritis
- Coarse, e.g. fractures
- Snap, e.g. snapping tendons.
  Remember it is unkind to elicit a crepitus in a fracture for fear of hurting the patient.

Categorization

Various clinical signs are described in fractures. They can be best represented as follows in order of their importance (Table 1.4).

Table 1.4: Clinical signs and their features	
Clinical signs	*Features*
Unfailing signs	• Abnormal mobility • Crepitus
Reliable signs	• Tenderness • Shortening
Important signs	• Bruise • Swelling
Other signs	• Loss of function • Deformity
Late or inconstant signs	• Blisters • Ecchymosis • Swelling due to callus

Clinical manifestations due to neurovascular injuries: Certain fractures are known to cause neurovascular damage quite frequently, e.g. supracondylar fracture of humerus in children. Impending vascular damage is detected by the familiar **five Ps** and nerve injuries are detected by the classical deformities and screening tests (as described in peripheral nerve injuries).

1

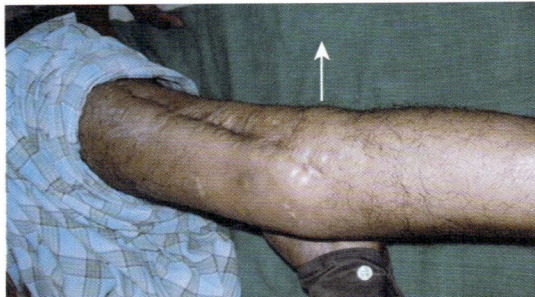

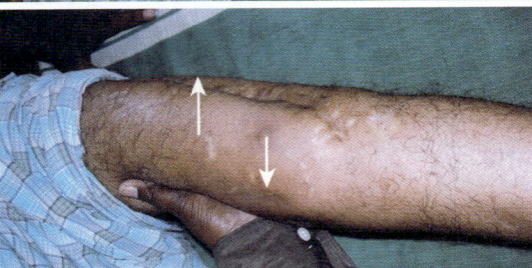

Fig. 1.6: Abnormal mobility in nonunion fracture of the shaft of femur

About Five Ps

In detecting impending vascular damage, following skeletal injuries remember the **5Ps** namely:

Pain
Pallor
Paraesthesia
Pulselessness
Paralysis

Note: Clinical manifestations in a fracture are due to:
- Fracture per se
- Its complications
- Or both

Investigations

Having made a clinical diagnosis of the musculoskeletal trauma by careful clinical examination methods enumerated above, patient needs to be subjected to judicious investigations for confirmation of the diagnosis and effective management of the injuries. The investigations recommended are plain X-rays (Gold standard) in almost all cases of fractures and CT scan, Doppler, MRI, etc. in certain special situations (Figs 1.7A to C). Laboratory investigations like Hb% BT, CT, blood group, HIV, HbSAg, etc. are commonly recommended.

Treatment

Treatment of fractures is by conservative and operative methods depending upon the type of fractures, extent of injuries, involvement of other systemic injuries, etc. First aid in fractures, management of simple fractures, open fractures, dislocations, soft tissue injuries, etc. are all dealt in relevant chapters.

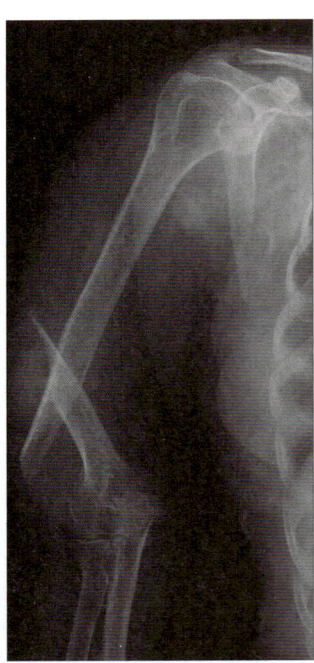

Fig. 1.7A: Investigations for fractures—Plain X-rays

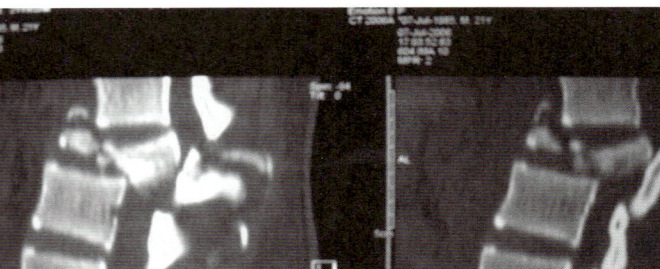

Fig. 1.7B: Investigations for fractures—CT scan

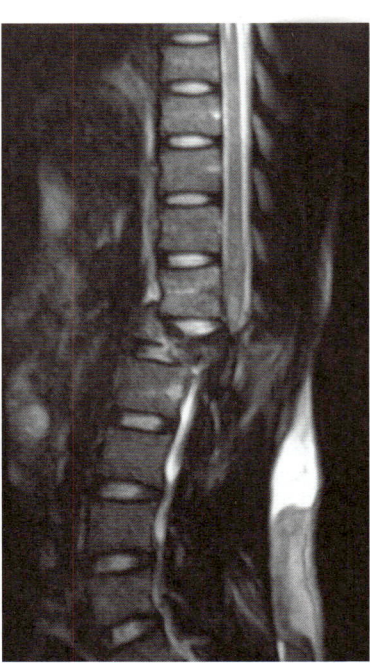

Fig. 1.7C: Investigations for fractures—MRIs

2 Atypical Fractures

These are special types of fractures that do not fail into the conventional types of fractures that we all know. Hence they are called 'atypical' and consist of the following types.

- *Hairline crack or fracture*: It is a very fine break in the bone, which is difficult to diagnose clinically. Radiology helps in identifying the crack (See Fig. 1.4F).
- *Greenstick fracture:* It is observed exclusively in children. Since the bone is elastic and usually bends due to buckling or breaking of one cortex when a force is applied (Fig. 2.1A).
- *Torus fracture*: This is just a buckling of the outer cortex of the bones in children (Fig. 2.1B).
- *Impacted fracture*: The fracture fragments impacted each other but are not separated and displaced.

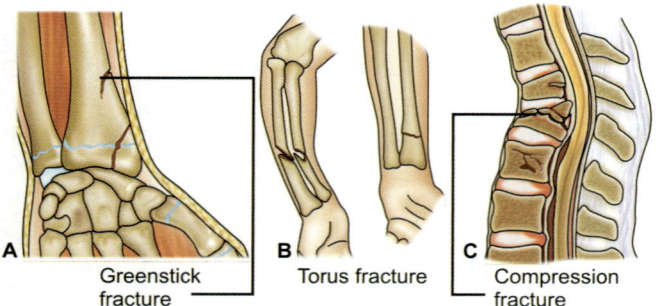

Figs 2.1A to C: Atypical fractures: (A) greenstick, (B) torus fractures, and (C) compression fracture

- *Stress or fatigue fracture*: This is usually an incomplete fracture commonly observed in athletes and in bones subjected to chronic and repetitive stress (e.g. third metatarsal fracture, tibia fracture, etc.) (Fig. 2.2).
- *Pathological fracture*: This occurs in a diseased bone and is usually spontaneous. The force required to bring about a pathological fracture is trivial.

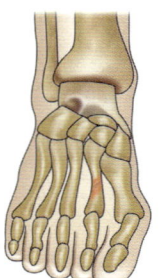

Fig. 2.2: Stress fracture of III metatarsal bone

PATHOLOGICAL FRACTURES

When a fracture occurs in a bone which has already been weakened by a generalized or localized skeletal disorder it is called a *pathological* fracture. Unlike traumatic fractures, these fractures take place either spontaneously or due to trivial trauma. Figure 2.3 shows the common sites of pathological fractures.

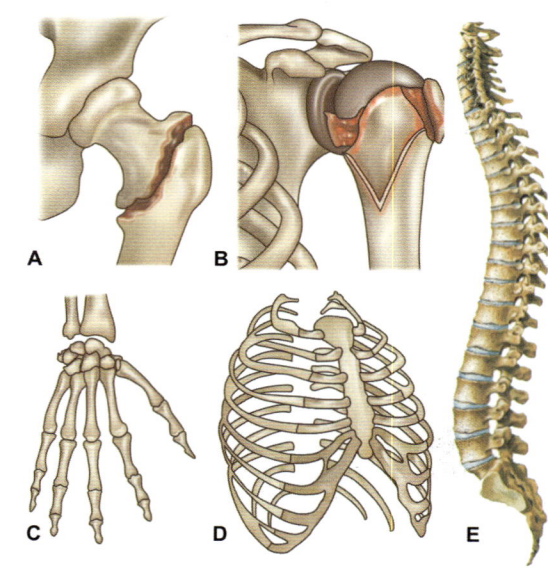

Figs 2.3A to E: Common sites of pathological fractures: (A) neck femur, (B) neck humerus, (C) lower end of radius, (D) ribs, and (E) spine.

Causes for Pathological Fractures

Localized Diseases

- *Infective disorders*
  - Chronic pyogenic osteomyelitis
  - Tubercular or syphilitic osteomyelitis
- *Neoplasms*

Benign	Malignant
• Chondroma	• Osteogenic sarcoma
• Giant cell tumor	• Ewing's sarcoma
• Hemangioma spine	• Solitary myeloma
• Tabes dorsalis, etc.	• Metastatic carcinoma
• Bone atrophy (e.g. polio)	• Metastatic sarcoma
	• Lung, breast prostate, kidney, etc.

- *Miscellaneous cause*
  - Simple bone cyst
  - Monostotic fibrous dysplasia
  - Eosinophilic granuloma.
- *General affections of bone*
- *Developmental disorders*
  - Osteogenesis imperfecta
  - Fibrous dysplasia
  - Gaucher's disease, etc.
- *Generalized rarefaction of bones*
  - Senile osteoporosis
  - Hyperparathyroidism
  - Osteomalacia
  - Nutritional rickets
  - Scurvy
- *Miscellaneous*
  - Multiple myeloma
  - Diffuse metastatic carcinoma
- *Disseminated tumors*
  - Paget's disease
  - Fibrous dysplasia
  - Gaucher's disease, etc.

Clinical Features

The patient usually complains of fracture following a trivial trauma. He or she complains of having suffered pain or discomfort in the region of the affected bone some time before the fracture. The cause could be either a generalized or a local skeletal disorder (See Box).

Radiology: Plain X-ray of the affected part helps to identify the pathological fracture (Fig. 2.4).

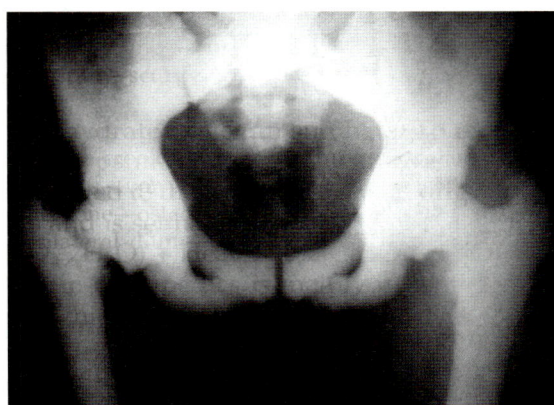

Fig. 2.4: Intracapsular femoral neck pathological fracture in osteopetrosis

Treatment

Conservative treatment has little role in the treatment of pathological fractures. The treatment recommended is open reduction, rigid internal fixation with or without cement and bone grafting. The aim is to obtain quick union and mobilize the patient early. Pathological fractures due to Paget's disease, osteogenesis imperfecta, etc. unite in the usual time, fractures due to osteomyelitis, bone cyst unite late but fractures due to malignancy, metastasis do not unite at all though union is possible after chemotherapy or radiotherapy.

FATIGUE OR STRESS FRACTURES

Fatigue or stress fractures occur due to repeated stress or minor trauma to a particular bone usually on the lower limbs. There is no single specific causative injury as in a traumatic fracture. The onset of pain is gradual or insidious. Activity increases the pain and rest relieves it. On examination, there is significant local tenderness, thickening of bone, local swelling, etc.

Radiology

Radiograph of the part at first may not reveal any fractures but may be seen after 3 to 4 weeks. The fracture itself will be hairline, transverse and undisplaced. More striking than the fracture is a zone of callus that surrounds it.

Treatment

Stress fractures usually heal by rest and support to the affected part.

3 Bone Structure and Fracture Healing

GENERAL STRUCTURE OF A BONE

The bone has an epiphysis, epiphyseal plate (which disappears with growth), metaphysis and diaphysis (Figs 3.1 and 3.2).

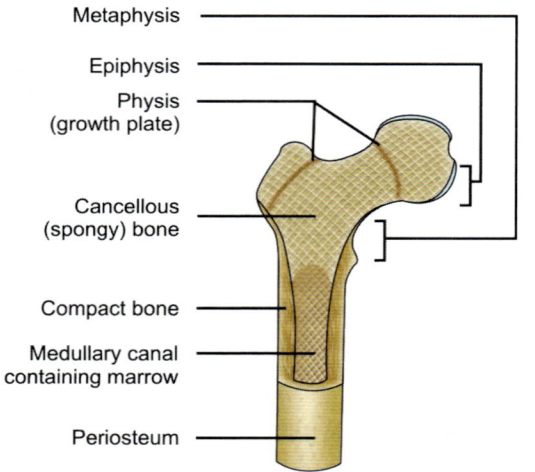

Fig. 3.1: Structure of a bone

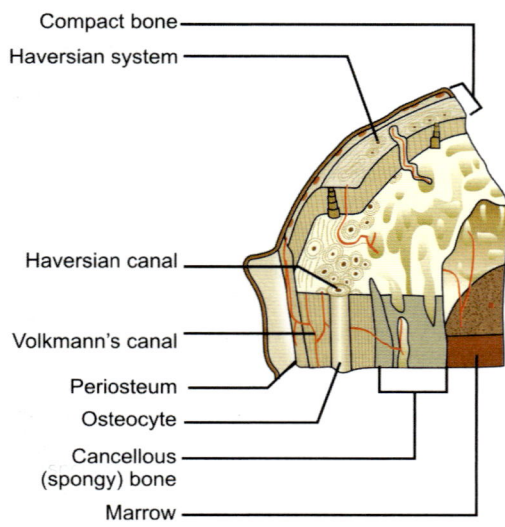

Fig. 3.2: Cross section of a bone.

Epiphysis: This is an expanded portion at the end of a bone developed under pressure and forms a support for the joint surface. It is easily affected by developmental problems like epiphyseal dysplasias, trauma, overuse, degeneration and damaged blood supply. The end result is a distorted joint due to avascular necrosis and degenerative changes.

Growth plate (physis): It is mechanically weak in nature but helps longitudinal growth. It responds to growth and sex hormones. It is affected by conditions like osteomyelitis, tumor, slipped epiphysis resulting in short stature, deformed growth or growth arrest.

Metaphysis: This is concerned with remodeling a bone. It is the cancellous portion that heals quickly. It gives attachment to ligament and tendons. It is vulnerable to develop osteomyelitis, dysplasias and tumors resulting in distorted growth and altered bone shapes.

Diaphysis: This is a significant compact cortical bone which is strong in compression and which gives origin to muscles. It forms shafts of the bones. Healing is slow when compared to metaphysis. In remodeling, it can remodel angulations but not rotation. It may develop fractures, dysplasias, infection and rarely tumors.

Organization of bones: They are 206 in number and are grouped into two subdivisions namely:
- Axial skeleton—80 bones.
- Appendicular skeleton—126 bones.

Axial skeleton forms the upright axis of the body and the *appendicular skeleton* forms the *appendages* and *girdles* that attach them to the axial skeleton (Table 3.1).

Out of these 206, some are short and some are long with different shapes. The shape and size depends upon the functions attributed to them.

Blood Supply to the Bones

Atypical long bone derives its blood supply through the following sources:
- *Peripheral:* This is through the periosteal vessels which penetrate the cortex in adults.
- *Central:* This is through the nutrient artery which seeks entry into a long bone at the middle, divides into two and proceeds to either ends of the bones. They divide into many branches near the ends of the growth plates.

3

Table 3.1: Bones		
Axial skeleton		
Skull		
• Cranium	8	
• Face	14	
Vertebral column		
• Cervical vertebrae	7	
• Thoracic vertebrae	12	
• Lumbar vertebrae	5	
• Sacrum	1	(5 fused bones)
• Coccyx	1	(3–5 fused bones)
Sternum		
• Manubrium	1	
• Body	12	pairs
• Xiphoid process	1	
• Ribs		
• Hyoid		
• Ear ossicles	2	
• Malleus	2	
• Incus	2	
• Stapes	2	
Total	**80**	
Appendicular skeleton		
Shoulder girdle		
• Clavicle	2	
• Scapula	2	
Upper extremities		
• Humerus	2	
• Ulna	2	
• Radius	2	
• Carpals	16	
• Metacarpals	10	
• Phalanges	28	
Hip girdle		
• Os coxa	2	
Lower extremity		
• Femur	2	
• Fibula	2	
• Tibia	2	
• Patella	2	
• Tarsals	14	
• Metatarsals	10	
• Phalanges	28	
Total	**126**	

- *Ends*: The blood supply is through two sources:
  - *Epiphyseal vessels*: The blood enters straight into the epiphysis through these vessels.
  - *Metaphyseal vessels*: The blood vessels in and around the vascular anastomosis near the joints pierce the metaphysis at their capsular attachments.

Thus, bones have abundant and rich blood supply which gets disrupted during injuries.

> **A 'QUICK VASCULAR RECAP'**
> A long bone has four important blood supplies:
> - Nutrient artery
> - Periosteal vessels
> - Metaphyseal vessels
> - Epiphyseal vessels.

Types of Bones

The following are the different types of bones (Fig. 3.3).

Long bones: These serve as levers for the muscle action, e.g. femur, tibia.

Short bones: Their major role is to provide strength.

Irregular bones: e.g. pelvic bones.

Flat bones: e.g. scapula, skull.

Sesamoid bones: Their name is derived from their resemblance to *sesame seeds*, e.g. patella (largest and most definitive of the sesamoid bones).

FRACTURE HEALING

Bone is repaired by *callus* which is a new tissue that may develop externally or internally. An *external* callus envelops around the outer aspect of the opposing ends of bone fragments while the *internal* callus forms between the bone ends.

During the first two days after fracture, the osteogenic cells proliferate and lift the fibrous layer of the periosteum away from the bone, a deep layer of periosteum, near the fracture site. Marrow cells also proliferate but to a lesser degree. These osteogenic cells differentiate into osteoblasts which form the bone trabeculae resembling the embryonic

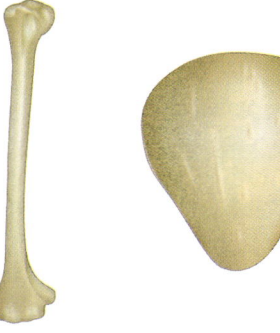
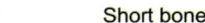
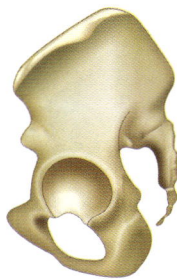
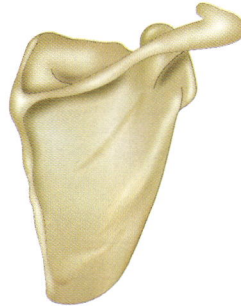

Long bone   Short bone   Irregular bone   Flat bone

Fig. 3.3: Types of bones

tissue. The osteogenic cells lying away from the fracture site due to inadequate vascularity differentiate into chondro-blasts and chondrocytes which form the cartilage. The cartilage is finally converted into bone by endochondral ossification.

The internal callus is formed by the mesenchymal cells which convert into pro-osteoblasts and later to osteoblasts laying down new bone. *Remodeling* is an activity of *osteoclasts* which slowly remove the necrotic bone and create cavities. Osteoblasts line these cavities and lay a new bone.

METHODS OF FRACTURE HEALING IN A CORTICAL BONE

A fracture in a cortical bone heals by three ways, viz.indirect, direct and distraction histogenesis as described by Ilizarov.

Indirect Fracture Healing

This is the common method of fracture healing where both external and internal callus are formed. Hunter has described six stages in this method of healing. Fractures treated by conservative methods heal by this method (Figs 3.4A to D).

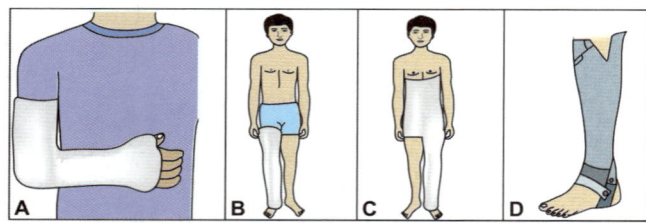

Figs 3.4A to D: An example of fracture healing by indirect methods: (A) above elbow cast, (B) above knee cast, (C) hip spica, (D) functional cast brace

Stage of impact: This stage extends from the moment of impact till the complete dissipation of energy causing fractures.

Stage of induction: Following fractures cells possessing osteogenic potential are activated. Other inducing factors are BMP (bone morphogenic protein), fall in oxygen tension and bioelectric effects (Fig. 3.5A).

Stage of inflammation: In this stage the disruption of blood supply results in necrosis of the bone ends. There is hemorrhage, cellular proliferation and vascular ingrowths (Fig. 3.5B).

Stage of soft callus: Here the hematoma is organized with fibrous tissue, cartilage and woven bone. Fragments are united with fibrous or cartilaginous tissue or both (Fig. 3.5C).

Stage of hard callus: Bone fragments are firmly united with bone. If immobilization is complete, membranous

bone healing takes place and if it is incomplete, healing happens by endochondral ossification (Fig. 3.5D).

Stage of remodeling: The fiber bone is converted to lamellar bone. Medullary canal is reconstituted and callus diameter begins to decrease in size which takes few months to several years. However, there will be no remodeling of rotational malalignment (Fig. 3.5E).

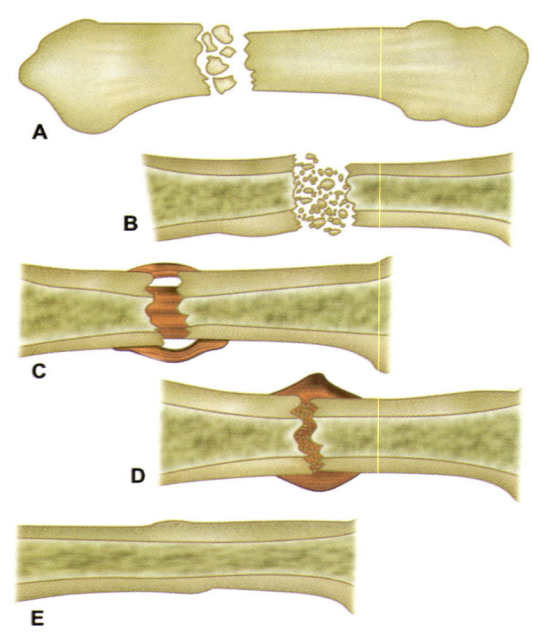

Figs 3.5A to E: Hunter' stages of fracture healing: (A) stage of induction, (B) stage of inflammation, (C) stage of soft callus, (D) stage of hard callus and remodeling, and (E) normal

Direct Fracture Healing (Primary bone healing, healing by primary intention)

This type of bone repair is seen when bone fragments are anatomically reduced by open methods and rigidly fixed. This cannot be obtained by closed methods of fracture treatment but can be achieved by operative reduction and fixation with special techniques of plates and screws. Ideally no external callus is formed and there is no interposing of fibrous tissue or cartilage tissue between the fracture sites. The fracture site is bridged by direct haversian remodeling which is almost a direct osteon to osteon hookup. The osteoclasts act as cutter heads to remove the bone and are in the forefront promptly followed by osteoblasts behind laying down new bone. This type of bone healing usually occurs in fractures treated by AO techniques developed by Swiss association for osteosynthesis (Fig. 3.6).

Factors Affecting Fracture Repair

Factors favoring union:
• Adequate circulation.

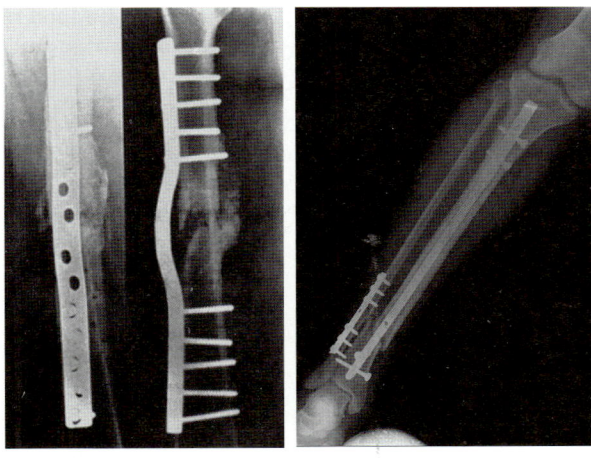

Fig. 3.6: Fractures fixed internally heal by direct methods

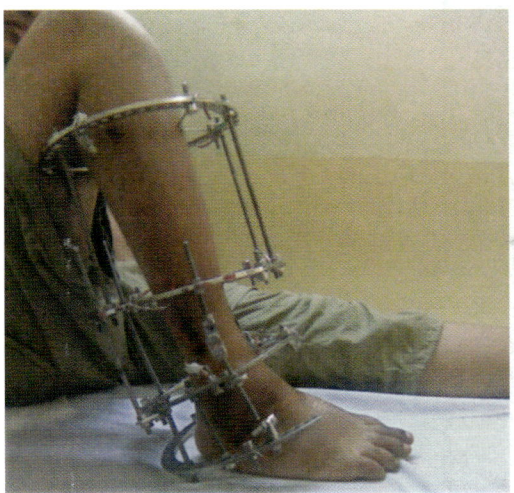

Fig. 3.7A: Ilizarov frame

- Good reduction and fixations.
- Hormones like growth hormone, parathormone, thyroxin.
- Good nutrition and mineral supplements help passively.
- Cancellous bone heal well.
- Bioelectric fixation.

Factors detrimental to union:
- Compound fractures
- Advanced age
- Poor circulation
- Infection
- Distraction
- Segmental fractures
- Comminution
- Osteoporosis
- Soft tissue interposition
- Inadequate and improper reduction and immo-bilization, etc.
- High and low velocity trauma.

Distraction Histogenesis

This is a recent concept described by Ilizarov. The bone under repair is induced by gradual distraction of osteotomies and fracture after an interval of induction, say 5 to 7 days. For osteogenesis to occur the fracture or osteotomy must be stabilized and slow distraction at the rate of 1 mm per day should be given (Figs 3.7A and B).

FRACTURE HEALING IN CANCELLOUS BONES

Mercifully fractures in cancellous bones generally unite well. The healing does not pass through the stage of callus but the bones unite readily. Unlike in the cortical bones, union in cancellous bones is direct and fast. The reasons being these bones have spongy constitution, have abundant blood supply and there is no medullary cavity. This increases the area of

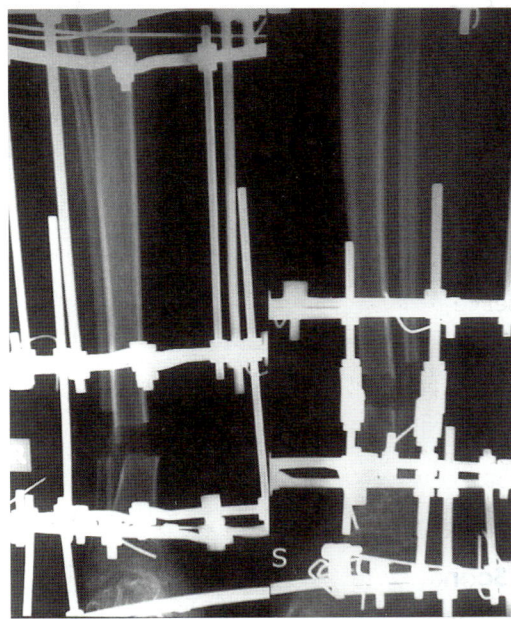

Fig. 3.7B: Distraction method by Ilizarov frame

contact between the trabecular ends of the bones. The fracture hematoma is converted directly into bone by the mature osteoblasts.

Factors Influencing Healing

Fracture healing is influenced by several factors, some are favorable while others are unfavorable. Few important factors are:
- *Age*: In children the fractures unite readily. (For reasons see chapters as fractures in children)
- *Type of fracture*: In terms of union, the incidence of good fractures union is as follows. Communited > segmented > oblige > transverse.
- *Type of bone*: Fracture in cancellous bones unite readily than cortical bones.

4 First Aid in Fractures

First aid is initial care offered to the injured at the scene of accident. Anyone can give first aid, but to carry out cardiopulmonary resuscitation measures, he/she should be trained in first aid and should possess a valid certificate issued by a competent body. First aid executed by a medical person is called a *medical aid*.

GOALS OF FIRST AID

First aid treatment goal is described by three **Ps:**
- **P**reserve life by carrying out appropriate resuscitative measures
- **P**revent further injuries by careful handling
- **P**romote recovery.
 To achieve the above goals, observe the following protocol under emergency.

INITIAL CARE FOR THE INJURED

At the Scene of Accident

Remove the victim from the accident spot.
- Check his or her vital parameters quickly (pulse, consciousness, etc.)
- Seek the help of bystanders if trained in first aid.
- Ensure that police and ambulance have been informed.
- Remember to carry out the first aid as per the modus operandi described below.
- Ensure personal safety.
- Arrange to shift the injured to a hospital at the earliest.

MODUS OPERANDI IN FIRST AID

Airway

Human brain cannot survive lack of oxygen for more than three minutes. Brain damage is irreversible, hence, a quick effort should be made to ensure that an accident victim breathes normally. For this, clear airway is necessary. In the event of a blocked airway, proceed as below:
- Clear the mouth of clots, dentures, loose teeth, etc.
- Extend the neck slightly as this opens up the pharynx.

Breathing

If the patient is not breathing, begin artificial respiration.
a. First keep a thin cloth over the patient's mouth, blow into the patients mouth keeping his or her nostrils closed. Blow at the rate of 16/min and see for the chest raise (Fig. 4.1).

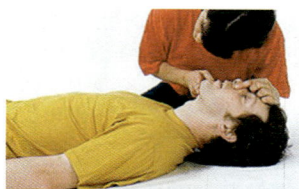

A. Clear the airway and extend the neck

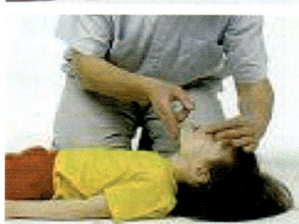

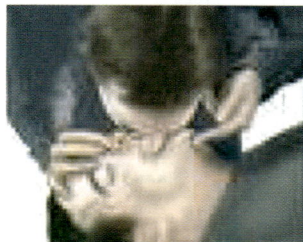

B. Close the nostrils and blow into the mouth

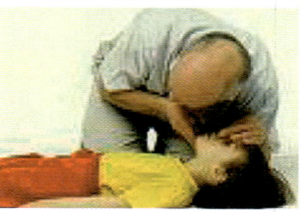

C. Feel and hear for the breath sounds

Fig. 4.1: Techniques of mouth-to-mouth and mouth-to-nose respiration to resuscitate a victim

b. Mouth-to-nose respiration is carried out if there is extensive injury to the mouth.

c. If the patient has suffered extensive facial injuries, put the patient prone, turn the face towards one side and apply pressure over the lower aspect of the chest (Holger-Nelson's method).

Cardia

Examine the radial pulse at the wrist and the carotid pulse at the neck for the function of cardia. If the pulse is absent initiate cardiac resuscitative measures as below:

- Ensure that the patient is lying on a hard surface.
- Apply pressure with the heel of the palm at the lower end of sternum.
- Optimum pressure should be applied and the depth of each pressure should be 1¼ inches.
- Perform external cardiac massage at the rate of 72/min (Figs 4.2A and B).
- It is preferable to carry out both external cardiac massage and artificial respiration simultaneously by two persons trained in first aid. But if there is no assistance available then cardiopulmonary resuscitation should be carried out by a single person as follows:
  – First artificial respiration is given once and then the same person should quickly change position and carry out external cardiac massage 5 times. So, this 1:5 ratio should be maintained throughout.

- The cardiopulmonary resuscitation (CPR) should be carried out until the patient recovers or at least for half an hour.

Bleeding

It is advisable to arrest the bleeding by direct application of pressure over the bleeding points. Tourniquet should be avoided and used as last option. Figures 4.3A to D show various method of arresting bleeding after injury.

Having ascertained that the patient is breathing, has satisfactory heart function and with the arrest of any bleeding points, carry out the below mentioned examinations of the vital structures.

Remember
The ABC in first aid treatment:
a. Airway management is the first priority.
b. Breathing is very vital for the patient to survive.
If the patient is not breathing, do the following:
• Mouth-to-mouth respiration.
• Mouth-to-mouth nose respiration.
• Holger Nelson method.
c. Cardia and circulation: Ensure that the heart beats and the bleeding stops.

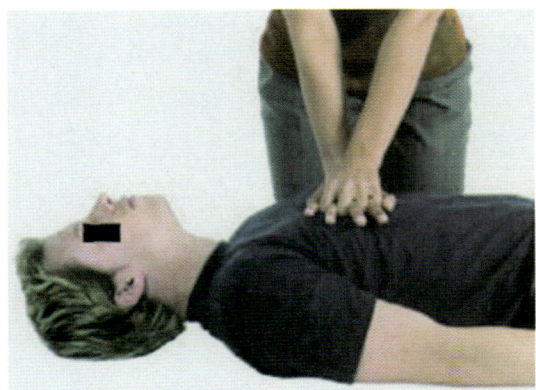
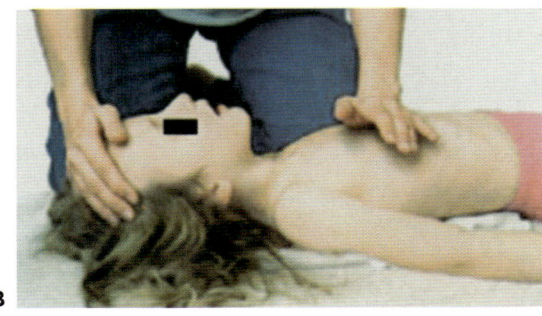

Figs 4.2A and B: Chest compression and technique of external cardiac massage: (A) adults , (B) children

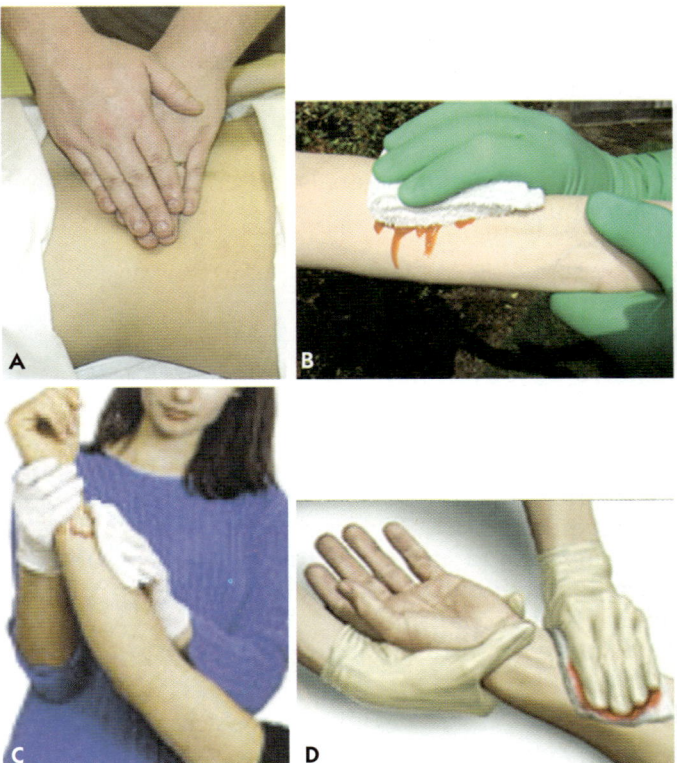

Figs 4.3A to D: Various measures to control bleeding: (A) direct compression over the femoral artery in case of lower limb injuries, (B) direct pressure over the injured site, (C) elevation of the limb, (D) direct compression over the injured area and application of compression bandage

After this initial aid, once you are sure that the patient's vital organs are stable, proceed to carry out examination of other parts of the body.

EXAMINATION OF VITAL STRUCTURES

Head Injuries

Examine the patient for head injuries. Cover the skull injuries with a clean cloth, and examine pupils and the level of consciousness.

Chest Injuries

Open chest injuries are dangerous as they may cause tension pneumothorax. Application of a clean cloth with firm pressure over the open wounds is required.

Abdominal Injuries

All injured patients should be examined for intra-abdominal injuries under emergency. Board-like rigid abdomen suggests blunt injury abdomen and there could be damage to liver, spleen, colon, etc. Arrangement should be made to shift the patient immediately to a hospital. In open wounds of the abdomen, firm pressure should be applied by a clean cloth.

Pelvic Fractures

Suspect pelvic fracture if the patient complains of pain during compression test or distraction test which is performed by applying pressure over the iliac bones. Tenderness over the symphysis pubis is also suggestive.

Injuries to the Genitourinary System

Suprapubic swelling indicates bladder injury, injury to the scrotum or perineal hematoma indicates urethral rupture.

Spine Injuries

Cervical spine injury should be suspected if the patient is lying still and loathes turning the neck. Injuries to the thoracic and lumbar spine should be suspected if the patient has developed paraplegia or complains of pain when individual spinous processes are palpated. Extreme care should be exercised in managing and shifting a patient with spinal injuries.

Fractures

Deformity, pain, swelling, loss of function of a limb are suggestive of fracture. Fracture needs to be splinted with whatever material is available at the scene of accident. The effective first aid measures during a bone and joint injuries are:

- Sling, strapping, etc. for clavicle and upper limb injuries.

- Splinting the injuries limb with make shift or regular splints or using patients own body (Figs 4.4A to D) at the scene of accidents.
- Rest to the patient
- Limb elevation
- Firm compression bandage
- Cold sponging
- Providing pain killers

They can be managed effectively after shifting the patient to the hospital.

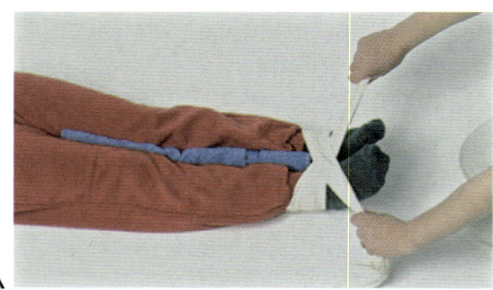

A

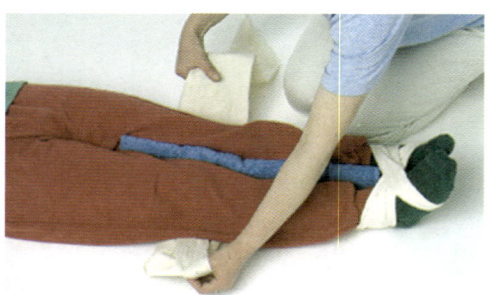

B

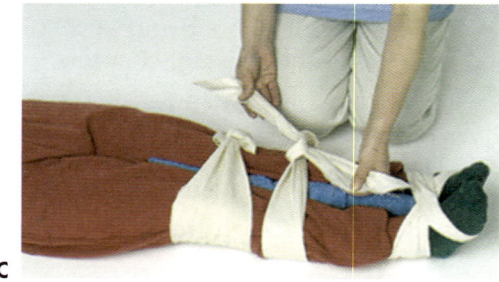

C

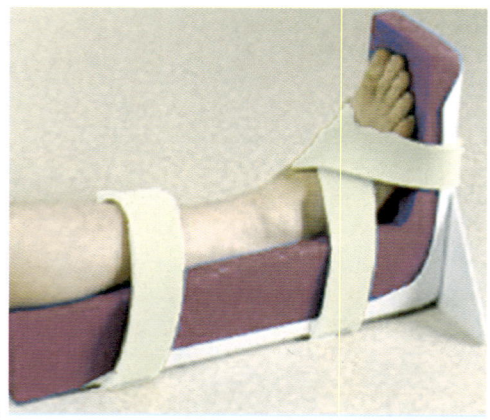

D

Figs 4.4A to D: Splinting of injured limbs by using patient's own body part

Remember
- Fracture is not an emergency.
- Most of them can be managed effectively at a later date.
- In A to F, management of injured fracture treatment comes last.
- Prepare and improvise splints with available materials at the scene of accident.

MANAGEMENT AT THE HOSPITAL

Once the injured reaches the hospital, the role of first aid ends and treatment at the hospital is not called first aid but *medical aid*. Trauma care at hospitals is given by various experts. Details of treatment are beyond the scope of this book. However, fracture management has been dealt in appropriate sections. An outline of the hospital treatment is given below. Mac Murthy has laid down the **A to F** management guidelines to be followed in the institutional care for an injured in the order of importance:

- **A**irway management
- **B**lood and fluid replacement
- **C**entral nervous system management
- **D**igestive system management
- **E**xcretory system management
- **F**racture management.

Other emergency measures like administration of antitoxin, antibiotics, antigasgangrene serum, and wound debridement should be carried out. Appropriate radiographs should be taken before treating the fractures. The treatment of bone and joint injuries are discussed in detail in the relevant chapters.

What are the pre-requisites to be a good first aider?
Anybody from an illiterate to an executive can be a first aider. The necessary qualities one should possess to become a good first aider is not academic degrees but human qualities like humanity, compassion, courage, and common sense.

Remember
Prerequisites for a good first aider:
- **Alertness**
- **Intelligence**
- **Decisions**

Mnemonic of a bad first aider:
- **A**pathy
- **I**ndecision
- **D**elay

In first aid:
- Delay is dangerous.
- If improperly executed, first aid will become the last aid!
- Always aid the patient to recovery and do not send him to mortuary by being apathetic.
- Shifting a patient to a hospital is extremely important.
- Terminate first aid measure once medical assistance arrives or after shifting the patient to the hospital.
- Value of do's during emergencies when offering first aid:
- Do not overdo: It may prove fatal to the victim.
- Do not underdo: This may also prove fatal.

The management of fractures at the scene of accident.
Five Ss
1. **S**ling for clavicle fractures, shoulder injuries, etc.
2. **S**trap for clavicle and rib fractures.
3. **S**plint, usually improvised. Best would be a Thomas splint or a pneumatic splint.
4. **S**hift the patient with utmost care.
5. **S**eek professional help at the earliest.

The priority in first aid
Three Ss
1. **S**hock to be corrected first.
2. **S**ystemic injuries to be tackled next.
3. **S**pine injuries call for extreme caution.
   Hence aid in emergency and act individually. Saving a life is an extremely noble act.

5 Management of Simple Fractures

DIFFERENT LEVELS OF FRACTURE TREATMENT

Fractures pass through different levels of treatment, namely:

- Treatment by unskilled people at the scene of accident. (Discussed in the previous chapter.)
- Treatment by semiskilled people at the emergency department.
- Treatment by skilled people, i.e. by the orthopedic surgeons.

Fracture treatment commences from the scene of the accident, progresses through various methods of treatment, operative and non-operative and finally concludes with rehabilitation. We shall discuss the treatment methodologies in three important stages.

Treatment by Unskilled People

In the accident scene, anyone from illiterate, to even a doctor could end up treating an accident victim. Nobody has any choice over treating persons during emergency. They are at the mercy of luck and god as to whom they end up being treated with. The principles of treatment at the accident site have to be:

- *Preserve life*: This takes precedence over the fracture management and consists of preserving life by ensuring proper respiration, circulation, heart functions and level of consciousness by various cardiopulmonary resuscitative measures.
- *Prevent further damage*: By judicious handling of the vital organs and immobilizing the fractures by appropriate splinting with whatever material is available at your disposal on the roads, e.g. newspapers, umbrella, sticks, cardboards, rods. All these materials can be used to prepare a make-shift splint.
- *Promote recovery:* By shifting the patient to the hospital at the earliest with utmost care, and entrusting, the patient to the trained personnel in

the hospital. Please refer chapter of First Aid for more details on emergency treatment of fractures.

Remember

Principles of fracture treatment at emergency site **4Ps**:
- **P**reserve life.
- **P**revent further damage.
- **P**romote recovery.
- **P**atient to be shifted to the hospital at the earliest.

The principle of fracture treatment at the scene of accident is splint, and splinting the fractures with whatever material you could lay your hands on!

Treatment by Semi-skilled People

Once the patient is shifted to the hospital, semi-skilled professionals, at the causality, like the duty doctors, junior residents, postgraduate students, nurses, and other paramedics now take up fracture treatment. Their job is to:

- Evaluate the whole body for injuries. Institute appropriate resuscitative measures to preserve and maintain life. Remove the tight bandages, tourniquets and make shift splints applied at the scene of accident.

After the general condition of the victim stabilizes:

- Apply proper splints like Thomas splints, BB splints, etc. to immobilize the fractures.
- Subject the patient to appropriate investigations like laboratory tests, X-ray, MRI, CT scan.
- Transfer the patient to the care of a specialist like orthosurgeon, neurosurgeon.

Remember

The principles of treatment at the emergency department:
- Evaluation.
- Resuscitation.
- Immobilization with proper splints.
- Investigations.
- Shifting the patient to the care of an orthopedic surgeon for the definitive treatment.

Treatment by Skilled Professionals (definitive treatment)

The role of an orthopedic surgeon in the fracture treatment begins now. With the life preserved and saved, his job is to tackle the fractures with a vast

armamentarium of choices of treatment methods available at his disposal and tailor to suit the needs of the individual patient. Fractures treatment may range from simple, compound, complicated, fractures, dislocations and multiple fractures. There could be multisystem injuries for which he needs to summon the services of other specialists like neurosurgeon, faciomaxillary surgeon, thoracic surgeon, vascular surgeon. Now he is part of a trauma team striving to restore the individual back to his pre-injury status. His role is discussed under the following headings:

- Appropriate investigations and decision-making.
- Management of simple fractures.
- Management of open fractures.
- Rehabilitation.

Appropriate Investigations in Orthotrauma

The surgeon can rely on the investigations already ordered by the junior surgeons or get the below mentioned investigations done again to evaluate the spectrum of the fracture pathology to his satisfaction before deciding the most appropriate treatment methods.

Radiography

It is an important diagnostic tool for fractures. Minimum two views, *anteroposterior* and *lateral*, are required since the bone is cylinder in shape. Sometimes an oblique view and other special view are required depending upon the clinical situations and the bone under study (see Fig. 1.7A).

CT Scan and MRI

These are the most sophisticated investigative methods available in orthopedics. Both are non-invasive and are extremely useful in evaluating both soft tissue and bony injuries. They are particularly useful in evaluating, spine, pelvis, and hip injuries (see Figs 1.7B and C).

Other Investigations

It includes laboratory investigations, arthroscopy especially for knee (see Fig. 65.1), shoulder, and ankle injuries, arthrography (see Fig. 40.13), bone scans, arteriogram, etc. Except laboratory investigations, and X-rays others are required under special situations and is entirely the choice of the treating orthopedic surgeon.

Goals of Fracture Treatment

The *goal* of an orthopedic surgeon in the fracture management is to restore the anatomy back to its normal or as near to normal as possible. The *responsibility* of an orthopedic surgeon is to ensure that there is no functional disability to the patient after the treatment for fracture. Management of fracture can be broadly classified and discussed as under.

Management of Undisplaced Fractures

Simple fractures are displaced or undisplaced and can be managed by conservative and operative methods. Treatment normally employed for undisplaced fractures, incomplete fractures, impacted fractures, etc. are rest and just immobilization seems to be enough and this can be achieved by (Figs 5.1A to D):

a. *Simple collar cuff and collar sling:* For upper limb fractures (Fig. 5.1A).

b. *Strapping* for fracture clavicle, ribs fracture, finger and toe fractures (Fig. 5.1B).

c. *Plaster slabs:* Plaster of Paris slabs can be used to support the injured limb in the initial stage (Fig. 5.1C).

d. *Rest and non-steroidal anti-inflammatory drugs (NSAIDs):* For impacted neck of femur fracture, etc.

e. *Splints:* Specialized splints like the Thomas splints, BB splints, Pneumatic splints, etc. can be used for immobilization of fractures of the femur, tibia, etc. (Fig. 5.1D).

Management of Displaced Fractures

Here the aim is to restore back the normal anatomy of the bones by either closed or open reduction. This consists of resuscitation, reduction, retention and rehabilitation (**4Rs**).

1. *Resuscitation* is highly prioritized if the patient is in shock following a fracture. A to F management proposed by MacMurthy is to be followed in all situations of emergencies (see page 16).

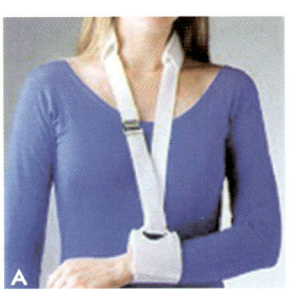
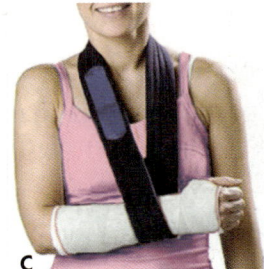
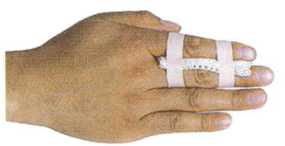
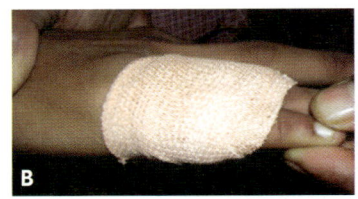
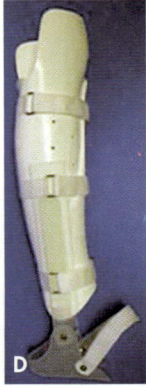

Figs 5.1A to D: Various conservative treatment methods in orthopedics: (A) simple cuff and collar sling, (B) strapping, (C) slab (D) splint for immobilization of fracture

2. *Reduction* of the fracture fragments is mandatory if displaced. It is usually done under general anesthesia after adequate radiographic study. Reduction methods consist of:
   a. *Closed reduction* technique consists of traction (given by the orthosurgeon) and countertraction (given by an assistant) methods (Fig. 5.2).
   b. *Continuous traction* is used for reduction of some fractures, e.g. Gallow's traction (for shaft femur fracture in children), (See Fig. 11.3) balanced skeletal traction (for adult shaft femur fractures, etc.). However traction as a primary method of fracture treatment is losing its importance and its mainly used as a first and measure or for initial stabilization.
   c. *Open reduction* is done when the above methods fail or if there are specific indications (See page 22).

3. *Retention*: Once the fracture fragments are reduced, it has to be retained in that position till the fracture unites, otherwise it tends to get displaced due to the action of muscles, gravity and other inherent factors. Retention methods after closed reduction are:
   a. *Plaster of Paris* is the most common splint employed for fracture treatment after reduction of displaced fractures (Fig. 5.2C).

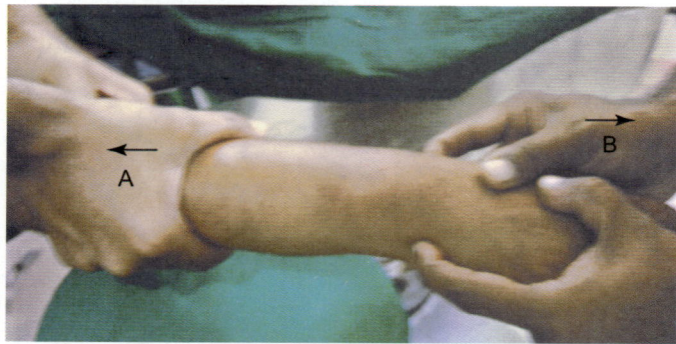

Figs 5.2A and B: Method of closed reduction: (A) traction and countertraction, (B) Plaster cast immobilization

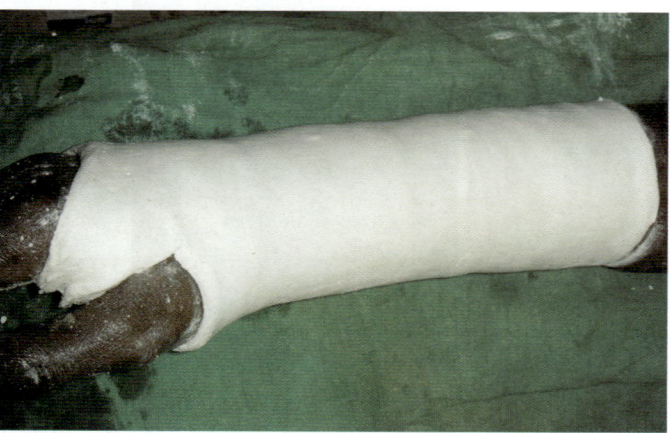

Fig. 5.2C: Plaster cast

b. *Continuous traction:* To overcome the muscle forces after closed reduction. The traction could be skin or skeletal traction and is employed as fixed, balanced or combined types of tractions (Figs 5.3 and 5.4).

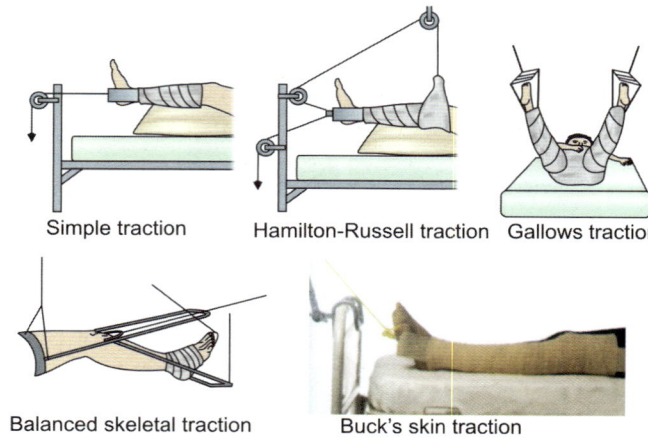

Simple traction   Hamilton-Russell traction   Gallows traction

Balanced skeletal traction   Buck's skin traction

Fig. 5.3: Methods of various skin and skeletal traction

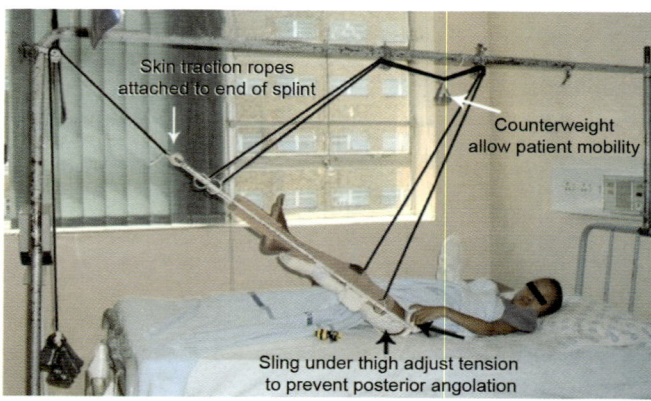

Skin traction ropes attached to end of splint

Counterweight allow patient mobility

Sling under thigh adjust tension to prevent posterior angolation

Fig. 5.4: Method of balanced traction

   c. *Use of functional brace:* This can be used after 3 weeks, once the fracture becomes sticky. This enables the patient to mobilize the joints early and thus prevent joint stiffness (Fig. 5.5).

4. *Rehabilitation* aims at restoring back the function of the affected limbs and this is achieved by the following exercises and physiotherapeutic methods.
   • Active exercises for the unimmobilized joints.
   • Isometric exercises for the immobilized joints.
   • Care for plaster splints to avoid loosening, breakage, tightness, skin excoriations, soiling, etc.
   • Training to carry out the functional activities with the unaffected limb.
   • Once the plaster is removed, mobilization of joints is done by appropriate active and passive exercises. Resistive exercises help to strengthen the muscles.

5

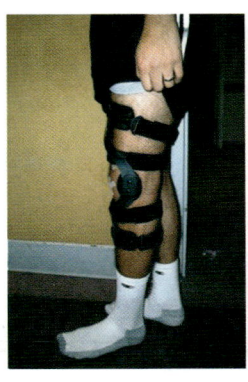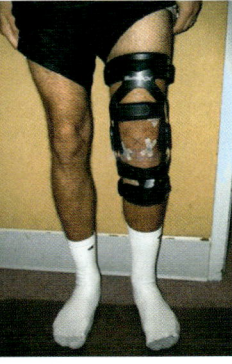

Fig. 5.5: Functional cast brace

- Heat therapy to alleviate pain, swelling and spasm.
- Massaging of the joints after application of pain relieving gel or oil helps to relax the muscles and relieve pain.
- Isotonic exercises help to strength on the muscles.
- Counseling to keep the depression and anxiety away.

Thus, rehabilitation begins soon after a fracture and ends once the functions are restored back completely.

Remember

Five Rs in the management of closed fractures treated by closed reductions:
- **R**esuscitations if the patient is in shock.
- **R**eduction of the fracture if displaced.
- **R**etention of the fragment by plasters, tractions, etc.
- **R**ehabilitation.
- **R**estoration of lost anatomy and functions.

Fracture Management by Open Reduction (operative management)

As mentioned earlier open method is indicated once the conservative methods fail and when there are specific indications. These indications could be absolute, relative or rare as mentioned below:

Indications

Absolute

- Failed/closed reduction.
- Displaced intraarticular fractures.
- Types III and IV epiphyseal injuries.
- Major avulsion fractures.
- Nonunion.
- Replantation of extremities.

Relative

- Multiple fractures.
- Delayed union.
- Loss of reduction.
- Pathological fractures.

- For better nursing care.
- To avoid prolonged bed rest.
- Closed methods ineffective in Galeazzi's fracture, Monteggia's fracture, femoral neck fracture, etc.

Questionable

- Neurovascular injury.
- Open fractures.
- Cosmetic reasons.
- Economic consideration.

Retention after Open Reduction

After open reduction the fracture fragment invariably needs to be fixed internally by suitable implants.

Choice of Implants

a. *K-wire*: For epiphyseal injuries and for small bones of hand and feet (diameter of the K-wires varies from 1–3 mm) (Fig. 5.6E).

b. *Screws*: For avulsion fractures and butterfly fragments.

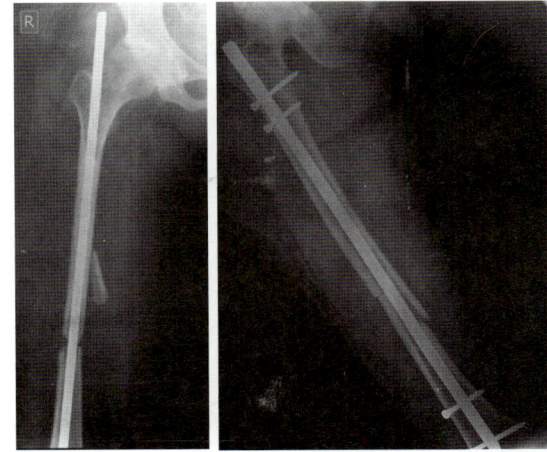

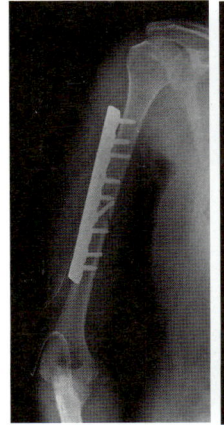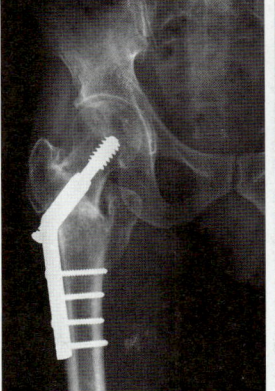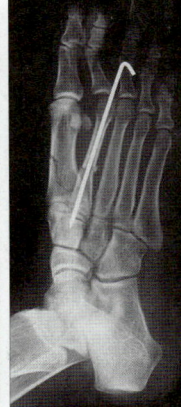

Figs 5.6A to E: Various internal fixations methods in orthopedics: (A) IM nail, (B) interlocking nail, (C) humerus plating, (D) DHS, (E) metatarsal fracture fixed with K-wire

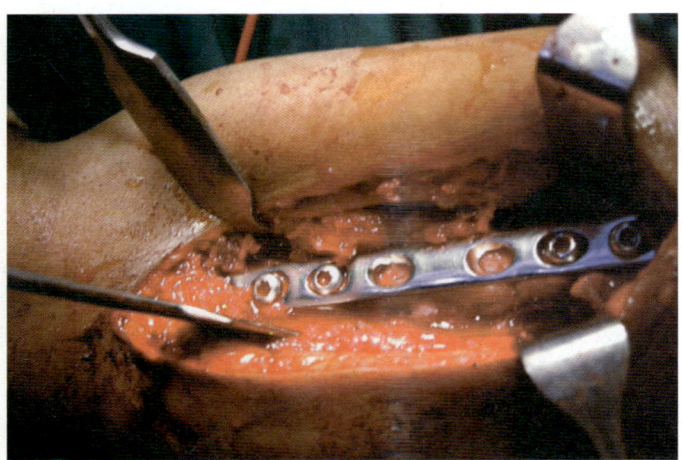

Fig. 5.7: Open reduction and internal fixation with DCP plate and screws in humerus fracture.

c. *Intramedullary nails*: For fracture through the narrowest portion of a medullary canal of a long bone (Fig. 5.6A).
d. *Interlocking nails*: For segmental fractures, comminuted fractures, etc. of long bones (Fig. 5.6B).
e. **Plate and screws:** For proximal and distal third fractures of long bones (Fig. 5.6C).
f. *Hip implants:* For neck femur fracture. Smith Peterson's nail, Richard's compression screw, multiple cannulated screws, etc. (Fig. 5.6D).
g. Condylo cephalic nails for supracondylar fracture of femur.
h. *Spine implants:* Steffee plate and screws (VSPs), Luque's rod, Hart shill frame, Harrington's rods, etc.
i. *Steel wires (No. 18–20 gauze):* Useful for tension band wiring for fracture of patella, olecranon, etc.

Contraindications for Open Reduction

- Infection
- Small fragments
- Weak and porotic bone
- Soft tissue damage
- Undisplaced or impacted fractures
- Poor general and medical condition.

Disadvantages of Open Reduction

- Closed fracture converted into an open fracture
- Fracture hematoma is disturbed
- Scar tissue
- Anesthetic problems
- Foreign body reaction due to metals

Rehabilitation of Fractures after Open Reduction

This proceeds on the same lines as that of the fractures treated by closed reduction except that wound care has to be followed meticulously. In cases of internal fixations, the joints can be mobilized early by appropriate physiotherapy techniques like electrotherapy and mobilization and strengthening exercises (Figs 5.8A and B).

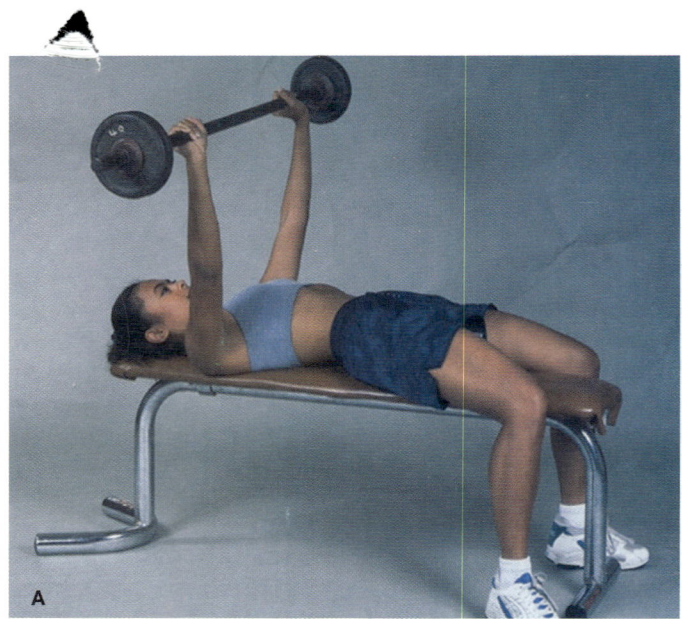

A

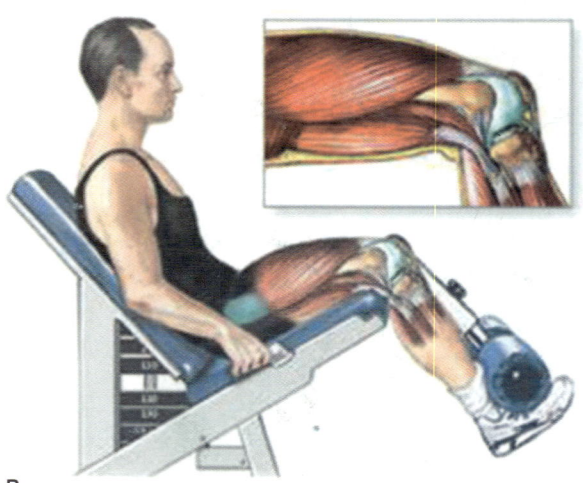

B

Figs 5.8A and B: Rehabilitation is the most essential part of fracture management: (A) isotonic exercises, and (B) isometric exercises

6 | Management of Open Fractures and Polytrauma

INTRODUCTION

Open fracture is a surgical emergency and presents as a problem which is much more difficult than closed fractures. It is defined as 'a fracture which communicates with the external atmosphere due to break in the soft tissue cover'. Open fractures 'open' up the possibility of 'infections' and 'closes' the options of internal fixations and plasters. It thus throws an 'open' challenge to the treating orthopedic surgeons in managing them. These fractures are also not 'open' for sound union and end mostly maluniting or nonuniting!

Mechanism of injury

Open fractures commonly occur due to high velocity RTA's violent falls, gunshot injuries crush injuries, etc. Tibia due to its subcutaneous location is notoriously susceptible for open fractures (Fig. 6.1).

Gustillo and Anderson's Classification

- *Type I*: Wound is less than 1 cm in size. It is usually due to a low-velocity trauma (Fig. 6.2A).

- *Type II*: Wound is more than 1 cm and less than 10 cm but there is no devitalization of soft tissue and is associated with very little contamination (Fig. 6.2B).
- *Type III*: Wounds moderate and severe in size (> 10 cm) and the soft tissues are devitalized and contaminated (Fig. 6.2C).
- *Type IIIA:* Extensive soft tissue injury but with adequate soft tissue to cover the fractured bone (Fig. 6.2D).
- *Type IIIB:* Extensive soft tissue damage and loss. Bone cannot be covered and is exposed to the atmosphere (Fig. 6.2E).
- *Type IIIC:* Compound fractures with arterial injuries.

APPROACH IN COMPOUND FRACTURES

Compound fractures are usually serious injuries and are due to high-velocity trauma. They may be associated with multisystem and multiskeletal injuries. The approach should be more cautious and the following protocol is recommended:

- *General physical examination:* This is of vital importance since the patient is usually in shock. Levels of consciousness, pulse, blood pressure, breathing, etc. should be recorded.
- *Examination of other systems:* Examinations should be carried out for head injury, neck and face injury, chest injury, blunt injury abdomen, pelvic fractures and spine fractures.

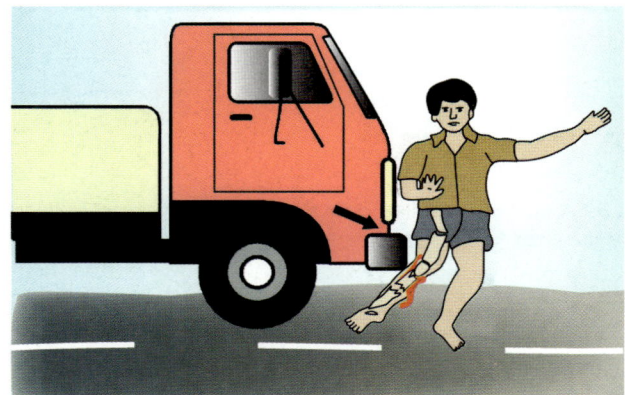

Fig. 6.1: Bumper injuries in RTA commonly cause open femur and tibia fracture.

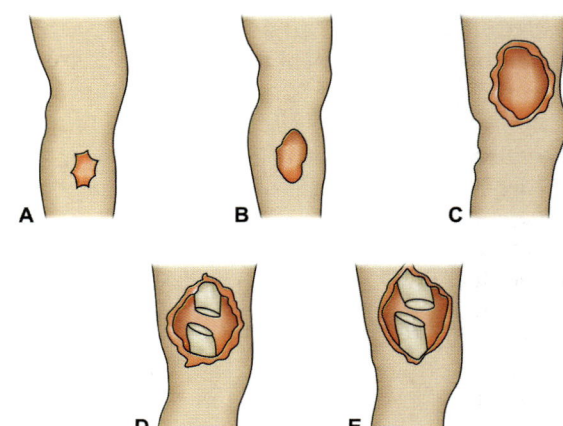

Figs 6.2A to E: Types of compound fractures: (A) type I (< 1 m), (B) type II (> 1 m), (C) type IIIA, (D) type IIIB, and (E) type IIIC

- *Examination of the compound injury:* Usually proceeds in the same line as mentioned in examination of closed fractures. In addition to the usual clinical features one should look for soft tissue injury and wound, bone loss, absence of bone pieces, distal neurovascular status of the limb, etc.

Investigations

Laboratory investigations like Hb percentage, blood group, bleeding time and clotting time, HIV, HbsAg urine examination, etc. are to be carried out.

Plain X-rays enable to study the fracture configuration and to look for missing pieces of bone in open fractures (Fig. 6.3).

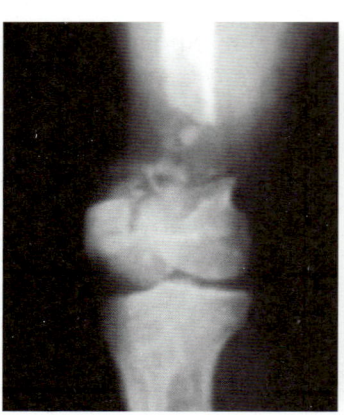 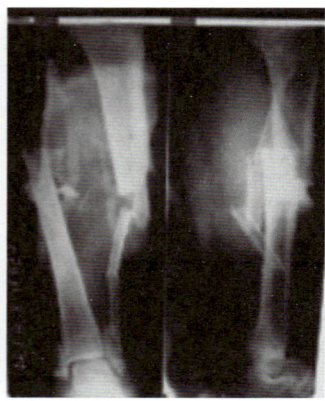

Fig. 6.3: Showing plain X-rays of the compound fractures of lower end of femur and both bones leg

Management Principles

The aims of the treatment are:
- To convert a contaminated wound into a clean wound and thus help to convert an open fracture into a closed one.
- To establish union in good position.
- To prevent pyogenic and clostridial infections.

Considerations
- First priority is to stabilize the general condition of the patient as the patient is usually in shock. This consists of resuscitation, blood transfusion, intravenous fluids, oxygen administration, etc.
- To keep the wound covered with proper sterile bandages till the patient is ready for surgery.
- Open fractures are surgical emergencies and surgery is to be done as soon as the patient is fit.
- Proper splintage by means of external fixators.
- ATS and AGGS to be given to avoid fatal complications like tetanus and gas gangrene.
- Appropriate broad spectrum antibiotics.

Treatment Plan

After stabilizing the general condition of the patient,

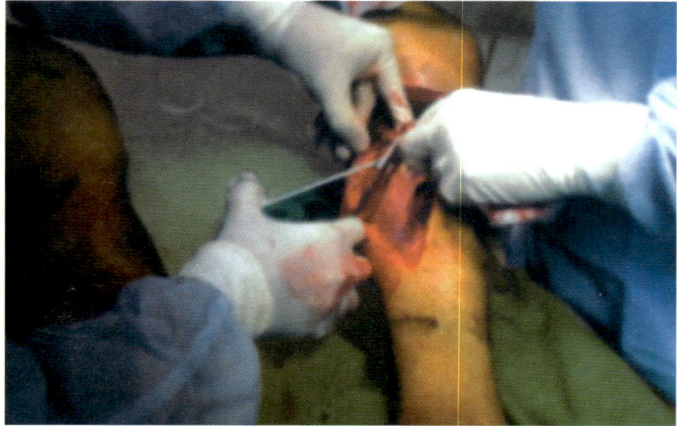

Fig. 6.4: Debridement is the mainstay of management in open fractures

surgical debridement is planned under strict aseptic measures in major operation theater.

DEBRIDEMENT

This is the most important step in the management of compound fractures. It consists of the following steps **(4 Es)**:
1. *Exploration of the wound:* The wound should be sufficiently explored proximally and distally to have a proper assessment of the extent of the damage.
2. *Excision of all non-viable structures:* A thorough excision of all the non-viable structures is important to prevent infection. The recognition of non-viable tissue before excision is of paramount importance. The tissues are dealt as follows:
   - *Skin:* The plan is to excise all the dead skin and yet be conservative.
   - *Muscle:* Non-viable muscle should be removed but often it is overlooked hence the axiom, *"when in doubt, take it out"*. **5Cs** help in deciding the muscle viability.

Features	Viable	Non-viable
Color	Pink	Pale
Consistency	Firm	Flabby
Capacity to bleed	Preserved	Lost
Circulation	Present	Absent
Contractility	Present	Absent

   - *Bones:* Small bits of loose bones devoid of soft tissues are removed. Large fragments with their soft tissue attachments are preserved.
   - *Nerves and vessels:* Primary repair is done if the wound is clean. In contaminated wounds they are dealt at a later stage.
3. *Evacuation of foreign bodies:* Like dirt, glass, stones, pebbles, etc. These foreign bodies are a source for infection and may invite a foreign body reaction. Hence, they have to be removed by a thorough irrigation (normal saline is used).

6

About irrigation
- Dilution is the solution of pollution.
- Single most essential step.
- Minimum 10 liters of saline is used.
- Forcible streams are avoided.
- Swirling movements of the irrigation fluid is preferred.
- Irrigation or wound toilet helps to clear the foreign bodies and clots minimizing the chances of contamination.

4. *External fixators* are used to fix the fracture fragment after debridement. Plaster of Paris and internal fixation devices have little and controversial role in the fracture management of compound fractures. External fixators help to stabilize fracture fragments, allow daily wound inspection and dressing, permit procedures like skin grafting, etc. to cover the wound, allow soft tissues to heal apart from providing early mobilization. In open tibial fracture, external fixator can be safely exchanged to internal fixation within 3 weeks with 5 percent incidence of deep infection (Fig. 6.5).

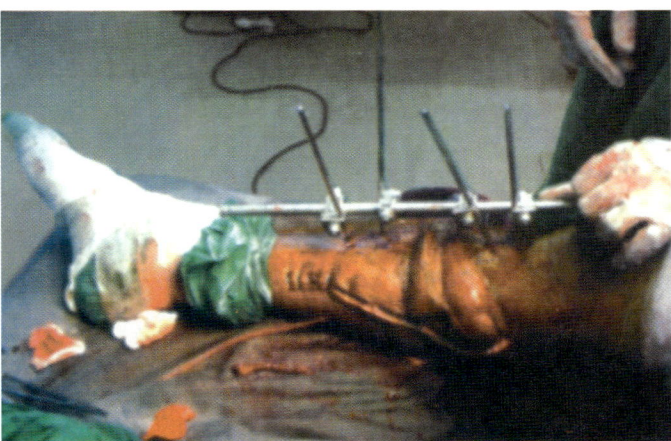

Fig. 6.5: Treatment of open fractures by external fixators

Other Forms of Fracture Immobilization

- *Pins and plasters:* The use is restricted and can be tried in type I fractures.
- *Limited internal fixation*: In grade I, grade II and grade IIIC fractures.
- *Skeletal traction*: Overhead olecranon traction for compound supracondylar fractures, Bohler-Braun skeletal traction for open femoral shaft fractures are few examples.
- *Plaster of paris:* Do not have any role.
- *Internal fixations* are slowly gaining ground in the primary fixations of open fractures. They are no longer a taboo. However a judicial selection has to be made regarding the choice of implants keeping in mind the fracture stability and the chance of infections.

Open facts in open fractures	
About fixation methods in open fracture:	
External fixators	Liberally used.
Internal fixators	Sparingly used.
Skeletal traction	Rarely used.
Plaster casts	Occasionally used (type I).
Functional brace	Never used.

Poetic Facts

James Learmanth's poem depicts the four major principles of debridement:

On the edges of the skin take a piece, very thin; the tenser the fascia, the more you should slasher; of muscles much more, until you see fresh gore; and the bundles contract at least the impact; hardly any of bone, only bits quite alone.

Remember

Problems peculiar to open fracture:
- In open fractures soft tissue injury is a dreaded problem than the fracture itself.
- A surgical emergency.
- Three problems:
  - Infection from the environment.
  - Problems of soft tissue loss.
  - Active infection.
- Effective immobilization rendered difficult.
- When bone repair is delayed speed is the watchword in treatment.
- Nonunion, malunion, chronic osteomyelitis are very common.
- Difficulty in using the standard internal fixation methods renders managing the fractures very difficult.

DEFINITIVE WOUND CARE

After resuscitation, debridement and application of external fixators, attention is now given to the definitive wound care. This is an extremely important step as the primary objective of treatment in open fracture is to convert an open wound into closed wound. The wound closure could be primary or secondary.

Criteria for Primary Closure

- All necrotic material should be removed.
- Circulation should be normal.
- Nerve supply should be intact.
- Patients general condition should be stable.
- Wound should be closed without tension.
- No dead space should be left after closure.
- There should be no multisystem injuries.

If all the above criterias are met, the wound is closed by primary suturing. Alternative measures considered in the event of above criteria not being met are:
- Split skin graft.
- Pedicle or flap graft.

- Secondary suturing after 2–3 weeks.
- Relaxing incisions to mobilize the neighboring skin.
- Biological dressings (homologous or heterologous skin).
- To leave it open and to follow by regular dressings, wound inspection and closure at a later date.

Role of antibiotics: It will not replace the wound debridement. Topical antibiotics have very little role. Parenteral administration is recommended. The choice of antibiotics is usually a broad spectrum, bactericidal hypoallergenic agent with adequate serum concentration.

Role of AGGS and ATS: Patient is to be protected against tetanus and gas gangrene by effective immunization against them.

Role of primary amputation: In open fractures. This is controversial but can be considered in type IIIC with neural injury and if the warm ischemia is more than 6 hours.

APPROACH TO A POLYTRAUMA CASE

Polytrauma injuries mean multiple (2 or more) traumatic injuries like head injuries, limb injuries, chest injuries, pelvic injuries. It presents a great challenge in managing these catastrophic injuries.

This is mentioned in the approach to a compound fracture. Speed is the watchword in approach towards a multiple trauma case and should proceed as follows:

- *Initial evaluation*: The ABCDEs of initial examination of a polytrauma case are as follows:
- A-airway, B-breathing, C-circulation, D-disability (neurological examination), E-exposure, F-fracture examination, G-go back to the beginning for a secondary survey and H-help.
- *Secondary evaluation* after the initial evaluation and resuscitation, is a more systematic and detailed evaluation of the injuries mentioned above. Fractures are splinted externally and managed at a later date. But in few cases primary internal fixation is recommended in ipsilateral fractures, multisystem injuries, etc. for faster rehabilitation. Dislocations are promptly reduced.
- *Fracture examination* is done systematically as mentioned in the previous discussions.
- *Investigation* includes routine blood examinations, radiographs of head, neck, chest, spine and affected parts. CT scan and MRI of injured structures are mandatory.
- *Management in polytrauma*: The cases are usually life-threatening and involves a multidisciplinary

approach. Depending upon the nature of injuries and systems affected, specialists and super specialists like fascio-maxillary surgeons, neurosurgeons, cardiothoracic surgeons, vascular surgeons, plastic surgeons, etc. are involved in the trauma team during management of these critical cases. As an important member of this team, an orthosurgeon gets to fix the bone and joint once the condition of the patient is stable.

Common Complications of Open Fractures

Immediate complications: This is similar to the ones described for closed fractures. However blood loss, loss of bone pieces, fat embolism, crush syndrome, gas gangrene, tetanus, etc. are peculiar to these injuries.

Delayed complications: These include:
- Malunion.
- Nonunion.
- Delayed union.
- Chronic osteomyelitis.
- Soft tissue contractures.
- Shortening and other body deformities.
- Joint stiffness.

Open Facts

Why is delayed union and nonunion common in compound fractures?

Reasons could be:
- Loss of small pieces of bones.
- Loss of important fracture hematoma.
- Loss of soft tissues.
- Troublesome infection.
- Less than rigid fixation.
- Soft tissue interposition.

Remember

In open fractures:
- Debridement is the mainstay of treatment
- The procedure is **4Es**:
  Exploration of the wound.
  Excision of the devitalized tissues.
  Evacuation of the foreign bodies.
  External fixators.
- Devitalized tissue recognized by **5Cs**.
- Wound irrigation is the most important step.
- Primary aim is to convert an open wound into a closed one.
- Wound closure is to be decided with caution.
- Antibiotics cannot replace wound debridement.
- External fixators have definite role.
- Internal fixators and plasters have limited role.
- Ultimate goal is to restore the patient's limb and function as early as and as full as possible.

6

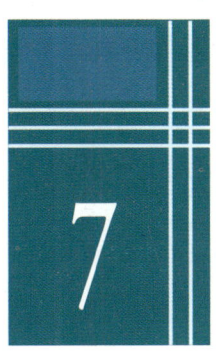

7 Injuries to the Joints and Soft Tissues

Dislocation

Subluxation

Sprain

Strain

Tendon injuries

DISLOCATION

Dislocation is defined as a total loss of contact between the two ends of bones. All dislocations are emergencies unlike fractures, delay in reduction may damage the articular surface, which are deprived of nutrition by the synovial fluid (Figs 7.1A and B).

Stability of the Joint

The stability of a joint comes from the following structures:
- Shape of the bone ends.
- Static stabilizers like ligaments, capsule.
- Dynamic stabilizers is provided by the surrounding muscles.

Pathology

In a dislocation, there could be damage to the capsule, articular cartilage, muscles, and ligaments in varying degrees. These could be osteochondral fractures and avulsion injuries.

Types of Dislocation

Congenital as in CDH (discussed in detail under chapter on CDH).

Acquired the following types are observed:

- Traumatic is common in young adults due to high velocity trauma.
- Pathological, e.g. TB hip, septic arthritis.
- Infective, e.g. Tom Smith arthritis in infants.
- Paralytic, e.g. poliomyelitis, cerebral palsy.
- Inflammatory disorders, e.g. rheumatoid arthritis.

Traumatic Dislocations

This is the most common type of all dislocations and considerable force is required to bring the joint out of its position. Capsules are invariably torn and the ligaments are avulsed. There could be damage to the articular cartilages, a fragment of which may break and form loose bodies within the joint.

Varieties of Traumatic Dislocations

- *Fresh dislocation:* Due to trauma, there could be acute dislocation of a joint. The more common ones are dislocations of the shoulder, patella, hip, and elbow, etc. (Fig. 7.1B).
- *Chronic unreduced dislocation*: In Asian countries, due to poverty, ignorance, illiteracy, apathy fresh dislocations are not promptly reduced and the patient lives with pain and disability. Due to secondary problems like pain, contractures, osteoarthritis, etc. patient may visit a doctor for treatment.
- *Repeated dislocations*: Due to inherent instability and other factors, some joints are prone for repeated dislocations. Topping the list in this group is the recurrent dislocations of the shoulder joint and the patella.
- *Fracture dislocations*: Along with the dislocation a piece of the neighboring bone is avulsed from its position or totally broken depending upon the

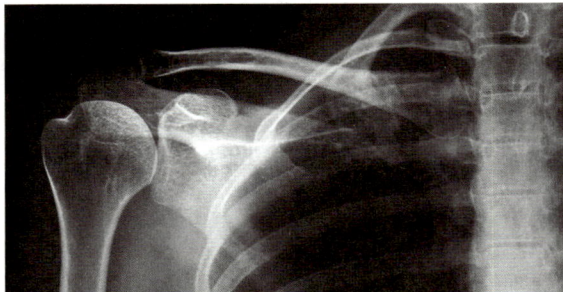
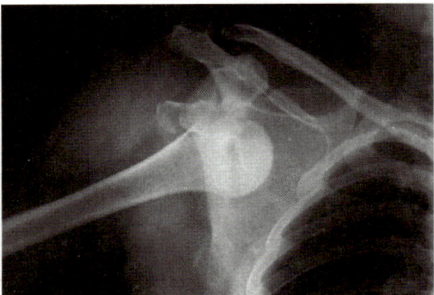

Figs 7.1A and B: (A) normal location, and (B) dislocation

severity of injury, e.g. posterior dislocation of the hip with acetabular fractures.

Clinical Features

Traumatic variety is the most common type of dislocation one encounters in clinical practice. Patient gives history of trauma usually a road traffic accident (RTA) or fall from heights following which there is pain, swelling deformity and loss of movements (Fig. 7.2). In dislocations of other varieties, clinical symptoms and signs pertaining to that particular disease are seen (e.g. TB).

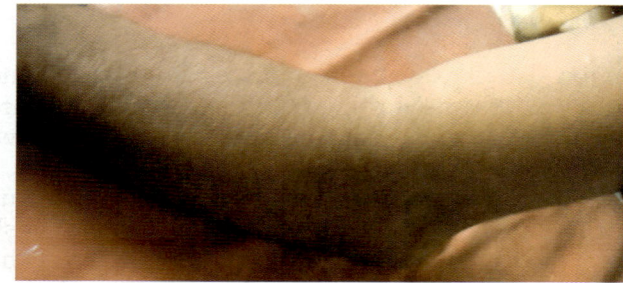

Fig. 7.2: Acquired traumatic dislocation in orthopedics: posterior dislocation of elbow

Investigations

Radiograph of the affected part should include anteroposterior and lateral views of the joints (Fig. 7.3). CT scan, MRI may be required in fractures and dislocations.

Treatment

Since dislocation is an orthopedic emergency, early closed reduction under general anesthesia is recommended. The part is immobilized for a period of 3 to 6 weeks to ensure adequate healing.

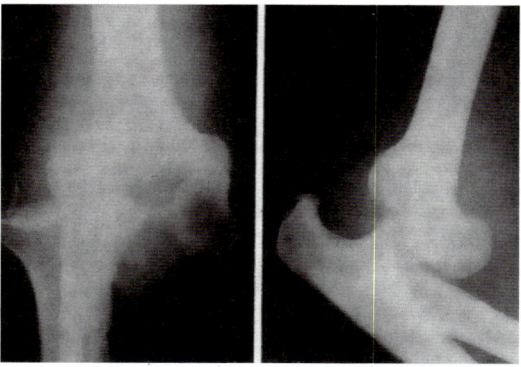

Fig. 7.3: Plain X-rays showing posterior dislocation of elbow

Operative reduction is rarely required and is reserved for:
- Failure of closed reduction
- Compound dislocations
- Irreducible dislocations
- Old unreduced dislocations
- Recurrent dislocations
- Fracture dislocations.

Do not be surprised to read about the story of *Missing Dislocations*! It is quite possible for some of the dislocations to elude the eyes of a discerning orthopedic surgeon. Here are a few examples:

1. *Some fracture dislocations:* Here the fractures are diagnosed but the dislocations are missed.
   - Monteggia's fracture.
   - Galeazzi's fracture.
   - Essex Lopressti fracture.
   - Fracture shaft or neck of femur with posterior dislocation of the hip joint.
   Reasons: Attention is diverted towards the fracture and the X-rays fail to include the neighboring joints and only include the fracture sites.

2. *Some serious situations:* There are situations where the life of the individual is at stake and the dislocations may get unnoticed or overshadowed by a greater tragedy like head injuries, unconscious patient, multiple fractures, polytrauma cases, ipsilateral fractures.

Complications of Dislocations

Acute injury to peripheral nerves and vessels can occur, e.g. sciatic nerve palsy in posterior dislocation of hip.

Chronic

- *Unreduced dislocation* which is common in Asian countries due to ignorance, delay in seeking treatment, etc.
- *Recurrent dislocation* due to inadequate and improper healing of soft tissues following initial trauma. Eg: RVS shoulder.
- *Traumatic osteoarthritis* due to damage to the articular cartilage following impaired nutrition by the synovial fluid.

7

- *Joint stiffness* due to capsular and other soft tissue injuries.
- *Avascular necrosis* due to injury to the vessels.
- *Myositis ossificans* more commonly seen in fractures due to greater perioseal strip.

Common Traumatic Dislocations

Area involved	Type of dislocation
1. *Spine*	Anterior, C5 over C6
2. *Upper limb*	
• Acromioclavicular joint	Type I/II/III
• Sternoclavicular joint	Anterior/posterior
• Shoulder joint	Anterior/posterior
• Elbow joint	Posterior
• Isolated dislocation of superior radioulnar joint	Anterior
• Fracture dislocation of superior radioulnar joint	Monteggia's fracture
• Fracture head of radius dislocation of inferior fracture	Essex
• Radioulnar joint	
• Wrist dislocations	Perilunar, lunar
• Kaplan injury	Carpometacarpal joint of the thumb
3. *Lower limb*	
• Hip dislocations	Anterior/posterior/central
• Knee joint	Posterior
• Patella	Lateral dislocations
• Ankle	Anterolateral
• Foot	Intertarsal
– Chopart's	
– Lisfranc's	Tarsometatarsal

SUBLUXATION

Subluxation is defined as partial loss of contact between the two ends of the bones. It poses a problem much less serious than dislocation.

SPRAIN

It is a tear in the ligaments. The severity varies from grade I to grade III (See Fig. 24.3). Mild sprains are more common and heal by conservative treatment, whereas grade III sprains cause joint instabilities and need to be repaired surgically. Sprains are commonly encountered in knee joints and ankle joints. They are discussed in detail in appropriate chapters. Mild sprains are treated by the PRICE regime.

STRAIN

It is tearing in the muscles, is more common in young athletes, and usually occurs due to sudden violent contractions (Figs 7.4A to C). Patient with acute muscular strain complains of agonising pain from muscle tightness due to spasm and inability to movse due to acute pain and spasm (Fig. 7.5).

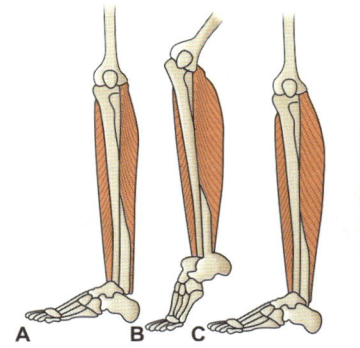 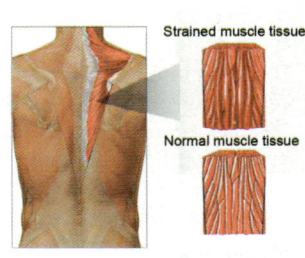

Figs 7.4A to C: Mechanism of muscle strain: (A) calf muscle at rest, (B) calf muscle contracts when flexed, (C) calf muscle does not relax causing cramp

Fig. 7.5: Clinicopathological manifestation of muscle strain

Treatment

It is essentially conservative and is denoted by the mnemonic **PRICEM**:

- **P**–pain killers
- **I**–ice
- **E**–elevation
- **R**–rest
- **C**–compression bandage
- **M**–mobilization

TENDON INJURIES

Tendon usually does not give way in young unless injured by a sharp cutting object like knife, chopper, etc. However, ironically in old age it does not hold its fort and gives way easily as it is rendered weak due to the efforts of relentless aging?

Treatment

In fresh cases, primary repair or tendon grafting is recommended. In old ruptures, if the disability is negligible no treatment is required. In the event of significant disability, tendon transfers may be contemplated.

Fracture Complications

Shock due to hypovolemia

ARDS

Acute Volkmann's ischemia

Volkmann's ischemic contracture

Delayed union and nonunion

Avascular necrosis

Traumatic myositis ossificans

Malunion

DVT

Injury to blood vessels

Injury to nerves

Crush syndrome

Other important delayed complications

IMMEDIATE COMPLICATIONS

SHOCK DUE TO HYPOVOLEMIA

In fracture of major long bones, pelvic fractures, multisystem injuries following road traffic accidents, etc. severe loss of blood may seriously threaten the life of a victim. Delay and apathy in attending a hypovolemic shock could prove fatal.

Source of Hemorrhage

This could be external or internal:
- *External hemorrhage*: This usually happens in compound fractures, pelvic fractures, etc.
- *Internal hemorrhage*: It is more often seen in blunt injury of abdomen, femur and pelvic fractures, etc. It could be much more in multiple fractures.

> **DO YOU KNOW A STAGGERING BLOOD LOSS IN FRACTURES**
> - *Femoral shaft fractures*: blood loss could range from 500 to 2000 ml.
> - *Pelvic fractures*: blood loss could range from 1000 to 2500 ml.

Clinical Features

Look for the classical features of shock apart from features of fractures (See box).

Look for the classical features of shock:
- Tongue-pale and dry
- Pale look
- Low BP
- Cold clammy skin
- Cold nose
- Peripheral pulses feeble or absent
- Drowsy or unconscious.

Investigations

Laboratory investigations like Hb%, blood group, bleeding and clotting time, HIV, HBsAg, etc. are of utmost importance. Plain X-rays of the affected limbs and other investigations like MRI, CT scan, etc. are done once the general condition of the patient is stabilized.

Treatment

Speed is the watchword in the treatment of shock which includes:
- Resuscitation.
- Immediate fluid replacement by:
  - IV fluids—normal saline, ringer lactate, etc.
  - Hemaccel.
  - Blood—is the best alternative.
- Administration of oxygen, etc.
- Splinting the fractures.
- Controlling the bleeding points.

ACUTE RESPIRATORY DISTRESS SYNDROME— FAT EMBOLISM

Acute respiratory distress syndrome (ARDS) is defined as a post-traumatic distress syndrome occurring within 72 hrs of skeletal trauma. It is seen in 10 to 45 percent cases of multiple fractures and is an important cause of morbidity and mortality (11%) in multiple fracture and multisystem injuries.

Etiology

Common etiological factor is a long bone fracture in young adult or a pelvic fracture in elderly.

Pathogenesis

Following injury, the bone marrow fats or the platelet agglutination are sucked into the injured vessels and are transported to various sites as emboli giving rise to varied clinical manifestation.

Source of fat: It could be from two sources:
- From bone marrow (accepted).
- From plasma by agglutination of chylomicrons which later acts as an embolus (less accepted).

Classification (Sevitt's) and Clinical Presentation

- *Classical type:* In this variety the onset is less than 24 hr, tachycardia is greater than 140/min, pyrexia is greater than 40°C, tachypnea, cyanosis, changing cerebral signs vary from confusion, restlessness and coma. Petechial rashes and in conjunctiva of lower lids, if present is pathognomonic (Fig. 8.1). In this type, the blood pressure is maintained throughout.
- *Fulminating type:* The sequence of events are very fast and there is no time for the rashes to develop. Patient is comatose within hours and throws repeated seizures. Patient rapidly collapses and death supervenes.
- *Incomplete type:* The manifestation is between the two types: unexplained tachycardia, fever and rash are its features.

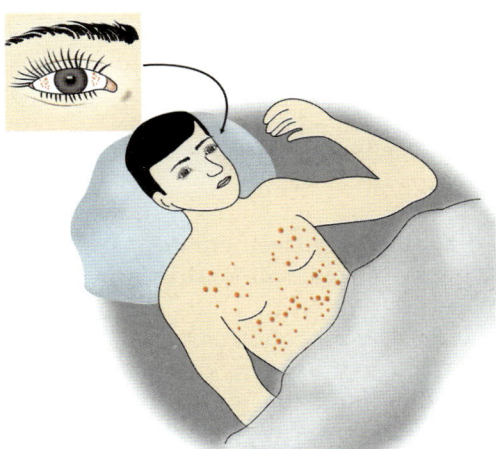

Fig. 8.1: Petechial rashes in ARDS (Condensed)

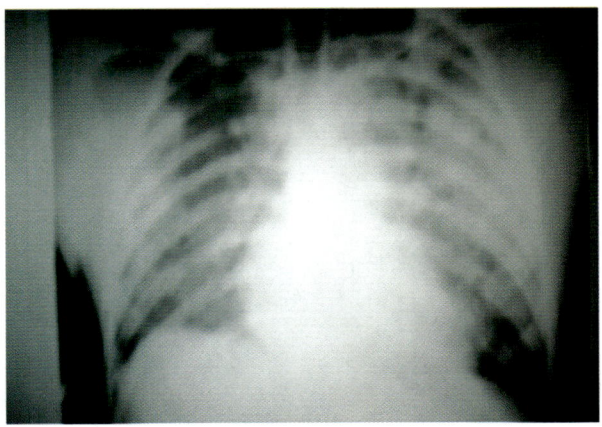

Fig. 8.2: Plain X-ray of the chest showing snowstorm appearance in ARDS

Investigations

- *X-ray of the chest* may show snowstorm appearance and if seen is pathognomonic (Fig. 8.2).
- PaO_2 less than 60 mm Hg.
- Platelet count is less than 1.5 lakh.
- ECG shows prominent S-wave.
- Gurd test: Isolation of fat emboli from the blood.
- There is no pathognomonic laboratory test.

The important diagnostic triad in ARDS is represented by the mnemonic **TPR**:
- **T**hrombocytopenia.
- **P**aO$_2$ < 60 mmHg.
- **R**ashes.

Management

There are two important steps in the management of ARDS. Specific and non-specific.
- *Non-specific* consists of three vital steps:
  - *Keep:* (a) airway patent, and (b) fracture immobilized by POP or external fixators.
  - *Restore:* (a) blood volume, (b) fluid, and (c) electrolyte balance.
  - *Avoid:* (a) careless handling of the injured, and (b) unnecessary transportation.
- *Specific* consists of three vital steps mentioned below:
  - Oxygen administration to restore back PaO_2.
  - *Drug therapy:* Steroids are given intravenously. These help gas exchange by decreasing inflammation in the lungs.
    - *Heparin*: This acts as a lipolytic and antiplatelet agent.
    - *Low molecular weight:* Dextran acts by increasing plasma volume.
    - *Intravenous alcohol* is not universally advocated.
    Antibiotics and other treatment.
  - *Definitive fracture treatment are* discussed in appropriate sections.

ADULT RESPIRATORY DISTRESS SYNDROME (ARDS)

This ARDS is slightly different from the ARDS discussed so far. Certain inflammatory mediators released during trauma are known to cause damage to the microvasculature structure of the pulmonary system leading to a condition of shock and trauma arising after 24 hrs or more after injury.

Clinical presentation: Patient presents with tachypnea and breathlessness.

Investigations: Arterial PO$_2$ is less than so and the chest radiograph shows diffuse pulmonary infiltrates.

Treatment: Consists of assisted ventilation and inhalation of 100% oxygen for 3–6 days. If undetected, it may prove fatal.

COMPARTMENTAL SYNDROME OF FOREARM

This is one of the most dreaded complications in orthopedics and ranges from mild ischemia to severe gangrene.

Definition

It is an ischemic necrosis of the structures contained within the volar compartment of the forearm (Fig. 8.3).

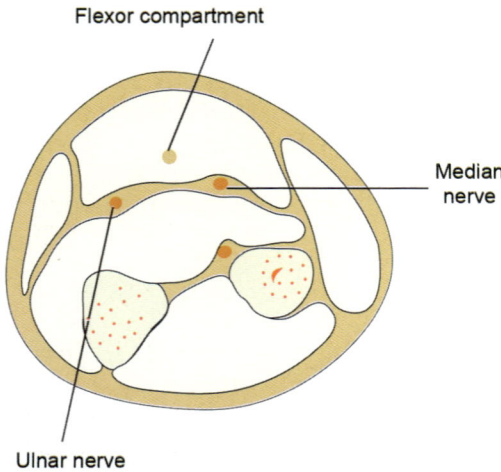

Fig. 8.3: Compartments of the forearm

Incidence and Etiology

It is common in children less than 10 years of age. Supracondylar fracture is the most common in children while crush injuries of the forearm are most common causes in adults. Occasionally fracture of both bones of forearm may be the cause. More recently intraarterial injections in drug addicts who lie on their forearm for prolonged periods in narcotized conditions are mooted to be a cause (Fig. 8.4). Improper application of splints is another important cause.

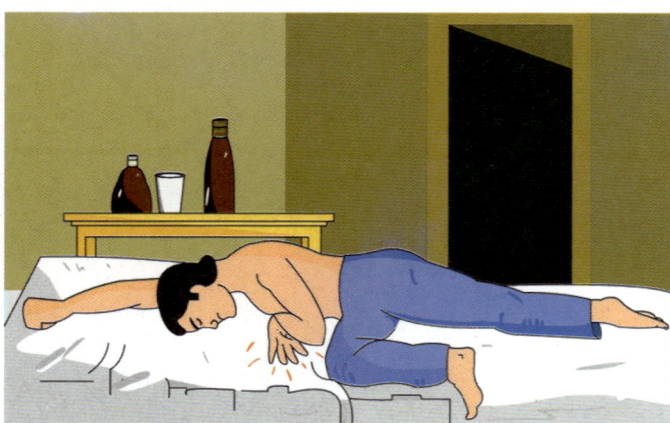

Fig. 8.4: Mechanism of compression of forearm in drug addicts

Pathophysiology

Usually the flexor muscles of the forearm, especially the flexor digitorum profundus and flexor pollicis longus and rarely flexor digitorum superficialis are involved.

External or internal constrictions → ↑ Arterial spasm or occlusion → Causes muscle ischemia → ↑ Capillary permeability → ↑ Intramuscular edema → ↑ Intramuscular pressure → Further arterial compromise →Muscle necrosis→Replaced by collagen → Contractures.

Pathology

An inelastic and unyielding deep fascia surrounds the forearm muscles. Rise in the intra-compartmental pressure due to any cause is not accommodated and the vessels are compressed resulting in muscle ischemia and consequent fibrosis.

Clinical Features

In the acute stages patient gives history of trauma and after an interval of few hours, severe, poorly localized pain develops in the forearm. The volar aspect of the forearm is swollen, red, warm, tender and tense. Fingers are held in flexion and attempt to extend the fingers, increase the pain (stretch pain) (Fig. 8.5). Peripheral pulses, which are present initially, disappear later. Median nerve is more commonly affected than the ulnar nerve. Impending acute Volkmann's ischemia is diagnosed by looking for the **6Ps** (See box).

Note: In compartment syndrome, patient complains of pain out of proportion to the injury.

Impending Volkmann's ischemia is detected by **6Ps**:
- **P**ain
- **P**allor
- **P**araesthesia
- **P**aralysis
- **P**ulselessness
- **P**ositive passive stretch test

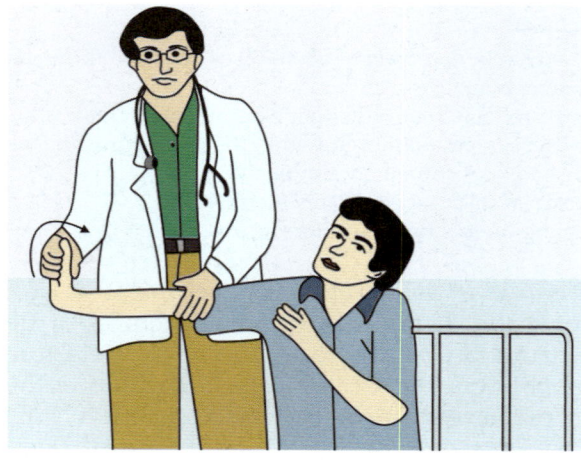

Fig. 8.5: Method of performing the passive stretch of fingers

8

Investigations

Plain X-ray of the affected part Doppler study, laboratory investigations, etc.

Management

It is a surgical emergency. All encircling tight bandages are removed, if present. If there is no improvement, record the pressure within the compartment (Fig. 8.6). If it is more than 30 mm Hg, an emergency surgical decompression is done by fasciotomy (Fig. 8.7). If the pressure is less than 30 mm Hg continuous monitoring is done.

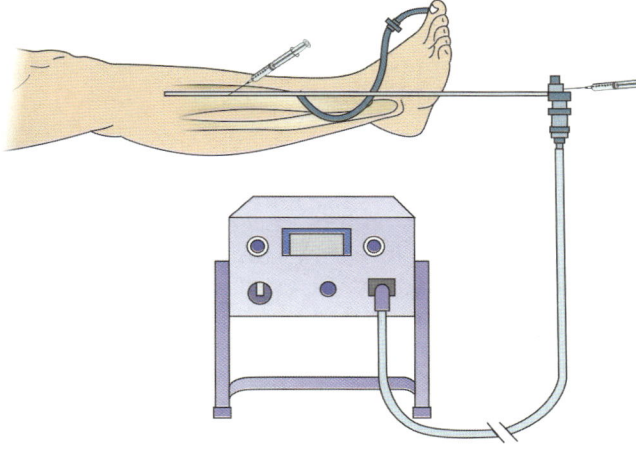

Fig. 8.6: Method of recording ICP

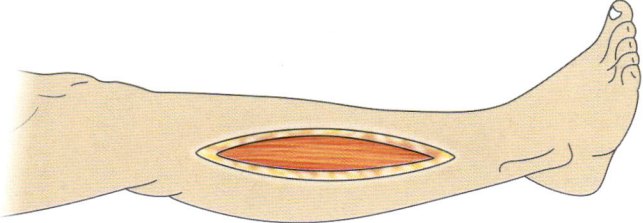

Fig. 8.7: A wide fasciotomy for acute compartmental syndrome ICP

Remember

If **5Ps** helps in detection of acute cases, 5Ps also form clue to the management:
- **P**ressure to be relieved either external or internal.
- **P**ressure to be monitored within the compartment.
- **P**ulse to be recorded continuously.
- **P**assive stretch test indicates the severity.
- **P**utting the fracture back into its position.

Volkmann's ischemic contracture: It is a late presentation. If mild, flexion contractures of flexor digitorum profundus and flexor pollicis longus develops but in severe cases all the finger flexors, thumb and wrist flexors are affected. The forearm is thin and fibrotic. Extensive scar tissue may be present. (Fig. 8.8) Peripheral nerves may be affected, amongst them

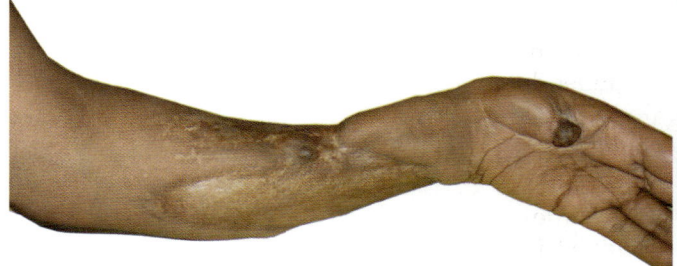

Fig. 8.8: Volkmann's ischemic contracture of the forearm

median nerve is the most commonly involved. A classical clawhand deformity results. Elicit *Volkmann's sign* in established VIC. This test consists of extending the wrist, which exaggerates the deformities, and on flexion, the deformities appear less prominent (Figs 8.9A and B). Joint contractures and gangrene may also be seen.

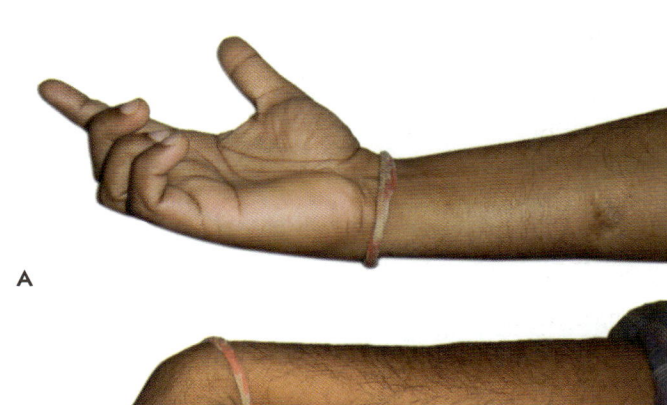

A

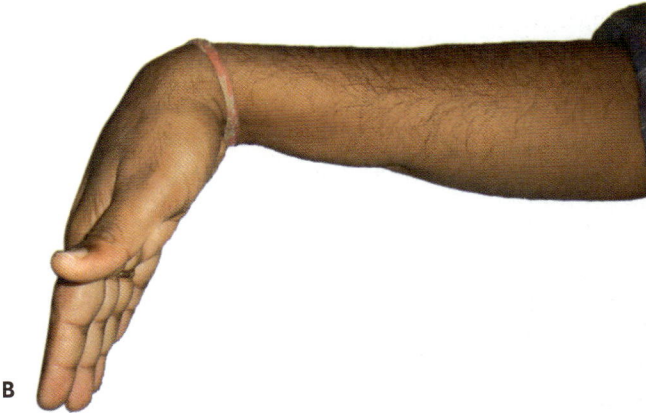

B

Figs 8.9A and B: Volkmann's sign: (A) deformity appears on extension, (B) disappears on flexion

In established VIC

Look for:
- Clawhand and deformity
- Volkmann's sign
- Extensive scarring of the forearm
- Joint and soft tissue contractures
- Neurological deficits
- Rarely gangrene
- Plain X-ray of the affected part is advised.

8

Treatment

The contractures are well established and the treatment plan depends upon the severity of VIC.

Mild Type

- Dynamic splinting
- Physiotherapy
- Total excision if single muscle is involved.

Moderate Type

- *Max page's muscle sliding operation:* This consists of releasing the common flexor origin from the medial epicondyle and passively stretching the fingers. This slides the origin of the muscle down and releases the contractures.
- *Excision of cicatrix*
- *Neurolysis:* It consists of freeing the peripheral nerves from the surrounding fibrous tissue.
- *Tendon transfers:* It is done if criterias for tendon transfers are met.

Severe Type

- Excision of the scar.
- *Seddon's carpectomy:* It consists of excising the proximal row of carpal bones thereby shortening the forearm to overcome the effects of contracted muscles.
- *Arthrodesis* of the wrist in functional position.
- *Amputation* for very severe cases of VIC with gangrene.

DELAYED COMPLICATIONS

DELAYED UNION AND NONUNION

In delayed union healing has *not advanced* at the average rate for location and type of fractures but healing can still take place if the limb is immobilized for a longer period.

In nonunion there is evidence to show clinically and radiologically that healing has ceased, union is improbable and needs surgery. Final status of nonunion is pseudoarthrosis.

Definition–FDA panel

Nonunion is said to be established when a minimum of nine months has elapsed since the injury and the fracture shows no radiologically visible progressive signs of healing continuously for three months.

Classification of Nonunion

Muller and Weber have classified nonunion depending on the amount of callus.

Hypervascular nonunion	*Avascular nonunion*
• Hypertrophic nonunion (Exuberant callus) • Horse hoof nonunion • Oligotrophic nonunion	• Comminuted nonunion • Torsion wedge nonunion • Atrophic nonunion • Defect nonunion

Hypervascular Nonunion

The fracture ends are viable and show biological reaction, hence, stable internal fixation is enough and no bone grafting is required (Figs 8.10A to C).

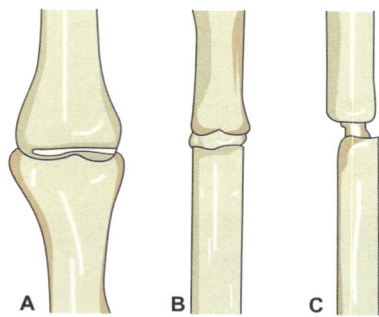

Figs 8.10A to C: Types of hypervascular nonunion: (A) elephant foot (B) horse hoof, (C) oligotrophic

Avascular Nonunion

The fracture ends are not viable due to poor blood supply. No biological reaction is seen, and this needs rigid internal fixation with bone grafting after decortications of non-viable ends (Figs 8.11A to D).

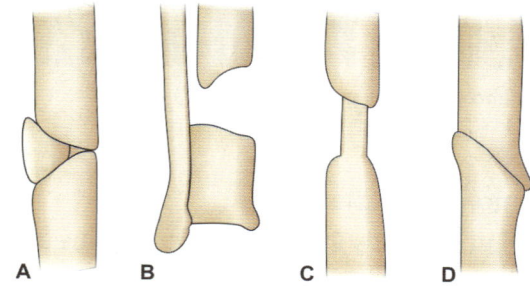

Figs 8.11A to D: Types of avascular nonunion: (A) comminuted non-union, (B) gap nonunion, (C) atrophic nonunion, (D) torsion wedge

Causes

Compound fractures infection, segmental fractures, distraction of fracture fragments, soft tissue interposition (it obstructs the growth of internal callus and thus jeopardizes union), ill-advised open reduction, insecure and inadequate fixation of fractures.

Apart from these local factors, the general factors which contribute to poor healing of fractures, are anemia, general debility, cachexia, steroid therapy, osteoporosis, malignancy, etc.

Clinical Features

Symptoms: Acute symptoms seen in fresh fractures are conspicuously absent in nonunion. There is usually history of no pain or minimal pain. There could be presence of a deformity or loss of function.

Signs: The important clinical signs are painless abnormal mobility, no crepitus, shortening, scars and sinuses, deformity, wasting of limb muscles, etc. (Fig. 8.12A).

Note: In delayed union, patient complains of dull pain at the fracture site, deep palpatation and clinical tenderness.

Investigation

Radiograph of the part in AP and lateral views (Fig. 8.12B) shows lack of callus in atrophic and excess callus in hypertrophic nonunion (Fig. 8.13).

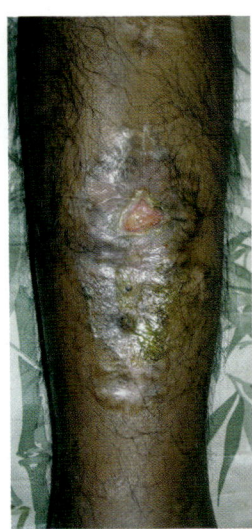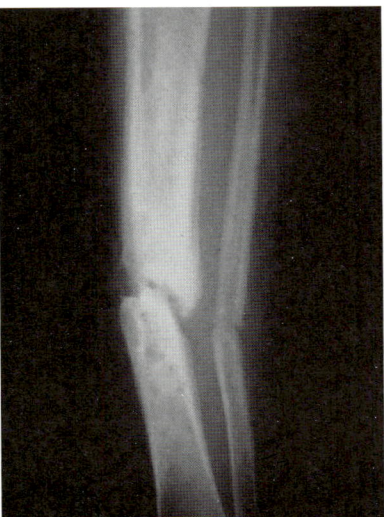

Figs 8.12A and B: Clinical photograph of (A) Infected nonunion of tibia and (B) plain X-ray showing of atrophic nonunion

Management Principles

- Nonunion is an absolute indication for surgery and it requires open reduction, rigid internal fixation and bone grafting.
- There is no role of conservative treatment.
- Other methods of treatment include electrical stimulation, interlocking nails, Ilizarov, excision, etc.
- In delayed union, most of the fractures unite when immobilization is further continued for several weeks. In complicated cases, surgery is the treatment of choice.

Other Measures

- *Masterly activity*: Do you remember the axiom *leave the sleeping tiger alone*? In certain situations (e.g. scaphoid nonunion) if it does not cause any significant functional impairment, it can be left alone.

- *Resection of the fragments*: Certain non-viable small bone pieces can be safely excised (e.g. distal end of ulna) and in some other situations like nonunion of fracture neck femur, the bone is excised and replaced with a prosthesis to make good the loss.
- *Role of Ilizarov in nonunion*: This allows simultaneous correction of all deformities and bone loss. In hypertrophy nonunion gradual compression helps union. In avascular nonunion, corticotomy, bone transport and compression helps. Ilizarov provides dramatic results but is technically very demanding. It is still the best way to treat cases of infected nonunion (Fig. 8.14).

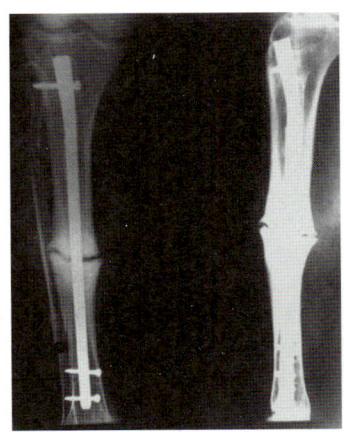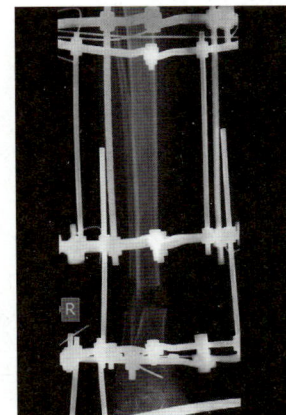

Fig. 8.13: Hypertrophic nonunion   **Fig. 8.14:** Ilizarov for nonunion tibia

AVASCULAR NECROSIS (AVN)

It is rare but severe complication of certain fractures. It occurs when the blood supply to a segment in a bone is affected.

Causes

- Extensive stripping of soft tissues, which damage the periosteal blood supply.
- In certain bones where the blood supply is unique and unidirectional, e.g. talus, scaphoid, neck of femur (Figs 8.15A to C).
- Other causes like steroid therapy, Caisson's disease, etc. which may cause on embolic block of the blood vessels.

Common Sites of AVN

They are head of femur in neck of femur fracture and dislocations of hip, body of the talus in fracture through the neck of talus, proximal pole of scaphoid in fracture through the waist of the scaphoid.

Problems in Avascular Necrosis

The loss of blood supply to a major bone segment impairs healing because the avascular segment cannot

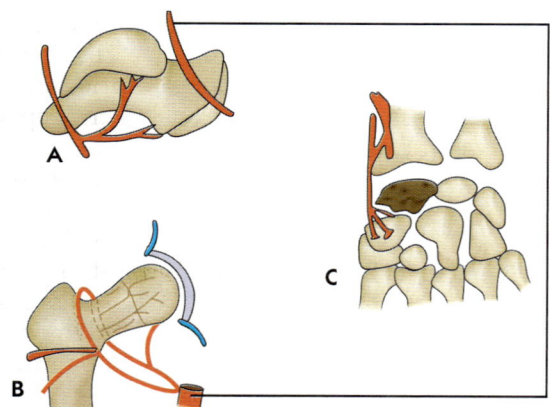

Figs 8.15A to C: Due to the peculiar blood supply, avascular necrosis is common in the above three bones: (A) talus, (B) scaphoid, and (C) femur of head

participate in the reparative process. This defective healing makes the bone weak and susceptible to external forces. This results in collapse of the bone and late osteoarthritic changes.

Clinical Features

Avascular necrosis of a bone is usually asymptomatic in the early stages. In the later stage patient may complain of pain, limp and slight loss of movements. In very advanced cases patient will show symptoms of secondary osteoarthritis.

Investigations

In the early stages, avascular necrosis can be detected by bone scan, radioisotope study. In the later stages, radiograph shows dense changes in the bone, collapse and osteoarthritic features (Fig. 8.16).

Treatment

Early stages require no treatment. Protective braces may be given to prevent bone collapse. Surgical decompres-

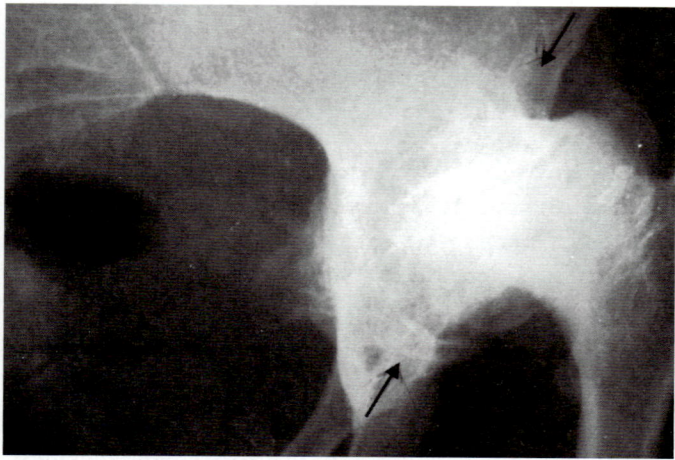

Fig. 8.16: AVN head of femur with features of Sec OA

sion has a doubtful role. In the later stages, total hip replacement is advocated for AVN head of the femur. AVN in scaphoid needs open reduction internal fixation with Herbert screws and bone grafting.

Other Measures

a. *Revascularization methods:* Meyer's muscle pedicle graft is a famous example of revascularization procedures for AVN head of femur following fracture of the neck of femur.
b. *Resection and Replacement (remember 2Rs):* Hemi replacement arthroplasty with AM prosthesis or Thompson's prosthesis is a popular example.
c. *Total joint replacement:* In hip and knee for advanced secondary osteoarthritis following AVN.

TRAUMATIC MYOSITIS OSSIFICANS

Introduction

It is a reactive lesion occurring in the soft tissues and at times in the bone periosteum. It is characterized by fibrous, osseous and cartilaginous proliferation of the subperiosteal hematoma. This is later followed by metaplastic changes.

Causes

- *Trauma:* This has a definitive role in the causation of myositis ossificans and could be simple blow or repeated minor trauma.
- *Dislocations and avulsion injuries:* That cause violent stripping of the periosteum and damage to the muscles.
- *Ill-advised massage:* This is by far the most common cause for myositis.

Interesting Facts about Myositis Ossificans

- It is more common is children due to loose periosteum attachment.
- Patients with head injury, paraplegia are more prone.
- Commonest cause is ill-advised massage.

Pathology

Muscle is commonly involved, but fascia, tendon and periosteum can also be affected. The process is a peculiar alteration within the ground substance of the connective tissue associated with proliferation of undifferentiated connective tissue.

Remember

In myositis ossificans, muscles commonly involved are:
- Brachialis anticus
- Quadratus femoris
- Adductor muscles of the thigh

Note: All these muscles take origin from a wide area-suggesting role of periosteum in its genesis.

8

Clinical Features

In the acute stages, patient may complain of pain, swelling and loss of movements. On examination, there may be tenderness. In the late stages, there is no pain and a bony hard lump may be palpated. This may act as a mechanical block to the movements.

> **Remember**
>
> Areas commonly affected:
> - Elbow joint common in young athletes
> - Ankle joint–known as footballer's ankle
> - Knee–known as Pellegrini-Stieda disease
> - Shoulder
> - Hip
> - More common in head injuries.

Investigations

Radiography has little role in the *acute stages* but in the late stages a bony growth may be evidently seen (Fig. 8.17).

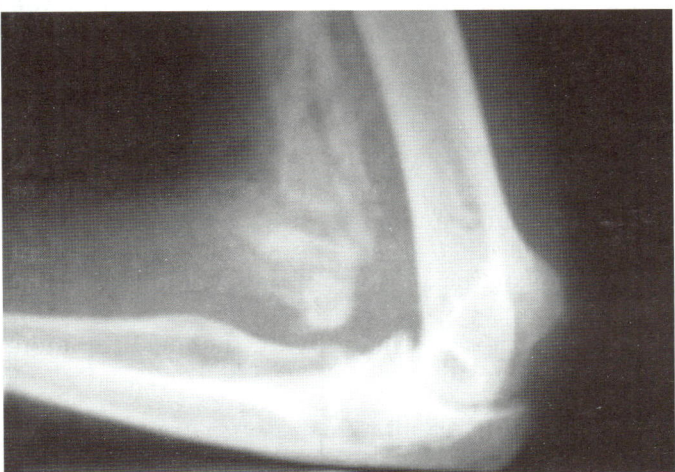

Fig. 8.17: Plain X-ray showing of the elbow showing myositis ossificans

Treatment

Remember the popular adage *"prevention is better than cure"* and it suits this condition aptly. Refraining from the ill-advised massage and handling the injured with care prevents this condition from raising its ugly head.

Curative Measures

Acute stages: Conservative treatment is the method of choice and consists of the following:
Immobilization of the part by splints, etc.
- *Drugs*: Diphosphonate therapy, calcitonin and non-steroidal anti-inflammatory drugs (NSAIDs).
- *Physiotherapy*: Active physiotherapy is encouraged and passive stretching is avoided.
- *Manipulation:* It is done under general anesthesia. It is double-edged sword and has to be performed very

carefully. Adhesions should snap abruptly and should not be broken gradually.

Chronic stages: Surgery is the treatment of choice and consists of soft tissue release and excision of bony spur when it is well formed.

> **Remember**
>
> - The term myositis ossificans is a *misnomer* because skeletal muscle is often not involved and inflammatory changes are rarely seen.
> - *Myositis ossificans progressiva:* A different condition and has nothing to do with trauma. It is a congenital condition affecting all the skeletal muscles.

MALUNION

When fracture fragments heal in an abnormal position, it is called malunion.

Causes

Improper treatment, improper immobilization techniques, treatment by quacks, multiple and multisystem injuries, etc.

Classification

Length malunion: This commonly results in shortening of the limb and may rarely give rise to lengthening.

Rotatory malunion: This may cause external or internal rotational deformities.

Angulatory malunion: This may cause varus or valgus deformities.

Of all the factors mentioned above, the one factor, which is not corrected by remodeling is rotation, while the other three are successfully overcome over the years by remodeling. Hence, all precautions should be taken to correct the rotation element during the initial treatment of fractures.

Clinical Features

A patient with malunion of bones may complain of deformity and/or loss of function of the affected extremities. There may be shortening and wasting of the involved limbs and restricted movements (see Fig. 23.12A).

Plain X-ray of the affected limb helps to diagnose the malunion of the bones in both the plan (see Fig. 23.12B).

Treatment

Masterly inactivity if patient has no functional problems. Certain malunion in children may be left alone as it is expected to remodel over a period of time.

Cosmesis alone does not form a sufficient indication for surgery unless the patient desires so. Nevertheless, operative treatment is highly justified when malunion

affects the function. This can be done by a *corrective osteotomy* at the old fracture site or a *compensatory procedure* may be necessary to restore functions (e.g. Darrach's operation in Malunited Colles). Sometimes pain may be the only predominant symptom necessitating fusion of the joint.

INTERESTING MALUNION FACTS (All M's)

a Malunion is due to:
   Mal-reduction;
   Mal-alignment;
   Mal-maintenance.
b. Made good in children courtesy remodeling.
c. Masterly inactivity in most cases.
d. Minimal interference if only cosmetic.
e. Maximum interference in functional impairment.

OTHER IMPORTANT ACUTE COMPLICATIONS OF FRACTURES

DEEP VEIN THROMBOSIS (DVT) AND PULMONARY EMBOLISM

It is an important complication seen after fractures of spine, pelvis, femur, tibia, etc. Virchow's triad of venous stasis, vascular damage and hypercoagulability are described in the pathogenesis.

Clinical Features

The patient complains of mild to severe calf pain, swelling, difficulty in standing or walking and cramps in the calf muscles or foot. The clinical signs include unilateral, leg swelling, increased temperature, tenderness, enlarged superficial veins, pitting edema, palpable cord along the involved veins, erythema (Fig. 8.18).

Homans' sign When forced ankle dorsiflexion produces calf pain, Homans' sign is said to be positive and is pathognomonic of DVT (Fig. 8.19).

Investigations

Laboratory tests consist of evaluating the bleeding time, clotting time, prothrombin time, etc. Venography helps in definitive diagnosis.

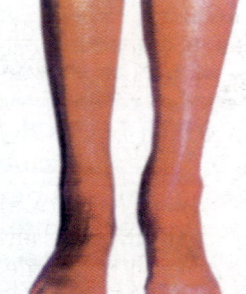

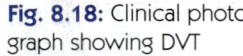

Fig. 8.18: Clinical photograph showing DVT

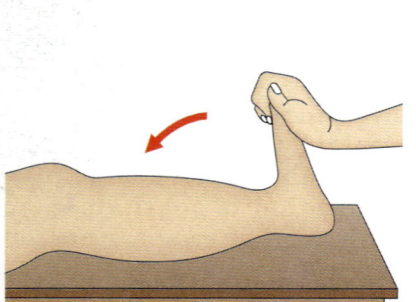

Fig. 8.19: Homans' sign

Treatment

Prophylactic methods consist of early ambulation, foot elevation, elastocrepe bandaging, ankle and foot exercises, etc.

Anticoagulant Therapy

This consists of aspirin (600–650 mg), heparin (low dose), low molecular weight dextran, low dose warfarin (2.5–16 mg/day daily orally), etc. Pulmonary thromboembolism is a serious complication of DVT. Patient with pulmonary embolism complains of unexplained dyspnea, pleurotic chest pain, hypoxia, tachypnea, tachycardia, signs of cor pulmonale, etc. Heparin therapy is the treatment of choice. Chronic venous insufficiency is the common long-term complication of DVT.

Disturbing DVT facts:
* *DVT*: It can occur as early as 48 hours after injury.
* *Embolism*: It can occur after 4–5 days
* *Pulmonary embolism*: It can occur usually after 4–5 days post accident.

Embolic facts
Other important predisposing factors for DVT:
* Surgery–orthopedic/thoracic/abdominal/GU systems
* Immobilization due to CCF, MI, Stroke, etc.
* Neoplasms
* Estrogen therapy
* Pregnancy
* Obesity
* Age > 40 years
* TAO, Behcet's disease, etc.
* Hypercoagulable states
* Total hip and knee replacement, etc.

Interesting facts about DVT and its detection:
* Keep and think DVT uppermost in the mind in high-risk cases
* Clinical diagnosis accurate
* Homan's sign-quite characteristic
* Vonography is the only definite diagnostic method

INJURY TO BLOOD VESSELS

Blood vessels in close proximity to the bones are injured during fractures and dislocations.

Injuries	*Blood vessel*
Upper limb trauma	
• Clavicle fracture	Subclavian vessels
• Proximal humeral fracture	Axillary vessels
• Supracondylar humerus fracture	Brachial vessels
• Posterior dislocation of elbow	Brachial vessels
• Fracture both bones forearm	Anterior interosseous artery
Lower limb trauma	
Dislocation of hip	Femoral vessels
Femur fracture	Femoral vessels

8

Supracondylar femur fracture	Popliteal vessels
Dislocation of knee	Popliteal vessels
Proximal tibial fracture	Posterior tibial vessels
Tibia and fibula fracture	Posterior tibial vessels
Ankle injuries	Posterior tibial vessels

Causes of Injury

The blood vessels may be injured in one of the following ways: reflex vasospasm, compression by the fracture fragments or hematoma, incomplete tear, complete tear, partial tear, internal thrombus, tight encircling bandages, etc. (See Fig. 17.12).

Effects of Injury

In the initial stages, it may range from mild ischemia to gangrene. In the late stages ischemic contractures may develop.

Clinical Features

Apart from the usual features of fractures, patient may show impending signs of vascular disaster recognized by **5P**s:
- **P**ain
- **P**ulselessness
- **P**araesthesia
- **P**allor
- **P**aralysis
  Cold extremities herald onset of gangrene.

Note: Absence of peripheral pulse is a pointer towards a vascular injury until proved otherwise.

Investigations

It consists of radiograph of the part, Doppler angiogram studies, etc.

Treatment

This consists of prompt reduction of fractures and dislocations and removal of all tight encircling bandages. Thrombectomy, direct end-to-end repair, injection of xylocaine, papaverine, sympathectomy to relieve the vasospasms are some of the commonly recommended methods of treatment. Amputation is considered in irreversible loss of blood supply.

INJURY TO NERVES

Forty percent of the bone and joint injuries are associated with peripheral nerve injuries quite a staggering figure.

Primary injury: The nerve is injured by the same trauma that resulted in the injury to bone and joint.

Secondary injury: This is due to involvement of the nerve in infection, scar, callus, etc.

Incidence

Radial nerve is the most commonly injured peripheral nerve (45%) (See Fig. 31.11), followed by ulnar nerve (30%), median nerve (15%), peroneal nerve, lumbosacral plexus (3%) and tibial nerve.

Mechanism of Injury

The nerve may be damaged by fracture fragments, entrapment between the fragments during fracture reduction, direct injury by the bullets, sharp cutting weapons, etc. In later stages, the nerve may be trapped in the callus or fibrous tissue.

Types of Nerve Injury

This may be neurapraxia, axonotmesis or neurotmesis depending upon the severity of injury.

Nerve Facts

Trauma	Nerves injured
Upper limb	
• Fracture clavicle	Brachial plexus
• Proximal humeral fracture	Axillary nerve
• Fracture humerus	Radial nerve
• Supracondylar fracture humerus	Radial nerve
• Posterior dislocation of elbow	Median nerve
• Monteggia's fracture nerve	Posterior interosseous nerve
• Hook of hamate	Deep branch of ulnar nerve
• Wrist injury	Median nerve
Lower limb	
• Dislocations of hip (posterior)	Sciatic nerve
• Anterior dislocation of hip and shaft femur	Femoral nerve
• Dislocation of knee	Common peroneal nerve
• Proximal tibial fractures and ankle injury	Posterior tibial nerve
• Fracture neck fibula	Lateral popliteal nerve

Classification, diagnosis, clinical features and treatment of individual nerve injuries are discussed in chapter on peripheral nerve injuries.

CRUSH SYNDROME

It is seen in severe crush injuries of the limbs and muscles, which results in massive release of myohemoglobin in the circulation, which blocks the renal tubules and leads to myoglobinuria and acute renal tubular necrosis. Prolonged and improper application of tourniquet, acute compartmental syndrome, gas gangrene are some of the other causes of crush syndrome. Treatment is directed towards managing acute renal failure in case patient develops oliguria or anuria.

OTHER IMPORTANT DELAYED COMPLICATIONS

JOINT STIFFNESS

This is due to improper technique during fracture immobilization which can be troublesome. Intra-articular fractures, periarticular adhesions of soft tissues, capsules and muscle contractures are some of the other important causes of joint stiffness. Physiotherapy, exercises, manipulation under anesthesia, surgical excision and lengthening of contractures are some of the important treatment methods.

REFLEX SYMPATHETIC DYSTROPHY

It is an abnormal sympathetic response following fractures. Commonly this is encountered in Colles' fracture (Page 97).

OSTEOMYELITIS

It is common in compound fractures. The other complications peculiar to open fractures are tetanus, gangrene and hypovolemic shock. It causes irregular bone, chromic discharging sinuses, etc.

IMPLANT FAILURE

It can occur due to defective manufacturing or biological reactions within the body. Sometimes it is due to premature weight bearing due to patient's non-compliance.

POST-TRAUMATIC OSTEOARTHRITIS

It is commonly seen in intraarticular fractures, malunion, etc. and it causes secondary osteoarthritis.

GROWTH ALTERATIONS

It is due to epiphyseal injuries in children and may lead to shortening, lengthening of limb, etc.

MISCELLANEOUS

The other complications peculiar to open fractures are tetanus, gangrene and hypovolemic shock.

SHORTENING

After nonunion and malunion, shortening of the long bones is another troublesome complication of fractures. Now the moot point is *why do the bones shorten*? Well the logical explanations could be one or all the points mentioned below:

In children: It could be due to disturbances in growth following the epiphyseal injuries.

In adults: The causes are slightly different and it could be due to:
a. *Loss of small pieces of bone*: This can happen in compound, comminuted fractures especially of the tibia.
b. *Malunion*: If there is excess angulation or overlapping during the union, it will translate into shortening.

After effects of shortening
- In the upper limbs, it normally goes unnoticed.
- In the lower limbs if the shortening is less than 2 cm it goes unnoticed but if it is more than 2 cm, patient has a limb and may develop secondary osteoarthritis of the knee or hip joints over the years due to the altered gait.

Treatment

Shortening of the long bones generally does not require any interference. Even in lower limbs, shortening do not need any treatment. However, interference is required in the following situations: If it is less than 2 cm, shoe raise is given. If it is more than 2 cm, limb lengthening procedures usually the Ilizarov's technique is advised.

COMPLICATION PECULIAR TO OPEN FRACTURES

This has been discussed in the chapter on open fractures (See page 22).

8

Plaster of Paris and its Role in Orthopedics

9

Introduction
Slab
Cast
Spica
Functional cast brace

INTRODUCTION

Mathysen, a Dutch surgeon in 1852, first used plaster of Paris in orthopedics. It is made from gypsum which is a naturally occurring mineral and is commercially available since 1931.

Chemical Formula

It is hemihydrated calcium sulphate. To make plaster of Paris, gypsum is heated to remove water. When water is added to the resulting powder original mineral reforms and is set hard.

$$2(CaSO_4\ 2H_2O) + Heat \longleftrightarrow 2(CaSO_4.\tfrac{1}{2}H_2O) + 3H_2O$$

Splint in orthopedics is mainly prepared from this wonder white mineral, the plaster of Paris.

Plaster of Paris is an Ideal Splint—Reasons

- It is cheap and easily available
- It is comfortable and easy to mold
- It sets quickly and easy to remove
- It is strong and light
- It is permeable to radiography, air and hence underlying skin can breathe.
- It is non-inflammable.

Types: Plaster of Paris is used in four forms as slab, cast, spica, and functional cast brace.

SLAB

It is a temporary splint used in the initial stages of fracture treatment and also during first aid. It is also useful to immobilize the limbs postoperatively and in infections. It is made up of half by POP and half by bandage roll and hence can accommodate the swelling in the initial stages of fractures. Slab is prepared according to the required length of the limb.

FAMOUS SLABS IN ORTHOPEDICS

Upper limbs
- *U-slab*: For fracture shaft humerus.
- *Above elbow slab*: For forearm injuries.
- *Below elbow slab*: For wrist and hand injuries.

Lower limbs
- *Above knee slab*: For knee and leg injuries.
- *Below knee slab*: For ankle and foot injuries.

Note: U-slab is the only slab in orthopedics used for definitive treatment of fracture. Rest of the slabs is used for temporary treatment of fractures and immobilization during first aid.

CAST

The POP roll completely encircles the limb. It is used as a definitive form of fracture treatment and to correct deformities. The technique of the application of a plaster cast is shown (Figs 9.1A to F).

Popular Casts in Orthopedics

Neck
- *Minerva cast:* For neck immobilization in cervical spine injuries and diseases.

Upper Limb
- *Hanging cast*: For lower third humeral fractures (Fig. 9.2A).
- *U-cast*: For proximal and middle third humeral fractures (Fig. 9.2B).
- *Colles cast*: For Colles' fractures (Fig. 9.2C).

Lower Limb
- *PTB cast*: For tibia fracture (See Fig. 23.8).
- *Cylindrical cast*: For patella fracture (Fig. 9.2D).
- *Boot plaster*: For calcaneal and ankle injuries
- *Calcaneal cast:* For calcaneal fractures
- *De-rotation boot*: For trochanteric fracture of the femur in very old people.

The casts of the upper limbs could be above or below elbow and in the lower limbs it could be above or below knee.

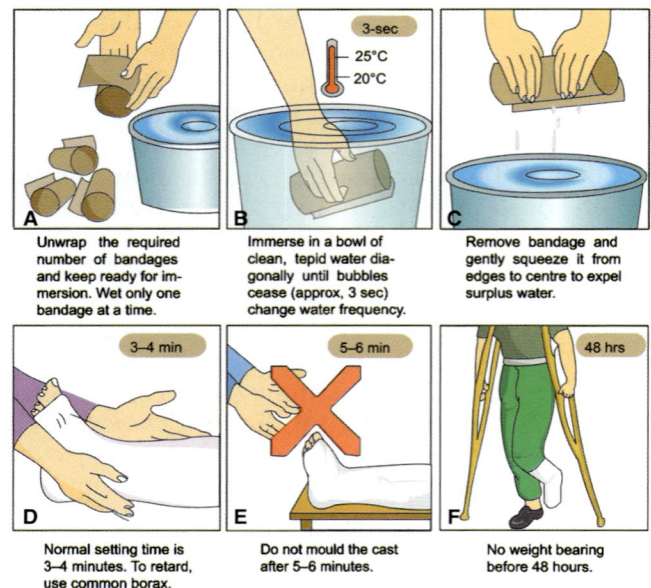

Figs 9.1A to F: Method of plaster preparation and application

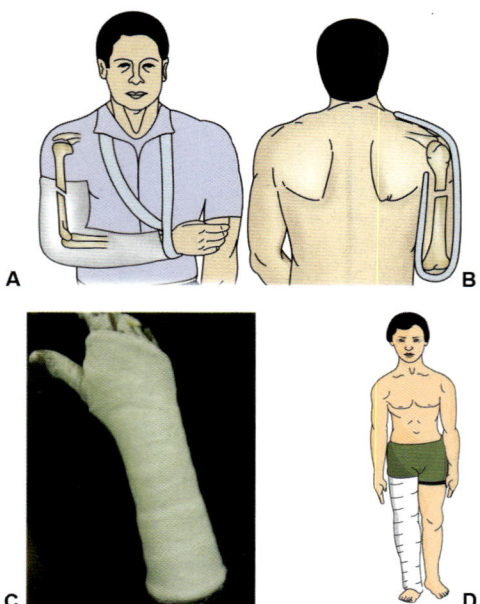

Figs 9.2A to D: Various types of plaster cast (A) above elbow cast (hanging cast), (B) U-cast, (C) below elbow cast, (D) cylindrical cast (above knee cast)

9

Thoracic Spine

- *Risser's cast*: For scoliosis correction.
- *Turn-buckle cast*: For scoliosis correction.

SPICA

This encircles a part of the body, e.g. hip spica for fracture around the hip, thumb spica for scaphoid fracture.

Popular Spicas in Orthopedics

Upper Limbs

- *Shoulder spica*: For injuries around the shoulder.
- *Thumb spica* (*Scaphoid cast*): For scaphoid fractures. (Fig. 9.3).

Lower Limbs

- *Hip spica*: For fracture femur in children (Fig. 9.4).

Rules of Application for POP Cast

- Choose the correct size, 8 inches for the thigh, 6 inches for the leg, and 4 inches for the forearm.
- A joint above and a joint below should be included. Accordingly, we have an above or below elbow POP cast or slab and above knee or below knee POP cast or slab. This is done to eliminate movements of the joints on either side of the fractures. However, this is not a hard-and-fast rule in certain fractures, like a below elbow cast in Colles's fracture which often suffices.
- It should be molded with the palm and not the fingers for fear of indentation.

- The joints should be immobilized in functional position.
- The plaster should just snugly fit and should not be too tight or too loose.
- Uniform thickness of the plaster is preferred.

After Care of the Plaster

Daily routine suggested after application of a cast:
- The plaster should not be made wet. Sponging of the body is preferable while taking regular baths.
- In the lower limbs patient should be instructed not to bear weight or walk on the plaster.
- A check has to be made for cracks and crevices and has to be promptly attended to.
- The plaster needs to be changed if there is loosening after the initial swelling has subsided.
- Patient should be instructed to take care to prevent small insects or ants from creeping through the plaster and the limbs. This may cause severe discomfort and itching.
- Joints not immobilized should be actively exercised, and for immobilized joints isometric exercises are advised.

Complications of POP

Due to tight fit:
- Pain.
- Pressure sores
- Compartmental syndromes
- Peripheral nerve injuries
- Cast syndrome

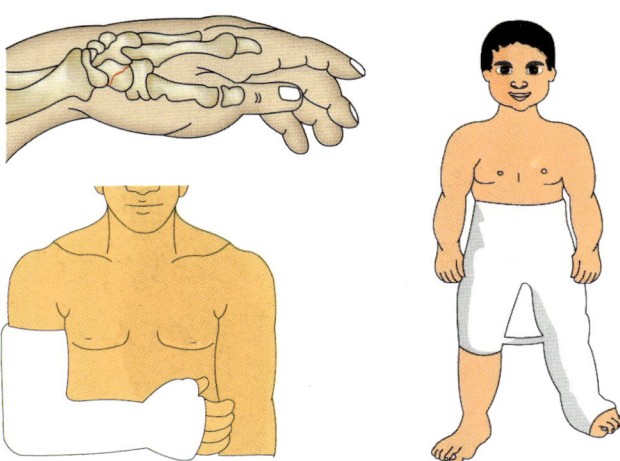

Fig. 9.3: Thumb spica for scaphoid fracture

Fig. 9.4: Hip spica for fracture femur in children

9

Caution: Bluish discoloration or excessive swelling of fingers or toes indicates too tight a plaster. Split it immediately. Perform passive stretch of fingers or toes. It should be painless. If painful, split the plaster.

Due to improper application:
• Joint stiffness.
• Plaster blisters and sores.
• Breakage.

Due to plaster allergy:
• Allergic dermatitis.
• Skin rashes.

Plaster sores are a troublesome complication of plasters. Early identification helps to prevent its undesirable effects. The following may give a clue on an impending sore:
• Unusual pain
• Wetting of the plaster
• Mild fever
• Restlessness and discomfort
• Swollen toes or fingers.

Split the plaster, clean the area with antiseptic solution and if the skin condition is good, carefully reapply the plaster.

FUNCTIONAL CAST BRACE

If function is allowed during closed method of fracture treatment, it has been observed that, this stimulates osteogenesis, promotes soft tissue healing and prevents development of joint stiffness thus hastening rehabilitation. This concept accepts loss of anatomic reduction to rapid healing. It compliments rather than replacing other forms of treatment. The observation that rib fractures still unite in spite of continued movements due to the action of intercostal muscles show that elimination of movements at fracture site are not mandatory for fracture to unite. It was on this concept that sarmiento devised functional bracing methods.

The mode of hydraulic action of muscles is brought into play. The fracture brace allows movements of the joints and permits the load to be transmitted through the muscles. The muscles which are surrounded by the inelastic deep fascia is encased in a hard plaster that cannot be stretched beyond the confines of the cast. On movements and bearing weight, the muscle forces are hence driven inwards towards the fracture and not outwards (Fig. 9.5A). This helps the fracture to be held firmly. These hydraulic forces control the fragments and resist overlap and angulations until callus forms. Rotation is also resisted by the brace and muscle contraction. In compound fractures due to severe disruption of soft tissues this principle will not work until soft tissues have healed. Functional cast brace is used for tibia and humerus fracture after initial immobilization (Fig. 9.5B).

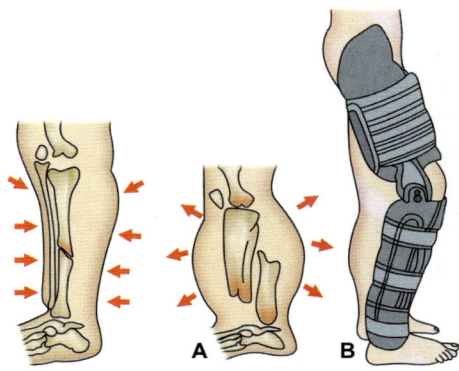

Figs 9.5A and B: (A) hydraulic principles of functional cast brace, (B) functional cast brace

---

Remember

About POP:
• It was used first in city of Paris
• An ideal splint
• Slab for temporary and initial treatment
• Cast for definitive treatment
• Spica for hip fracture, etc.
• Functional cast brace for early mobilization

About functional cast brace:
• Fracture ribs indicate that absolute immobility for fracture healing is not required
• It is a secondary form of fracture treatment
• Muscle action favors osteogenesis
• Hydraulic action of muscles stabilizes the fracture in a closed compartment
• Eliminates fracture disease like in AO technique
• Not useful in compound fractures
• Popularized by Sarmiento
• Useful in long bone fractures like humerus, tibia and femur fractures.

Important Splints in Orthopedics Other POP

INTRODUCTION

The most dramatic discovery ever made in the treatment of fractures or orthopedic disorders is *splints*. *Any substance used to immobilize a fracture or inflamed joint is called the splint.* The credit of refining the splints from a crude variety to that of finesse and quality deservingly goes to the Father of British Orthopedic Surgeon, HO Thomas. His epoch making discovery of a knee splint, named after him, as the Thomas splint has stood the test of time and still finds a pride place in the treatment armamentarium of orthopedics. Thus, he proudly deserves to be called *Father of Splints*.

Uses

The splint has the following uses:
- It is used to immobilize the fractures.
- It is used to transport the injured patient and rest an inflamed joint.
- It is used to correct or prevent deformities.
- It also finds place in definitive treatment of fractures.

SPLINTS USED IN DIFFERENT REGIONS

Neck

- *Cervical collar* (See Fig. 63.7).
- *Four post-collar* (See Fig. 63.8).
  It is used to immobilize the neck in painful conditions.

Upper Limb

- *Aeroplane splint*: Brachial plexus injury.
- *Carpal tunnel splint:* For carpal tunnel syndrome (See Fig. 37.7)
- *Cock-up splint:* Used in wrist drop (See Fig. 31.15).
- *Mallet splint*: For mallet injuries (See Fig. 20.8B).
- *Finger splint:* Phalangeal fractures (See Fig. 5.1B).
- *Knuckle benders splint:* Ulnar nerve palsy.
- Volkmann's splint for VIC.

Spine

- *Dorsal region:* Milwaukee brace, Boston brace, used for correction of scoliosis (See Fig. 63.6).
- *Dorsolumbar region:* Anterior spinal hyperextension brace, ASHE Taylor brace. Used to immobilize the thoracolumbar spine (See Fig. 42.20).
- *Lumbar region:* Belts and corsets. Used to immobilize the lumbar spine in low backache (See Fig. 63.5).

Lower Limb Splints

- Thomas splint to immobilize the knee joint.
- *Bohler-Braun splint*: To immobilize femur fracture.
- *CTEV splint (Denis Browne splint):* For CTEV correction (See Fig. 47.13).
- *Foot drop splint:*For foot drop condition (See Fig. 31.25).
  Now let us focus our attention to some of the commonly used splints in orthopedics.

THOMAS SPLINT
(also called Thomas knee-bed Splint)

This is one of the very commonly used splints in orthopedics described by HO Thomas in 1876 to assist ambulatory treatment of TB knee. It is now widely used for the first aid treatment of shaft fractures of femur (Fig. 10.1).

Parts of a Thomas Splint

A Thomas splint consists of four parts:
- A padded metal oval ring with soft leather set at an angle of 120° to the inner bar.
- Two side bars, one inner and another outer of equal length. They bisect the oval ring. The outer bar has a curve to accommodate greater trochanter.
- Distal end where the two side bars are joined in the form of 'W'.
- Outer side bar is angled 2 inches below the padded ring to clear the prominent greater trochanter.

Uses of Thomas Splint

- To immobilize femur fracture anywhere.
- As a first aid measure for lower limb injuries.
- For transportation of an injured patient.
- In the treatment of joint diseases like TB knee, septic arthritis.

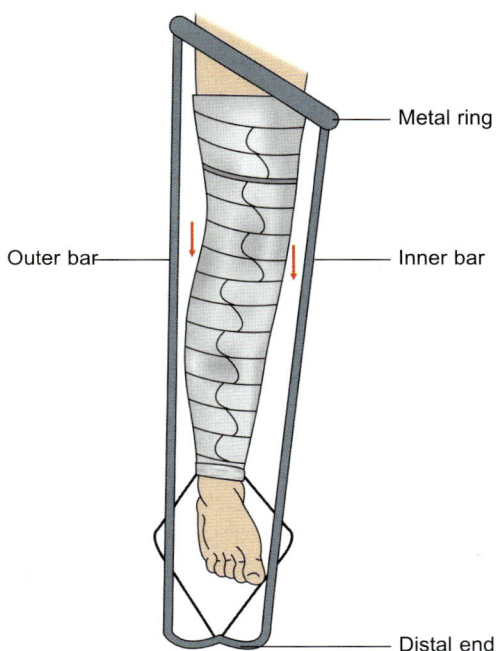

Fig. 10.1: Parts of a Thomas splint (the most famous splint in orthopedics)

used for the treatment of fracture shaft femur and supracondylar fractures of the femur. Rarely it can be used for fracture shaft of tibia and fibula.

One important precaution, which should be taken while using the BB splint, is to provide support at the fracture site and not at the knee joint to prevent angulations especially in supracondylar fractures of femur (Fig. 10.2). This helps prevent troublesome knee stiffness.

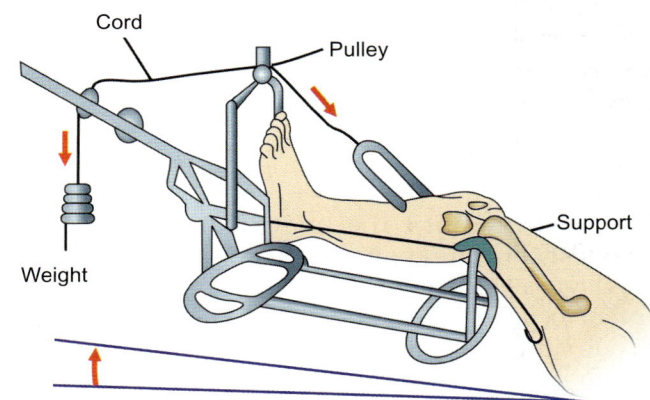

Fig. 10.2: Böhler-Braun splint (support provided at the fracture site)

Vital Thomas Splint Facts

- *How to choose the proper ring size:* Measure the thigh circumference at the highest point of the groin and add 2 inches.
- *How to choose the correct length:* Measure the highest point on the medial side of the groin to heel and then add 6 inches.

BÖHLER-BRAUN (BB) SPLINT

This is Böhler's modification of Braun splint. It consists of a heavy metallic frame with four pulleys.
- Proximal pulley prevents foot drop.
- Second pulley to apply traction in the line of femur.
- Third pulley to apply traction in the line of supracondylar area of femur.
- Fourth pulley to apply traction in line of the legs.

Indications of BB Splint

Skeletal traction is applied through this frame for comminuted trochanteric fractures of the femur. It is also

Problems due to BB Splint

- Makes nursing care difficult.
- It is a heavy and cumbersome frame.
- It is associated with recumbent problems like bed sores, hypostatic pneumonia, renal calculi.

Care of the Splints

- *Padding:* The splint should be well padded at the bony prominences and at the injury sites.
- *Bandage:* This should be tied with optimum pressure.
- *Exercises:* Active exercises of the joints and muscles should be permitted within the splints.
- *Checking:* Daily regular checking and adjustments of the splints are recommended.
- *Neurovascular status:* Distal neurovascular status should be assessed daily.

Traction in Orthopedics

INTRODUCTION

Traction is a unique method of treatment in orthopedics. It plays multiple roles like providing stretching effect on the muscles, ligaments, other soft tissue structures including the bones and the discs. It helps in providing relaxation of the above structures. It also helps to keep the patient on the bed and thereby ensures total rest to the body which is otherwise not possible. It is mainly useful in the regional conditions like low backache, cervical spondylosis. Traction also plays an important role in the management of fractures in orthopedics. Let us find out how?

Uses of Traction in Fractures and Dislocations

- To reduce a fracture or a dislocation
- To retain the fracture after reduction
- To overcome the muscle spasm
- To control movement of an injured part of the body and to aid in healing.

METHODS OF TRACTION

There are four methods of applying traction, namely skin, skeletal, pelvic, and spinal.

SKIN TRACTION

The traction is applied over a large area of skin. Maximum weight that can be applied through skin traction is 15 lb or 6.7 kg. If the weight used is more than this, the traction will slide down peeling off the skin. When used in fracture, skin traction is applied from the limb distal to the fracture site.

Types of Skin Traction

Adhesive skin traction: The adhesive material is used for strapping which is applied anteromedial and posterolateral on either side of the lower limbs.

Nonadhesive skin traction: Useful in thin and atrophic skin and in patients sensitive to adhesive strap. It is less secure than the former.

Contraindications: Abrasions, lacerations, impaired circulation, dermatitis, marked shortening, allergy to plaster are some of the important contraindications for skin tractions.

Complications: Allergy, excoriations, pressure sores around the malleoli, common peroneal nerve palsy, etc. are some of the known complications in skin tractions.

> **Remember**
>
> Rotation of the limb is difficult to control with skin traction.

Important Skin Traction

Buck's extension skin traction: This is the commonest type of traction employed for lower limbs. It is used for temporary treatment of neck femur fracture, undisplaced fractures of acetabulum, after reduction of hip dislocation, to correct minor fixed flexion deformity of the hip and knee for low backache, etc. (Fig. 11.1).

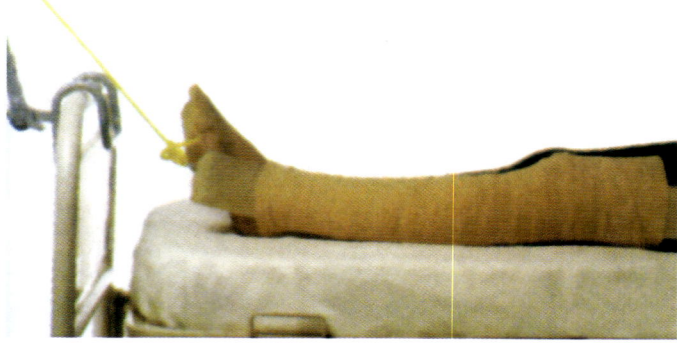

Fig. 11.1: Skin traction: Buck's extension skin traction

Dunlop's traction: Used in upper limbs and is indicated for supracondylar fractures, intercondylar fractures of humerus where elbow flexion causes circulatory embarrassment (Fig. 11.2).

Gallow's traction or *Bryant's traction:* Used for shaft femur fracture in children less than two years. If used

45

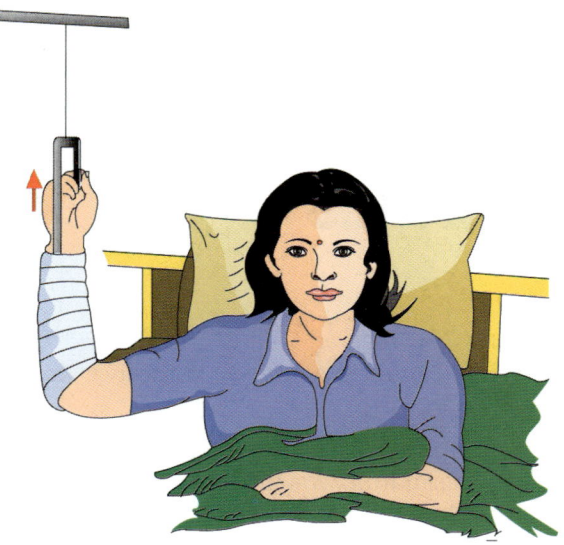

Fig. 11.2: Dunlop's traction

in children above 2 years, it causes vascular complications (Fig. 11.3).

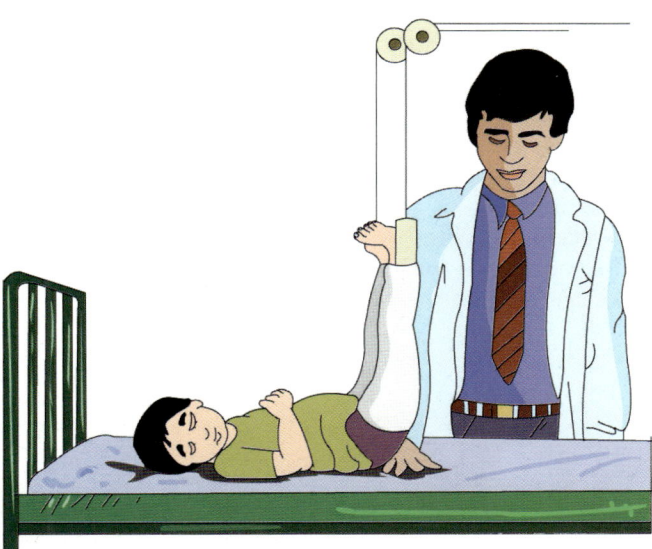

Fig. 11.3: Gallow's traction

SKELETAL TRACTION

The traction is given through a metal or pin driven through the bone. It is seldom necessary for upper limb fractures but useful in lower limb fractures for reducing and maintaining the fracture reduction. It is reserved for those cases in which skin traction is contraindicated and where the need to be applied weight is more than 5 kg. It is commonly indicated in trochanteric fractures, central fracture dislocation, fracture femur, etc. (Fig. 11.4).

Pins used for Skeletal Traction

Steinmann pin: It is a rigid stainless steel pin 4 to 6 mm in diameter. Böhler's stirrup allows the direction of the traction to be varied without turning the pin in the bones.

Denham pin: The pin is threaded in the center and engages the bony cortex. It reduces the risk of pin sliding and is useful in cancellous bone like calcaneum and osteoporotic bones.

K-wire: It is of small diameter and is often used in upper limbs for olecranon traction and through the metacarpal and metatarsal bones.

Rules of Application

- Skeletal traction should be applied in a Major OT under local anesthesia.
- Follow strict aseptic measures.
- Drive the pin from lateral to medial in case of upper tibial traction, to avoid injuring the lateral popliteal nerve.
- Pin should be at right angles to the limb and parallel to the ground.
- Cover the sharp tip on the medial side with a stopper bottle to prevent damage to the normal limb.

Complications

During application:
- Injury to the nerves (lateral popliteal nerve).
- Injury to the vessels.
- Injury to the muscles, ligaments, and tendons.
- Injury to epiphysis in children (upper tibial epiphysis).

When pin is in situ:
- *Infection*: due to improper aseptic measures.
- *Migration*: due to loosening.
- *Breakage*: thin pin or more weight.
- *Bending*: same reasons as above.
- *Loosening*: due to osteoporosis, infection, etc.
- *Distraction of fracture fragments*: due to excessive weight.

Late effects:
- Pin tract infection.
- Chronic osteomyelitis with ring sequestra at the site.
- Genu recurvatum due to damage to the anterior epiphysis of tibia in children.
- Depressed scar.

Precautions during Traction

- Carefully watch the pin tract sites everyday. Cleaning these sites with aseptic solutions should be a daily routine.
- Bedsores should be prevented at all costs. For this regular back care, use of waterbeds, turning the

patient over for every 2 hours are some of the effective time tested methods to prevent bedsores.
- The feet should not be left touching the pulleys.
- The suspended weight of the traction unit should not touch the ground.
- Ensure that the bandages are not too tight.
- Prevent chest complications by proper chest physiotherapy measures.
- To prevent stiffness, active exercises of the unimmobilized joints should be initiated at the earliest.
- Proper bowel and bladder care is mandatory to prevent urinary tract infections and constipation.

Traction Points

Tractions	Indications
1. *Head or cervical traction*	
• Crutchfield or garden wells	Cervical spine injuries
• Head halter	Cervical spine injuries
• Halo pelvic	Scoliosis
2. *Upper limb traction*	
• Dunlop's traction	Supracondylar fracture of humerus
• Metacarpal traction	Compound forearm injuries
3. *Lower limb traction*	
• Gallow's or Bryant's	Shaft femur fracture (less than 2 years)
• Russel's traction	Trochanteric fracture
• Perkin's traction	Shaft femur fracture in adults
• 90–90° traction	Shaft femur fracture in children
• Agnes hunt traction	Correction of hip deformity
• Well leg traction	To correct abduction and adduction deformity of hip
• Calcaneal traction distal traction	Compound fractures of leg and ankle
• Buck's traction	Low backache etc.
• Pelvic traction	Low backache etc.

COUNTER TRACTION

A force will overcome muscle spasm only if another force is acting in the opposite direction as counter traction.

Fixed traction: The counter traction is achieved through an appliance, which obtains a firm purchase on a part of the body. This can maintain but cannot obtain reduction, e.g. fixed traction on a Thomas splint for a shaft femur fracture (See Fig. 10.1).

Sliding or balanced traction: The weight of all or part of the body acting under the influence of gravity is utilized to provide counter traction. This can be achieved by raising the foot end of the bed. Unlike in a fixed traction, both reduction and maintenance of a fracture can be obtained (Fig. 11.4).

PELVIC TRACTION

This is mainly indicated in the conservative treatment of pelvic fractures. A detailed account of this is discussed in chapter on pelvic injuries.

SPINAL TRACTION

Cervical Traction

This could a head halter or chin halter traction (Fig. 11.6) or skull traction through the Crutchfield tongs or garden wells tongs (Fig. 11.5). The purpose of these

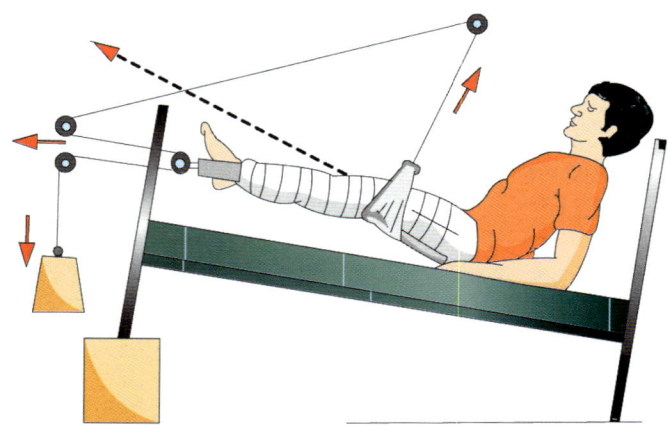

Fig. 11.4: Sliding or balanced traction

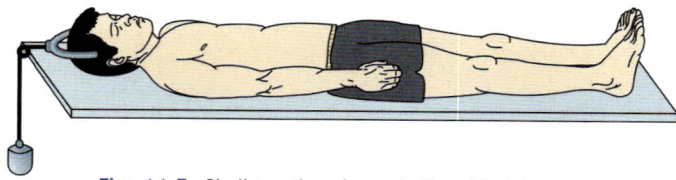

Fig. 11.5: Skull traction through Crutchfield tongs

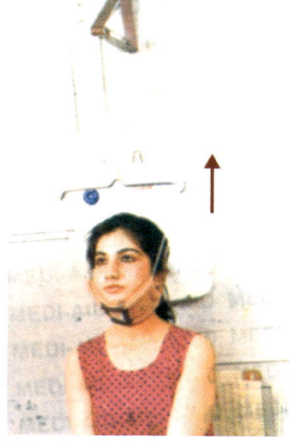

Fig. 11.6: Cervical traction in sitting position

11

traction is to immobile the neck in fractures or dislocations of the cervical spine. It could be used as first aid, reducing the fracture or dislocation, maintenance of reduction, postoperative immobilization, etc.

> **Remember**
> - Utility of a cervical traction in neck injuries.
> - As a first aid measure for transport of the patient.
> - For reduction of fracture and dislocation and maintenance of the reduction.
> - To relieve the neck muscle spasm.
> - For postoperative immobilization.

Cervical traction is also extensively used for common neck pains due to cervical spondylosis, to relieve pain, muscle spasm, stiffness, etc. (Fig. 11.6).

Lumbar Traction

Traction to the lower back can be used in acute low backache situations like muscle strain or ligament sprain. It can also be used as a first aid measure to transport a patient in fractures and dislocations of the lumbar spine (Fig. 11.7).

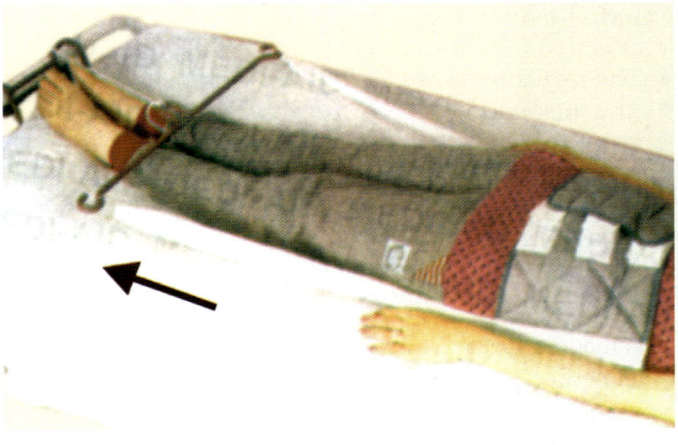

Fig. 11.7: Lumbar traction in low backache

Note: Lumbar and cervical tractions are most often used in treatment of the regional conditions of the neck, spine and lower back.

Implants in Orthopedics

12

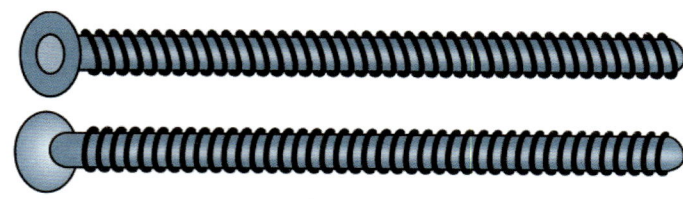

Fig. 12.1: Cortical screws—threaded whole length and not self-tapping

INTRODUCTION

An implant is defined as a material inserted or grafted into intact tissues or body cavity with some specific purpose.

Indications: This is the same as described for the indications in the open reductions. Most of the open reductions are followed by internal fixation.

Types of Implants

Metallic implants: Generally, alloys such as iron based stainless steel, cobalt based and titanium alloys are used.

Nonmetallic implants: Usually they are made up of plastic materials such as polyethylene, polymethyl methacrylate (PMMA), silicones and are the commonly used nonmetallic implants.

> *Note:* Corrosion is a chronic reaction that weakens the implants. Addition of chromium and nickel makes the implant corrosion resistant.

Commonly used implants in orthopedics are screws, plates, intramedullary nails, K-wires, special implants, and spinal implants.

SCREWS

It is widely used for fixation of small fracture fragments, avulsion fractures, interfragmentary compression and along with plates for fixation to the bone surfaces. The commonly used screws in orthopedics are cortical screws (threaded whole length) (Fig. 12.1), cancellous (threaded half-length) and malleolar screws (like cancellous screws but with a sharp tip) (Fig. 12.2). The screws can provide compression at the fracture site.

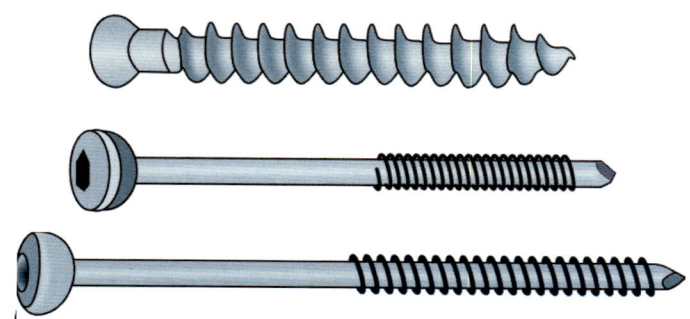

Fig. 12.2: Cancellous screw above and malleolar screw below

Compression by Screws

Lag effect to provide compression at the fracture site when cortical screws are used, one has to over drill the proximal cortex so that the screw will slide down through the hole pulling the far fragment towards the near fragment.

Cancellous screws provide a lag effect without over drilling of the proximal cortex since it is half threaded and pulls the far fragment towards the near fragment (Fig. 12.3).

PLATES

They are widely used for internal fixation of diaphyseal fractures.

Types of Plates

Ordinary Plates

These just function as positional plate to hold the fractures but will not bring about any compression between

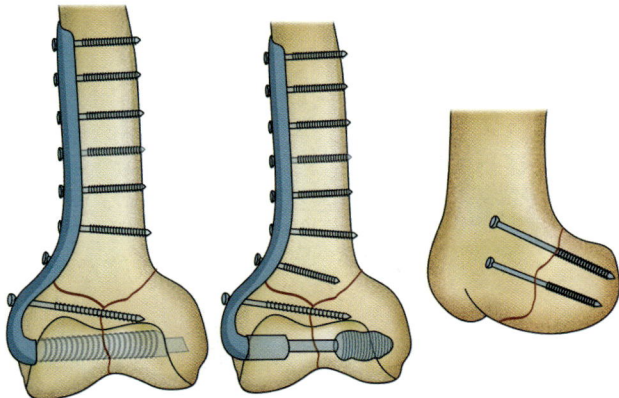

Fig. 12.3: Lag effect produced by cancellous screws

12

the fracture sites. They are used in subcutaneous locations for forearm bones, clavicle, fibula, etc. or where extreme rigidity is not required. The patients need prolonged immobilization once this plate is used, e.g. semi tubular plate, Scheuermann plate (Fig. 12.4A).

> **Remember**
>
> *About ordinary plates*:
> • Functions as merely a positional plate.
> • Useful in subcutaneous situations.
> • Needs prolonged immobilization.
> • Role is limited and has given way to compression plating.

AO Plates

AO techniques aim at early mobilization of the limb by providing a rigid compression at the fracture site and thereby prevent the possibility of fracture disease. Rigid fixation at the fracture site can be obtained by providing compression at the fracture site (Fig. 12.4B).

Dynamic Compression Plates (DCP)

The screw holes are designed to utilize spherical gliding principle with inclined contour of screw holes and the slope on under side of the screw head. As the screw is tightened, its head is guided by the contours of the screw hole in such a way that the head glides towards the centre of the plate until the deepest portion of the hole is reached. Result is that bone fragment into which screw is being driven is displaced at the same time, in the same direction providing rigid compression. It is called dynamic because the bone fragment moves while the screw is being tightened (Fig. 12.4C).

Advantages of DCP

• Less surgical exposure than the conventional AO surgery.
• Screw and plate fit congruently in any position.
• Screw may be inserted at any angle.
• All other advantages of rigid fixation.

Special Plates

For example, T-plates, L-plates, etc. are used for condylar fractures of tibia, distal femoral fractures, proximal humeral fractures, etc. (Figs 12.4D and E).

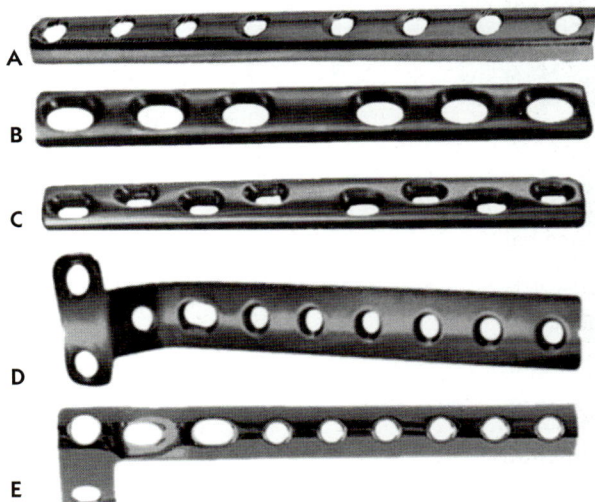

Figs 12.4A to E: (A) semi tubular plate, (B) AO plate, (C) dynamic compression plate (DCP), (D) special shaped T-plates, and (E) L-plates

INTRAMEDULLARY NAILS

The standard intramedullary (IM) nails called the Kuntscher's nail (K-nail) are cylindrical rods placed inside the medullary canals of long bones. Originally discovered by G. Kuntscher for fixing shaft femur fracture, now it is being used for other long bones fractures as well. Its modification of interlocking nails have ushered in a new era of internal fixation and are currently being cited as the gold standard of internal fixations of long bone fractures.

Mode of Action of Intramedullary Nails

• It is a load-sharing device unlike a plate, which is a load-bearing device.
• It fills the medullary cavity.
• It provides three-point fixation (at the ends of nail and at the point where curve of the nail is in contact with the opposite cortex).
• It resists bending movement but is poor against torsional forces.

Regarding techniques of insertion and complications refer chapter on Instruments.

> **Remember**
>
> *IM nails used in different bones*:
> • Humerus fracture.
> • Femur fracture (most common).
> • Tibia fracture.
> • Radius and ulna fracture (out of vogue now).

Different Varieties of IM Nails

Upper limbs

Types	Indications
K-nail	Humerus fracture
Rush nail	Radius fracture
Square nail	Radius fracture
Talwalkars nail	Fracture in both bones forearm

Lower limbs

Types	Indications
K-nail	Femur fracture
SP nail	Neck femur fracture
GK nail	Proximal femur fracture
Gamma nail	Proximal femoral fracture
Sirus nail	Proximal femoral fracture
Reconstruction nail	Proximal femoral fracture
Ender's nail	Supracondylar or intertro-chanteric femur fracture

INTERLOCKING NAILS

It is no exaggeration if we say that interlocking nailing has revolutionized the treatment of long bone fractures. (See Figs 13.3A and B). The fever of ILN has become so infectious that every orthopedic surgeon seems to be gripped by this epidemic. What is this ILN, which is so appealing? This is described in detail in chapter on Recent Advances of Internal Fixation.

SPECIAL IMPLANTS

Other than the conventional implants there are certain unconventional implants used in special situations in orthopedics. However, they do not have wider applications.

About Special Implants

- *DHS*: Intertrochanteric fracture of femur (See Fig. 21.19)
- *SP nail and plate*: Neck femur of fracture.
- *L-plate or condylar blade plate*: Supracondylar fracture of femur (Fig. 12.3).
- *Cobra plate:* For hip arthrodesis.
- *Spoon plate:* Lower end fracture of tibia.
- PFN Proximal femoral nail (See Fig. 21.6B).
- LCP Locked compression plate (See Fig. 16.4C).
- TENS titanium elastic nails (See Fig. 22.11D).
- T or L buttress plates (Fig. 12.5).

MISCELLANEOUS IMPLANTS

Stainless steel wires: Used for the tension band wiring for patella fracture, fracture of olecranon, etc. It is also used for anchoring pieces of bones to the rod or plate in comminuted fractures.

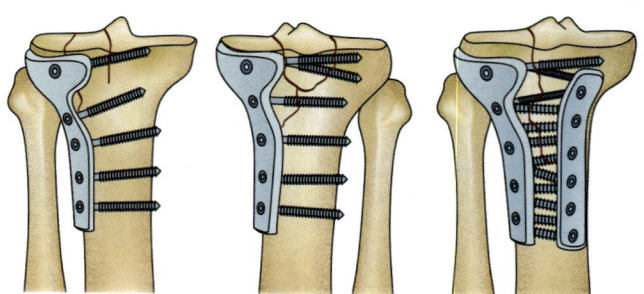

Fig. 12.5: Buttress plate for proximal tibial fractures

Kirschner's wires: This is widely used for fixation of fractures of smaller bones of the hands or feet.

> **Remember**
>
> *Stainless steel wire is widely used for tension band wiring in:*
> - Fracture olecranon
> - Fracture patella
> - Fracture medial malleolus

SPINE IMPLANTS

This needs a special mention as it has different connotations than the usual implants. Here are some of the few important spinal implants:
- VSP plates (variable stabilization plates).
- Luque's rod.
- Harrington's rod.
- Hart shill frame.

These implants are useful in stabilizing the spine following vertebral fractures and also for correction and maintenance of spire deformities like scoliosis, spondylisthesis, etc.

A detailed description of these implants is not within the scope of this book.

> **Remember**
>
> *Benefits of internal fixation with implants:*
> - It helps to rigidly fix those fractures, which cannot be immobilized by external means.
> - It permits early mobilization of the patients.
> - It overcomes confinement problems like bed sores, DVT, chest complications.
>
> *Drawbacks of internal fixation:*
> - It opens up the possibility of infections.
> - Fracture hematoma is lost.
> - It leaves a scar.
> - Another surgery is required to remove the implants.
> - Tissue trauma may slow down rehabilitation program.
> - It needs good infrastructure and training.

Nevertheless, internal fixation with implants when done in specific indications gives excellent results and has an important place in the treatment methodology of orthopedics.

12

13 Recent Advances in Fracture Treatment

Fiberglass plaster
Functional cast brace
LCDCP
Locked compression plates
Interlocking nails
Improvements in external fixation
Minimally invasive surgeries
Other advances

FIBERGLASS PLASTER

Now, the days are of ultra short setting plaster casts or slabs made up of a material called *polyurethane*. It sets very fast, lightweight, more esthetic, waterproof and more appealing. However, its high cost is prohibitive. It is also available in different colors and is very firm (Fig. 13.1).

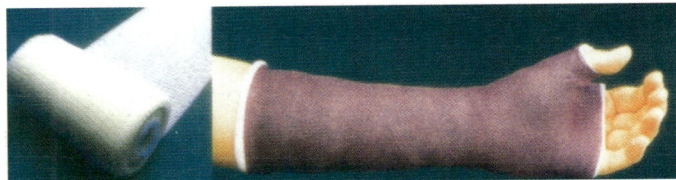

Fig. 13.1: Fiberglass plaster casts

FUNCTIONAL CAST BRACE

Earlier application of cast or slab confined the patient to the bed till the fracture united. Now, the concept is to mobilize the patient on the plaster cast by using the functional cast brace, an idea developed by Sarmiento. This has been discussed earlier.

AO TECHNIQUE

The principles and techniques of AO method of treatment have been previously discussed in chapter on Implants. Now, let us try to know more about the improvements made in AO.

LCDCP (LIMITED CONTACT DCP)

It is considered as a step in the improvement of rigid fixation by AO technique. Unlike conventional plates, these plates are in limited contact with the bone surfaces. This enables better healing as the vascularization is less damaged. Moreover, these plates are made up of titanium which is better than the stainless steel but is certainly more expensive (Fig. 13.2).

LOCKED COMPRESSION PLATES (LCP)

These are now in vogue. The plate has both the conventional oval hole and a hole for locked screws. This plate fixation is a boon in osteoporotic fractures, complicated fractures of the long bones. It gives better fixation and stability and helps in faster rehabilitation (Fig. 13.3).

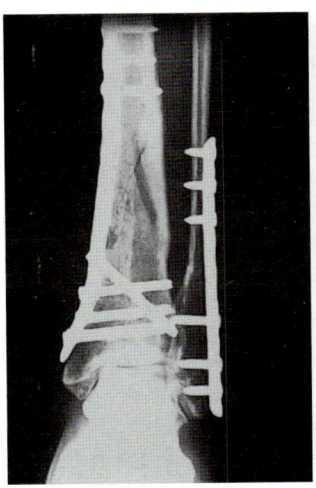 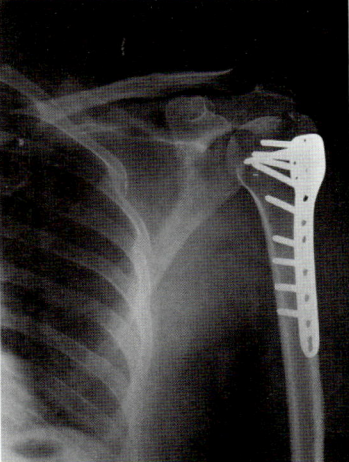

Fig. 13.2: Fixation with LCDCP   **Fig. 13.3:** Proximal humeral fracture fixed with locked plate

IMPROVEMENTS IN INTRAMEDULLARY NAILS

These are the days of interlocking nails. Earlier intramedullary nails could not be used in proximal and distal third fractures because the wider medullary canal in these areas rendered it difficult to control the rotation of the nail. The only alternative left was to use a plate and screw. Nevertheless, the problems associated with plate and screws necessitated the discovery of newer intramedullary nail with the problem of rotation eliminated by locking. Thus, the concept of interlocking nail was born and has made greater strides in the management of complicated fractures.

INTERLOCKING NAILS

Standard IM nails designed by Küntscher for shaft fractures leaves two unresolved problems, which are detrimental to healing namely, rotation of the fracture fragments and telescoping at the fracture site. By locking the nail into the bone by means of self-tapping screw driven through holes located at both the ends, the above two problems are solved. Gross and Kempf locking nail is found to be successful (Figs 13.4A and B).

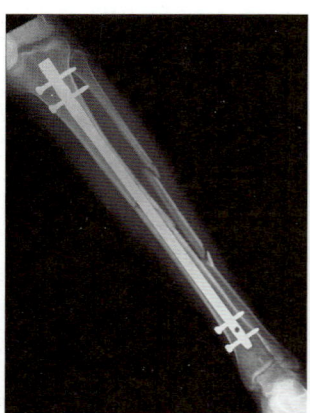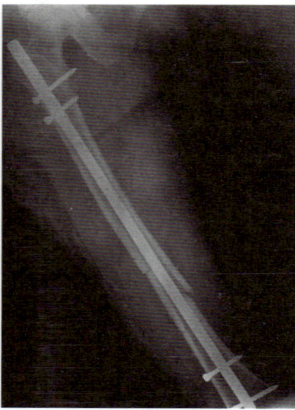

Figs 13.4A and B: (A) ILN tibia (B) ILN femur

Advantages

- It can be used for both simple and compound shaft fracture from subtrochanteric to supracondylar area in the femur and from upper third to supramalleolar area in the tibia.
- It can be used in the treatment of segmental frac-tures, comminuted fractures, bone loss, etc.
- It can be used for the treatment of nonunion.
- For reconstructive surgery following tumor excision.
- Low blood loss, low risk of infection.
- Short operative time.

Principles

Static locking: The screws are placed both proximal and distal on either sides of the fracture. This neutralizes the rotation and restricts telescopy.

Dynamic locking: The screws are placed either proximal or distal depending on the site of fracture. It neutralizes rotational movements but allows certain movements at the fracture site favoring osteogenesis. It allows immediate mobilization and early weight bearing.

Remember

About interlocking nail:
- It is modification of standard IM nail
- It extends the indication of IM nail and can be used for a wide range of shaft fractures

- Low blood loss and low rate of infection
- Less operative time
- Technically demanding
- Requires sophisticated equipment

IMPROVEMENTS IN EXTERNAL FIXATION

Ilizarov technique: Hippocrates first described the use of external fixators in the management of fractures 2400 years ago. Conventionally, there are two types of external fixator: pin fixator, and ring fixator. Ilizarov developed the ring fixator in 1951 (Figs 13.5A and B).

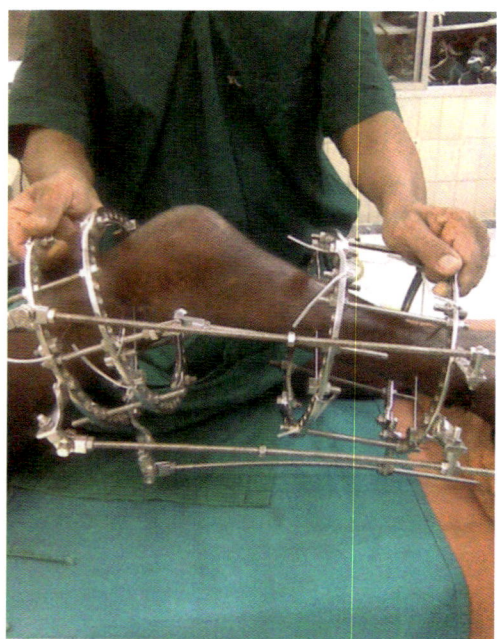

A

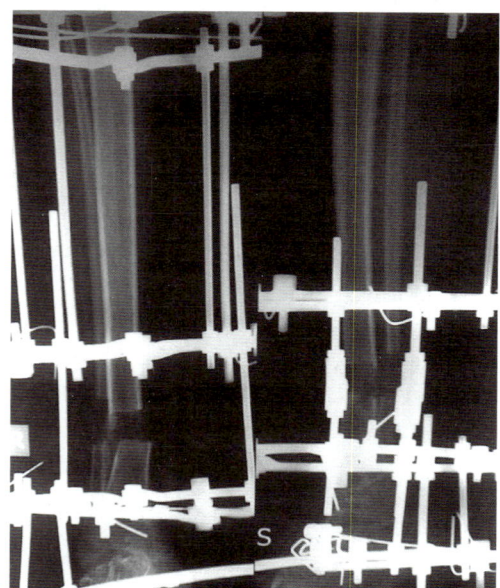

B

Figs 13.5A and B: (A) Ilizarov frame, (B) X-rays of the Ilizarov assembly

13

Principle: An important law of nature, which was not known to the biologists, was "distraction or pulling apart of living tissue creates a new tissue of its own kind". It was the beginning of a new era of successfully treating unsolved orthopedic problems. The following are the principles of his method:

Law of tension force: When a living tissue is slowly pulled apart at the rate of 1 mm/day, it creates a new tissue. This is called distraction osteogenesis.

Use of a unique ring: The fixator which is multilevel, multidirectional, multiplane external fixator and hence it is superior to other external fixators.

Corticotomy: The cortex of the bone is cut subperiosteally and intramedullary circulation is left intact. Preservation of periosteum and intramedullary circulation produces a better quality of new bone.

Indications

Complex fractures: Ilizarov is very useful in treating very complex fractures like open fractures, comminuted fractures, intraarticular fractures, etc.

Nonunion: Ilizarov gives excellent result in the management of both infected and uninfected nonunion. It simultaneously attends to all the components of nonunion.

Limb lengthening as in achondroplasia and in other shortenings.

Deformity corrections due to polio, cerebral palsy, etc.

Other Important Indications

- Congenital pseudoarthrosis of tibia
- Stump lengthening
- TAO
- Tumor excision and lengthening
- Foot deformities.

Complications

- Poor patient compliance
- Damage to nerves and vessels during insertion
- Wire tract infection, loosening or breakage
- Joint contractures.

- Inadvertent injury to the patient or operating room personnel caused by K-wire.

Remember

About Ilizarov
- Makes use of the hitherto unknown principle that distraction stimulates osteogenesis
- A single frame by arranging it in different combinations can be useful to solve 65 percent of orthopedic problems
- The greatest boon is early ambulation and weight-bearing
- Low rates of complications
- Virtually a bloodless surgery
- Very effective in the treatment of nonunion
- Cost-effective.

Minimally Invasive Surgeries

These surgeries are gaining lots of importance now for their obvious advantages:

- Less blood loss
- Quicker operating time
- Lesser operating time
- Lesser tissue trauma
- Faster recovery
- Faster rehabilitation
- Shorter hospital stay
- Socio-economic advantages.

Almost all surgeries in orthopedics are going the minimally invasive way and the examples are:
- Minimally invasive plate osteosynthesis (MIPPO).
- This is now being increasingly employed in fractures of humerus, tibia; femur, etc.
- Minimally invasive spine surgeries through endoscope and microscopes.
- Minimally invasive hip and knee replacement surgeries.

Other advances: Computer assisted and navigation techniques are the fast advancing techniques and invasion of computers promise much improved methods of orthopedic diagnosis and management. We are now practicing a more sophisticated hi-tech orthopedics. Some of the examples are LASER treatment for disc prolapse, spinal endoscopy, artificial replacement of discs, etc.

13

14 Fractures in Children

INTRODUCTION

Fractures in children are different from fracture in adults for the following reasons:

- Complete fractures are rare due to thick periosteal sleeve and greater elasticity.
- For the above reasons, buckle (Torus fractures) and greenstick fractures are more common.
- Fracture displacements are relatively less common.
- Fracture bleeding is also less.
- Avulsion fractures are more common because bone gives way earlier than the ligaments.
- Disruptions of the epiphyseal plate are relatively more common because they form the weakest portion of the bone in the children and account for nearly one-third of all childhood fractures.
- A pediatric fracture unites faster.
- Differential periosteal activity causes better remodeling which is more likely in: (a) younger the child (b) the nearer the fracture to the epiphyseal plate and (c) if the deformity is angulated in the plane of the joint movement.

PECULIAR FACTS IN CHILDREN

Fracture heals faster: This is due to loose periosteum, which strips for a considerable distance, and the blood, which collects beneath the periosteum over a wider area, is calcified and thus the fracture unites faster.

Complete fractures and deformities are uncommon: This is due to the thick periosteum and greater elasticity of the bones.

Epiphyseal injuries are more common: It is the growing ends of the bones and thus is the potential weak spot in children bones.

Incidence

- Fracture accounts for 10 to 25 percent of all injuries in childhood.
- Common between 11 and 14 years of age.
- Boys account for 62 percent of all cases.
- Fracture distal end of forearm is the most common skeletal injury in children contributing 25 percent of all fractures in them.

Remember

P the *Periosteum* in Pediatric fractures. Periosteum is thick in children:
- **P**revents displacements
- **P**revents complete fractures
- **P**ools blood below periosteum
- **P**eriosteum artery helps with remodeling.

Etiology

- *Falls* are the most predominant cause in children (See Fig. 17.6).
- *Traffic accidents* especially bicycle accidents account for 12 percent of cases (See Fig. 18.3).
- *Sporting activities* contribute 21 percent.
- *Birth fractures*: The clavicle is the most commonly injured bone during birth (accounts for 40–50% of all birth injuries), followed by brachial plexus injury (usually during instrumental rotation of the vertex), the humerus (injured during breech delivery) and the femur in that order.
- *Pathological fractures*: The conditions leading to pathological fractures could be:
  - Generalized, e.g. osteogenesis imperfecta, metabolic disorders.
  - Localized to one limb, e.g. fibrous dysplasia.
  - Localized to the lesion, e.g. benign cystic condition of the bone, infection, benign and malignant neoplasm. Pathological fractures usually result from trivial trauma (See Fig. 18.4).
- *Child abuse* (battered baby syndrome): Eight percent of child abuse takes place less than two years of age.
- *Stress fractures* are not very common. Seen in tibia, neck of femur, etc.

Fracture Facts in Children

Common	Uncommon
• Clavicle fracture	Fractures of the hand
• Supracondylar humerus fracture	Fractures of the feet

- Forearm bone fractures   Dislocations
- Lateral condyle of   Hip fracture
  humerus fracture
- Tibial spiral factures   Spine fracture
- Epiphyseal injuries

14

Types of Fractures

Greenstick fracture are incomplete fracture seen exclusively in children. Sometimes the bones are just bent and this is possible only in greenstick fractures in children (Fig. 14.1). Here one cortex is broken and the other is intact (Fig. 14.2).

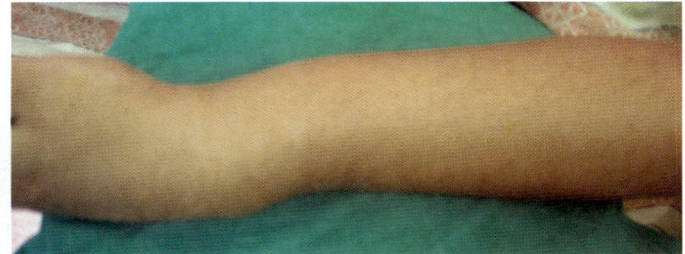

Fig. 14.1: Clinical photograph of greenstick fracture forearm

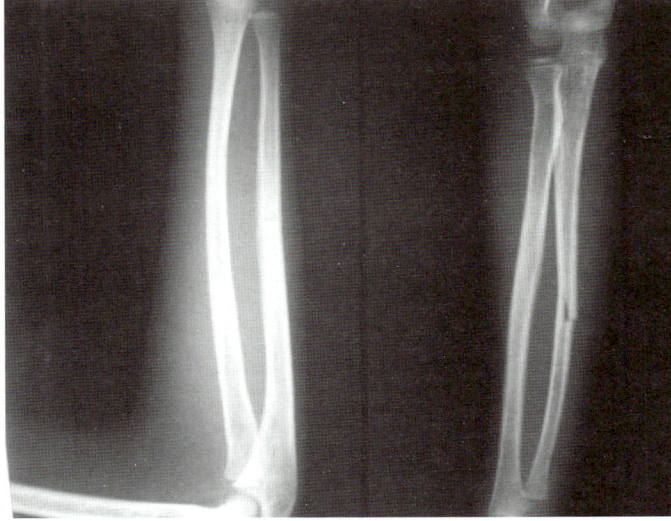

Fig. 14.2: Plain of a X-ray showing greenstick bend of radius and the unicortical break of ulna

Plastic bowing: The bone deforms but does not break. It is seen in paired bones. There is a micro fracture on the concave side (Fig. 14.3).

Buckle fracture (Torus fracture): This is common in metaphyseal region and is due to compressive force. The fracture cortex is buckled and not broken (Fig. 14.4).

Epiphyseal Injuries

Epiphyseal injuries are seen in children. Since the junction between the metaphysis and the epiphysis is

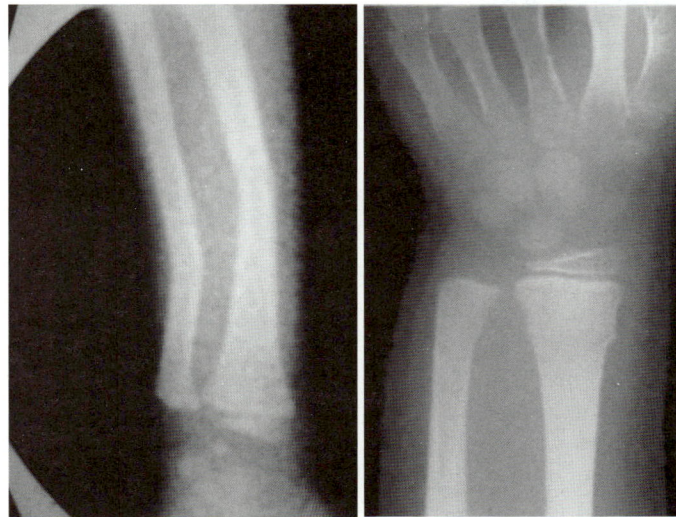

Fig. 14.3: Plain X-ray showing green-stick bend   **Fig. 14.4:** Plain of a X-ray showing Torus fracture

weakest, the point of a long bone in children is most vulnerable to shearing forces.

Salter and *Harris* have classified epiphyseal injuries into 5 types and *Rang* has added the 6th variety (Fig. 14.5).

Type I: The complete separation of epiphysis from the metaphysis without fracture. It is common in rickets, scurvy and osteomyelitis.

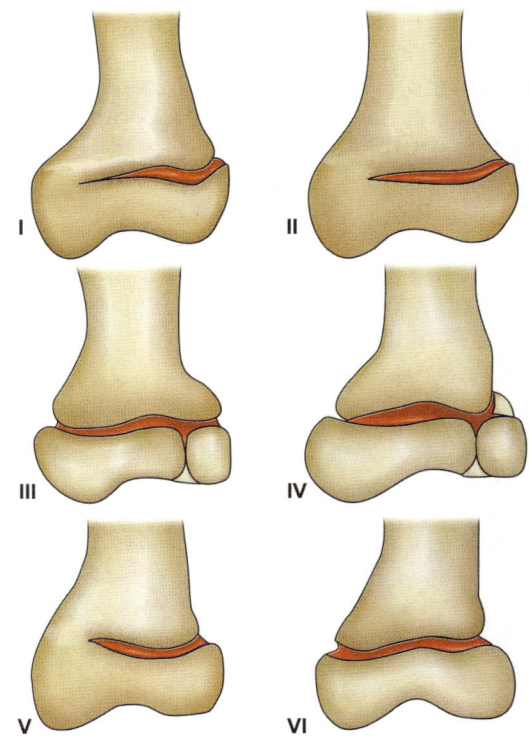

Fig. 14.5: Salter and Harris classification types of epiphyseal injuries

Type II: The fracture involves the physis and a triangle of metaphyseal bone (*Thurston Holland sign*). This is the commonest type of epiphyseal injury accounting for 73 percent of cases over 10 years of age.

Type III: The fracture is intraarticular and extends along the physis and then along the growth plate. This injury is relatively uncommon.

Type IV: The fracture is intraarticular and extends through the epiphysis, physis, and metaphysis. Perfect reduction is necessary and open reduction is more often necessary to prevent growth arrest.

Type V: It is a crushing of the epiphysis followed by growth arrest.

Type VI: There is a peripheral physis lesion and is described by Rang.

Clinical Features

The child complains of pain, deformity, swelling, loss of movements in the affected joints. But features of crepitus, loss of transmitted movements, etc. are not quite elicitable because displaced fractures are not common in children. On the other hand, deformity is a major complaint because the bone bends in greenstick fractures and does not break completely (Fig. 14.6A).

Plain X-ray of the affected bones helps to study the type of fractures whether greenstick, torus, incomplete or epiphyseal (Fig. 14.6B).

Treatment

Challenges of treatment in children
- The younger child is fretful and difficult to examine fully.
- Worried parents and a crying child pose problems.
- Many fractures are difficult to see on radiographs and need X-rays of good quality.
- General anesthesia is required for manipulation.
- Circulatory compromise is relatively common.
- Redisplacement after reduction is common during the first week.
- Wound care should be the same as in adults.
- Overgrowth after long bone fracture is a very common problem and an overlap of 1 cm should be allowed.

> **Remember**
>
> The general rules in treatment of fractures in children:
> - Angulations > 10° are unacceptable.
> - Rotation will not be compensated and hence it is not acceptable.
> - Overlap of the fracture site by 1 to 2 cm is acceptable as there is overgrowth following a long bone fracture.
> - Correction occurs at the average rate of 1° per month.

Treatment Options

Conservative: NSAIDs, crepe bandage, and plaster slabs slings, etc. for undisplaced fractures.

Closed reduction and plaster immobilization: This is preferred if fracture is displaced or if the bones are bent as in greenstick fractures. Retention is usually by slab, cast and rarely by traction (Fig. 14.6C). Hip spica immobilization is usually done in shaft femur fracture.

Closed reduction by traction: This can also be attempted in certain situations, e.g. Dunlop's traction (See Fig. 11.2) or overhead olecranon skeletal traction in difficult supracondylar humerus of fracture, Gallows traction in shaft femur fracture, etc. (Fig. 11.3).

Open reduction and internal fixation: This is rarely done in children. Indications being failed closed reduction, redisplacement, multiple injuries, neurovascular injuries, delayed union and soft tissue interposition.

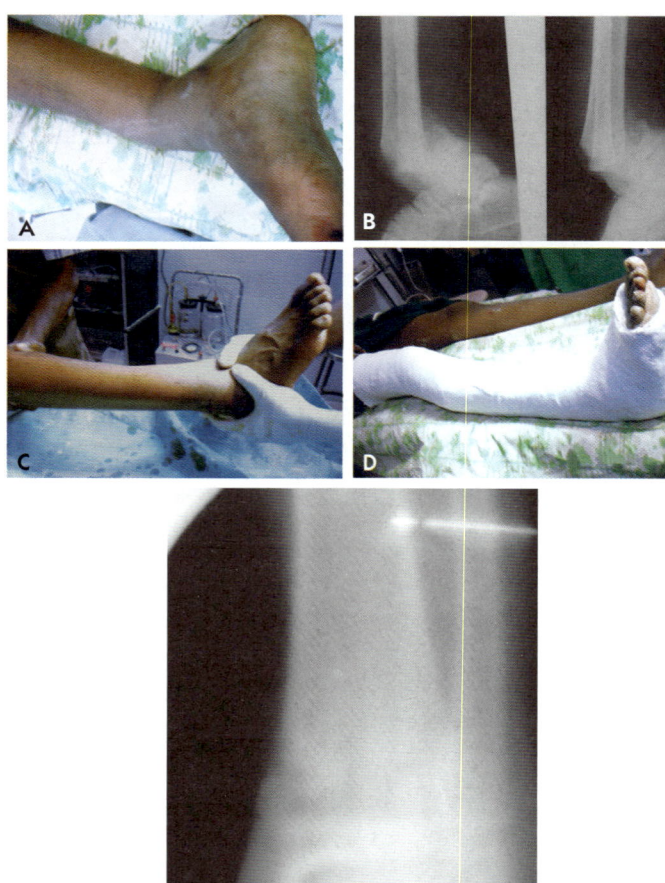

Figs 14.6A to E: Reduction of epiphyseal injury by traction and counter traction methods: (A) clinical photograph showing deformity of epiphyseal injury of tibia lower end, (B) plain X-ray showing epiphyseal injury, (C) reduction by traction and countertraction methods, (D) application of an above knee cast, (E) post-reduction plain X-ray

14

Treatment of Epiphyseal Injuries

Type I and II injuries can be managed conservatively. *Type III and IV injuries* usually require closed or open reduction. Angular deformity and shortening are the consequences of premature growth arrest.

Some specific fractures in children which require open reduction and internal fixation:
- Lateral condyle of humerus fracture.
- Neck of femur fracture (displaced).
- Epiphyseal injuries of the medial malleolus.
- Shaft femur fracture in the 14–16 age group (See Fig. 22.11D).

Corrective osteotomy: This is required in malunited fractures like cubitus varus deformity due to malunited supracondylar fracture and is usually done after skeletal maturity (Fig. 14.7).

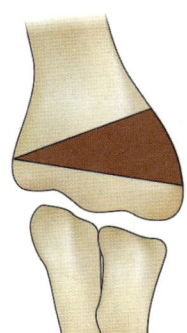 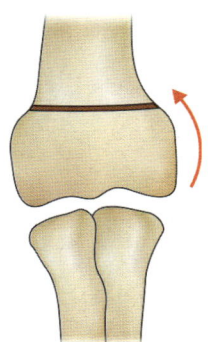

Fig. 14.7: Corrective osteotomy in supracondylar fracture of humerus in children (Lateral closed wedge osteotomy)

Remember

The principles of treatment in children. Three **R**s:
- **R**ealign the fracture.
- **R**espect the soft tissues.
- **R**emember the child.

COMPLICATIONS

- *Overgrowth* is due to stimulation and hypervascularity after epiphyseal injury.
- *Deformities* are due to unequal damage of the epiphyseal plate.
- *Growth disturbances* are due to crushing of the growth plate.
- *Growth arrest* is due to damage of the growth plate.
- *Shortening* is due to crushing of the growth plate.
- *AVN* is seen in the neck of femur fracture.
- *Myositis ossificans* is commonly seen in injuries around the elbow joint.

IMPORTANT FRACTURES IN CHILDREN
- Monteggia's fracture.
- Supracondylar humerus fractures.
- Greenstick fractures and torus fractures.
- Radial neck fractures.
- Clavicle fractures.
- Neck femur fractures.
- Epiphyseal injuries of the ankle and distal end of radius, etc.

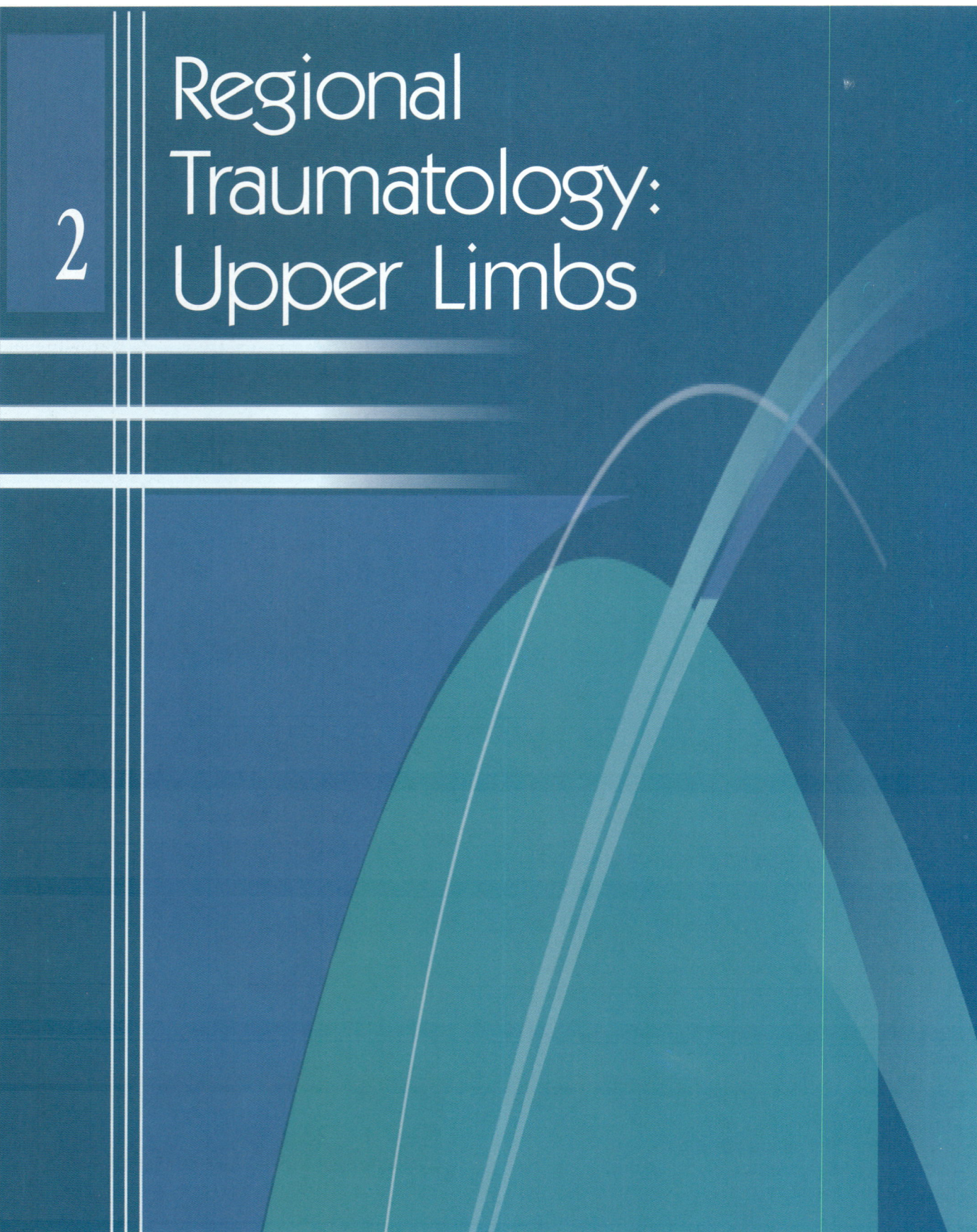

2

Regional Traumatology: Upper Limbs

Injuries Around the Shoulder

The shoulder joint complex consists of glenohumeral joint, the acromioclavicular joint and sternoclavicular joint. The injuries concerning all the three joints and the fractures involving the clavicle, proximal humerus are discussed in this chapter.

RELEVANT ANATOMY

Glenohumeral Joint

It is a multiaxial ball and socket joint and the most mobile joint in the body. Various parts of the joint are detailed below.

- *Humeral head*: It is approximately one-third of a sphere and is oriented at 45° from the long axis of the shaft and retroverted 30°. The indistinct anatomical neck consists two important landmarks, the lesser tuberosity anteromedially and the greater tuberosity superolaterally separated by the bicipital groove. The shallow shaped glenoid cavity is retroverted approximately and inferiorly angulated 5° from the long axis of the scapula.
- *Labrum:* It is a fibrocartilage, which is triangular in cross-section and is attached to the outer perimeter of the glenoid. It increases the contact area by 70 percent and helps in stability.
- *Ligaments*: The fibrous capsule is attached peripherally to the margins of glenoid cavity and anatomic neck. It has three intrinsic capsular ligaments called the glenohumeral ligaments, which reinforce together. The coracohumeral ligament assists the capsule in supporting the arm.
- *Rotator cuff*: Infraspinatus, supraspinatus, subscapularis, and teres minor are four inter-related muscles. The coordinated activity provides support during finer adjustments of the humeral head within the glenoid cavity.
- *Bursae*: It provides smooth movements aided by numerous bursae of which subdeltoid or subacromial bursa is most important. It helps to carry out various activities like flexion, extension, adduction, abduction, internal and external rotation and circumduction with ease.

FRACTURE CLAVICLE

The term clavicle is derived from the Latin root *Clavis* meaning *Key*.

Mechanism of Injury

Direct: Due to fall on the point of the shoulder. This is the most common mode of injury accounting for 91 percent of the cases. Trauma over the clavicle due to RTA, etc. accounts for 8 percent of the cases (Fig. 15.1).

Indirect: Due to fall on the outstretched hands accounts for 1 percent of the cases.

Sites of Fracture

- Eighty percent of the fracture clavicle occurs at the junction of middle and outer third.
- One percent at medial end of the clavicle (5%).
- Lateral end fracture is uncommon (15%).

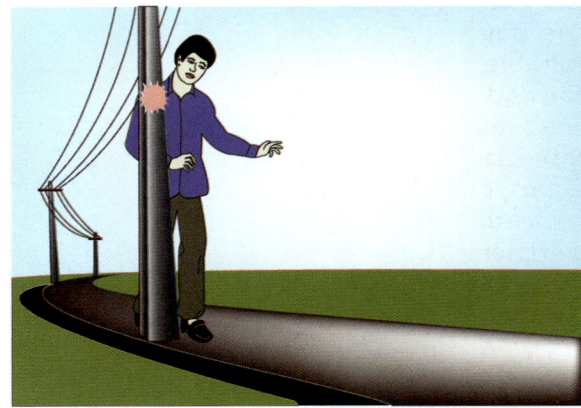

Fig. 15.1: Direct injury causes fracture clavicle

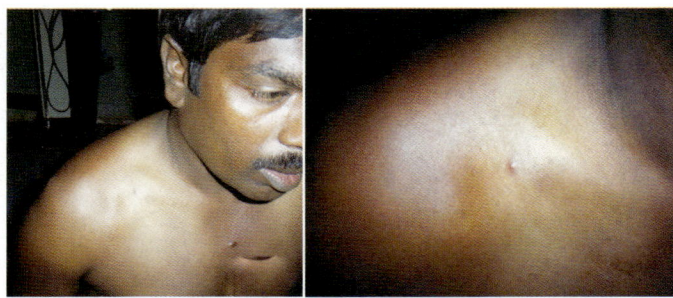

Fig. 15.2: Classical deformity in fracture of the clavicle

Clinical Features

Patient presents with pain, swelling, deformity and inability to raise the shoulder (Fig. 15.2). Rarely patient may present with pseudo paralysis of the affected arm.

Radiology: Routine antero-posterior view of the clavicle is sufficient to make the diagnosis (Fig. 15.3).

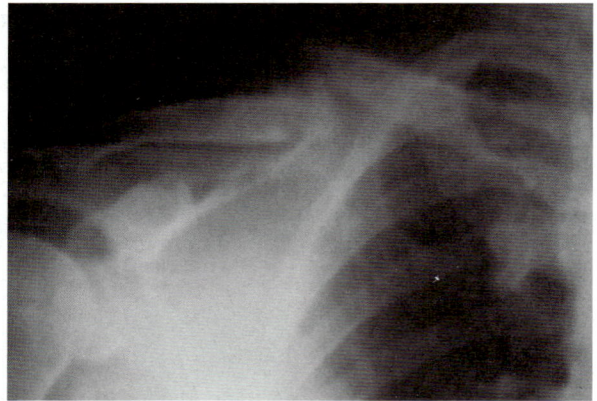

Fig. 15.3: X-ray showing fracture clavicle of middle-third

Treatment

Before proceeding to the treatment proper one needs to understand the two distracting forces acting on the fracture fragments in clavicle making the treatment difficult. Sternocleidomastoid muscle attached at the medial and of the clavicle pulls it up, while the pectoralis major muscles under gravity pulls the lateral end of the clavicle down (Fig. 15.4). Successful treatment of fracture clavicle depends on how effectively one overcomes these displacing forces. To counter the above two detrimental forces, the shoulder should be elevated and braced back and the arm should be supported while treating fracture clavicle.

Conservative methods: This is the treatment of choice in fracture clavicle and consists of the following methods.
- *Cuff and collar:* Sling for undisplaced fractures (Fig. 15.5A).

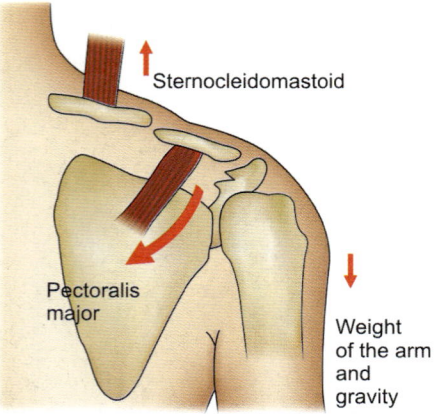

Fig. 15.4: Various displacing forces in fracture clavicle

- *Strapping:* The fracture site using dynaplast gives good results especially in children and young adults (Fig. 15.5B).
- *Figure of 8:* This is popularly used and it acts by retracting the shoulder girdle, minimizes the overlap and allows more anatomical healing (Fig. 15.5C).

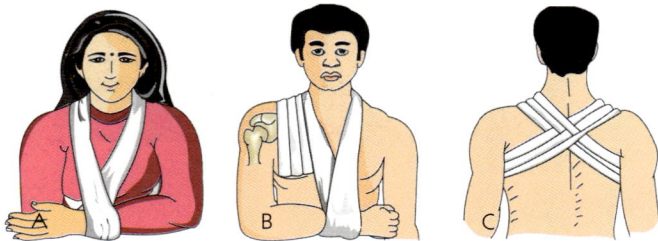

Figs 15.5A to C: Methods of conservative treatment of fractures clavicle: (A) collar and cuff sling, (B) strapping and sling suspension, (C) figure of 8 bandaging

Surgery is rarely indicated and is considered in the following situations. Open fractures, injury to neurovascular bundle, the fracture is threatening to penetrate the skin, non-union, fracture near acromioclavicular joint and displaced epiphysis in children.

Fixation methods: This could be either by plate and screws (Figs 15.6A and B) or by special intramedullary rods or by K-wire.

Complications

- *Neurovascular injury:* The structures commonly injured are subclavian vessels and the medial cord of the brachial plexus through which the ulnar nerve is derived.

15

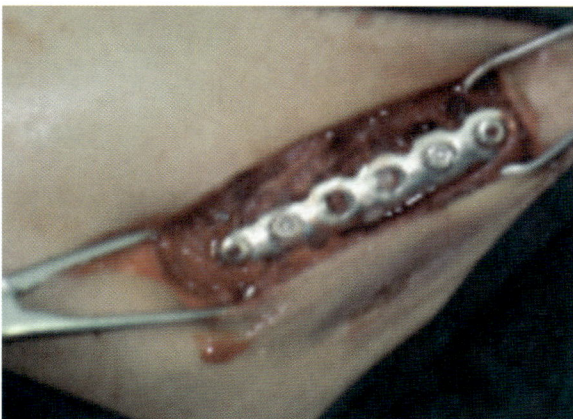

Fig. 15.6A: Operative photograph, showing open reduction and internal fixation with plate and screws is rarely indicated in fracture clavicle

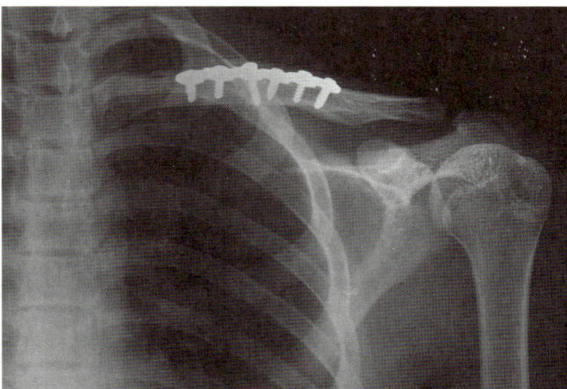

Fig. 15.6B: Plating of the clavicle

- *Malunion*: It is very common, causes only a cosmetic problem and does not usually impair function. Hence no treatment is required in most situations.
- *Nonunion*: It is rare and requires open reduction, rigid internal fixation and bone grafting.
- *Frozen shoulder*: It is due to periarthritis of the shoulder joint following prolonged immobilization.

Remember
- Most common fracture in children
- Common mode of injury is direct
- 80% break at junction of middle and distal third
- Nearly all fractures are treated closed
- Open reduction for specific indications
- Malunion is a rule, but no functional disability

ACROMIOCLAVICULAR JOINT INJURIES

Acromioclavicular joint is a diarthrodial joint with a fibrocartilaginous disc between the two bones (similar to a meniscus).

Mechanism of Injury

- *Direct force*: This is the most common mechanism of injury as in RTA, assault, fall, etc. (Fig. 15.7).
- *Indirect force*: It is due to fall in outstretched hands.

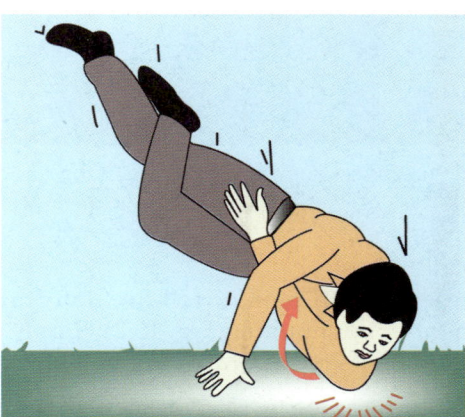

Fig. 15.7: Common mechanism of acromioclavicular joint injury

Classification: Depending upon the severity of the tear of acromioclavicular and coracoclavicular ligaments, the injury is classified as Grades I to III.

Clinical Features

Patient complains of pain, swelling, and difficulty in raising the arm up. On examination there is tenderness over the lateral end of clavicle and is prominently felt (Fig. 15.8A).

Radiology: Routine anteroposterior view helps clinch the diagnosis while sometimes special views are called for (Fig. 15.8B).

Treatment

Conservative methods: Fortunately, most of the ACM injuries are mild and hence can be effectively managed by conservative methods like rest to the part, collar and cuff sling, ice and heat packs, adhesive strapping.

Surgery: Either persistent pain or more severe ligament tears needs to be tackled surgically by repair, reinforcement and fixation with K-wires (Fig. 15.8C) or reconstruction of the ligaments or by excision of the lateral end of clavicle in more troublesome cases.

STERNOCLAVICULAR JOINT INJURIES

This is the least commonly dislocated joint because of its strong ligament.

Mechanism of Injury

Causes: Road traffic accidents (RTA) are responsible for 80 percent of the cases, sports related injuries account for the remaining 20 percent (Fig. 15.9).

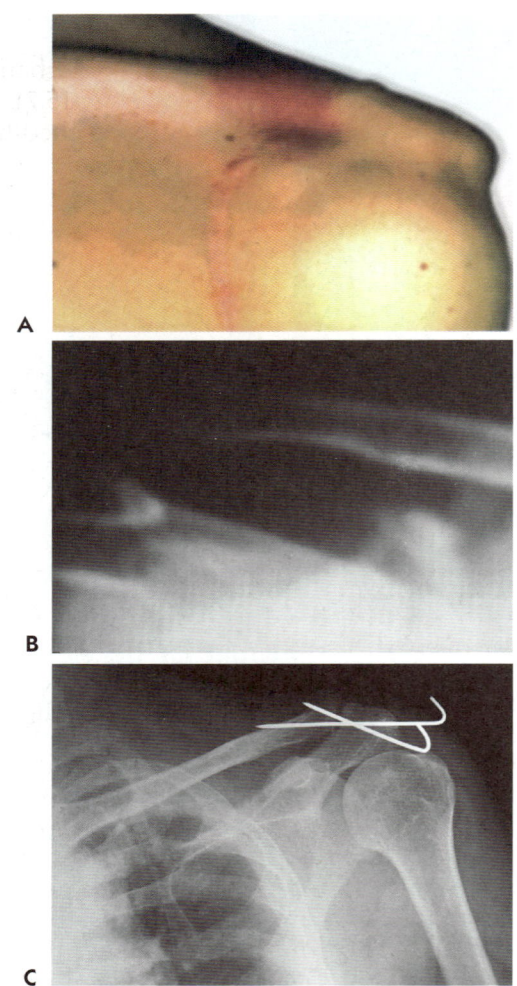

Figs 15.8A to C: (A) ACM dislocation, (B) Plain X-ray showing ACM joint subluxation, (C) Fixation with K-wires

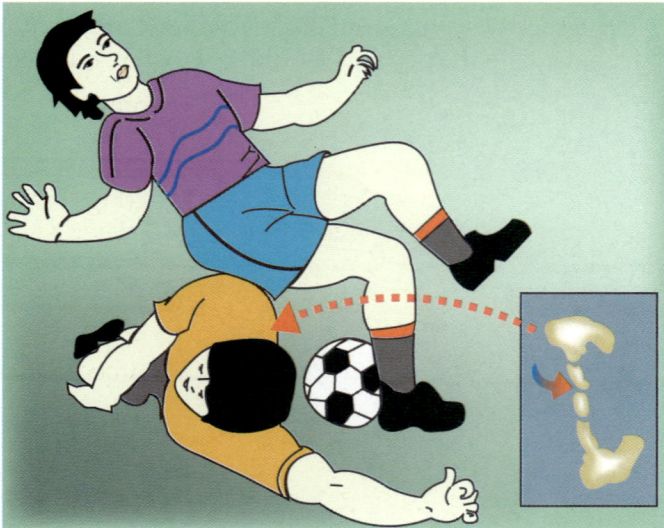

Fig. 15.9: Common mechanism of injury in sternoclavicular injuries

Clinical Features

Patient complains of pain and swelling over the sternoclavicular joint. Medial end of the clavicle is prominently seen and felt in anterior dislocation. When the affected shoulder is short the lateral shoulder compression test would prove positive.

Radiology: It is difficult to interpret the routine AP views in these cases. The special views are called for. CT scans and MRI are more helpful in making an accurate diagnosis.

Management

Mild sprain: The treatment method consists of ice, sling, pain killers, etc.

Subluxation: The treatment methods are ice for first 12 hrs, warmth for 24–48 hrs, clavicle strap, figure of '8' and excision of medial end of the clavicle if pain persists.

Dislocation: The treatment is closed reduction followed by figure of '8', clavicle strap, sling. If it proves futile, open reduction and internal fixation using K-wire is necessary.

PROXIMAL HUMERAL FRACTURES

This is common in elderly patients and accounts for 4 to 5 percent of all fractures.

Mechanism

- Fall on outstretched hands is the classical history.
- Blow on the lateral side of the arm is the other mode of injury.

Classification: Neer has proposed a classification for fractures of the proximal humerus based on this 4-segment concept and could involve the:

1. Anatomical neck
2. Greater tuberosity
3. Lesser tuberosity
4. Shaft or surgical neck of the humerus.

The fragments tend to get displaced depending on the direction of the pull of the surrounding muscles (Fig. 15.10).

Fracture is said to be displaced if there is displacement of > 1 cm or rotation > 45° (Neer)/Depending upon the fragments involved it is called 2 part, 3 part or 4 part fractures.

Clinical Features

The patient complains of pain, swelling and other features of fractures. Movements of the shoulder joint are grossly restricted.

15

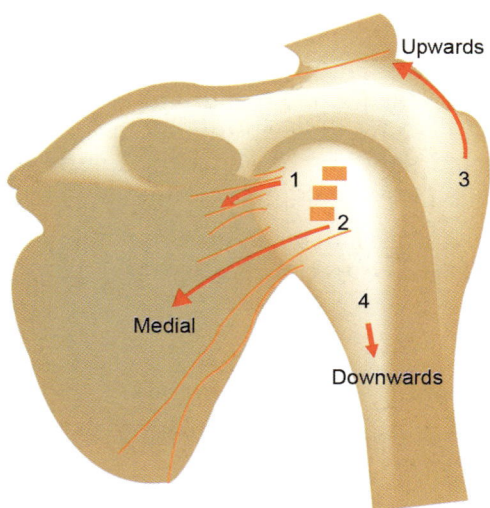

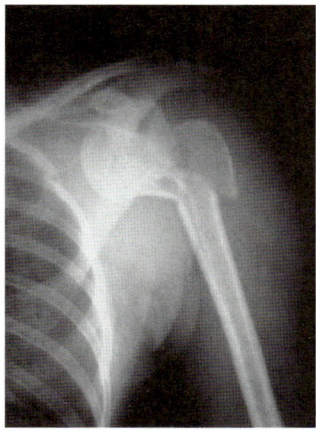

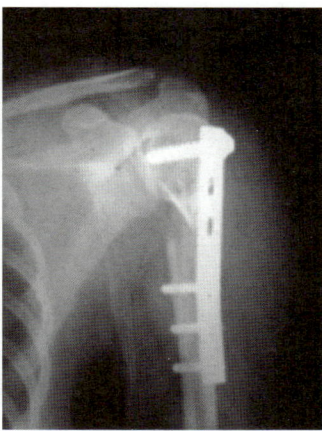

Fig. 15.11A: Four part proximal humeral fracture

Fig. 15.11B: Internal fixation with blade plate device

Fig. 15.10: Various displacing forces an acting in proximal humeral fracture: (1) Suprascapularis pull, (2) P major pull, (3) Supra and infraspinatus pull, (4) Gravity

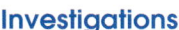

15

HUMERAL FRACTURES OF SPECIAL INTEREST

GREATER TUBEROSITY FRACTURE OF THE HUMERUS

This fracture is more commonly seen in adults and is due to the fall on the joint of the shoulder. Rarely it could be due to avulsion of the supraspinatus muscle. (Fig. 15.12A). Patient complains of pain, swelling and inability or difficulty to abduct the shoulder. Plain X-rays help to study the displacement and angulation of tuberosity (Fig. 15.12B). Conservative treatment is by cuff and collar, sling, etc. and it suffices for undisplaced or minimally displaced fractures. Abduction splints or ORIF is reserved for displaced fractures. Frozen shoulder could be a troublesome complication.

SURGICAL NECK FRACTURES

It is commonly seen in frail elderly women and is due to trivial fall on the point of shoulder. However, unlike

Investigations

- *Plain X-rays of the shoulder*: Trauma series consists of AP, lateral, and axillary view of shoulder joint in scapular plane (Fig. 15.11A).
- Laminagrams to judge the articular defects.
- CT scan helps to study the fracture lines with greater accuracy.

Management

Conservative treatment: It consists of rest, NSAIDs, sling, ice and heat therapy in the initial stages. Since 80 percent of the fractures are minimally displaced, early motion of the shoulder is the mainstay of treatment to prevent stiffness of the joint. Pendulum exercises, elevation, pulley, external and internal rotation and wall climbing exercises are some of the recommended methods in the later stages.

Operative treatment: It consists of rigid internal fixation of displaced fracture of the proximal humerus in older patients with a blade-plate device or locked plates (Fig. 15.11B) and this provides sufficient primary stability to allow early functional treatment. Badly comminuted fractures need Neer's prosthetic replacement or total shoulder arthroplasty.

Fracture of the greater tuberosity, surgical neck of humerus and shaft are discussed in the following chapter.

Complications

Malunion nonunion, AVN , periarthritis, etc. are some of the important complications.

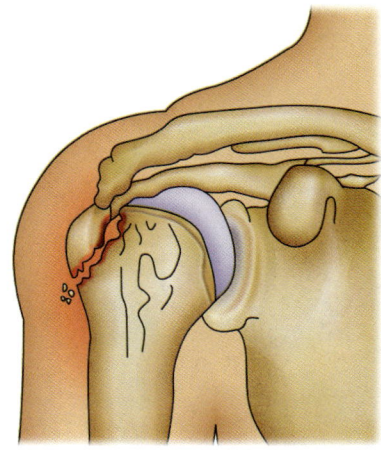

Fig. 15.12A: Avulsion fracture of greater tuberosity of humerus

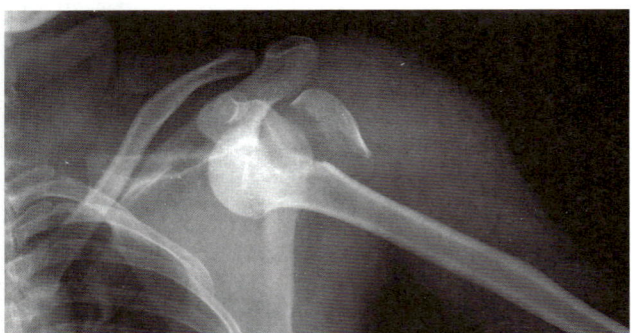

Fig. 15.12B: Greater tuberosity fracture

fracture neck of femur, this fracture is frequently impacted and generally heals well by simple conservative methods like sling. Displaced fractures (Fig. 15.13) required closed reduction and percutaneous K-wire fixation or rarely open reduction and rigid internal fixation. Axillary nerve injury may occur and is identified by the loss of sensation in the regiment bandage area. Frozen shoulder is another important complication.

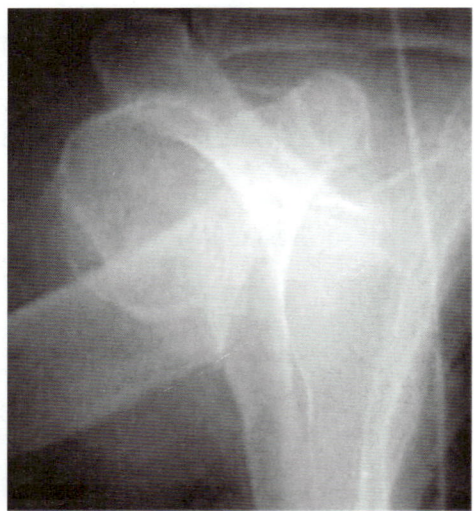

Fig. 15.13: Surgical neck humerus fracture

ANTERIOR DISLOCATION OF THE SHOULDER (ADS)

Shoulder joint is vulnerable for dislocation more often than any other joint in the body. Anterior dislocation is more common than the posterior dislocation and accounts for more than 95% of the cases (Figs 15.14A to E).

Mechanism of Injury

- *Direct force:* A violent direct blow on the posterior aspect of the shoulder can lead to ADS. However, this is not very common.

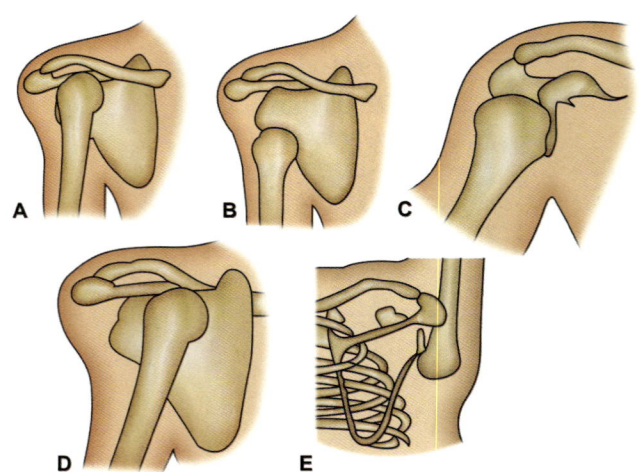

Figs 15.14A to E: Various types of anterior dislocation of shoulder: (A) subcoracoid, (B) subglenoid (commonest), (C) infraclavicular, (D) posterior, and (E) inferior (luxatio erecta)

15

- *Indirect force:* A fall on an outstretched hand with the shoulder in abduction and external rotation dislocates the shoulder anteriorly. This is the common method of dislocation.

Clinical Features

An ADS victim writhes with agonizing pain, holds the drooping, abducted and externally rotated shoulder in the opposite hand (Fig. 15.15). The more unlucky patients may complain of loss of sensation on the outer aspect of the upper arm (Regiment badge sign) due to the injury of the circumflex nerve (Fig. 15.16). The ADS presents a spectrum of interesting, unmistakable and classical clinical signs.

- Loss of normal spherical counter shoulder. An in-elegant flat shoulder replaces this.

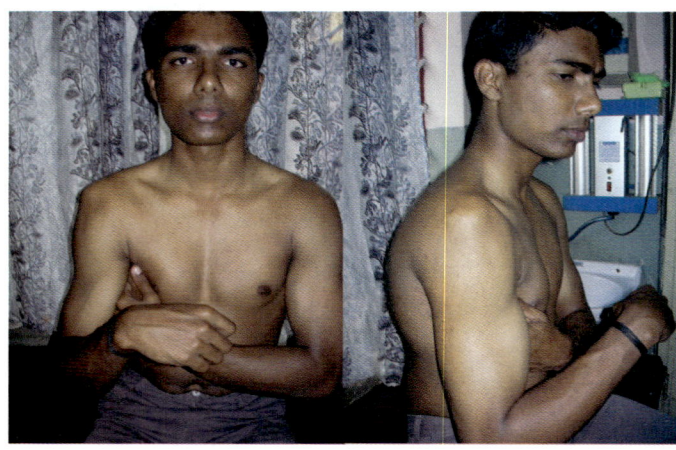

Figs 15.15: Classical presentation of anterior dislocation of the shoulder

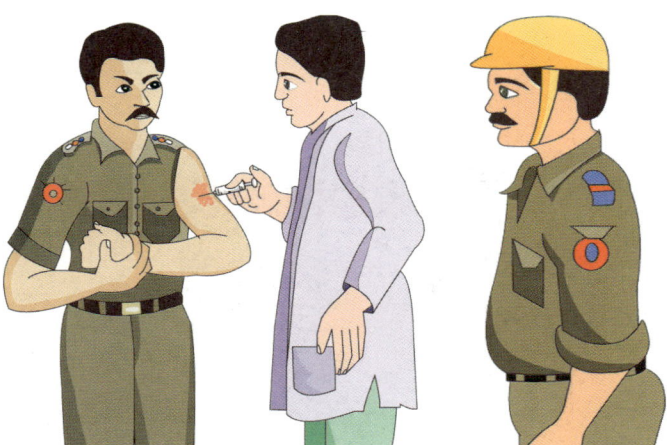

Fig. 15.16: Regiment badge test

- An anterior shoulder prominence.
- ADS make it possible for a ruler to be placed straight touching the acromion and the lateral epicondyle of the humerus (Hamilton ruler test).
- Girth of the axilla is increased (Callaway's test).
- Anterior axillary fold is lower than the posterior (Bryant's test).

Radiology: Proper radiographic techniques help to identify these above mentioned dislocations (Fig. 15.17).

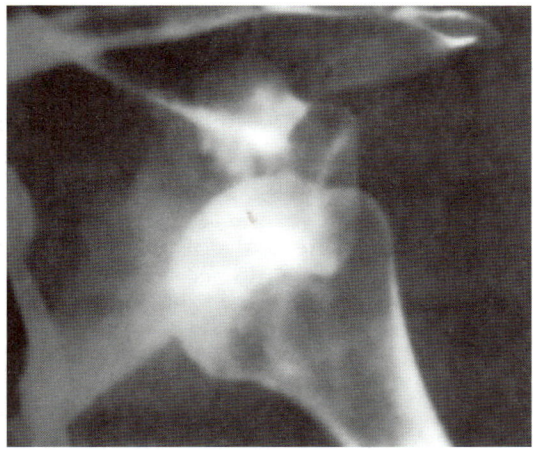

Fig. 15.17: Plain X-ray of the shoulder showing anterior dislocation

Management

All dislocations are emergencies and they need to be put back immediately without any delay and shoulder dislocation is no exception. Closed reduction under general anesthesia is preferred as it not only keeps the patient quiet but also ensures adequate muscular relaxation for smoother reduction.

Methods of closed reduction: As the forces dislocating the shoulder are many, similarly there are many methods

to put back into same position. Our ancestors deprived of today's advanced technical gadgetries, crudely placed a foot into the axial and pulled the shoulder back into position (*Hippocrates method*). Nowadays, a more refined and scientific technique is in *vogue*, the *Kocher method* (Figs 15.18A to C).

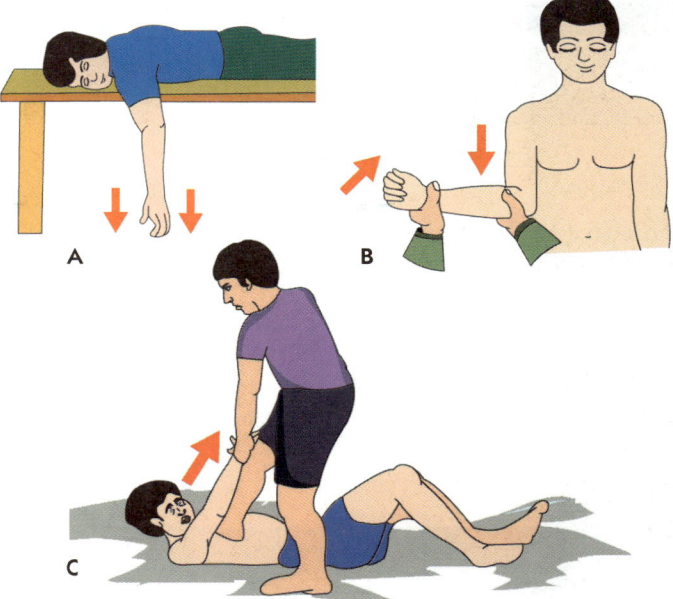

Figs 15.18A to C: (A) Stimson's gravity method, (B) Kocher's method, (C) Showing the outdated Hippocratic method of reduction of anterior dislocation of shoulder

Kocher's Method of Reduction

Mnemonic **TEAM** helps to remember the various steps involved in this method:

T Traction in the line of the humerus by the surgeon.
E External rotation of the arm is done next.
A Abduction of the arm.
M Medial rotation of the arm is slowly done last.

If the reduction is successful, the patient's hand can be placed now on the opposite shoulder quite easily (Figs 15.19A to E).

Note: It is imperative that following the reduction, the shoulder needs to be immobilized for a minimum period of three weeks (Fig. 15.20). Failure to do so leads to improper healing of the shoulder capsule and other structures resulting in recurrent dislocation of the shoulder.

Open reduction is rarely required and is reserved for specific indications like failed closed reduction.

Complications: These could be recurrent dislocation of shoulder or old unreduced dislocation of the shoulder, frozen shoulder, acute problems like injury to the axillary nerve.

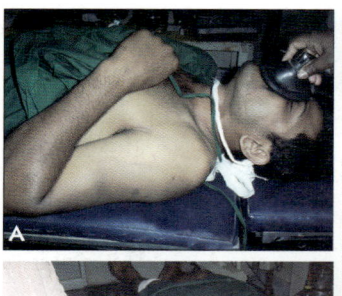
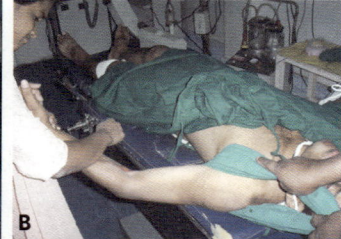
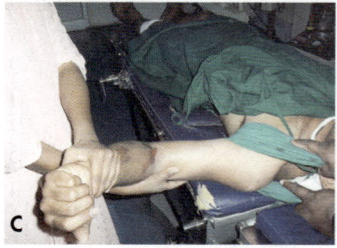
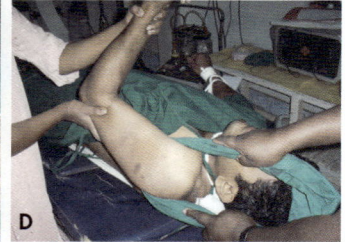
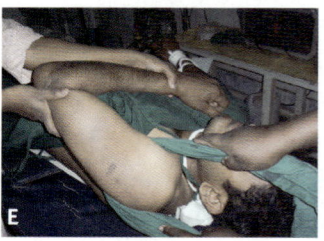

Figs 15.19A to E: Kocher's method of reduction of the anterior dislocation of the shoulder joint: (A) Patient is in general anesthesia, (B) Traction in line of humerus, (C) External rotation, (D) Adduction of the arm, (E) Internal rotation of the arm

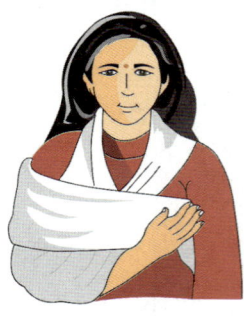

Fig. 15.20: Method of shoulder immobilization after reduction of ADS (failure to do this for at least 3 weeks is the prime cause of RDS)

Remember

- Most common dislocation.
- Subcoracoid and subglenoid account for 99% of cases.
- Capsular injury in 30%; labral lesion in 60%.
- Prompt reduction required. Kocher's method is the best.
- Check for axillary nerve injury before reduction.
- Immobilize for three weeks and relative immobilization for further three weeks.
- Prolonged rehabilitation.
- Avoid provocative positions for 6 weeks.

Recurrent Anterior Dislocation of the Shoulder (RDS)

This is a very common complication of anterior dislocation of shoulder and accounts for greater than 80 percent of dislocations of the upper extremity. Age at the time of initial dislocation is an important prognostic factor, recurrence rate being 55 percent in patients 12–

22 years old, 37 percent in 23–29 years, and 12 percent in 30–40 years.

Pathological Anatomy

Due to the initial acute dislocation there could be three classical injuries which can later lead to recurrence of dislocation. No single deformity is responsible for recurrent dislocation of shoulder. Three important reasons have been cited and they have been called as *essential lesions*.

Triad of Essential Lesion

Hill-Sachs lesion: It is a posterolateral defect in the head of the humerus. This is produced due to the impact of the posterolateral part of the head of the humerus against the sharp anterior margin of the glenoid rim.

Bankart's lesion: Perthes first described this as defect in the anterior part of the glenoid labrum and the anterior capsule. If this defect does not heal properly or heals in elongated position, it results in RDS.

Erosion of anterior rim of glenoid cavity

Mechanism of RDS: External rotation of the shoulder in abducted position pops out the head of humerus from the glenoid cavity due to lax anterior capsular structures. The posterolateral defect now encounters glenoid rim and is levered out of the socket, producing dislocation. Since no single factor is responsible for recurrent dislocation, no single operative procedure can be applied to the patient either.

Clinical Features

During the abduction activities of the shoulder, the joint may suddenly and unexpectedly give way and all the features of anterior dislocation of the shoulder mentioned earlier could be seen however with lesser intensity.

Investigations

Plain X-ray of the shoulder, CT scan, MRI, etc. helps to study the triad of lesion in RDS.

Treatment

There is no role of conservative treatment in recurrent dislocation of shoulder. Patient is advised to avoid abduction and external rotation of the shoulder. However, surgery is the treatment of choice and is indicated if the patient has more than three episodes of RDS. More than 150 operations are devised. A few are mentioned in Table 15.1. All the surgeries aim at correction of the essential lesions and prevent external rotation of the arm.

15

Table 15.1

Name of the surgery	What is done
Bankart's operation	Detached anterior structures are attached to the rim of the glenoid cavity with sutures.
Staple capsulorrhaphy Destot and Roux	Bankart lesion attached to labrum with staples.
Putti–Platt's operation	Subscapularis tendon and capsule is overlapped and tightened.
Magnuson and stack	Subscapularis tendon and capsule is advanced laterally on the humerus.
Eden Hybinette	Bone graft is placed against the anterior aspect of neck of scapula and rim of glenoid cavity.
Bristow's	Transplantation of coracoid process with its attachments to the anterior rim of glenoid.
McLaughlin's	Tendon of subscapularis is transplanted into the posterolateral defect.

Arthroscopic repair: These are the days of minimally invasive surgeries. It is possible now to carry out the Bankart's repair through arthroscopy. It is less invasive leading to less morbidity and faster recovery and rehabilitation.

FRACTURE OF SCAPULA

Scapula is a flat bone thickly covered by muscles. From above downwards, the scapula may be fractured as follows (Figs 15.21A and B):
a. The coracoid process
b. The spine of the scapula
c. The neck
d. The body
e. Acromion
f. Glenoid

Mechanism of injury: The scapula may be fractured due to:

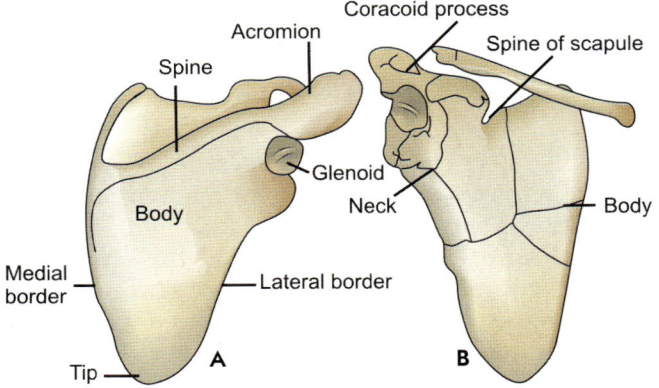

Figs 15.21A and B: (A) Normal anatomy, (B) types of scapular fractures

a. Direct injury to the shoulder blade (Fig. 15.22).
b. Fall on outstretched hands.
  Whatever may be the mechanism of injury, scapular fractures are seldom displaced, thanks to the thick muscles surrounding it.

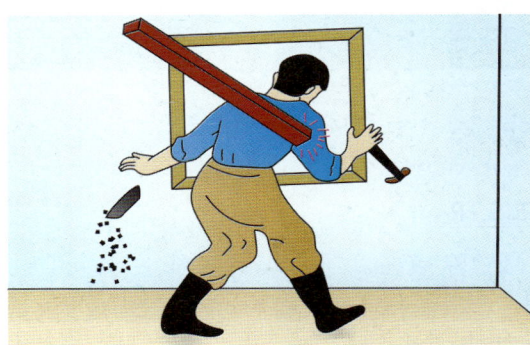

Fig. 15.22: Common mechanism of injury to scapula by direct force

Clinical Features

Patient will complain of pain swelling, tenderness and painful shoulder movements.

X-ray of the scapula: The routine and special scapula radiological views help in making the diagnosis (Fig. 15.23).

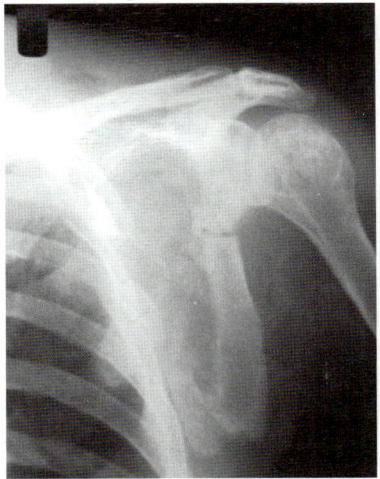

Fig. 15.23: Plain X-ray showing fracture of the body of the scapula

Treatment

Conservative treatment by sling for a period of 2–3 weeks forms the mainstay of treatment. Surgery is seldom required. Early mobilization of shoulder is the 'mantra' in scapular fractures.

Rehabilitation program: Aims to restore back the shoulder movements to normal or to achieve at least the functional range of moments.

16 Injuries of the Arm

HUMERUS FRACTURE

Shaft humerus fracture is more common in adults than in children, though it can appear in any age group.

Mechanism of Injury

Three important mechanisms are described:
- *Direct force:* This may produce a transverse or comminuted fracture as in RTA, assault, etc. (Fig. 16.1).
- *Indirect force:* It is due to fall on an outstretched hand and this will produce an oblique or spiral fracture.
- *Birth injuries:* This is the second most common birth fracture after clavicle.

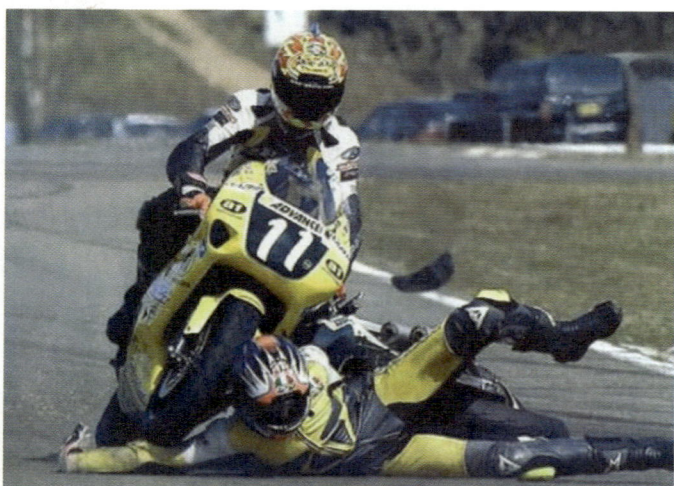

Fig. 16.1: Direct injury in RTA's common cause of humeral shaft fractures

Anatomic considerations: The deformity is influenced by the muscles of the upper arm. If the fracture is between pectoralis major and deltoid, the proximal fragment is adducted by pectoralis major, teres minor and latissimus dorsi, while the distal fragment is pulled upwards by the deltoid. If the fracture is below the insertion of deltoid, the proximal fragment is abducted by the deltoid while the coracobrachialis, biceps and triceps pull the distal fragment upward (Figs 16.2A and B).

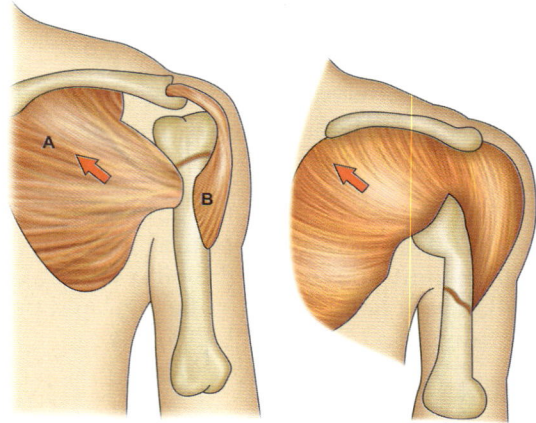

Figs 16.2A and B: Muscle forces causing deformity in humerus shaft fracture: (A) pull of pectoralis major muscle, (B) pull of deltoid muscle

Clinical Features

Clinical features show all signs and symptoms of fractures like pain, swelling, deformity, abnormal mobility depending on the extent and severity of fracture (Fig. 16.3). A careful neurological and vascular assessment is important. Injury to radial nerve is common in fractures at the spiral groove or lower one-third of humerus and this could lead to the wrist drop.

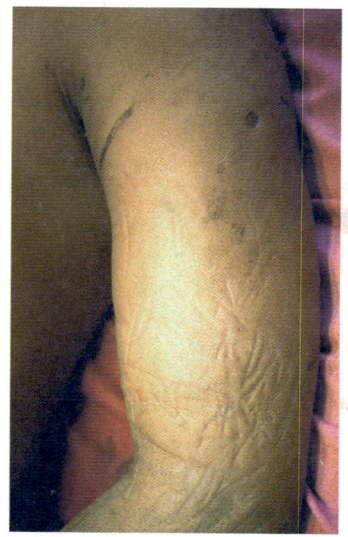

Fig. 16.3: Fracture shaft of humerus

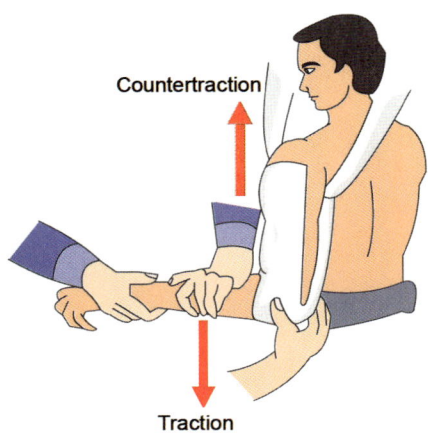

Fig. 16.4: Method of closed reduction and application of U-slab

Radiology

Radiography of the entire upper arm including both the shoulder joint above and the elbow joint below should be taken. It helps to study the level and pattern of the fracture (Figs 16.6A and 16.7A).

Treatment

Conservative Methods

This is the mainstay of treatment of although it is seldom practised.

1. **Undisplaced fractures:**
   - *Simple U-splint* in birth fractures.
   - *Simple sling* may be sufficient in young children.
   - *Chest arm bandage*: The arm is strapped to the side of the chest with bandages. It can be considered in children less than 5 years of age.
2. **Displaced fractures:**
   - *Hanging cast:* This is useful in older children and adolescents. The gravity aids in reduction of the fracture. They are not suitable if the level of fracture corresponds to the upper limit of the cast, because of the deforming effect of the proximal end of the cast. It is indicated in comminuted fractures of the distal third. If the cast is too heavy it may cause distraction and consequent delayed or nonunion (Fig. 16.5A).
   - *Plaster U-splint or cast:* It is sufficient in most of the situations of fractures of proximal, middle third portion of the humerus. The method of closed reduction and application of U-slab as shown in Fig. 16.4. U-slab covers the following areas of the upper arm:
     - *Inner arm of the U*: It supports the inner side of the arm just beneath the axilla.
     - *U-turn*: It supports the medial epicondyle, olecranon tip and the lateral epicondyles.
     - *Outer arm of the U*: It supports the outer aspect of the arm, shoulder, and extends up to the base of the neck (Fig. 16.5B).

- Functional cast brace gives good results (Fig. 16.5C).

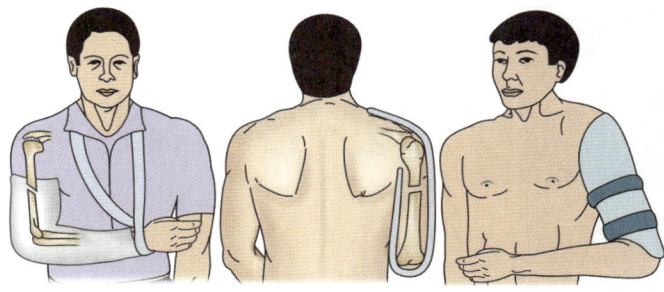

Figs 16.5A to C: Conservative methods of treating fracture shaft humerus: (A) Hanging arm cast, (B) U-slab, (C) Functional cast brace

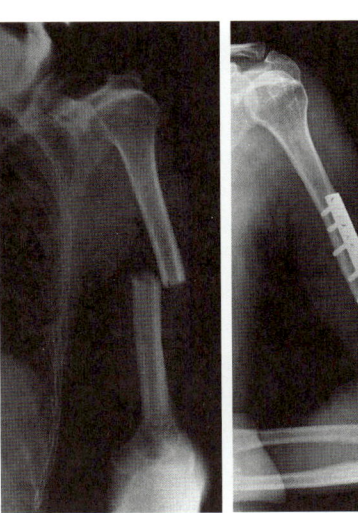 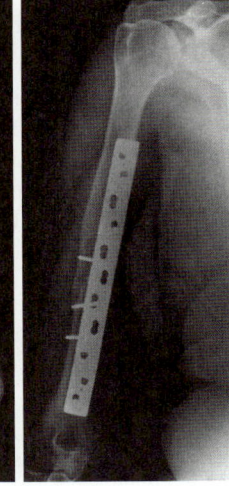

Fig. 16.6A: Fracture shaft humerus | **Fig. 16.6B:** Fracture humerus fixed with DCP | **Fig. 16.6C:** Fracture shaft fixed with locking plate

Operative treatment: Fortunately, the incidence of surgical treatment in humerus fracture is reduced to a miniscule in few cases with the following specific indications:
- Failed conservative treatment.
- Multiple fractures and unstable fractures.
- Multi-system injuries.
- Radial nerve palsy after closed reduction.
- Segmental fracture.

Methods

- DCP plating or locked compression plating for fractures at all levels (Figs 16.6A and B)
- Intramedullary fixation at middle third fractures.
- Of late locked compression plate has gained important (Fig. 16.6C).
- Recently interlocking nailing is also being tried with varied success (Figs 16.7A and B).

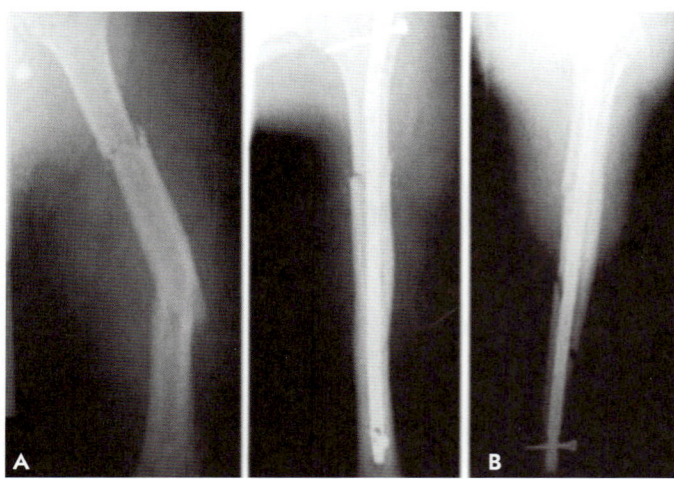

Figs 16.7A and B: (A) A segmental fracture humerus, (B) fixation with interlocking nails

Complications

Radial nerve injury: This is common in lower one-third fractures and is usually of a high variety. It may also be damaged in the spiral groove. Closed fractures need observation, splinting of wrist and fingers. If a radial nerve deficit occurs after closed manipulation, immediate exploration is necessary (See Fig. 31.11).

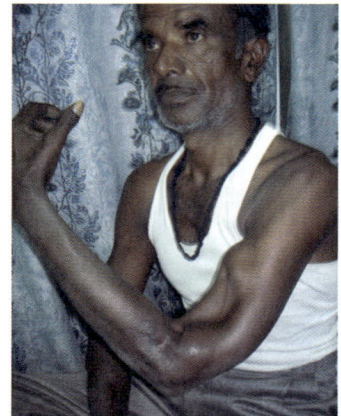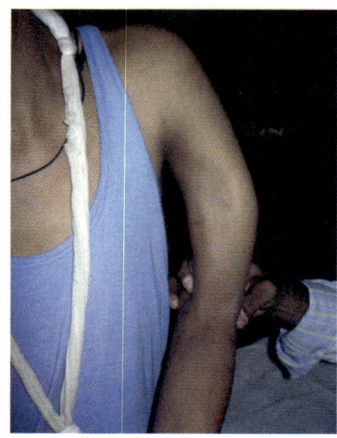

Fig. 16.8: Malunion humerus   **Fig. 16.9:** Nonunion humerus

Vascular injury: Injury to the brachial vessels is unusual. It requires repeated assessment and prompt treatment.

Malunion: In humeral fractures, angular deformity of 20° is acceptable in the middle and distal one-third; while in the proximal one-third, 30° is acceptable. Thick muscles in the upper arm usually conceal the malunion (Fig. 16.8).

Nonunion: This is not very common but may be seen due to over-weight hanging cast. This requires open reduction, rigid plating and bone grafting (Fig. 16.9).

16

Injuries Around the Elbow

BRIEF ANATOMY

Elbow joint is the most important joint in the body for it is associated with many complications mainly stiffness, following injury or trauma to the elbow. It easily becomes stiff and offers stiff resistance to the efforts of treating doctors to make it mobile again.

Elbow joint is a hinge joint formed by the lower end of the humerus and the upper end of ulna (humeroulnar joint) and with the head of radius (humero radial joint). Bony anatomy of the elbow is seen in Fig. 17.1.

Posterior Elbow Geometry

The relation between the three bony points around the elbow namely lateral epicondyle, medial epicondyle and olecranon is important to differentiate between fractures around the elbow and dislocations. In flexion, these three bony points almost form an equilateral triangle. This is maintained in supracondylar fractures and is disturbed in posterior dislocation of the elbow. In extension, these three bony points lie in the same straight line normally. In posterior dislocation of the elbow, the olecranon process of the ulna lies above the line joining the medial and lateral epicondyle (Figs 17.2A and B).

Carrying angle (Normal vs. Abnormal) In full extension of the elbow joint and with the forearm fully supinated, the long axis of the arm and the long axis of the forearm, do not lie in the same straight line. The latter forms a valgus angle of 11° with the former in males and 14° in females. This is slightly more in the females due to wide pelvis and is called the carrying angle. The carrying angle helps the elbow to clear the pelvis when the arm swings while walking. Increase in this angle results in

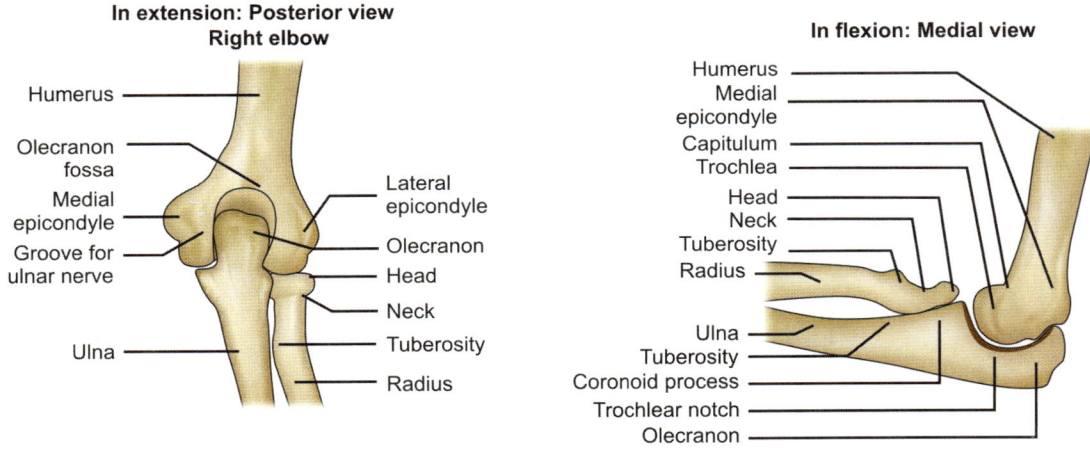

Fig. 17.1: Bony anatomy of the elbow joint

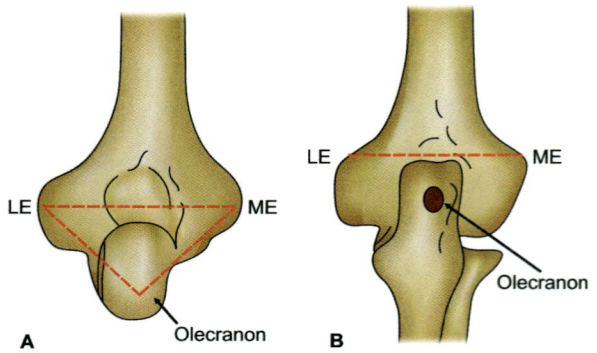

Figs 17.2A and B: Relationship between the three points of the elbow in flexion and extension are: LE–lateral epicondyle, ME–medial epicondyle, and olecranon

cubitus valgus deformity and decrease in the angle forms the cubitus varus deformity (Fig. 17.3). However, the carrying angle disappears with full flexion of the elbow, and it is in this position that the long axis of the forearm and long axis of arm lie parallel to each other.

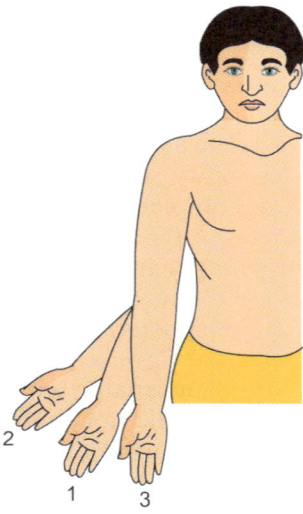

Fig. 17.3: (1) Normal carrying angle, (2) increased carrying angle (cabitus valgus), (3) cubitus varus (decreased carriying angle)

Note: Carrying angle is nature's plan to prevent collusion of your arm with the pelvis while walking.

Ossification Centers of the Elbow

An elbow has multiple ossification centers and can be easily remembered as multiples of 2 and 3 (Fig. 17.4).

Multiples of '2' (CHT)		Multiples of '3' (MOL)	
	YOA		YOA
C Capitulum	2	M Medial epicondyle	3
H Head of radius	4	O Olecranon	9
T Trochlea	8	L Lateral epicondyle	12

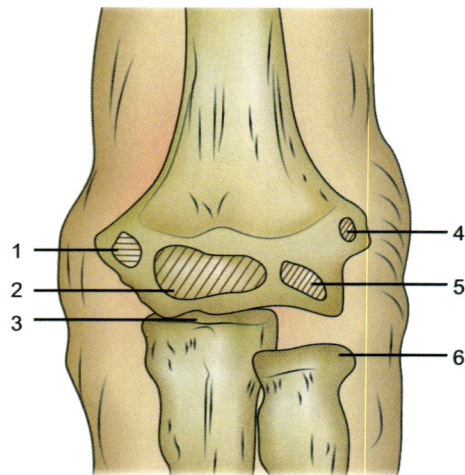

Fig. 17.4: Secondary centers of ossifications: (1) medial epicondyle, (2) capitulum, (3) olecranon, (4) lateral epicondyle, (5) trochlea, (6) head of radius

Note: In children, these ossification centers can be mistaken for a fracture. Hence, its importance. YOA—year of appearance.

Mechanism of Injury

Elbow injuries in children mostly occur due to fall on outstretched hand (indirect trauma). In contrast, elbow injuries, in adults is mostly due to direct trauma following RTA, assault, fall on pointed elbows, etc.

Elbow trauma	
Direct trauma (*Common in adults*)	*Indirect trauma* (*Common in children*)
Olecranon fractures	Lateral condyle fracture (varus force)
Condylar fractures of lower end of humerus Head and neck of radius fracture	Medial Condyle fracture (valgus force)
Side swipe fractures	Supracondylar fractures (hyperextension force) Capitulum fractures, dislocation of elbow (longitudinal force)

Fall on outstretched hands is more common in children because they are more playful and hence more prone to fall. Sixty-five to seventy-five percent of all fractures sustained by children are seen in the upper limbs.

SUPRACONDYLAR FRACTURE

Supracondylar fractures of the humerus are very common in children. The reason lies in the weak bony architecture of the supracondylar area in children. The mechanism of injury and certain predisposing factors exploit this potential weakness in this area and break it more often than any other bone in children (Fig. 17.5).

17

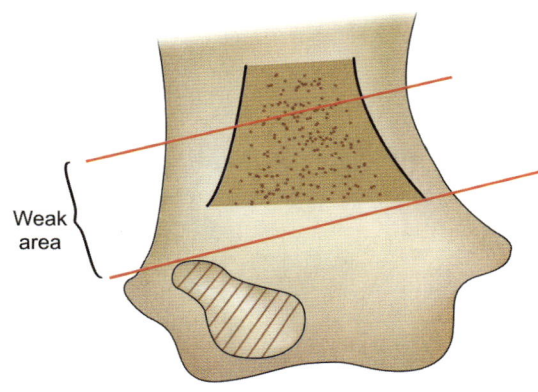

Fig. 17.5: Supracondylar area in children

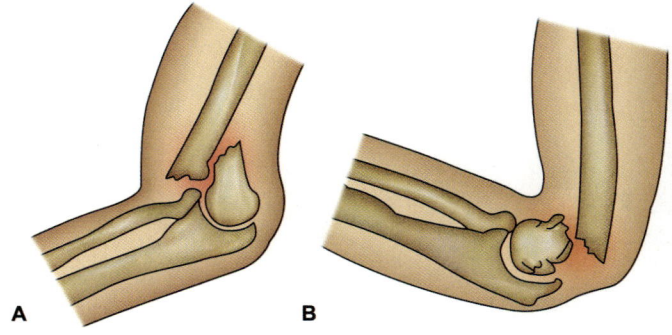

Figs 17.7A and B: Types of supracondylar (SC) fracture: (A) flexion type 2.3%, and (B) extension type 97.7%

Mechanism of Injury

Fall on outstretched hand with hyperextension at the elbow with abduction or adduction, with hand dorsiflexed. It is more common in boys as they tend to be more mischievous and hence more prone to falls (Fig. 17.6).

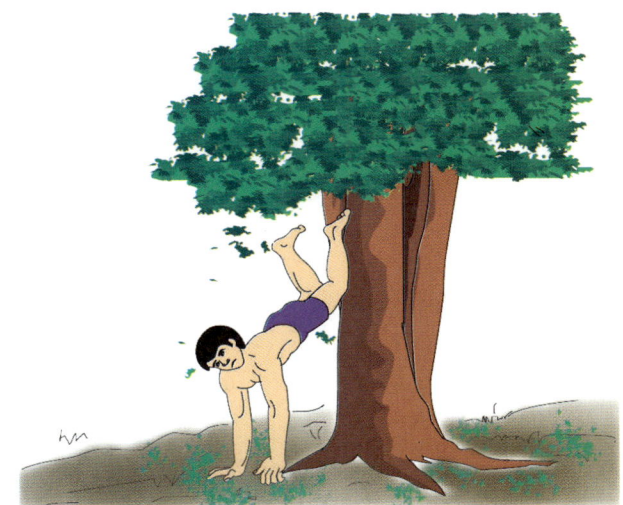

Fig. 17.6: Fall on outstretched hands is a common mechanism of upper limb fractures in children

Side prediction: Left side (58.6%) is more common than the right (42.4%) for the simple reason that it is the non-dominant hand in most individuals.

Classification: Supracondylar fracture is broadly classified into extension type (97.7%) and flexion type (2.3%). In extension type, the fracture line runs upward and backward and in flexion type, it runs downward and forward (Figs 17.7A and B).

Gartland's classification: Extension type of supracondylar fracture is further classified into following subtypes depending on the displacement of distal fragment.

- *Type I:* Undisplaced.
- *Type II:* Displaced, but posterior cortex is intact.
- *Type III:* Displaced, but no intact, posterior cortex and the distal fragment could be displaced either posteromedially or posterolaterally.
- *Type IV:* Completely displaced fracture with no periosteal contact.

Clinical Features

The patient complains of pain and swelling which is gross, *S*-shaped deformity of the upper arm and there is loss of movements of the elbow. Symptoms relating to vascular and nerve injury may be seen *(impending VIC).* Patient may also complain of pseudo paralysis. Tests should be carried out for brachial artery and all the three nerves of the upper limb, namely the radial nerve, the median nerve and the ulnar nerve. The following are the other characteristic clinical signs in supracondylar fracture:

- Arm is short, forearm is normal in length.
- Crepitus is present but should not be elicited for fear of increasing the pain and damaging the neighboring neurovascular structures.
- Dimple sign due to one of the spikes of proximal fragment penetrating the muscle and tethering the skin.
- Relationship between three bony points is maintained.
- "Soft spots" is an effusion beneath anconeus muscle.

Radiology: Subjecting a child to radiological examination of the elbow is a painful process. However, a good X-ray of the elbow in both anteroposterior and lateral views is necessary. It is not just to make an accurate study of the fracture anatomy, but also to study the efficacy of reduction methods (Figs 17.8A and B). An error now embarrasses with an ugly deformity in later childhood.

Radiological illusions: Keep a vigil on the radiological illusions thrown at you by the ossification centers in children.

17

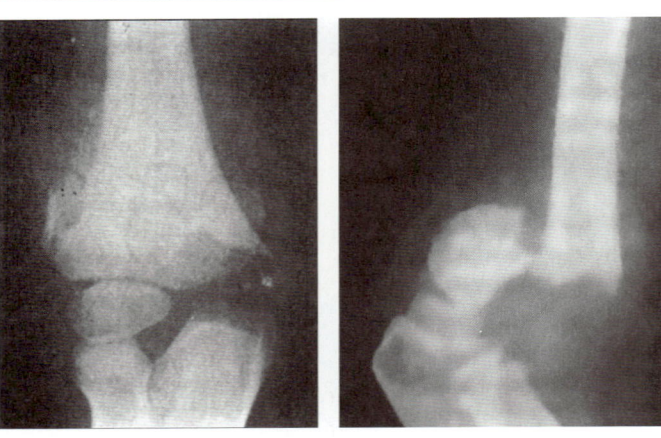

Figs 17.8A and B: Extension type of supracondylar fractures: (A) AP, and (B) lateral views

Management

Conservative management: Initially closed reduction and POP casting or slab application is tried under general anesthesia by traction and countertraction methods. The medial and lateral tilt is corrected first and posterior displacement next (Fig. 17.9). An immediate check can be made whether the reduction has been successful by noting the long axis of the forearm and arm which should be parallel to each other in flexion. Any deviation from the normal indicates residual uncorrected deformities. Two to three attempts under the same anesthesia can be made and the elbow is

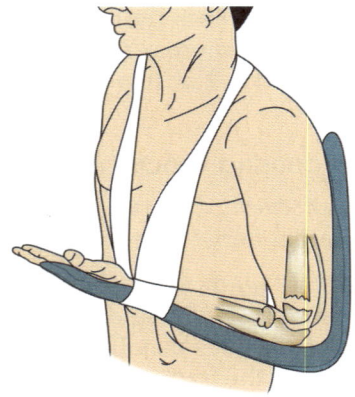

Fig. 17.10: Triceps muscle acts as an internal splint in supracondylar humerus fracture when flexed beyond 90°

immobilized in hyperflexion, as in this position the posterior periosteum tightens up and the triceps acts as an internal splint (Fig. 17.10).

Operative management: This is reserved for some difficult situations. The method usually followed is an open reduction and internal fixation with K-wires. However, more recently closed reduction and percutaneous fixation with K-wires under C-arm control has gained popularity due to simple technique and superior results (Fig. 17.11).

Traction methods: Though it is not a popular method of treating supracondylar fracture of the humerus, it does have a role in specific instances. Traction methods could be either below elbow skin traction (Dunlop's traction) (See Fig. 11.2) or an overhead skeletal traction (Smith traction). Depending upon the traction methods chosen, this form of treatment requires the patient to stay in hospital for longer periods (a definite present-day taboo) and needs constant monitoring by treating doctors.

Complications: They are broadly divided into two categories, viz.

17

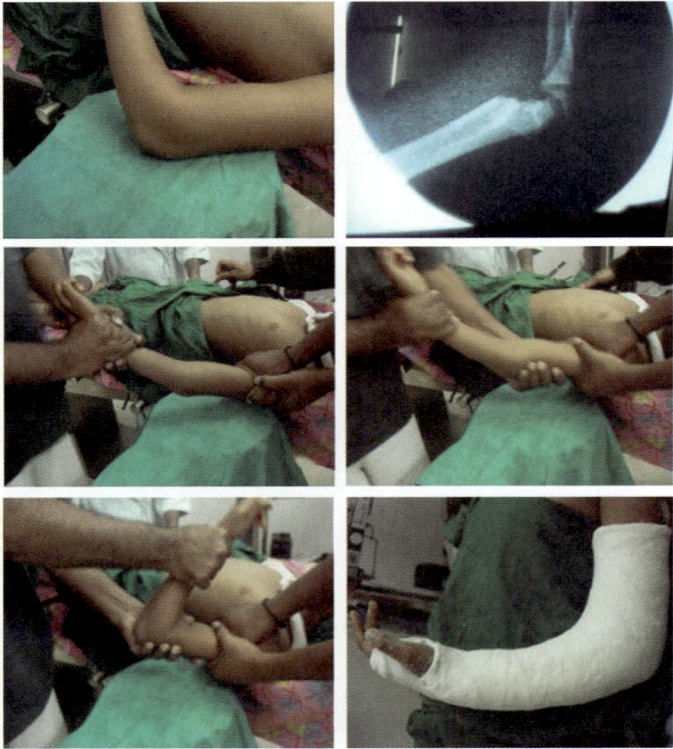

Fig. 17.9: Steps of reduction of supracondylar fracture by traction and countertraction methods

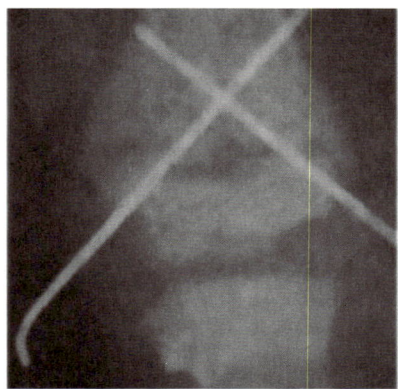

Fig. 17.11: Percutaneous fixation with K-wire of supracondylar humerus fracture

- The category that causes functional impairment of the extremity and is more serious.
- The other category that produces only cosmetic sequelae.

Complications causing Functional Impairment

Neurological involvement: Overall incidence is around 7 percent and radial nerve is more commonly injured.

Vascular injury: It leads to Volkmann's ischemia. The incidence is between 0.5 and 1 percent. Common with extension type and is usually due to direct injury of brachial artery by the fracture (Fig. 17.12). The other causes are internal thrombus, intimal tear, brachial artery spasm, external compression by proximal fracture fragment of the humerus, fracture hematoma, partial or complete rupture of brachial artery. If acute Volkmann's ischemia is not detected and treated properly during initial stages, it may lead to VIC, a dreaded forearm complication, which writes its obituary (See Section on VIC for details).

Loss of mobility: Average loss of flexion is by 4° and is usually due to posterior displacement, which unites in that position causing mechanical block for flexion.

Myositis ossificans: It is rare and is seen in manipulative closed reduction and open reduction.

Complications that Produce Cosmetic Abnormalities

Cubitus varus (Gunstock elbow): This is the most common complication of supracondylar fracture and the incidence varies from 9 to 58 percent (Fig. 17.13).

Treatment

Cubitus varus is only a cosmetic disability with no functional impairment of the elbow (Figs 17.14A and B). Treatment of choice is corrective osteotomy and is deferred until skeletal maturity as cosmetic gains importance at this age. There is fear of recurrence of deformity, if surgery is done before the growth stops, since there is still potential for growth left. A modified

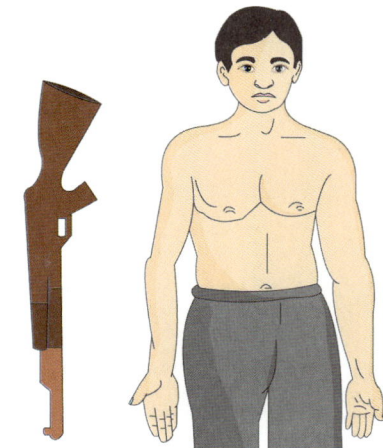

Fig. 17.13: Cubitus varus deformity (also called gunstock deformity)

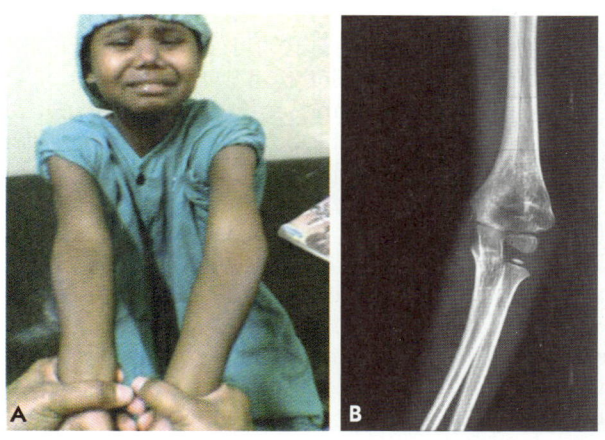

Figs 17.14A and B: Cubitus varus deformity: (A) clinical photo, (B) plan X-ray showing deformity

lateral closed wedge osteotomy (popularly called as French osteotomy) is the surgical method of choice (Figs 17.15A and B).

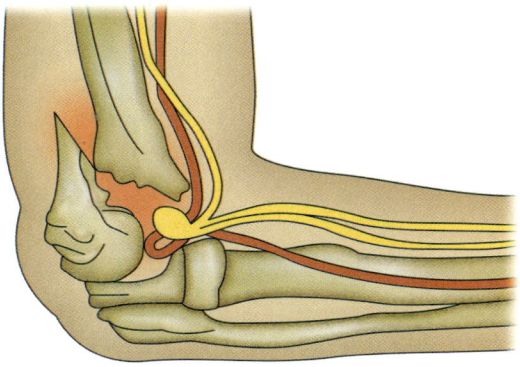

Fig. 17.12: Supracondylar fracture causing injury to neurovascular structures

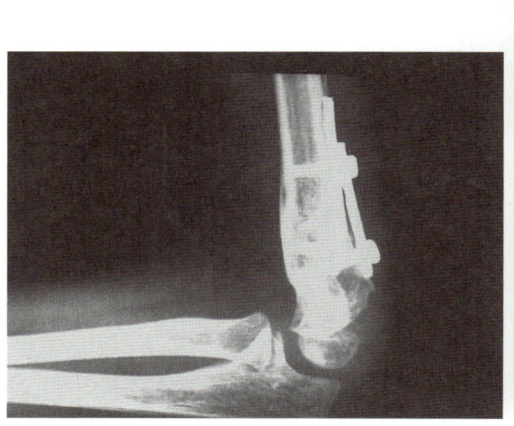
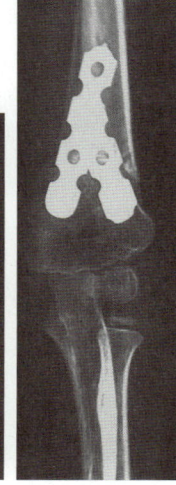

Figs 17.15A and B: French osteotomy

Cubitus valgus: This is rare and may be seen in post lateral displacement in the extension type of supracondylar fracture. Unlike cubitus varus, it is cosmetically acceptable and the treatment is by medial closed wedge osteotomy. Tardy ulnar nerve palsy is a distinct possibility in cubitus valgus deformity.

> **Remember**
> - Supracondylar fracture of humerus:
> - Second most common injury next to forearm fractures in children.
> - Characteristic pathological anatomy.
> - Extension type accounts for 98 percent.
> - Study and restoration of radiological anatomy is very vital.
> - Closed reduction difficult.
> - Open reduction in specific indications.
> - Cubitus varus is the most common complication.

EPICONDYLE FRACTURES

Medial and epicondylar fractures are mainly epiphyseal injuries common children and are due to avulsion of common flexor and extensor muscle origin. They need to be anatomically fixed either by cast or K-wires after reduction.

FRACTURE LATERAL CONDYLE OF HUMERUS

It accounts for 16.8 percent fractures of distal humerus can be associated with dislocation of elbow and fracture olecranon. This is a common fracture in children and is due a severe varus force. This fracture usually involves the lateral epicondyle and capitulum and fracture line may extend to either the capitulo-trochlear groove or apex of the trochlea (Figs 17.16A and B). The distal fragment may be undisplaced, displaced or displaced and rotated due to the pull of the common extensor group of muscles.

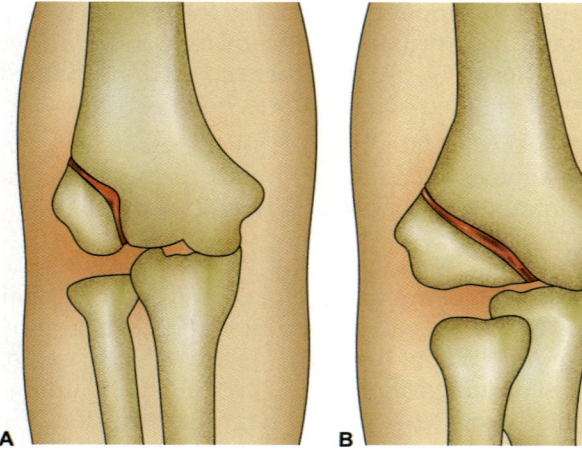

Figs 17.16A and B: Types of lateral condyle fracture of the humerus

Clinical Features

This consists of little distortion of the elbow, less swelling, tenderness and crepitus is present over the lateral condyle.

Radiology: It helps in confirming the diagnosis and study the pattern of fractures (Fig. 17.17).

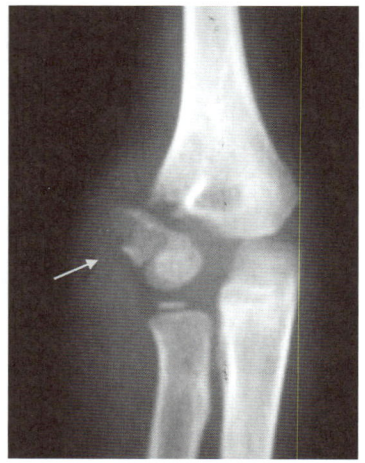

Fig. 17.17: Radiograph showing fracture of the lateral condyle

Treatment

It consists of immobilization with slab in undisplaced fractures, in displaced fractures closed reduction and percutaneous pinning with K-wire, if the fracture is > 24–48 hours old, open reduction and K-wire fixation is advised.

Complications

- Lateral condylar overgrowth.
- Delayed union and nonunion can occur if fracture is undetected or left untreated. The cause for nonunion could be the constant force exerted by the common extensor tendon. In early stages, it is treated by open reduction and internal fixation and in late stages by osteotomy.
- *Cubitus valgus*: This is a common complication.
- *Tardy ulnar nerve palsy*: This is noticed after several years.

FRACTURE MEDIAL CONDYLE OF HUMERUS

This is less common than the lateral condyle fracture. It is commonly due to avulsion of common flexor origin (Fig. 17.18), or due to direct postero-medial trauma. They are common in children frequently intraarticular and need reduction either by closed or open methods and internal fixation with K-wires or screws.

INTERCONDYLAR HUMERUS FRACTURE

This fracture is a disaster for the elbow joint. It normally occurs when one falls on a pointed elbow resulting in

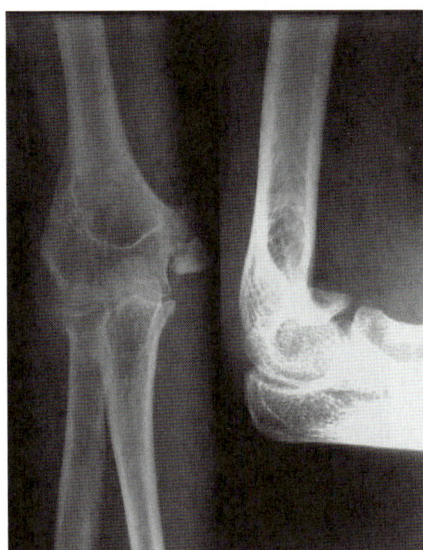

Fig. 17.18: Medial condyle fracture

the olecranon slicing through the condyles of the humerus like a sledge hammer. Mostly these fractures are grossly comminuted and there lies the difficulty.

Fracture pattern: The mechanism of injury in this fracture is such that either you get a T- or Y- shaped comminuted fractures. If the fall is severe, there could be gross communition.

Clinical Features

Diagnosis is easy since the history is classical, there is marked swelling, gross swelling, broadening of the elbow width, tenderness, crepitus and loss of movements of the elbow joint (Fig. 17.19A).

Radiology: It helps to confirm the diagnosis, study the fracture patterns and plan the method of treatment (Fig. 17.19B).

Treatment

Conservative: In the rare event of this fracture being undisplaced, immobilization in the above elbow slab or cast for a period of three weeks usually suffices.

Surgery: In adults, in displaced fractures, open reduction and internal fixation with either plate and screws or sometimes only screws is the treatment method of choice (Fig. 17.19C).

Complications

- *Elbow stiffness:* Inevitably, considering this fracture is usually intraarticular and comminuted.
- *Myositis ossificans:* Vigorous or ill-advised treatment or massage may result in this complication.
- *Malunion:* Due to cancellous nature of the bone, non-union is rare but there could be malunion either in valgus or in varus position.

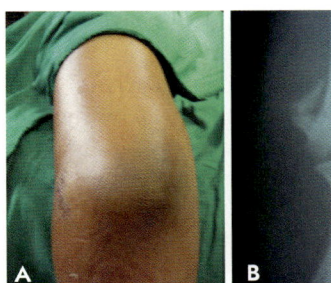
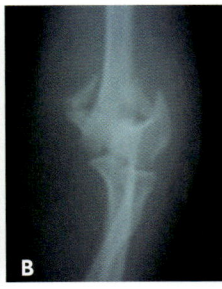
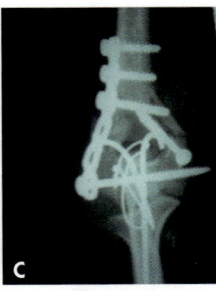

Figs 17.19A to C: Deformity in intercondylar fracture, plain X-ray showing the fracture and reconstruction of the fracture: (A) Clinical photo, (B) Plain X-ray showing fracture, (C) Reconstruction

- *Osteoarthritis of the elbow:* In the later stages, secondary osteoarthritis changes may set in making matters further worse.

DISLOCATION OF THE ELBOW JOINT

Posterior dislocation of the elbow joint is an unfortunate event, which throws the joint mechanism totally out of gear. It is rare in children below 10 years of age.
- *Incidence:* 3 to 6 percent.
- *Males:* 71 percent.
- *Nondominant extremity:* 62 percent.

Fifty percent of all elbow dislocations occur in patients less than 20 years of age.

Mechanism of Injury

This is frequently due to fall on outstretched hands with elbow slightly flexed. A valgus twist is added to the longitudinal force by the projecting trochlea and thus the dislocation is usually posterolateral. Commonly seen in sporting events and in RTA.

Clinical Features

Less pain, moderate swelling but severe restriction of movements of the elbow is the hallmark of this injury. The posterior elbow geometry is disturbed and the forearm is short (Fig. 17.20A). There could be features suggesting injury to the brachial artery and injuries to the nerves of the upper limbs mainly the median nerve. There could be a prominent triceps tendon (*called the Bowstrings sign*) (Fig. 17.20B). There could be associated fractures of the medial epicondyle, head of radius, etc.

Radiology: AP and lateral views of the elbow help to make a diagnosis and identify fracture dislocations that are so commonly associated (Figs 17.21A and B).

Treatment

Conservative treatment by closed reduction under general anesthesia is attempted first and reduction by operative methods is reserved for those rare cases of failed closed reduction (Figs 17.22A to D). The limb is immobilized with elbow in 90 degrees of flexion and midpronation of above elbow with plaster of Paris slab for three weeks.

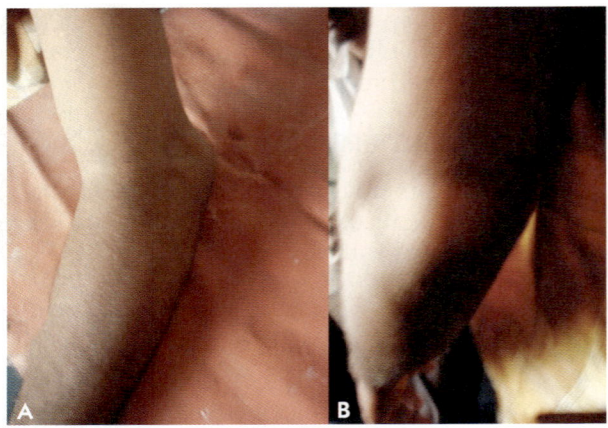

Figs 17.20A and B: Posterior dislocation of elbow

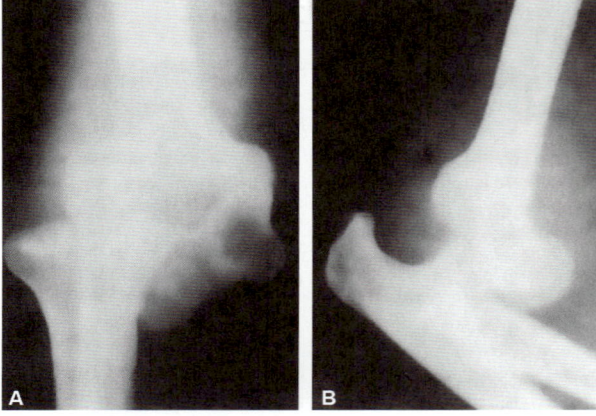

Figs 17.21A and B: Posterior dislocation of elbow joint: (A) AP, and (B) lateral views

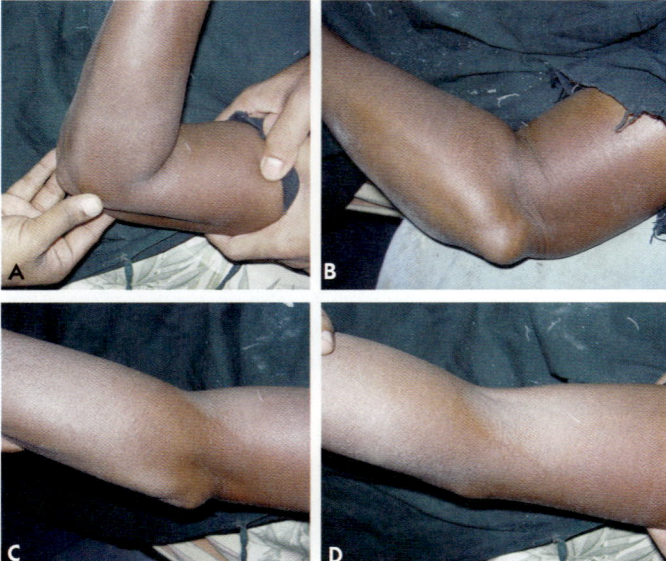

Figs 17.22A to D: (A) Deformity from the side, (B) traction and countertraction, (C) method of reduction traction, (D) reduction successful

Complications

- *Neurological injuries*: The ulnar nerve is very commonly injured, followed by radial and median nerve in that order.
- *Myositis ossificans*: This has an incidence of 5 to 18 percent and is generally not due to the injury *per se* but due to the manner in which it is treated.
- *Causes:* Delay during initial treatment use of hyperextension force during reduction, vigorous active physiotherapy and massage are some of the common causes.
- *Arterial injuries:* These are rare but brachial artery injury may be seen in open fractures.
- *Recurrent dislocation* This is relatively rare but can be seen in males and is usually found to be confined to pediatric age groups.
- *Unreduced dislocations*: Strange but true. There are some shocking instances wherein a dislocated elbow is allowed to remain dislocated for years! However, on the decline, this is a situation peculiar to the underprivileged people in underdeveloped countries. Thanks to illeteracy, ignorance, apathy and poverty.
- *Osteoarthritis of the elbow joint*: This is a troublesome complication which gives rise to a long-term disability.

Differential Diagnosis

Posterior dislocation of the elbow joint is often confused with supracondylar humerus fracture in children

Remember
About posterior dislocation of the elbow: • Slightly older child • Disturbed posterior elbow geometry • Forearm is short • Gross elbow movements restriction • Positive bow string sign • Median nerve injury.

RADIAL HEAD FRACTURE

It is a common injury in adults and rare in children. However, radial neck fractures are common in children.

Mechanism

- Indirect trauma due to fall on an outstretched hand with valgus force.
- Direct trauma to the elbow, usually a blow on the lateral side of elbow.
- Based on the extent and severity of fracture it is classified from I to III (Fig. 17.23) (Masson's types).

Clinical Features

A patient with radial head fracture complains of pain on the lateral side of the elbow, minimal swelling and restriction of elbow movements and supination,

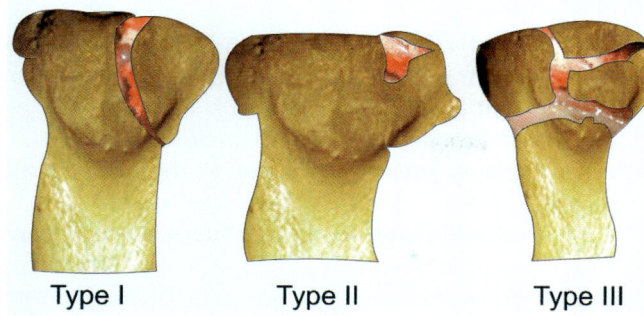

Type I   Type II   Type III

Fig. 17.23: Fracture head of the radius. Type III fracture with posterior dislocation of the elbow is called as Type IV

pronation of the forearm. There is tenderness over the radial head and crepitus can be elicited.

Diagnostic Facts

- Tenderness over the radial head
- Painful forearm rotation.

Radiograph

An anteroposterior and lateral radiographs of the elbow help to study the fracture anatomy and displacements. Additional oblique radiograph delineates the fracture line better (Fig. 17.24).

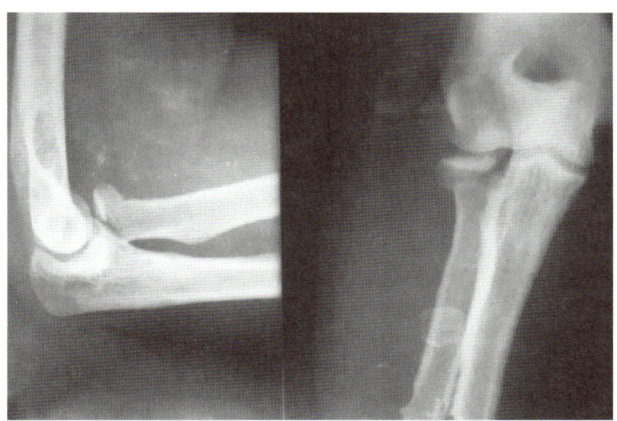

Fig. 17.24: Plain X-ray fracture of the radial head

Treatment

Conservative management: An undisplaced radial head fracture and the involvement of the displaced fragment is less than one-third of the size of the head of radius. These fractures can be treated by an elbow plaster scast or slab for 3–4 weeks, with the elbow in 90 degrees of flexion and the forearm in mid-pronation.

Operative management: If the involvement of the fragment is more than one-third of the size of the head of the radius, such fractures are treated by excision of the head of radius.

Complications: Injury to posterior interosseous nerve, osteoarthritis and elbow stiffness are the common complications of radial head fractures.

RADIAL NECK FRACTURES

Children suffer from this fracture more than adults. The mechanism of injury is usually a fall on the outstretched hands with a valgus force.

Clinical Features

Mild pain, tenderness and mild swelling on the lateral aspect of the elbow and painful supination and pronation of the forearm are the usual features. There is no obvious deformity.

Radiology: X-ray of the elbow plays a greater role in the diagnosis due to minimal clinical findings (Fig. 17.25).

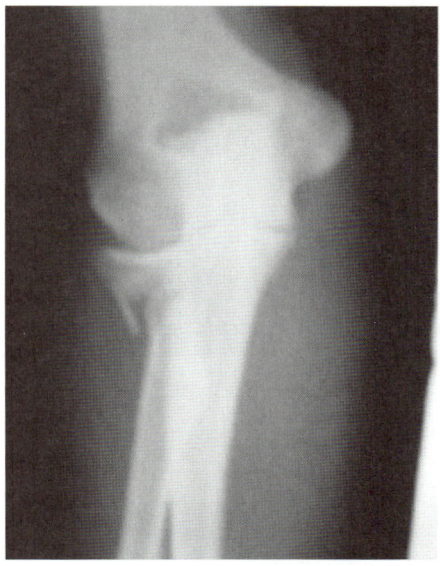

Fig. 17.25: Plain X-ray showing radial neck fracture

Treatment

Treatment of this fracture is relatively simple. In undisplaced fractures, immobilize the above elbow plaster slab or cast for a period of 3–4 weeks. However, displaced fractures need closed reduction under general anesthesia before being immobilized.

FRACTURE OF OLECRANON

It is uncommon in children. Olecranon fracture in adults is comparable to fracture patella
- *Direct:* Trauma due to fall on the point of below. This is the frequent cause (Fig. 17.26).
- *Indirect:* Due to forcible triceps contraction.
- *Classification:* It is classifed as undisplaced (Cotton's) displaced or comminuted fracture (Figs 17.27A to C).

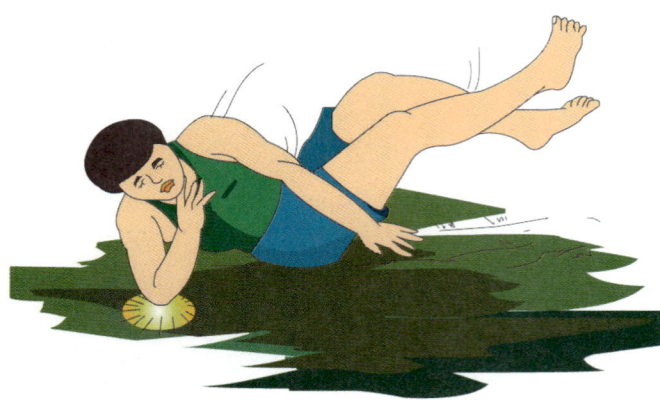

Fig. 17.26: Common mechanism of injury direct trauma due to fall on the point of elbow

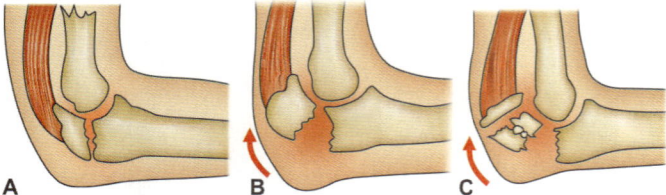

Figs 17.27A to C: Undisplaced fracture: (A) displaced, (B) comminuted, (C) olecranon fracture.

Clinical Features

The patient complains of pain, swelling, deformity and inability to extend the elbow. Clinically, tenderness and crepitus can be elicited.

Radiology: Routine AP and lateral views of the elbow help in confirmation of the diagnosis (Fig. 17.28).

Treatment

In undisplaced fractures: Immobilization of the elbow in the above elbow plaster slab or cast with the elbow in 30–40 degrees flexion (as immobilization usually in 90 degrees position may cause displacement due to the pull of triceps muscle) is the recommended method of treatment.

In displaced fractures: In children, closed reduction under general anesthesia and immobilization in the elbow plaster cast of slab is done and is often successful.

Surgery: In adults, however, there is no place for conservative treatment, because closed reduction needs immobilization of extension for 6 to 8 weeks, which except in children causes permanent stiffness. Hence, surgery is the treatment of choice in adults.

Methods of operative treatment for comminuted fractures: Open reduction and internal fixation with figure of 8-wire loop is recommended (Figs 17.29A and B).

17

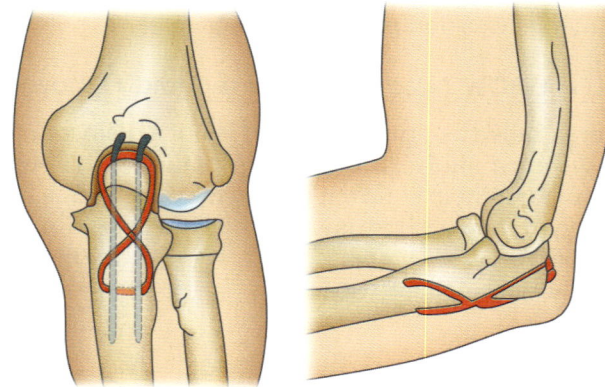

Fig. 17.29A: Figure of '8' tension band wiring in olecranon fracture

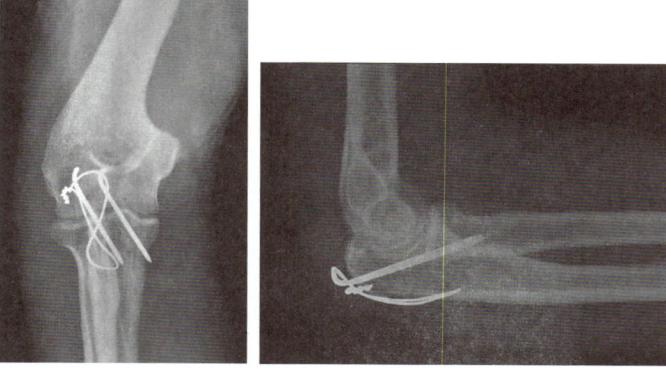

Fig. 17.29B: TBW of olecranon

Comminuted fractures: If undisplaced generally, the above elbow plaster slab is sufficient, but if displaced, tension band wiring or excision of the loose fragments is the operative methods of choice.

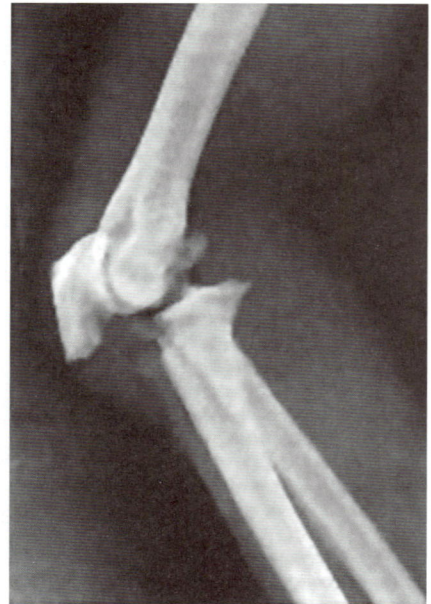

Fig. 17.28: Olecranon fracture

Complications: Nonunion, osteoarthritis of elbow, triceps insufficiency and restricted movements of the elbow are the common complications of olecranon fracture.

CAPITULUM FRACTURE

Of all the fractures occurring around the elbow, capitulum fracture is always intraarticular.

Mechanism of Injury

It is due to fall on an outstretched and the head of the radius slices through the capitula. It is rare and is seen in adults.

Radiology of the elbow: A lateral X-ray of the elbow usually helps to diagnose it. Any fragment seen lying superior to the capitellum is indicative of capitellar fracture (Fig. 17.30).

Management: If the trochlea is involved, the fragment is large, and if the patient is relatively young then open reduction and internal fixation with AO lag screws is recommended. In other cases, small and comminuted fragments, excision is the choice.

PULLED ELBOW (Also called Nurse Maid's Elbow)

Though called as pulled elbow, it is not a dislocation of elbow but a subluxation, or dislocation of superior radioulnar joint in children less than 5 years of age. This happens when a child is suddenly lifted holding the hand (Fig. 17.31). Conservative management is commonly indicated.

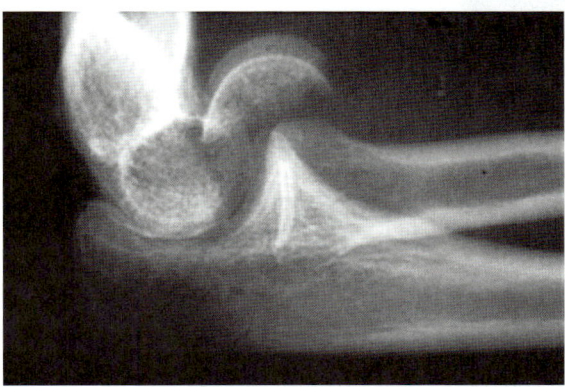

Fig. 17.30: Fracture of the capitellum

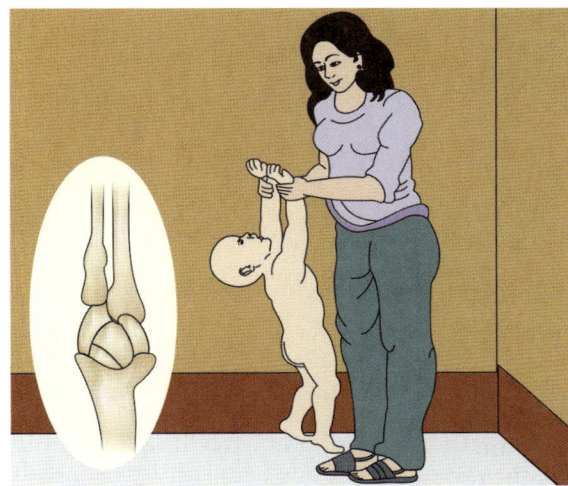

Fig. 17.31: Mechanism of pulled elbow. Inset showing the lesion

18 Injuries of the Forearm

- Brief anatomy
- Fracture both bones of forearm
- Monteggia's fracture
- Galeazzi fracture
- Isolated fracture of ulna
- Essex-Lopresti fracture

Injuries of the forearm presents an interesting combination of injuries like fracture both bones of forearm, Monteggia's fracture, Galeazzi's fracture, Essex-Lopresti fracture, etc.

BRIEF ANATOMY

Pathoanatomy of the Forearm Muscles

The muscle attachments of the forearm make the treatment of these fractures difficult. The supinator of the forearm, biceps muscles, is inserted in the proximal third of the radius and supinates this part of the forearm after the fracture. The middle third of the radius gives attachment to the pronator teres muscle and the distal third to the pronator quadratus.

When the fracture occurs in the middle third, the forearm is held in the position of mid-pronation due to the balancing action of supinators and pronator quadratus muscle. In fractures of the distal third, the forearm is pronated due to the action of pronator quadratus. Hence, the treating physician should be aware of the various muscular forces acting in the forearm to effectively neutralize them and bring about proper union between the fracture fragments. Immobilizing the forearm in *supination* in upper third fractures, *midpronation* in middle third fractures and *pronation* in distal third fracture is found to effectively counter the muscular forces, which resist to displace the fracture fragments (Figs. 18.1 A and B).

Articulation between radius and ulna: Radius and ulna are the twin forearm bones meet at three levels: upper at the superior radioulnar joint, middle connected by the interosseous membrane and lower at the inferior radioulna joint.

Monteggia's fracture along with Galeazzi's fracture forms a rare and interesting combination of injuries where there is fracture of one bone with dislocation of the other. Curiously, both are described in the forearm

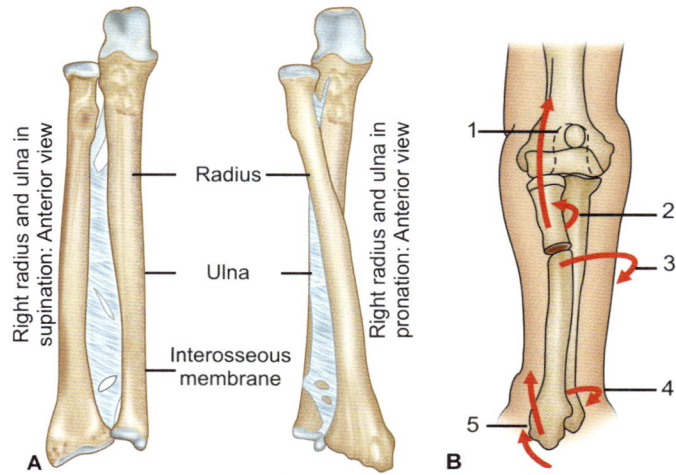

Figs 18.1A and B: (A) Anatomy of radius and ulna (B) Muscle forces in fracture both bones of forearm: (1) biceps, (2) supinator, (3) pronator teres, (4) pronator quadratus and (5) brachoradialis

with the former involving the upper and middle forearm, and the latter involving the distal forearm.

FRACTURE BOTH BONES OF FOREARM

This is a complex problem especially in adults. The complex muscle arrangements already described makes retention of the fracture fragments very difficult. The fracture could be due to either direct or indirect trauma (Figs 18.2A and B).

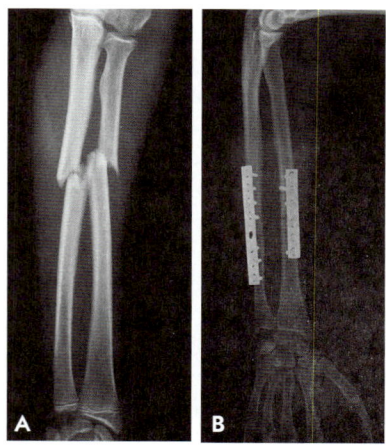

Figs18.2A and B: (A) Fracture both bones forearm, (B) DC Plating both bones forearm

Clinical Features

Patient presents with pain, swelling, deformity and other features of fractures. Tenderness can be elicited and the functions of the forearm, elbow and wrist are usually affected.

Radiology: It plays an important role in the diagnosis of fracture and a routine AP and lateral views including both elbow and wrist joints help in diagnosis (Fig. 18.2A).

Treatment

Conservative treatment: It consists of closed reduction by traction and countertraction methods under general anesthesia followed by an above elbow plaster cast immobilization and is usually successful in children (Fig. 18.3).

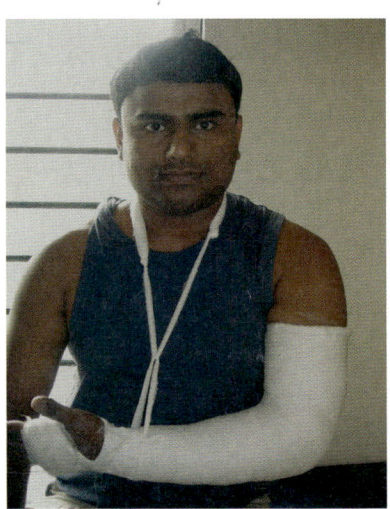

Fig. 18.3: Above elbow plaster cast

Surgery: In adults open reduction and internal fixation is often indicated because it is difficult to regain length, apposition, axial and normal rotational alignment in adults by closed reduction. Open reduction is by two approaches, one for the radius and the other for the ulna. The choice of implants for ulna is either a medullary nail or plate and screws but for fracture radius, rigid compression plating is usually desired (Figs 18.2B). Cancellous bone grafting is done if the comminution is more than one-third of the circumference of the bone.

Complications of Fracture both Bones of Forearm

- *Volkmann's ischemia:* Because of the tight fascial compartment, a patient with fracture both bones forearm is more prone to develop acute compartmental syndrome (See Fig. 8.3).
- *Malunion:* Due to the complex muscular forces, it is difficult to retain the position of the bones in perfect

alignment after closed reduction. It is in this situation that malunion commonly results (Fig. 18.4). It is treated by corrective osteotomy, plating and bone grafting.

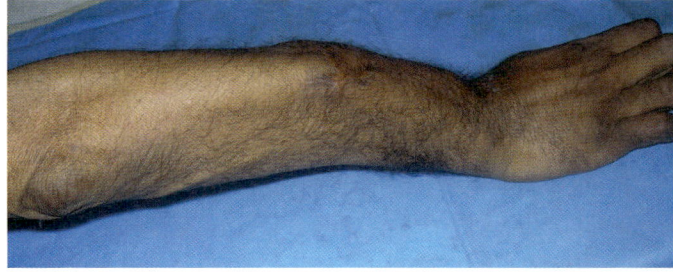

Fig. 18.4: Malunion forearm

- *Delayed union and nonunion:* This can be encountered due to soft tissue interposition, inadequate immobilization, etc. It has to be treated by open reduction, rigid internal fixation and cancellous bone grafting (Fig. 18.5).

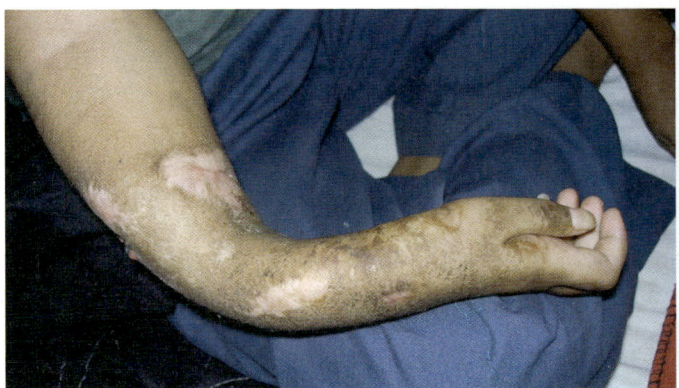

Fig. 18.5: Nonunion forearm bones

- *Cross union:* This is due to malunion of a radial fracture in a medially deviated position, which occupies the interosseous space and blocks pronation and supination. If the cross union takes place in the middle third of the forearm, it can be left alone as the forearm is held in midpronation with less functional damage. In other situations it needs corrective osteotomy and rigid internal fixation.

MONTEGGIA'S FRACTURE

The fracture is in the upper third of ulna with dislocation of the head of the radius. This is usually called a *treacherous lesion* because the dislocation is often missed. Monteggia first described it in 1881.

Classification: Bado's classification is employed in adults and John Wein's classification in children and which takes into consideration the greenstick fractures in them (Table 18.1 and Figs 18.7A to E).

Table 18.1: Bado's classification (adults)

Type I (60%)	Anterior dislocation of head of the radius with fracture ulna at upper third and with anterior angulation.
Type II (5%)	Posterior dislocation head of the radius and fracture proximal ulna with posterior angulation.
Type III (20%)	Lateral dislocation head of the radius and fracture proximal ulna with lateral angulation.
Type IV (15%)	Fracture radius and ulna in their upper one-third and anterior dislocation of head of the radius with anterior angulation.

Note: Hume's fracture occurs in children and is a variant of Monteggia as the fracture of the ulna occurs at a higher level.

Mechanism of Injury

Monteggia's fractures are caused by fall on the outstretched hands with hyperpronation (common) or hyperextension (Fig. 18.6). A direct blow over the forearm can also result in such an injury.

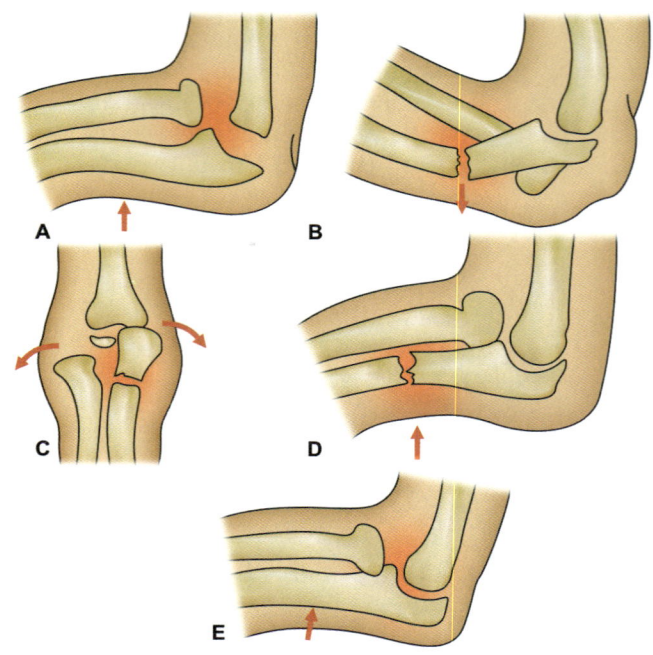

Figs 18.7A to E: Bado's varieties of Monteggia's fracture: (A) anterior, (B) posterior, (C) lateral, (D and E) Monteggia equivalents

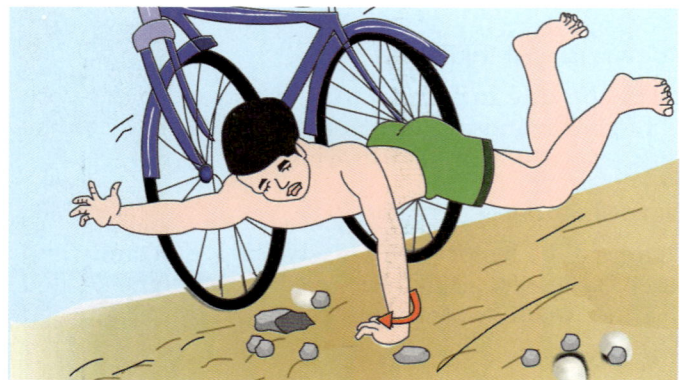

Fig. 18.6: Mechanism of injury in Monteggia's (hyperpronation injuries)

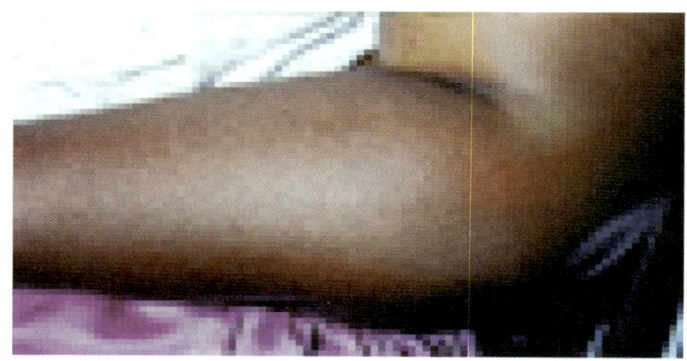

Fig. 18.8: Clinical photograph Monteggia's fracture

Clinical Features

All varieties of Monteggia's fractures may show marked pain and swelling over forearm and elbow (Fig. 18.8). There may be severe loss of forearm function. Depending upon the type of Monteggia's fractures, the head of the radius and the fracture angulations of the ulna may be felt either anteriorly, posteriorly or laterally. Features suggestive of injury to the posterior interosseous nerves may also be present (See page 185).

Radiology: This plays a very important role in the diagnosis of these fractures. A routine anteroposterior and lateral views of the forearm including the elbow joint above are the recommended views. These views help to study the fracture angulations and the direction of dislocation of the head of the radius (Figs 18.9A and B).

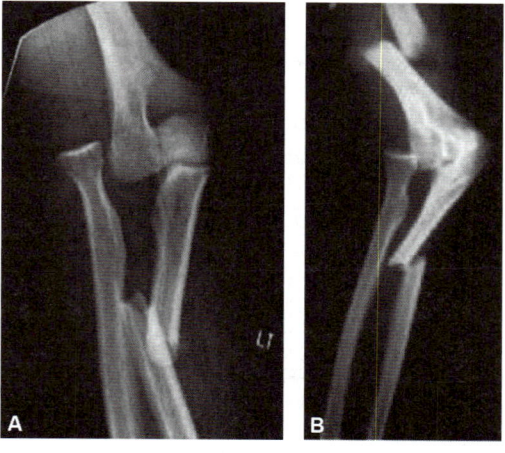

Figs 18.9A and B: Radiograph showing Monteggia's fracture: (A) lateral, (B) anterior

18

18

In order to avoid missing the diagnosis of dislocation of the head of radius, in a few doubtful cases, McLaughlin's line is employed as described below. A straight line drawn along the center of the shaft of the radius cuts the capitula in the center irrespective of the position of the elbow (Fig. 18.10). If this does not

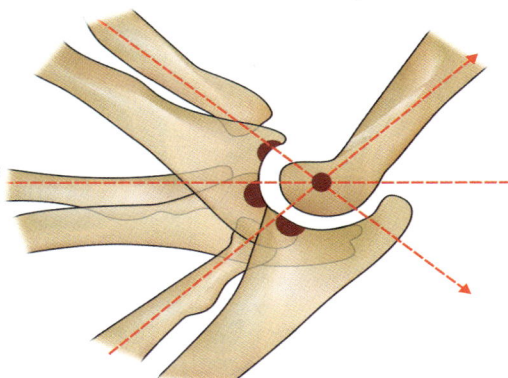

Fig. 18.10: McLaughlin's line

happen, then a strong suspicion of the missing dislocation has to be borne in mind.

Remember

Monteggia's fracture is dangerous because dislocation of the head of radius is often missed:
- *Missed by patient:* When the victim reflexly pulls the elbow after fall and reduces the dislocation unknowingly.
- *Missed by quack:* Due to ignorance
- *Missed by physician:* He fails to order to include the elbow in radiographs of forearm bone fractures.
- *Missed by radiologist:* If he or she fails to utilize the McLaughlin's line.

Treatment

In children, closed reduction under general anesthesia is tried first. If successful, the forearm is immobilized in an above elbow plaster cast or slab for a period of 4–6 weeks. If closed reduction fails, then open reduction of the head of the radius and repair of the annular ligament is carried out. In adults, open reduction and rigid internal fixation for ulnar fracture with plate and screws is the treatment method of choice.

Complications of Monteggia's fractures are listed below:
- Unreduced dislocation head of the radius
- Posterior interosseous nerve palsy
- Malunion of ulna fracture
- Nonunion of ulna fracture
- Myositis ossificans
- Synostosis between radial head and proximal ulna
- Tardy posterior interosseous nerve palsy
- Proximal migration of radius
- Dislocation of inferior radioulnar joint
- Cubitus valgus deformity.

GALEAZZI FRACTURE

This is otherwise called Piedmont fracture after Piedmont Orthopedic Society. This is a fracture of radius at the junction of middle and distal third with associated subluxation or dislocation of the distal radioulnar joint. Subluxation of this joint may be present initially or occur during treatment. French call this fracture reverse Monteggia's, while Campbell calls it as fracture of necessity since it always requires open reduction and internal fixation (ORIF).

The following are the major deforming forces causing loss of reduction and difficulty in reduction (Fig. 18.11).
- Gravity acting through the hand.
- Insertion of pronator quadratus pulls the distal fragment in proximal and volar direction.
- Brachioradialis uses the distal radioulnar joint as a pivot and causes shortening.
- Abductors and extensors of the thumb cause shortening and relaxation of the radio carpal ligament.

Incidence: This is three times as common as Monteggia's fracture. The fracture occurs between bicipital tuberosity and within 5 cm of the distal radial articular surface.

Mechanism of Injury

It may be due to fall on an outstretched hand with marked pronation of the forearm or direct blow on the dorsolateral side of the forearm.

Clinical Features

There will be history of pain, swelling, deformity and other features of a fracture. Tenderness can be elicited and the function of the wrist is usually not affected (Fig. 18.12).

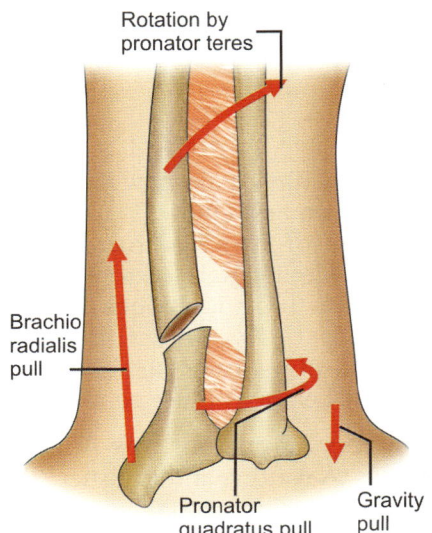
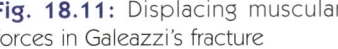

Fig. 18.11: Displacing muscular forces in Galeazzi's fracture

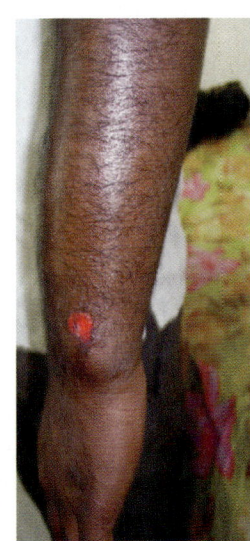

Fig. 18.12: Clinical photograph Galeazzi's fracture

Radiology: It plays an important role in the diagnosis of this fracture and a routine AP and lateral views including distal radio ulnar joint helps (Fig. 18.13A).

Treatment

Closed reduction is usually not successful due to the deforming forces of the muscles, hence, ORIF is the preferred method of treatment. Intramedullary nails and small plates do not provide adequate fixation, hence long plate and screws (DCP or LCDCP) are used, the dislocated distal radioulnar joint may be fixed with K-wire (Fig. 18.13B).

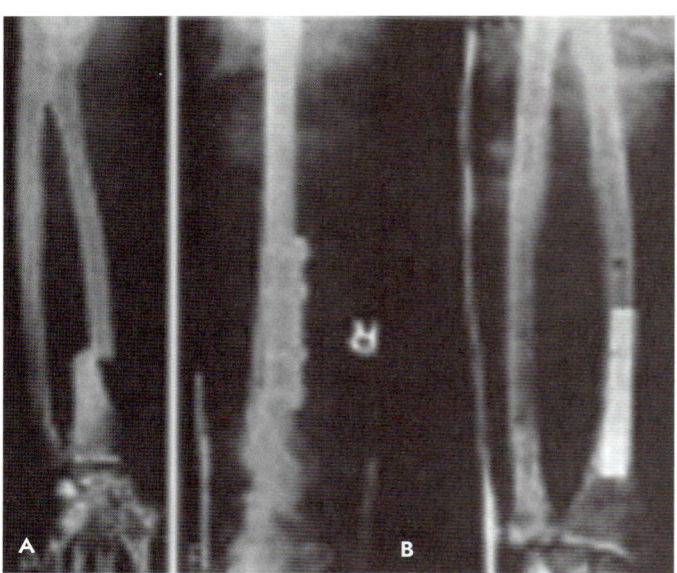

Figs 18.13A and B: (A) Galeazzi's fracture, (B) ORIF with DCP plate and screws (preferred method)

Complications of Galeazzi fracture are nonunion, malunion, loss of rotation movements of forearm, instability of DRUJ, etc.

ISOLATED FRACTURE OF ULNA

In a remarkable show of unity, the twin bones of the forearm, radius and ulna stay together and usually break together. Nevertheless, in some strange instances the shaft of the ulna may break singly due to direct blow and is infamously called *nightstick fracture.* Radiograph of the forearm helps in the diagnosis and the management is by open reduction and rigid internal fixation with plates and screws.

Interesting facts mystery behind nightstick fracture: A burglars night out may end up in a nightmare if he is caught with the booty by a patrolling police officer. When he tries to ward off the raining blows from the cops *lathi,* a direct blow over the medial border of the forearm could result in this fracture. Hence the name (Fig. 18.14).

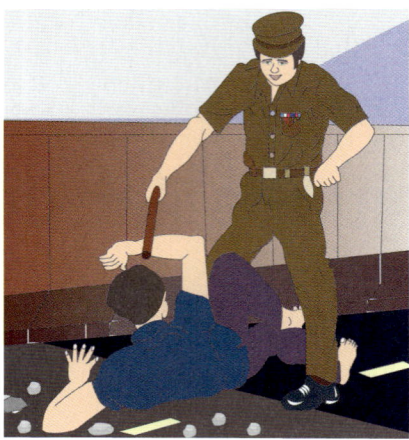

Fig. 18.14: Common mechanism of nightstick fracture

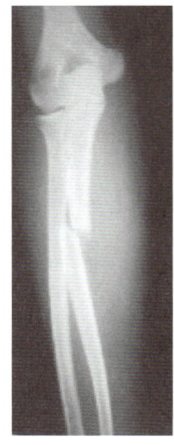

Fig. 18.15: Isolated fracture of ulna fracture

Plain X-ray of the forearm helps in making the diagnosis (Fig. 18.15).

Complications: Nonunion and malunion are notorious complications. Angulations of the fracture and subluxation of the distal radioulnar joint can also occur. Rarely entrapment of extensor carpi ulnaris tendon in distal radioulnar joint is encountered.

ESSEX-LOPRESTI FRACTURE

This is a fracture of the radial head with injury to the distal radioulnar joint. It is a relatively rare fracture and in order to avoid missing it, radiograph of the wrist joint should be taken in all cases of fracture of the head of the radius (Fig. 18.16). If there is disruption of distal radio ulnar joint, excision head of the radius is likely to aggravate the proximal migration of the radius. Hence, if fracture radial head needs excision, it has to be replaced by silastic prosthesis.

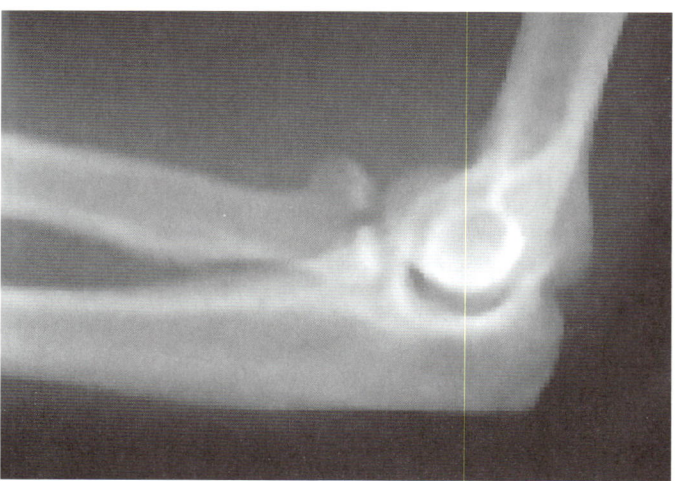

Fig. 18.16: Essex-Lopresti fracture

18

19 | Injuries Around the Wrist

BRIEF ANATOMY

Wrist Joint

Wrist is not a single joint but made up of radiocarpal, midcarpal, and intercarpal joints. The middle finger, the third metacarpal and the capitate are the axial bones of the hand. The midcarpal component of wrist allows flexion and extension as this being a hinge joint. The main flexors are flexor carpi ulnaris and radialis aided by finger flexors. It extends mainly by the action of extensor carpi radialis, longus and brevis supported by extensor digitorum and extensor carpi ulnaris. This movement occurs at radiocarpal joint. It abducts mostly at radiocarpal joint by the action of flexor and extensor carpi ulnaris and entirely at the radiocarpal joint due to the combined action of extensor carpi radialis longus, extensor pollicis brevis, abductor pollicis longus and flexor carpi radialis. The normal range of movement includes flexion 80°, extension 70°, radial deviation 20°, and ulnar deviation 30° and the functional position is 30° dorsiflexion.

RADIAL STYLOID FRACTURE

It is otherwise called as chauffeurs fracture, backfire fracture or Hutchinson's fracture. It is similar to the posterior marginal fracture of the radius.

Mechanism

It usually happens when the starting crank of an engine suddenly reversed by backfire and strikes the wrist with a force. It is common in chauffeurs and is an avulsion fracture of the radiocarpal ligament (Fig. 19.1).

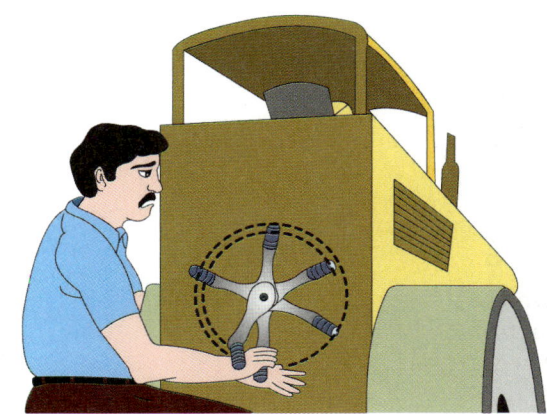

Fig. 19.1: Mechanism of chauffeurs fracture

Clinical Features

Pain, swelling, tenderness, painful restricted movements of the wrist are some of the important clinical features.

Radiology: Radiograph AP views of the wrist shows it as a transverse fracture of the posterior margin of the radius.

Treatment

This fracture is undisplaced and best treated by immobilization in a plaster cast or slab and if displaced it is treated by closed reduction and above elbow plaster cast. However, unstable fractures need percutaneous fixation with K-wire after closed reduction obviously under C-Arm control (Fig. 19.2).

SMITH'S FRACTURE

This is a fracture of distal one-third of radius with palmar displacement. Hence it is called as reverse Colles' fracture. However, it is less common than Colles' and is readily confused with Colles' fracture. It has a clear fracture line dorsally with comminution of the palmar surface.

Mechanism

There are three modes of injury that cause this fracture like fall on the back of the dorsum of the hand, fall on the forearm in supination and a direct blow to the flexed hand.

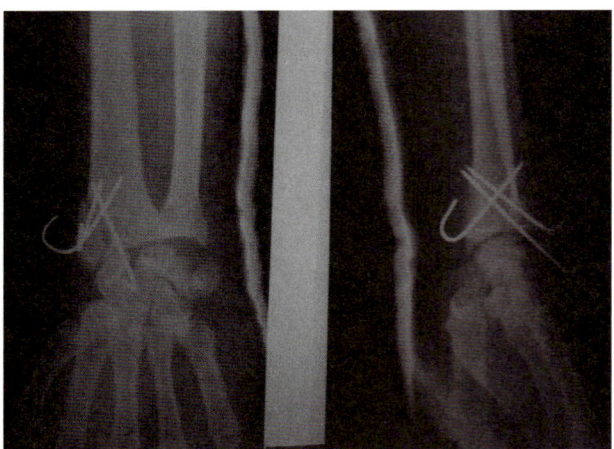

Fig. 19.2: Radial styloid fracture

Clinical Features

Pain, swelling, deformity and all other features of a fresh fracture are present. The deformity in Smith's fracture is called 'garden spade' deformity.

Radiography: Anteroposterior view of the wrist shows the carpus proximally displaced. There will be anterior displacement of the fragment with palmar angulation of distal radial articular surface (Fig. 19.3). The ulnar styloid process is frequently fractured.

Treatment

The treatment of choice is closed reduction and immobilization in a long arm cast with forearm in supination and wrist in flexion. For unstable fractures, fixation with percutaneous K-wire may be required.
Complications: Misinterpretation of radiographs for Colles' and other complication of Colles'.

BARTON'S FRACTURE (RADIOCARPAL INJURIES)

Rim fractures of the distal radius are called Barton's fracture. Dorsal or volar rim could be involved and these fractures are invariably intraarticular.

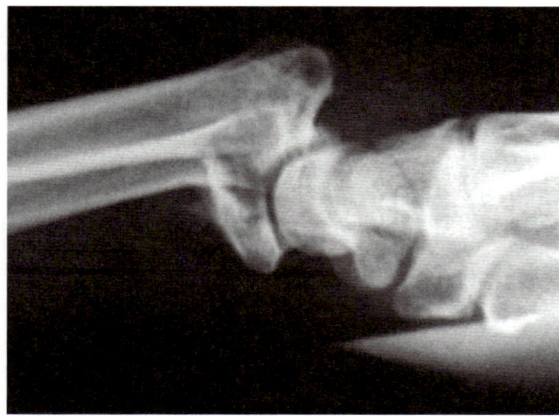

Fig. 19.3: Smith's fracture

DORSAL BARTON

It is a dorsal rim fracture of distal radius and is a variant of Colles' fracture.

Mechanism

Fall with dorsiflexion and pronation of the distal forearm on a flexed wrist.

Clinical Features

Patient complains of pain, swelling, tenderness, deformity and painful restrictions of the wrist joint movements.

Radiology: It is best seen on the lateral view. Dorsal lip of distal radial articular surface is displaced proximally and posteriorly and may be associated with dorsal subluxation of the wrist.

Treatment

Conservative short arm cast with wrist in neutral position.
Surgery: Unstable fracture is fixed by percutaneous pins or with small plate and screws. Healing, prognosis complications remain similar.

VOLAR BARTON

Palmar rim dislocation is otherwise called palmar rim fracture of distal radius.

Mechanism

It is due to palmar tensile stress and dorsal sheer stress and is usually combined with radial styloid fracture.

Clinical Features

The patient complains of pain, swelling, tenderness, deformity and painful restrictions of the wrist joint movements.

Radiology: Palmar rim of distal radial articular surface is displaced dorsally, proximally, posteriorly and may be associated with dorsal subluxation of the wrist (Fig. 19.4).

Treatment

Conservative: Reduction is simple, but retention is difficult. Long arm cast is used.

Surgery: If reduction does not remain satisfactorily stable with wrist in neutral or slight palmar flexion, fixation with K-wire, external fixators and buttress plate, etc. may be required (Fig. 19.5).

COLLES' FRACTURE

This is also called as *Poutteau's* fracture in different parts of the globe. It was first described by Abraham Colles in 1814. It is not just fracture of lower end of radius but

19

19

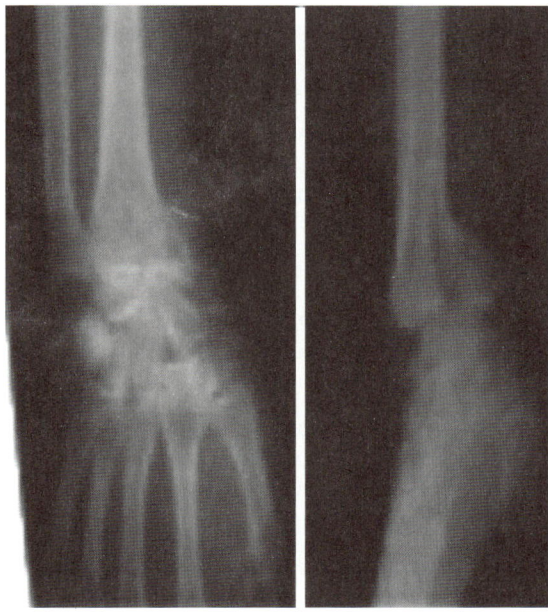

Fig. 19.4: Plain X-ray showing volar barton fracture

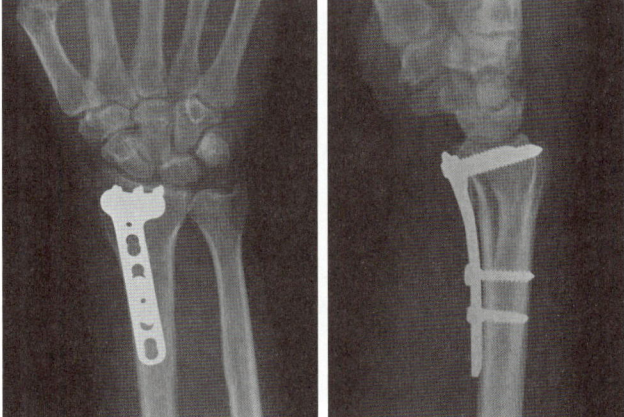

Fig. 19.5: Volar Barton fracture plate fixation

a fracture dislocation of the inferior radioulnar joint. The fracture occurs about 1" (about 2.5 cm) above the carpal extremity of the radius. Following this fracture, some deformity will remain throughout life but pain decreases and movements increase gradually.

Mechanism

The common mode of injury is fall on outstretched hands with dorsiflexion ranging from 40 to 90° (average 60°). The force required to cause this fracture is 192 kg in women and 282 kg in men.

Clinical Features

Usually the patient is an elderly female in her sixties and the history given is a trivial fall on an outstretched hand (Fig. 19.6). The patient complains of pain, swelling, deformity and other usual features of fracture

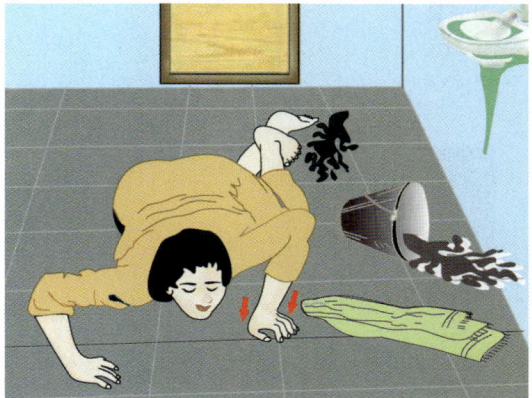

Fig. 19.6: Common mechanism of Colles' fracture is old women

at the lower end of radius. Though *dinner fork* deformity is a classical deformity in Colles' fracture, however, it is not found in all cases but seen only if there is a dorsal tilt or rotation of the distal fragment. However, the styloid process test is more reliable. There are six classical displacements in Colles' fracture; however, the most common is the dorsal displacement (Fig. 19.7).

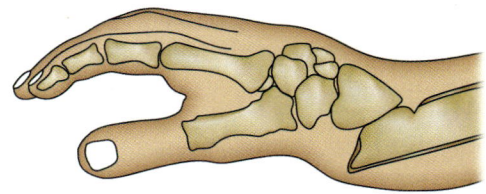

Fig. 19.7: Colles' fracture (A dinner fork deformity)

Styloid process test: The radial styloid process is lower by 1.3 cm when compared to the ulnar styloid process. In Colles' both radial and ulnar styloid processes are at the same level and are found in all displacements of Colles' fracture. Hence, this is a more reliable sign than the dinner fork deformity (Fig. 19.8).

Note: Dinner fork deformity is seen only in dorsal displacement and dorsal tilt in a Colles' fracture (note the d's).

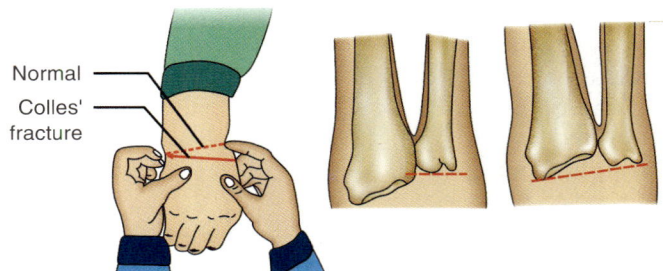

Normal
Colles' fracture

Figs 19.8: Styloid process test

Radiology: Radiograph of the wrist both AP and lateral views of the affected wrist and lower end of the radius helps in evaluating the fracture (Figs 19.9A and B).

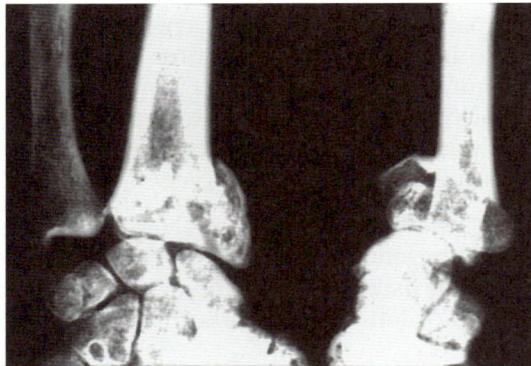

Figs 19.9A and B: Colles' fracture: (A) AP view, and (B) lateral view

Treatment

The aim of treatment is to restore fully functional hand with no residual deformity. The treatment methods include conservative methods, operative methods and external fixators.

Conservative methods: The fracture reduction is carried out by closed methods under general anesthesia (GA) or local anesthesia (LA). The examiner holds the hand of the patient as if to shake hand. With an assistant giving counteraction by holding the forearm or arm of the patient, the examiner gives traction in the line of the forearm. This disimpacts the fracture and the examiner corrects the other displacements of the fracture. At the end of the procedure, styloid process test is carried out to check the accuracy of reduction. If the level of the styloid processes is restored back to normal, it indicates that the reduction has been achieved satisfactorily. Then a below elbow an above elbow cast is put and check radiograph is taken (Figs 19.10A to D). The plaster cast is removed after 6 to 8 weeks and physiotherapy is begun. However the common method of immobilization is the *Colles' cast* (Figs 19.11A and B).

The common causes for failure of reduction are incomplete reduction of the palmar fracture line and dorsal comminution of the lower end of radius.

Closed reduction and percutaneous fixation: However, more recently for comminuted Colles' fracture, closed reduction and percutaneous K-wire fixation under C-arm or X-ray control is fast emerging as the treatment method of choice. The technique is simple and the results seem to be good (Fig. 19.12).

Operative methods: This consists of ORIF with plate and screws (Fig. 19.13). However, operative treatment is rarely required for Colles' fracture except in few special situations.

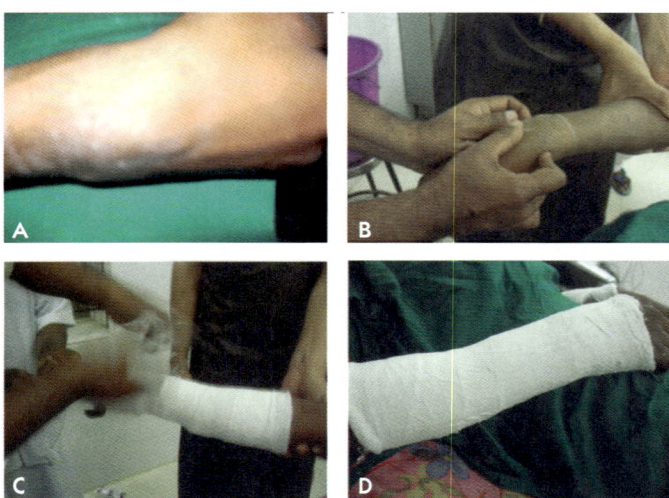

Figs 19.10A to D: The steps of closed reduction and application of a below elbow cast in displaced Colles' fracture. (A) dinner-fork deformity, (B) traction and counter traction, (C) application of cast, (D) final cast Colles's

19

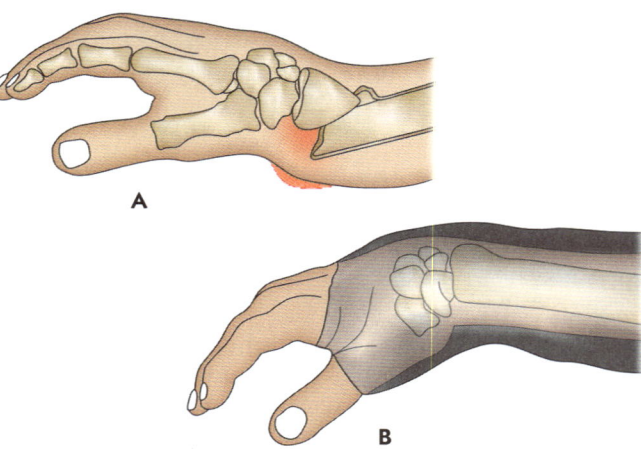

Figs 19.11A and B: Retention of a Colles' fracture by a Colles' cast (a below elbow cast)

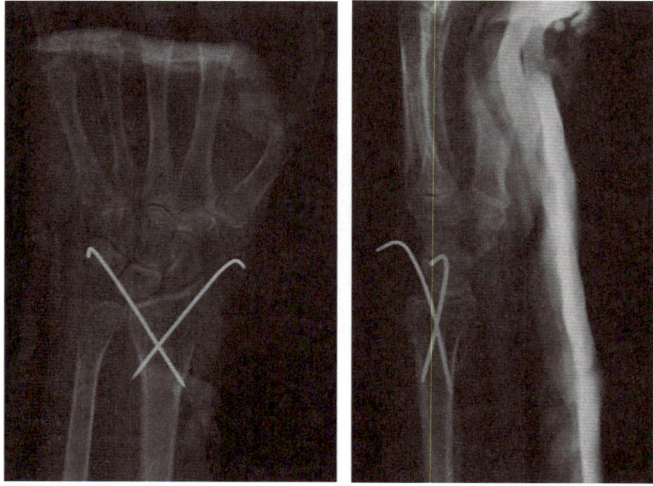

Fig. 19.12: Percutaneous fixation of a Colles' fracture

Indications: Operative treatment may be required in the following situations: extensive comminution, impaction, median nerve entrapment and associated injuries in adults.

External fixators: These are found to be extremely useful in highly comminuted fractures, unstable fractures, compound fractures and bilateral Colles' fracture (Fig. 19.14).

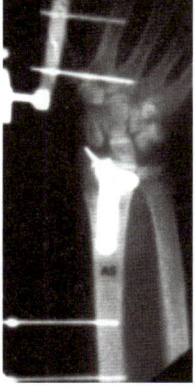

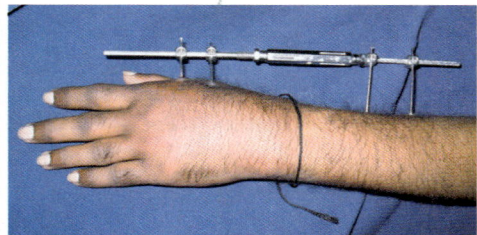

Fig. 19.13: Plate fixation of a Colles' fracture   **Fig. 19.14:** External fixation of a Colles' fracture

Complications

Colles' fractures may be associated with many complications. However, a few significant ones are discussed here.

Malunion: This is the most common complication of Colles' fracture. It may be due to improper reduction, inadequate immobilization or recurrence due to communition, etc. Plain X-ray helps reveal malnunion (Fig. 19.15).

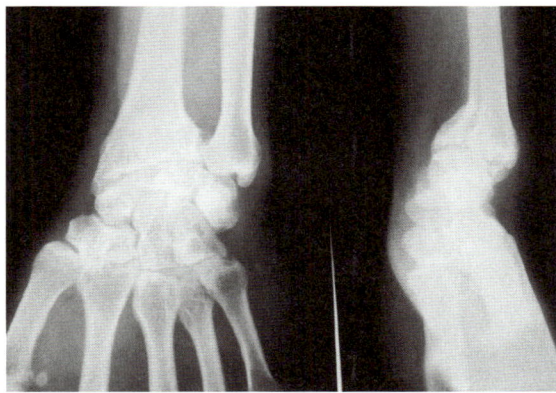

Fig. 19.15: Malunion of Colles' fracture

Treatment

The options of treatment in a malunited Colles' fracture are:

- No treatment is required if the patient has no functional abnormality.
- Darrach's operation is more often indicated if the patient complains of functional disability.
- Corrective osteotomy and grafting is recommended if the patient wants cosmetic correction.
- Arthrodesis (for intraarticular fracture) Patient complains of pain in the wrist joint due to traumatic osteoarthritis following an intraarticular fracture. In these patients arthrodesis of wrist in functional position is the surgery of choice.

Rupture of extensor pollicis tendon: This occurs due to the attrition of the tendon as it glides over the sharp fracture surfaces. This usually occurs after 4 to 6 weeks and may be repaired or left alone with no residual disability.

Sudeck's osteodystrophy: This is due to abnormal sympathetic response which causes vasodilatation and osteoporosis at the fracture site. The patient complains of pain, swelling, painful wrist movements and red stretched shiny skin. Treatment consists of immobilization of the affected part with plaster splints, injection of local anesthetics near the sympathetic ganglion in the axilla or cervical sympathectomy in extreme cases (Fig. 19.16).

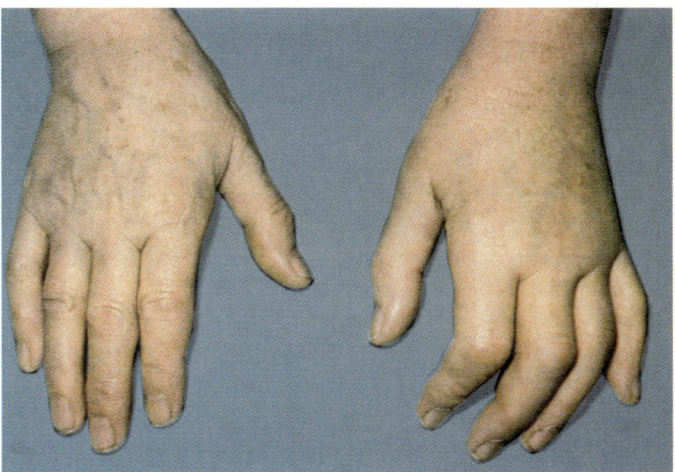

Fig. 19.16: Sudeck's dystrophy

Frozen hand shoulder syndrome: This is a troublesome complication, which develops due to unnecessary voluntary shoulder immobilization by the patient on the affected side for fear of fracture displacements. It is said that the patient has performed a mental amputation and kept the limb still.

Carpal tunnel syndrome: Malunion of Colles' fracture crowds the carpal tunnel and compresses the median nerve.

Nonunion: This is extremely rare in Colles' fracture because of the cancellous nature of the bone which

enables the fracture to unite well. However, soft tissue interposition may cause this problem. The treatment consists of open reduction, rigid internal fixation and bone grafting (Flow chart 19.1).

Note: Darrach's is the most common surgery done for malunited Colles' fracture. It improves the function more than cosmesis but still it is preferred because Colles' fracture usually occurs in elderly women for whom function is important rather than cosmetics. If cosmetics is the priority, corrective osteotomy is done at the radial fracture site and gives good results.

CARPAL INJURIES

Do you remember the famous mnemonic *"she looks too pretty, try to catch her"* learnt in first MBBS? The starting letter of each word denotes the names of the eight carpal bones (scaphoid, lunate, triquetral, pisiform, trapezoid, trapezium, capitate and hamate). Their order of arrangement and placement are at the proximal and distal rows. A brief discussion of scaphoid and lunate is done here as they are the commonly injured wrist bones. Carpal injuries have an overall incidence of 6 percent.

Remember
- Scaphoid fracture–60 percent.
- Dorsal chip radius fracture–10 percent.
- Post-traumatic carpal instability with/without dislocations –10 percent.
- Lunate fracture–3 percent.
- All other carpal bone fracture–7 percent.

SCAPHOID FRACTURE

Scaphoid fractures usually result from fall on outstretched hands. Frequently misdiagnosed, it is known for complications like early avascular necrosis, late carpal instability and arthritis. Hence, prompt and correct treatment is mandatory. Lack of callus in fractures in this region makes judgment about the progress of union difficult.

Remember
- This bone forms the radial part of the carpus.
- It lies obliquely at 45° to longitudinal axes of 2 rows.
- It articulates with five bones (radius, lunate, triquetral, trapezium, capitulum).
- The central indentation is called waist.
- Since it crosses 2 rows of carpus, it is more susceptible to fractures.

Anatomical Peculiarities

- It articulates with distal radius and with four carpal bones. It moves in all the movements of the wrist.

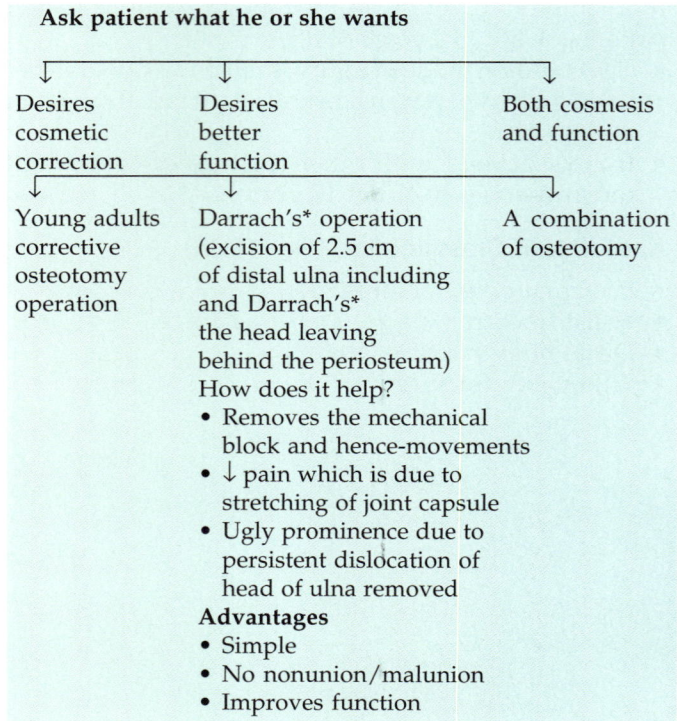

Flow chart 19.1: Approach to a patient with malunited Colles' fracture

Ask patient what he or she wants

Desires cosmetic correction	Desires better function	Both cosmesis and function
Young adults corrective osteotomy operation	Darrach's* operation (excision of 2.5 cm of distal ulna including and Darrach's* the head leaving behind the periosteum) How does it help? • Removes the mechanical block and hence-movements • ↓ pain which is due to stretching of joint capsule • Ugly prominence due to persistent dislocation of head of ulna removed **Advantages** • Simple • No nonunion/malunion • Improves function	A combination of osteotomy

- It has a precarious blood supply.
  - Sixty-seven percent of scaphoid have arterial foramina throughout its length.
  - Thirteen percent have predominant blood supply in the distal one-third.
  - In about 20 percent most of the foramina are in the waist with no foramina in the proximal one-third.
  - This suggests that one-third of the fractures occur in proximal and one-third without adequate blood supply resulting in avascular necrosis. It is present in 35 percent of cases at this level (Fig. 19.17).

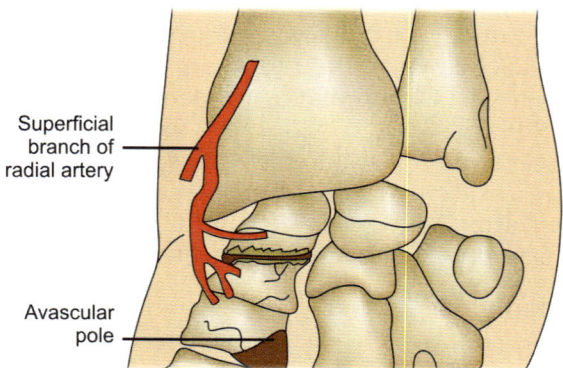

Superficial branch of radial artery

Avascular pole

Fig. 19.17: Fracture of scaphoid and its peculiar blood supply

Etiology and Mechanism

It is common in young adults though it can be seen in patients of 10 to 70 years of age.

- The common mode of injury is fall on an outstretched hand with hyperextension and slight radial deviation at the wrist.
- It is associated with other fracture of carpus and forearm bones in about 17 percent.

Anatomical Classification (Fig. 19.18)

- Proximal pole fracture (20%)
- Waist fracture (70%)
- Distal body fracture (10%)
- Tuberosity fracture

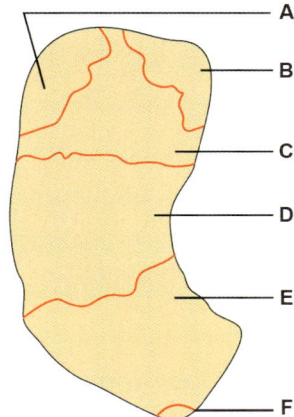

Fig. 19.18: Different levels of scaphoid fracture (Mayo's types): (A) fractures of the tuberosity, (B) distal articular fracture, (C) distal one-third fractures, (D) waist fractures, and (E) fractures of the proximal pole (F) osteochondral fracture

Clinical Features

Patient complains of pain and swelling of the wrist, tenderness in the anatomical snuff box is a characteristic, finding. The movements of the wrist may be painful. The other significant clinical tests are tenderness over the scaphoid compression test.

Radiology

Routine radiograph of the wrist with the PA and lateral views. PA views in the radial and ulnar deviated positions (Stress view) helps to identity this fracture (Fig. 19.19).

However, in few cases, the X-rays may not show a fracture in the initial stages, hence repeat X-rays should be done after 2–3 weeks. MRI and CT scan are better options in undisplaced or incomplete fractures.

Treatment

Undisplaced fracture: The treatment for this fracture is essentially conservative. It consists of a below elbow cast applied to the level of metacarpal heads of the

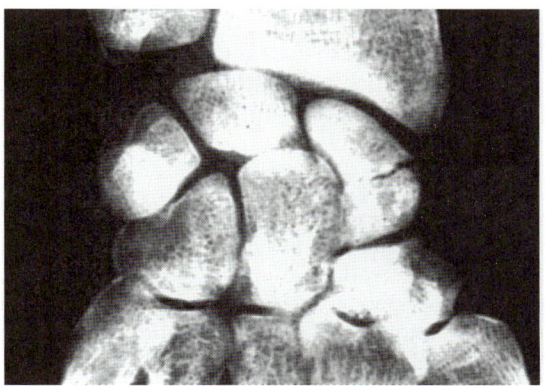

Fig. 19.19: Scaphoid fracture

index, middle, ring, and little fingers. In the thumb, it extends up to the level of PIP joints. The wrist is held in sight dorsiflexion (151) and radial deviation (50). The whole position assumes a *glass-holding* and is popularly called the *Scaphoid cast* (Fig. 19.20).

Displaced fractures: Initially closed reduction under general anesthesia or regional anesthesia and immobilization with scaphoid cast is tried. If it fails, open reduction and internal fixation with Herbert screws is indicated (Fig. 19.21).

Note: Union rate is around 95% after 10 weeks' time in undisplaced fracture while 54% in displaced fracture.

Complications

- Nonunion and delayed union due to delayed diagnosis, displacement and associated carpal injuries and requires open reduction internal fixation and bone grafting.

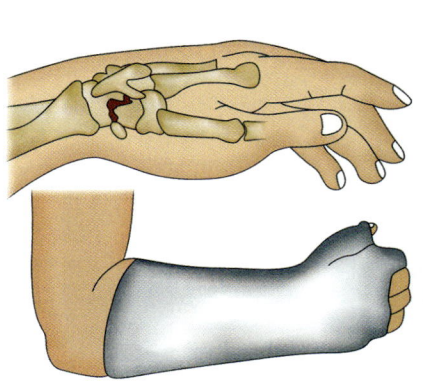

Fig. 19.20: Scaphoid fracture which commonly occurs at the wrist being treated by a "scaphoid cast"

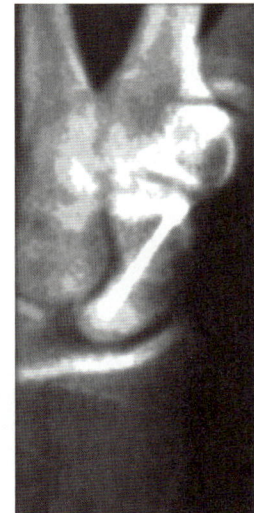

Fig. 19.21: Herbert screw fixation for scaphoid fracture

- Forty percent cases are undiagnosed in the initial stages of fracture.
- Incidence of avascular necrosis is as high as 40 percent.
- Radiocarpal joint secondary OA.

Remember about scaphoid fracture

- Accounts for 70 percent of carpal injuries.
- Frequently missed
- High incidence of AVN.
- Fracture may not be seen on initial radiograph.
- Treat according to symptoms and repeat radiograph after 10 to 14 days.
- If pain still persists, cast it.
- If undisplaced, cast it including the thumb.
- If displaced, cast after manipulation.
- Open reduction is required if gap is more than 2 mm or if still a step remains after reduction. If union is slow or if AVN develops open reduction, internal fixation and bone grafting is done. It is a common carpal dislocation.

LUNATE FRACTURE AND DISLOCATION

Mechanism

This is almost similar to scaphoid fractures.

Clinical Features

Patient complains of pain, swelling, painful restricted wrist movements in the proximal part of the wrist.

Radiology: It is easily diagnosed by the radiograph of the wrist, as in the lateral view lunate normally forms a half moon shape. This is lost in dislocation. In the anteroposterior view the normal rectangular profile is lost (Fig. 19.22).

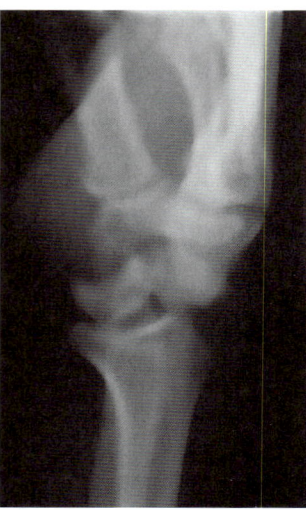

Fig. 19.22: Dislocation of the lunate bone

Problems

This may cause compression of the median nerve (See Fig. 20.21). If left untreated, it may cause permanent palsy, hence reduction should be carried out under emergency.

Treatment

- If seen early, reduction is easy and immobilization for 3 weeks with wrist in slight flexion usually gives good result.
- If seen after 3 weeks, open reduction is done.
- If lunate cannot be reduced by open reduction, resection of the proximal carpal bones or arthrodesis of the wrist may be necessary.

19

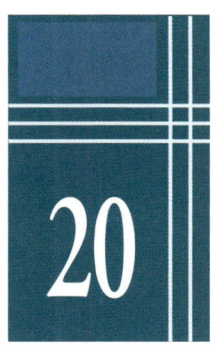

20 Injuries of the Hand

Hand is the most dexterous part of the human body. Anatomically though made up of small bones functionally it performs a wide array of unbelievable functions. Few important injuries of the hand are discussed here.

BENNETT'S FRACTURE

Bennett's fracture is a fracture dislocation of the base of the first metacarpal bone of the thumb with either subluxation or dislocation of the first carpometacarpal joint. It was described by Edward Bennett in 1882. It is an intraarticular fracture.

Mechanism of Injury

The common mechanism of injury is an axial blow directed against the partially flexed metacarpal, in most cases during "fist fights."

Clinical Features

Patient complains of pain and swelling at the base of the thumb. Tenderness could be elicited. Movements of the thumb are painful and restricted.

Peculiarity of this fracture: Base of the thumb metacarpal is pulled dorsally and medially by the abductor pollicis longus, while the distal attachment of adductor further levers the base into abduction. Hence, though reduction can be obtained, retention is difficult (Fig. 20.1).

Radiology: Plain X-ray of the hand helps to identify the fracture (Fig. 20.2).

Treatment

Like all other intraarticular fractures, it needs accurate reduction and retention to prevent future post-

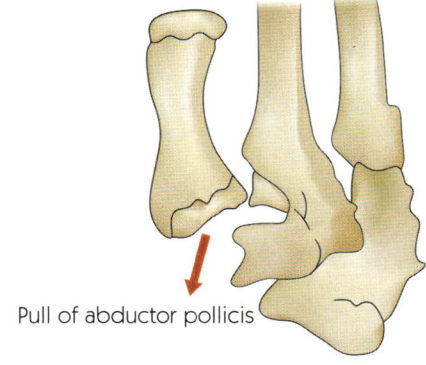

Pull of abductor pollicis

Fig. 20.1: Bennett's fracture (Displacing force)

traumatic osteoarthritis. A single attempt at closed reduction is tried first and a percutaneous fixation under C-arm or X-ray control with K-wire is usually performed (Fig. 20.3). If it fails, ORIF with K-wire or a small screw is carried out.

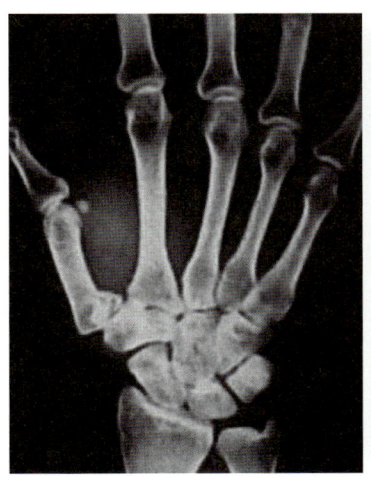

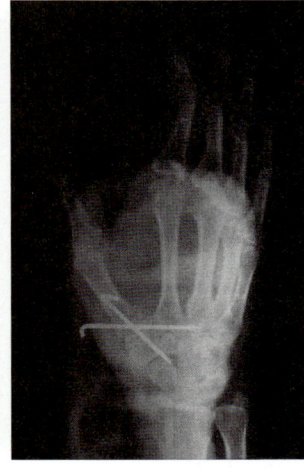

Fig. 20.2: Bennett's fracture

Fig. 20.3: Bennett's fracture fixed with K-wire

ROLANDO FRACTURE

This was first described by Rolando in the year 1910. Though this is also a fracture of the base of the first metacarpal, but unlike Bennett's fracture, it is extra-articular in nature (Fig. 20.4). Absence of the notorious

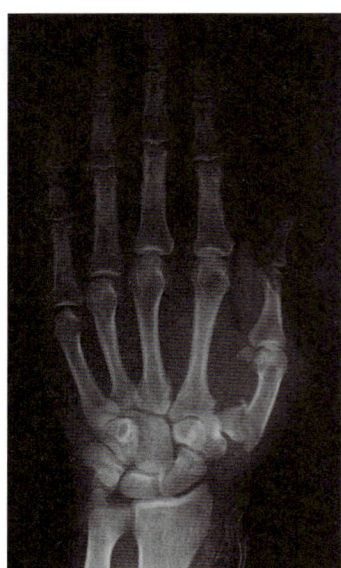

Fig. 20.4: Rolando fracture

distracting muscle forces as in Bennett has, makes this fracture simpler to treat. Closed reduction and retention with a thumb spica for 2–3 weeks is the recommended method of treatment. If it fails, open reduction and fixation with K-wires or miniplates is indicated.

> **Remember**
>
> Rolando fracture in comparison with the Bennett's fracture:
> • Extraarticular
> • No displacing muscle forces
> • Since extraarticular perfect reduction is not a must
> • Conservative treatment suffices.

Complications: Both Bennett's and Rolando fractures could lead to secondary OA of the carpometacarpal joint stiffness of the CMC joint of the thumb and rarely damage of sensory branch of the radial nerve during surgical intervention.

KAPLAN'S LESION

Dorsal Metacarpophalangeal (MP) Joint Dislocation

Kaplan described a hyperextension injury due to buttonholing of the metacarpal head through the volar capsule into the palm. Here there is an interposition of volar plate between the base of the proximal phalanx and the head of the metacarpal.

Incidence

This is commonly seen in the index finger, thumb and little finger in that order of frequency. It is rarely seen in the middle and ring fingers.

Clinical Features

Patient complains of pain, swelling, deformity and loss of moments of the affected finger. A puckered scar could be seen at the Volar surface of the hand (Fig. 20.5).

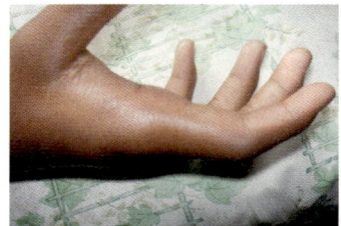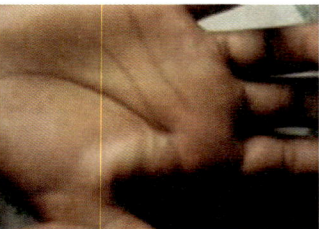

Fig. 20.5: A clinical photograph of dislocation of II MP joint (Kaplan's lesion)

Plain X-ray of the Hand

Presence of the sesamoid bone within the MCP joint virtually clinches the diagnosis (Fig. 20.6).

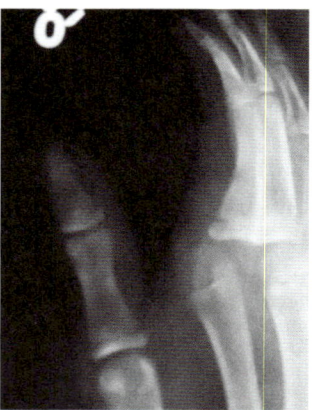

Fig. 20.6: Kaplan's lesion

Treatment

A single attempt at closed reduction is made and if this fails surgical reduction either by the volar (Kaplan's operation) approach or by the dorsal approach and fixation with cast or K-wire is done.

MALLET FINGER (Syn: baseball finger, drop finger)

Mallet finger is a common finger injury and is due to avulsion or avulsion fracture of the extensor tendon from its insertion at the base of the distal phalanx.

Mechanism

This injury occurs when the finger is forcibly flexed, while the extensor tendon is taut, e.g. while tucking the bed, catching a ball, striking an object with extended finger (Figs 20.7A and B).

20

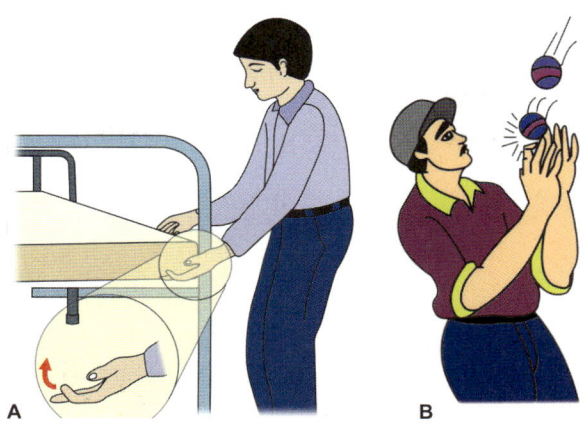

Figs 20.7A and B: Common mechanism of mallet injury: (A) tucking the bed, (B) catching a ball

Clinical Features

Pain, swelling, tenderness, flexion deformity of the tip of the finger and inability of the patient to actively extend the finger at the distal PIP joint (Fig. 20.8).

Plain X-ray of the finger AP and lateral views may show an avulsion fracture (Fig. 20.9).

Treatment

Distal inter-phalangeal joint is immobilized in hyperextension by using:
- Simple volar unpadded aluminum splint, which provides three-point pressure (Figs 20.10A and B).
- Dorsal padded aluminum splint.
- A stack plastic mallet finger splint.

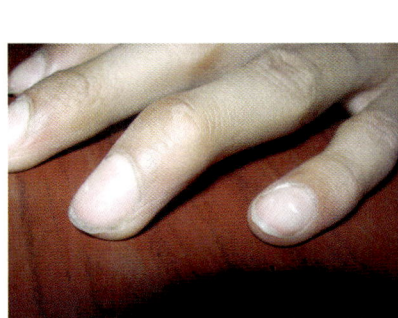

Fig. 20.8: Clinical photograph of mallet finger

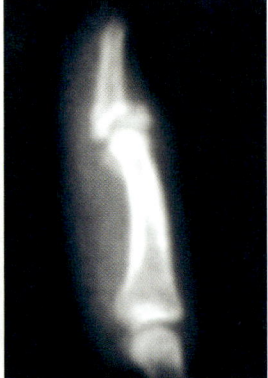

Fig. 20.9: Avulsion fracture in mallet injury

JERSEY FINGER

It is due to avulsion of flexor digitorum profundus from its insertion on distal phalanx. This is the opposite of 'Mallet finger' and the patient is unable to flex the distal interphalangeal joint. It is seen in football and rugby players (Fig. 20.11).

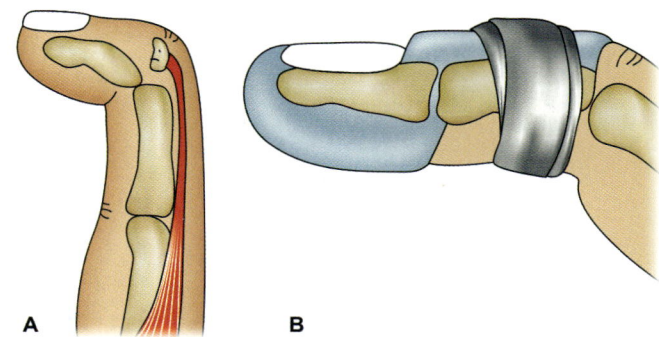

Figs 20.10A and B: (A) Mallet finger, and (B) treatment by a Dorsal splint

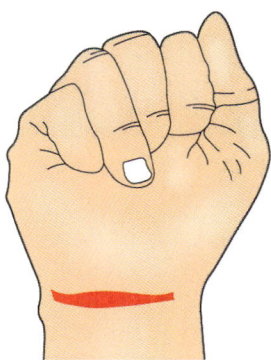

Fig. 20.11: Jersey finger

METACARPAL BONE FRACTURES

The common causes for these injuries are direct hit on the dorsum of the hand as in assault, boxing, fall, road traffic accident (RTA), etc. Plain X-ray of the hand helps to diagnose the fractures (Figs 20.12A and B). These fractures should be accurately reduced with no rotational malalignment and immobilized with either plaster (common) or percutaneous or open K-wire or plate fixation (less common) (Fig. 20.14A).

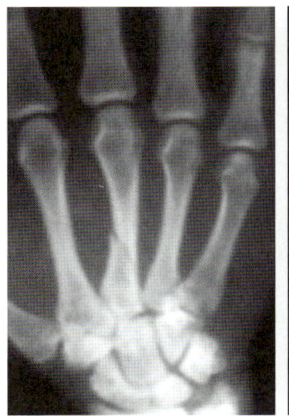
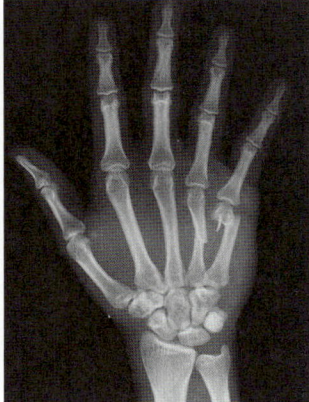

Figs 20.12A and B: (A) Metacarpal fracture, (B) Multiple metacarpal fractures

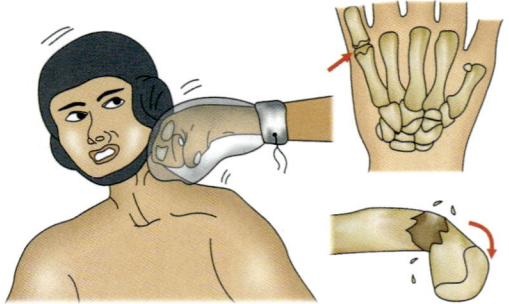

Fig. 20.13: Common mechanism of fracture neck of 5th metacarpal bone (Boxer's fracture)

METACARPAL NECK FRACTURE

Fracture of the fifth metacarpal neck is known as boxer's fracture. It occurs when a closed fist hits against a hard object, in this case, the jaw of the opponent! (Fig. 20.13). Treatment is by closed reduction and percutaneous fixation with K-wires (Fig. 20.14A to C) or external fixator (Fig 20.14D).

METACARPAL HEAD FRACTURE

These are also known as 'fist bite' fractures as they occur when the patient srikes an opponent's teeth in a fist fight. They are frequently intraarticular and need open reduction and internal fixation with K-wire.

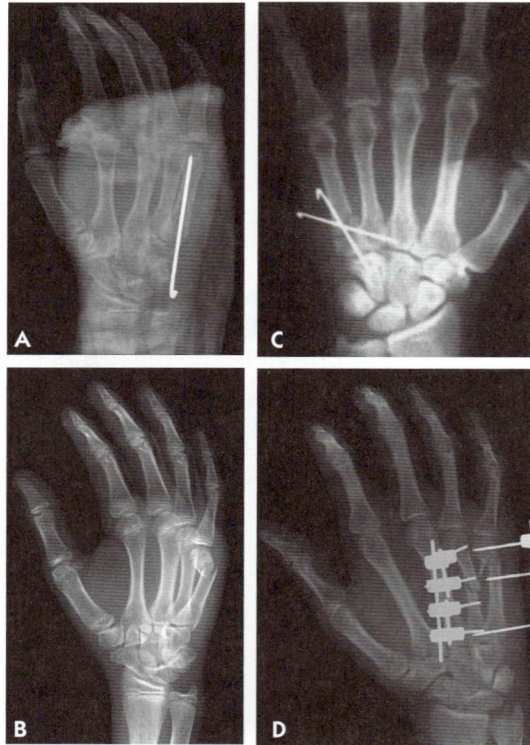

Figs 20.14A to D: (A to C) 5th Metacarpal fracture fixed with K-wire, (D) fracture fixed with an external fixator

PHALANGES FRACTURE

Fracture of distal phalanx: These fractures are usually caused by crushing injuries, they are frequently comminuted and require only splinting. K-wire fixation may be required for unstable or open injuries.

Fracture of middle or proximal phalanx: These are due to direct blow on the dorsum of fingers. The fracture is angulated towards the palm. Plain X-ray helps study of the type of fracture (Figs 20.15A and B). Rotational malalignment should be strictly avoided. Undisplaced fractures are best managed by conservative methods by buddy taping (here, the unaffected finger is used as the supporting external splint) (See Fig. 5.1B) while highly unstable oblique fracture require open reduction and K-wire fixation (Fig. 20.16A). Severely comminuted fractures are aligned best by external fixators (Fig. 20.16B).

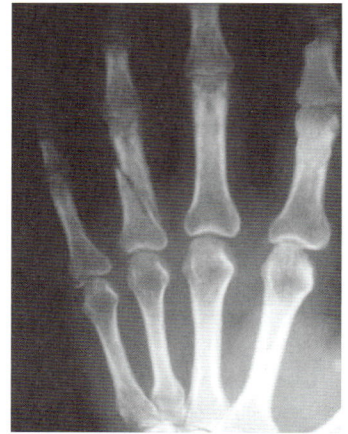 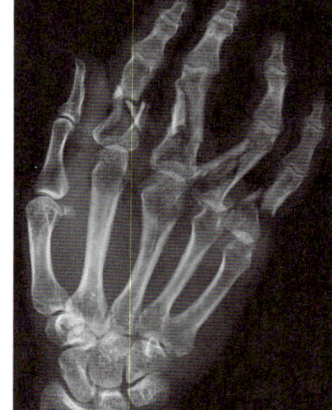

Fig. 20.15A: Oblique phalangeal fracture   **Fig. 20.15B:** Multiple phalangeal fracture

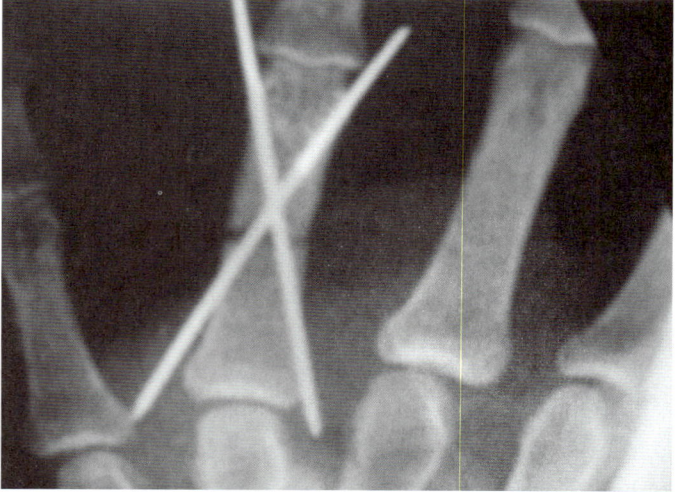

Fig. 20.16A: Phalanx fracture K-wire fixation

20

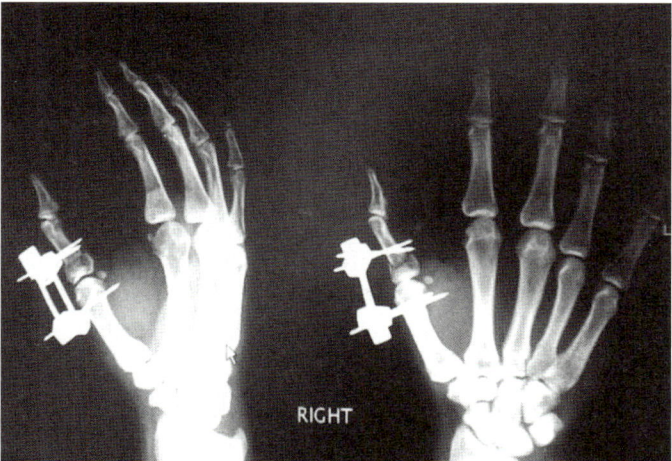

Fig. 20.16B: Phalanx fracture fixed with external fixation

Complications

The important complications of finger bone fractures are nonunion, malunion, tendon adhesions, joint stiffness, infection, etc.

TENDON INJURIES

Either flexor or extensor tendons of the hand can be injured when the patient sustains hand injuries by a sharp cutting object. Flexor tendons are more commonly injured than the extensors (Fig. 20.17). The clinician who treats it, if he or she does not explore the hand or the wrist wounds and look for the possibility of tendons being severed more often misses these tendons injuries. Old healed scars over the hand or wrist with loss of function of the injured tendon confirms the diagnosis.

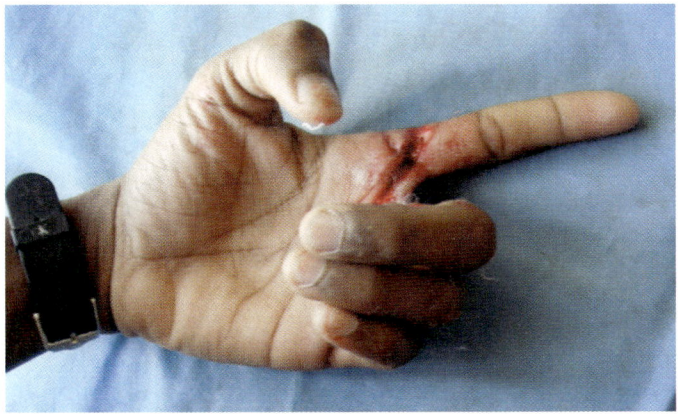

Fig. 20.17: If the flexor tendon is injured, the finger does not flex but remains straight

FLEXOR TENDON INJURIES

Flexors tendon injuries of the wrist, fingers and thumb are discussed here.

Wrist flexors: The main wrist flexors are the flexor carpi radialis and flexor carpi ulnaris. They together bring about palmar flexion of the wrist in the midline. If the flexor carpi radialis is cut, wrist deviates medially towards the intact flexor carpi ulnaris and laterally towards intact flexor carpi radialis if flexor carpi ulnaris is cut.

Finger flexors: Flexion of the proximal inter-phalangeal joint of the fingers is brought about mainly by FDS and since FDP crosses this joint, it also aids FDS but FDP is solely responsible for the flexion of distal inter-phalangeal joint. Both flexor digitorum superficialis (FDS) and flexor digitorum profundus (FDP) could be injured single or together and the injured finger does not flex but remains straight (Fig. 20.18).

FDP: Instruct the patient to actively flex the DIP joint while you stabilize the PIP joint. If he or she can flex it, there is no injury to FDP tendon (Fig. 20.18).

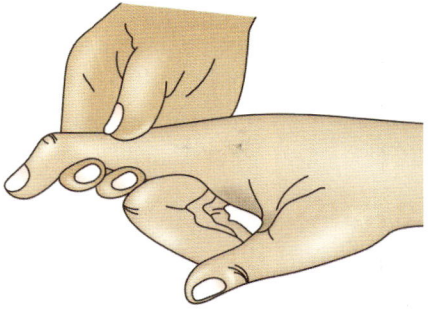

Fig. 20.18: Clinical method of testing FDP

FDS: Hold the two adjacent fingers in complete extension. This anchors the FDP tendon in the extended position and prevents it from flexing the PIP joint. Now instruct the patient to flex the finger at the PIP joint, if he or she can do it FDS is intact (Fig. 20.19).

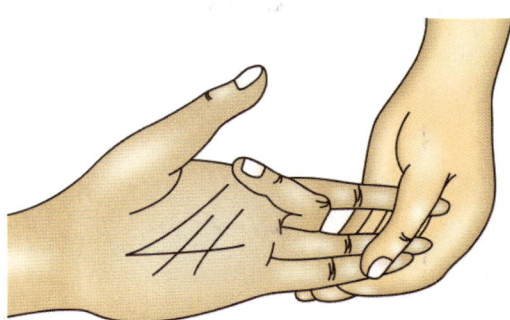

Fig. 20.19: Clinical test to test FDS

Both FDS and FDP: Stabilize the metacarpo-phalangeal joint and instruct the patient to flex the finger. If he or she cannot flex either the DIP or the PIP joints, both the tendons are cut.

Flexor pollicis longus: Stabilize the MP joint of the thumb and instruct the patient to actively flex the IP joint, if he or she can do it FPL is intact.

Flexor zones of the hand: It is extremely important to know the zones of injury with regard to flexor tendon injuries of the hand and wrist. There are five zones: (Fig. 20.20).

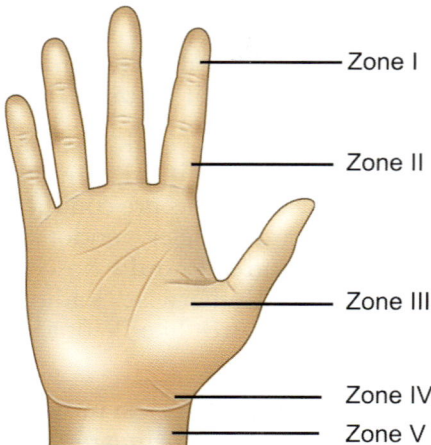

Fig. 20.20: The flexor zones of the hand

Zone I: This extends from the tip of the finger to the middle of the middle phalanx.
Zone II: This extends from the middle of the middle phalanx to the distal palmar crease. Zone
Zone III: This overlies the palm.
Zone IV: Overlies the transverse carpal ligament of the wrist.
Zone V: Extends from the wrist crease to the level of the musculocutaneous junction of the flexor tendons.

Importance of the zones: Bunnel has labeled Zone II as *no-man's land* and is a critical area of pulleys. These pulleys help in the tendon movements. Primary repair at this level invariably fails due to the adhesions in the area of pulleys.

Methods of Treatment

Primary repair: This is indicated in fresh, clean-cut wounds. Here the tendons are primarily sutured end to end, end to side or by various special suturing techniques.

Secondary repair: This may be necessary in severe hand injury, contamination, skin loss, etc. Here after the initial debridement tendons are secondarily repaired after 2 to 3 weeks.

Tendon transfers: This can be thought of if the patient comes to the treatment late or the previous measures have not been successful. In this, a normal functioning tendon is used to replace the damaged tendon and for this to happen all the necessary criteria for tendon transfers should be fulfilled.

Tendon grafting: In the event of loss of tendons due to crush injury, tendon grafting can be considered. Donor tendons for grafting in order of preference are the palmaris longus, the plantaris, the long extensors of the toes, etc.

EXTENSOR TENDON INJURIES

Extensor tendons of the hand are less commonly injured than the flexor tendons.

Tests: Instruct the patient to extend the metacarpo-phalangeal joint. If the long extensors are severed, he or she will not be able to do so. However, he or she can extend the IP joints due to the action of the intrinsic muscles of the hand.

Treatment

The extensor surface of the hand is also divided into six zones. However, unlike in the flexor tendons, extensor tendons can be primarily repaired at almost any level if the injury is clean-cut. In contaminated or crushed injuries, secondary repair after 2 to 3 weeks can be done with good results.

Remember

Tendon injuries:
- Flexor tendons are more commonly injured than extensors.
- Primary flexor tendon injury repair is unsuccessful in Zone II
- It is likely that tendon injuries can be missed during the initial evaluation and treatment of hand injuries
- Primary repair is done in clean-cut injuries while secondary repair is done in contaminated wounds
- Extensor tendons can be successfully sutured in any zone.

CRUSH INJURIES OF THE HAND AND AMPUTATIONS

Crush injuries of the hand are very serious injuries seen in industrial accidents, RTAs, fire-cracker injuries, machine tool injuries, etc. Amputation of the fingers or hand is not readily advocated and then following considerations are taken into account before making this painful decision (Fig. 20.21):
- Is the part injured suffering from absolute or irrever-sible loss of blood supply? If so, this is the only absolute indication for primary amputation.

20

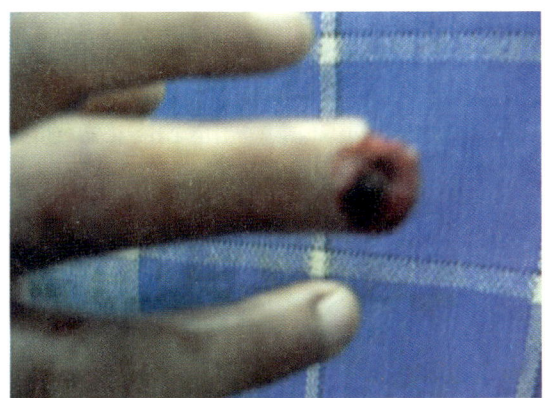

Fig. 20.21: Finger tip crush injury

- Are the other fingers normal? If not, delay the amputation of the affected finger.
- If the finger is left unamputated, will the ultimate function of the hand be good?
- What is the status of the five tissue areas namely the skin, tendon, nerve, bone and joint. If three or more than three of these five areas require special procedures like grafting, etc. give a serious thought about the possibility of amputation.
- Is the victim a child? If so exercise caution.
- If both the flexor tendons and digital nerves are damaged and if the patient is an adult consider amputation.
- Is the thumb badly injured, do everything to salvage the thumb.

Thus in badly crushed hand injuries it is advisable to avoid radical amputation and to be as conservative as possible in excising the vital parts of all the important hand.

Principles of amputation of fingers: After thorough debridement and removal of all the foreign bodies, amputation is planned keeping the following principles in mind:
- The volar skin flap should be long enough to cover the stump and join the dorsal flap.
- The digital nerves should be resected at least 6 mm proximal to its end and allowed to retract back.
- The digital arteries should be cauterized.
- The flexor and extensor tendons should be pulled distally, cut and allowed to retract.
- If the amputation is through the joint, the flares of the bony condyles are excised.

- No much consideration should be given to the dog ears.
- Tourniquet should be released before closing the wound and all the bleeders should be cauterized.
- Small interrupted sutures are used to close the flaps.

Treatment protocol in crush injuries: Whatever treatment protocol is followed it should aim to fulfill the following objectives:
- It should promote primary healing.
- The injured parts should be salvaged.
- It should aim to prevent infection.
  The recommended protocol are follows:

First aid: These measures include covering the wound with a sterile dressing, hand elevation and judicious application of a tourniquet if required.

First examination: Here status of the skin is assessed in sterile conditions without probing the deeper structures. After the skin, tests are conducted to assess the damages to bones, muscles, tendons and nerves. Each of these structures should be considered as damaged until proved otherwise. Radiograph of the hand and general measures like IV fluids, antibiotics, etc. is then done.

Second examination: This is the most important step and is done in a major operation theater under general anesthesia or a regional block. After a thorough debridement all the structures are very carefully inspected again. Skin is examined for viability, bones, nerves, tendons; vessels are inspected for crushing, loss, viability, etc. All the nonviable structures are excised and loose small pieces of bones are removed.

If the wound is clean all the structures are primarily repaired and the bone is fixed either by K-wire or Joshi's external fixators. If the wound is contaminated, secondary repair of the tendons, nerves, etc. are planned after 2 to 3 weeks. If the wound is badly crushed and nonviable, then primary amputation is considered as discussed above.

Postopertive Considerations

After the surgical procedures mentioned above the hand is splinted in functional position and is kept elevated. Active and passive physiotherapy, wax bath, and other rehabilitative measures are planned and appliances given if necessary.

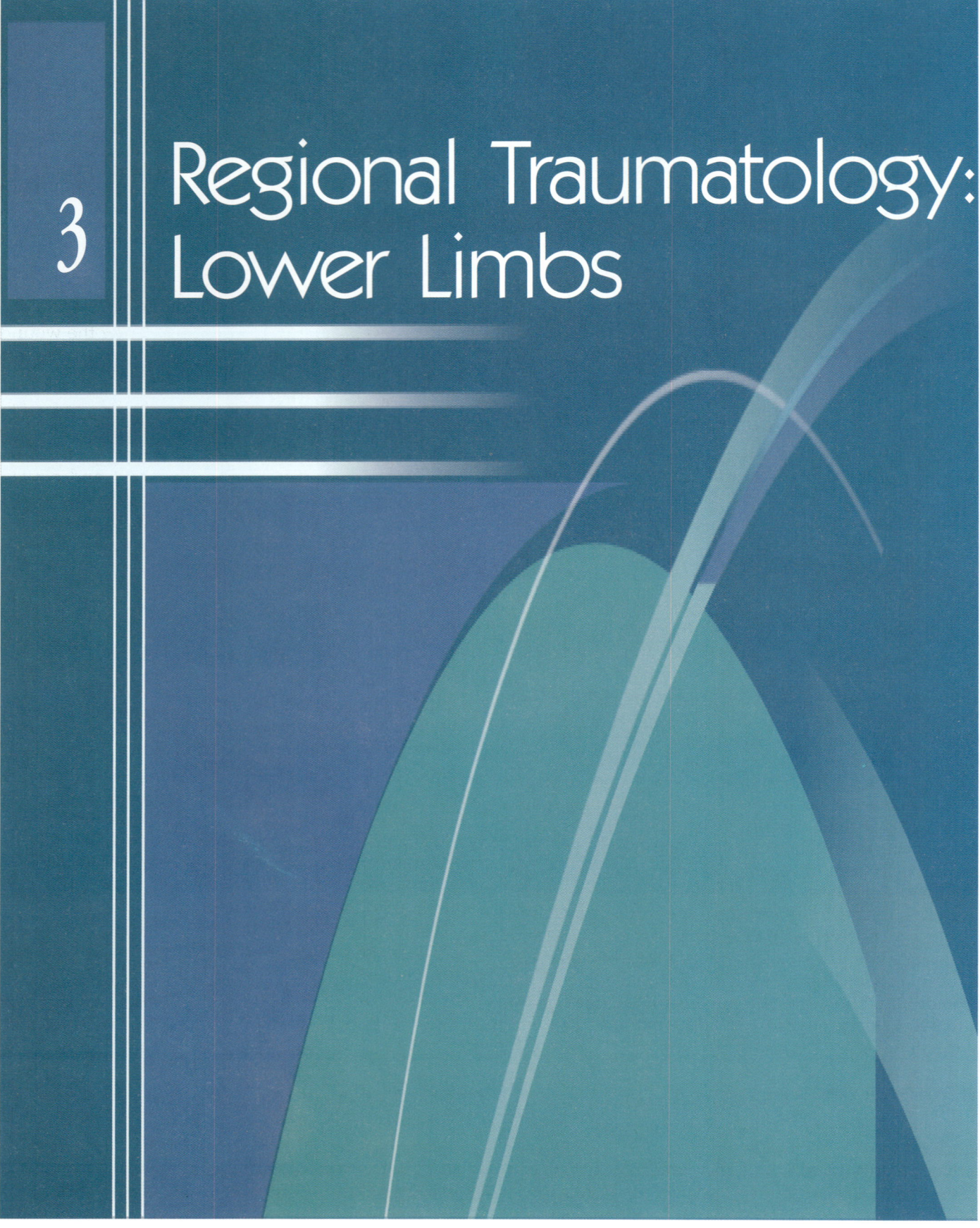

3

Regional Traumatology: Lower Limbs

Injuries Around the Hip

Brief anatomy
Neck femur fracture
Subtrochanteric fracture
Intertrochanteric fracture
Dislocations of hip

Injuries to the hip are one of the most catastrophic events for both the patient and the treating orthopedic surgeons. Being the biggest weight bearing joint in the body, it is prone to lots of complications. It indeed needs a great clinical acumen to put the house in order as far as hip joint is concerned. Let us begin by knowing first about this fabulous joint.

Brief Anatomy

Hip joint is an articulation between the femoral head and the acetabulum. It is a ball and socket variety of joint with a high degree of stability and an excellent range of movements exceeded only by the shoulder joint. The ball is formed by the head of the femur which has a small fovea in the center. This gives attachment to the ligamentum teres which carries a small artery to the head. The deep socket is formed by the acetabulum which is lined by a horseshoe-shaped articular cartilage. Its inferior aspect is formed by the acetabular notch which is devoid of hyaline cartilage. The socket is completed by the transverse ligament inferiorly.

The neck of femur is placed at an angle of 135° to the shaft and it projects 10 to 12° anteriorly to the coronal plane. Its inherent strength depends upon the trabecular pattern which consists of primary and secondary compression and tensile trabeculae. These trabeculae are continuous with the trabeculae of the acetabulum. The degree of movements include flexion 0 to 140°, extension 0 to 15°, adduction 0 to 25°, and abduction 0 to 30°.

NECK FEMUR FRACTURE

"We come to the world under the brim of pelvis and go out of the world through the neck of femur fracture."

Neck femur fracture could be intracapsular or extra-capsular. Intracapsular fracture neck femur is notoriously known as an orthopedic enigma, since a permanent solution for its treatment still eludes the orthopedic surgeons. Hence, it is infamously termed as an unsolved problem. Fracture neck of femur does not unite readily and this makes it a difficult problem to tackle.

> **Remember**
> Problems of healing, why?
> • No cambium layer in the intracapsular area, so no peripheral callus. Healing is only by endosteal callus.
> • Synovial fluid lyses blood clot at the fracture site and thereby destroys another mode of secondary healing.
> • Displaced fracture leads to avascularity.

Clinical significance of vascular anatomy: Avascular necrosis of femoral head and nonunion neck femur fracture are the two very important and common complications of intracapsular neck femur fracture. A thorough knowledge of the vascular anatomy is necessary to understand the reasons behind. Femoral head circulation is through three sources:

1. Intraosseous cervical vessels.
2. Artery of ligamentum teres.
3. Retinacular vessels (main supply).

In neck femur fracture, intraosseous cervical vessels are disrupted and blood supply is dependent on artery of ligamentum teres and retinacular vessels only. Artery of ligamentum teres supplies only a small portion of head, hence, avascular necrosis of the head of the femur occurs if retinacular vessels, the only main source, are damaged in neck femur fracture (Fig. 21.1).

"Therefore the aim of treatment is early anatomical reduction, impaction and rigid internal fixation to protect the existing circulation and to allow revascularization to take place before late segmental collapse can occur."

Etiology

Indirect Trauma

• It is common in older patients with osteoporosis or osteomalacia (12%) and in them usually it is fracture through a pathological bone. According to Sir Astley Cooper the patient falls due to fracture in an osteoporotic bone and not vice versa.

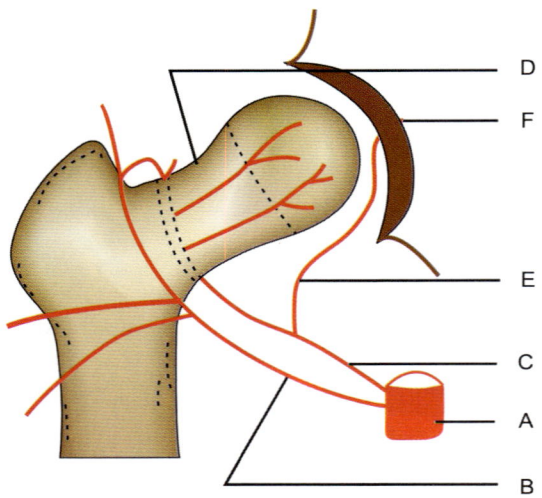

Fig. 21.1: Vascular anatomy of femoral head: (A) profunda femoris artery, (B) lateral circumflex artery, (C) medial circumflex artery, (D) ascending retinacular vessels, (E) obturator branch of medial circumflex artery, and (F) artery of the ligamentum teres

- It is common in elderly women secondary to senile osteoporosis. It also causes marked comminution of the posterior cortex and thus decreases the quality of reduction.
- Direct trauma to the trochanter.

Mechanism of Injury

Majority are due to trivial fall, because of direct blow over the greater trochanter (Fig. 21.2). Major trauma in young adults like road traffic accident (RTA) fall, etc. cause femoral neck fracture. These are due to axial loading.

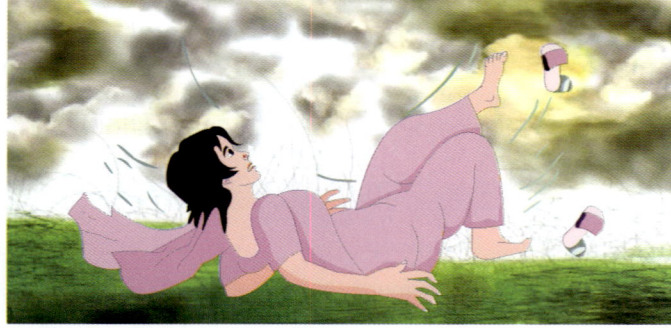

Fig. 21.2: Neck femur fracture is common in elderly females due to trivial fall like a slip in the bathroom

Classification

Many classifications are proposed for neck femur fracture. Few important ones are mentioned here.
1. *Broad classification:*
   Intracapsular—from subcapital area to the middle of the neck (Figs 21.3A and B)

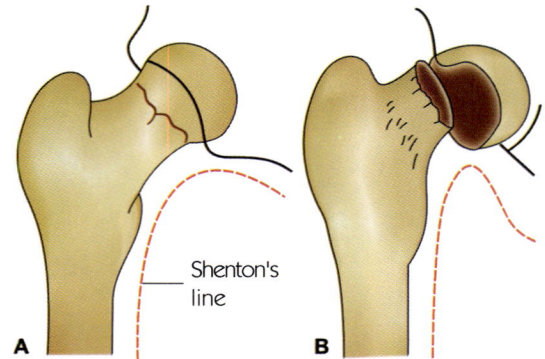

Figs 21.3A and B: Intracapsular neck femur fracture (A) undisplaced, and (B) displaced

Extracapsular—from base of the neck to the pertro-chanteric region.
2. *Based on fracture character:*
   a. Anatomical location
      1. Subcapital—beneath the neck.
      2. Transcervical—in the middle of the neck.
      3. Basal—at the base of the neck.
   b. Fracture angle

Pauwel's classification: Angle the fracture line forms with respect to horizontal line (Fig. 21.4).
   I: 30°
   II: 50°
   III: 70°

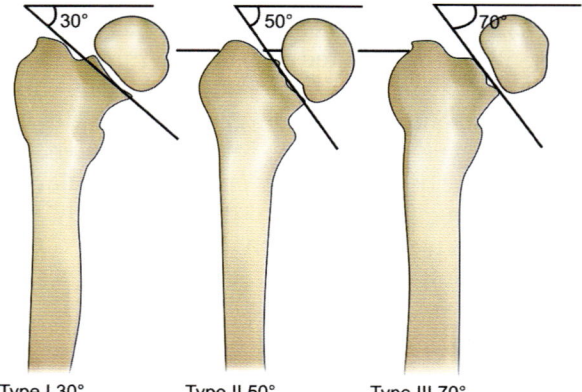

Type I 30°   Type II 50°   Type III 70°

Fig. 21.4: Pauwel's classification of neck femur fracture more the angle more is it likely to be unstable

Perlington's classification: Angle the fracture line forms with respect to the vertical line.
   I: 70°
   II: 50°
   III: 30°

Garden's classification: This is the most accepted classification and is based on the pattern of fracture line and the displacement of the fracture (Fig. 21.5):

21

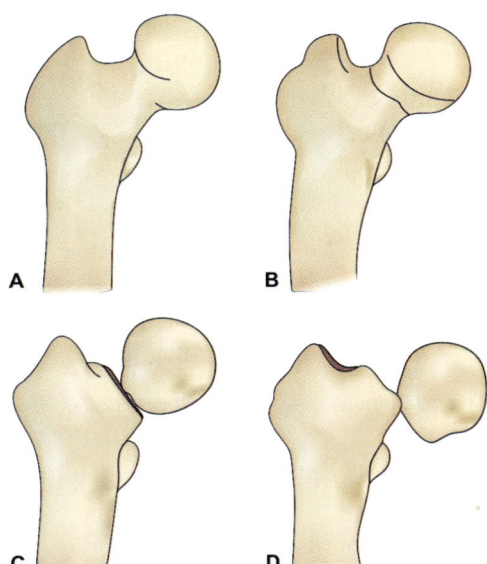

Figs 21.5A to D: Garden's classification showing four varieties of Intracapsular fracture neck of femur

1. Incomplete fracture.
2. Complete fracture but undisplaced.
3. Complete fracture with partial displacement.
4. Complete fracture with total displacement.

Clinical Features

Usually patient is an elderly female and gives history of trivial trauma like slip and fall in a bathroom (Fig. 21.2). Patient complains of pain and restriction of movements of the affected hip. On examination, there is tenderness over the anterior hip joint line. There is minimal shortening and external rotational deformity of the affected limb due to the fracture being intracapsular. The capsule prevents the muscular forces from displacing the fracture fragments grossly. Active straight leg rising is difficult. In impacted fracture neck of femur, patient complains of groin pain, antalgic gait and restriction of hip movements.

Radiography: It consists of routine AP and lateral views of the hip joint (Fig. 21.6). The following points are noted:
- The extent of fracture line whether complete or incomplete.
- The fracture angle.
- Break in the Shenton's line.
- Posterior wall comminution of the neck is best seen in the lateral view.
- Prominent lesser trochantar.
- The degree of osteoporosis (Singh's index).
- Shenton's line is a line drawn from the superior margin of the obturator foramen to the inferior margin of the neck which is continuous (Fig. 21.7).

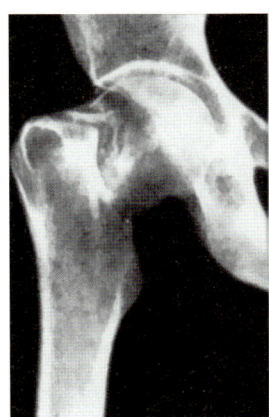

Fig. 21.6: Intracapsular neck femur fracture

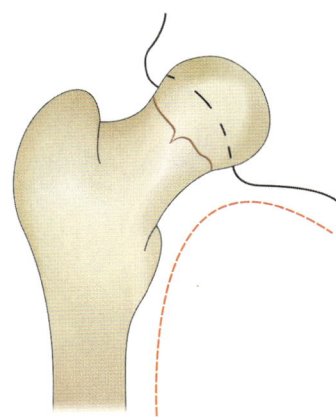

Fig. 21.7: Shenton's line

- *Singh's index:* This is a classification system that measures the degree of osteoporosis in the proximal femur based on radiographic evaluation of the trabecular pattern. This helps to decide the choice of implants.

Treatment

Fracture neck femur is an orthopedic emergency, which needs to be reduced and fixed within 24 hours to get an optimum result. Hence *speed is the watchword* in managing neck femur fracture and invariably needs to be operated. Because of the small proximal fragment an accurate reduction is required, which is usually not possible by conservative methods.

Aims of Treatment

- Early anatomical reduction, which helps, prevents further vascular damage.
- Impaction of the fracture fragments.
- Rigid internal fixation: enables revascularization from the surrounding soft tissues and uninjured bones, which helps in early callus formation.

Table 21.1: Broad treatment guidelines		
Age group	*Undisplaced*	*Displaced*
>70 years	• Dynamic hip screws (DHS)	• Prosthesis • Total hip replacement (THR)
Young adults	• PFN • DHS • Cannulated screws (ASNIS)	• PFN • DHS • Later osteotomy or prosthesis
Children	• HIP spica • Multiple Moore's	• Multiple Moore's pinning • Osteotomy pinning • Arthrodesis

Treatment Plans as per Garden's Classification

Garden I

a. *Conservative:* Hip spica is applied in children and in adults if fracture is several weeks old and if the patient is unfit for surgery or if the fracture is impacted.
b. *Surgical:* Multiple pins by Moore, Knowles, Cannulated screws, etc.

Garden II

Here the fracture is complete and may get displaced. Hence, it is fixed with either DHS or multiple cannulated AO screws.

Garden III/IV

Conservative treatment is rarely indicated except in severely ill patients and mentally ill patients, e.g. hip spica and well leg traction. Surgery is the treatment of choice.

Aim of Surgery

Goal of surgery is anatomical reduction, impaction and stable internal fixation.

Techniques of internal fixation for the neck of femur fracture: Though there are many choices for internal fixation in fracture neck femur, the principles of preoperative preparation, reduction of the fracture, C-arm or radiographic control, surgical approaches and methods of insertion of fixations are the same.

Procedure: The patient is fixed to the fracture table after anesthesia. Closed reduction of the fracture is done under radiograph or C-arm control. If the reduction is satisfactory, the greater trochanter and upper end of femur is exposed through a lateral incision. Midway between the anterior and posterior cortices of the lateral femur and about 2 cm distal to the edge of the greater trochanter drill a hole and insert a guide pin at an angle of 45° to the shaft and parallel to the ground. Check the positions of the guidewires by lateral radiograph or C-arm. If satisfactory, insert the cannulated screws or Moore's pins parallel to the guidewire and if Richard's screw is used through the guidewire. Confirm the position of all the pins as mentioned above and close the wound in layers (Fig. 21.8). Postoperatively patient is mobilized early.

Methods of internal fixation: After having accurately reduced the fracture and ascertained the accuracy, the fracture neck femur can be fixed by any one of the methods mentioned below. However, no ideal internal fixation methods are available. The factors that determine the choice and method of internal fixation are age, duration type and the quantity of bone as determined by "Singh's Index".

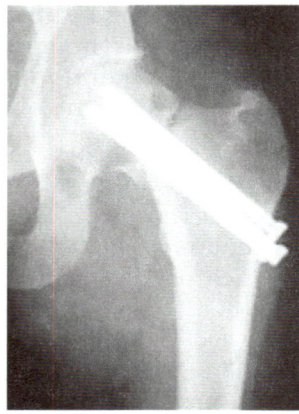

Fig. 21.8: Intracapsular neck femur fracture fixed with multiple cannulated screws

Multiple pins (Knowles, Moore): For impacted fracture, percutaneously for medically unfit persons, and for fractures in children (Fig. 21.9A).

ASNIS: This is a system of cannulated screws that provide improved pullout and bending and torque strengths as compared to Knowles pins. These are the commonly preferred screws for the intracapsular variety.

Fixed angle nail: It has fallen into disrepute because the nail is rigid and may penetrate the joint (Fig. 21.9B).

Sliding or telescoping nails (dynamic hip screws): It has replaced the fixed angle nail. The nail offers collapsibility which ensures continuous impaction at the fracture site and which lessens the chance of nail penetration through the femoral head. *This is the most commonly employed fixation method for fracture neck femur* especially the extracapsular variety (Fig. 21.9C).

Meyer's muscle pedicle graft: A mention has to be made about the posterior muscle pedicle grafting technique.

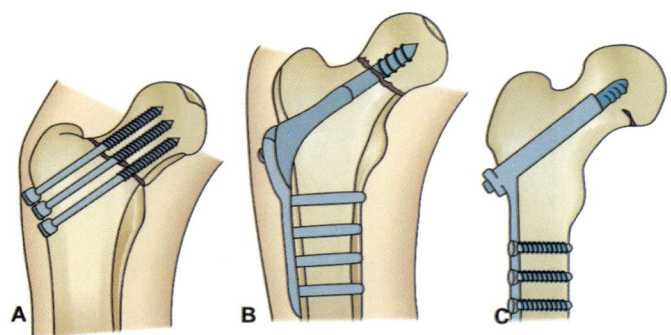

Figs 21.9A to C: Methods of internal fixation of intracapsular neck of femur fracture: (A) Multiple pins, (B) blade plate fixation, and (C) Dynamic hip screw

21

Muscle pedicle graft from the gluteus maximus or quadratus femoris (Meyer's technique), is particularly useful in posterior wall comminution. Dr Bakshi of Kolkata has popularized this technique.

Other treatment options: These include hemi replacement arthroplasty, osteotomy and very rarely THR. However, they are not recommended as the primary modality of treatment in fresh fracture neck of femur. They are also indicated in special situations like nonunion, AVN.

COMPLICATIONS OF FEMORAL NECK FRACTURE

Thromboembolism

It is a leading cause of death within first 7 days. Incidence is 40 percent.

Nonunion

21

Only one-third of the fracture neck femur are known to heal with OR + IF. Nonunion rate is 85 to 95 percent. If there is no evidence of radiological healing between 6 and 12 months at treatment on a radiograph, it is declared as nonunion.

Causes

- Inaccurate reduction.
- Poor internal fixation.
- Lack of cambium layer in the periosteum of the neck.
- Avascularity of femoral head.
- Posterior wall comminution.

Clinical Features

Patient presents with pain in the hip and is unable to bear weight on the affected side. Trendelenburg test, telescopic test will be positive. Wasting of the muscles and minimal shortening of the affected lower limb are the other features.

Radiology: Radiographs of the hip reveals ununited fracture neck of femur and there may be avascular changes in the head (Fig. 21.10).

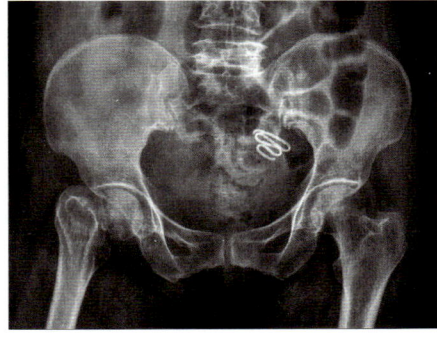

Fig. 21.10: Nonunion fracture neck of femur

Treatment

Surgery is the treatment of choice. The method chosen takes into account the viability of the head (Flow chart 21.1).

Flow chart 21.1: Plan of surgical treatment

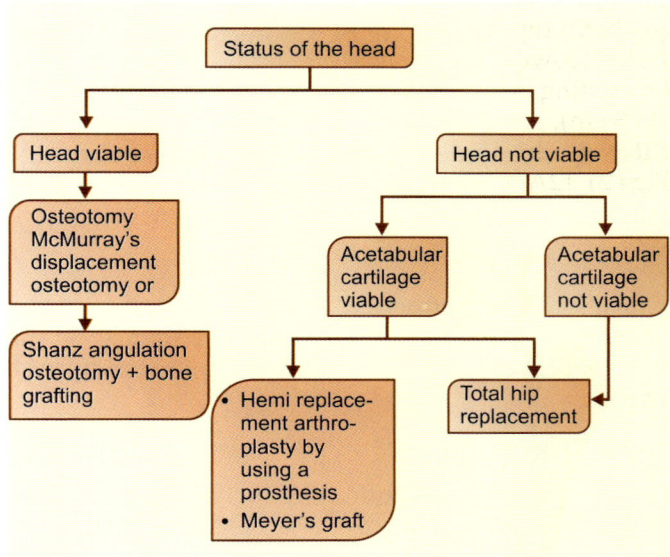

Osteotomy: To treat nonunion of fracture neck femur, two types of osteotomies and their modifications have been described and they are as follows:

McMurray's displacement osteotomy: In this the osteotomy is made just proximal to the lesser trochanter and the distal fragment is pushed medially and fixed internally (Fig. 21.11A).

Shanz angulation osteotomy: In this the osteotomy is made through or just distal to the lesser trochanter. A laterally based wedge of bone is removed and the varus angulation is corrected and fixed with plate and screws (Fig. 21.11B).

Role of osteotomy: Displacement or angulation osteotomy helps to convert the shearing force at the fracture site into compression force by changing the line of weight bearing and thereby enhances the chances of fracture union (Figs 21.11C and D).

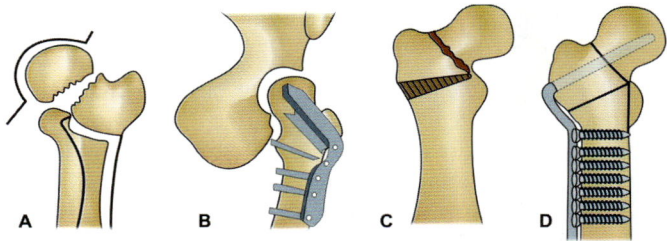

Figs 21.11A to D: (A) McMurray osteotomy, (B) Shanz angulation osteotomy, (C) Angulation osteotomy, and (D) Pauwell osteotomy

Osteotomy as a treatment for nonunion fracture neck femur has a role only if the head of the femur is viable otherwise, hemiarthroplasty is preferable.

Hemi replacement arthroplasty (HRA): As mentioned earlier if the head is not viable but the acetabular cartilage is viable, and if the patient is over 60 years of age, hemi replacement arthroplasty is the treatment of choice. However, the choice of prosthesis depends upon the existing calcar femori. If sufficiently present (at least 1 to 3 cm), Austin Moore's prosthesis is the choice and if it is inadequate Thompson prosthesis is preferred (Figs 21.12A and B).

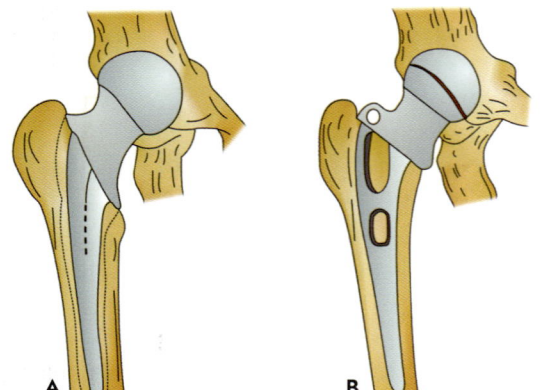

Figs 21.12A and B: Types of HRA: (A) Thompson's prosthesis, and (B) Austin Moore's prosthesis

Bipolar arthroplasty is another effective option in patients who are young (Figs 21.13A and B).

Total hip replacement: If both the femoral head and the acetabular cartilage are not viable and if the patient is more than 60 years old total hip replacement is the surgery of choice (Fig. 21.14).

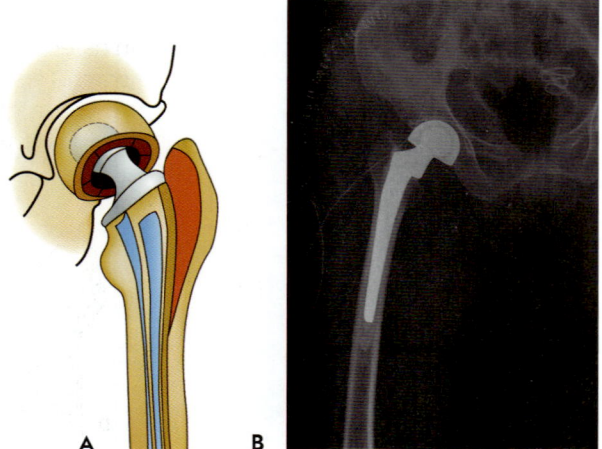

Figs 21.13A and B: (A) Bipolar arthroplasty, (B) Bipolar arthroplasty for nonunion fracture neck of femur

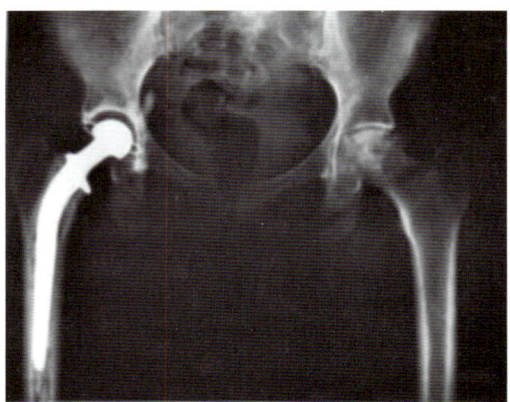

Figs.21.14: Total hip replacement

Avascular Necrosis

It is the next important complication and is a tragic sequel, which writes the obituary of the hip joint, and all this happens due to the total disruption of the precarious blood supply to the femoral head. The natural fall out of AVN is collapse of the head and the inevitable secondary osteoarthritis of the hip.

Clinical Features

Patient presents with pain in the hip and has difficulty to bear weight on the affected side. There could be minimal wasting of the muscles and minimal shortening of the affected lower limb.

Investigations

Radiograph shows increased density of the femoral head and this may take 6 months to 2 years to be seen on radiograph (Fig. 21.15).

Bone scan: Early and accurate determination of avascularity can be made, but it is not 100 percent accurate.

Treatment

- Symptomatic treatment like bed rest, nonsteroidal anti-inflammatory drugs (NSAIDs).

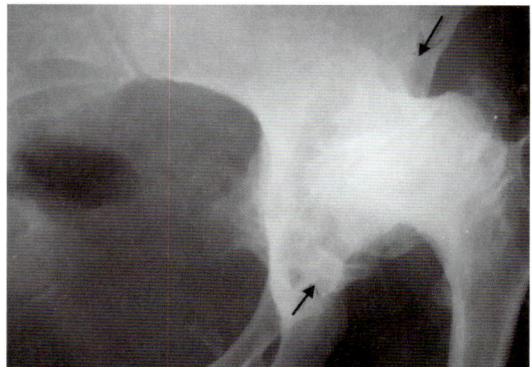

Fig. 21.15: Plain X-ray of the hip showing AVN

- Displacement or angulation osteotomy in early stages.
- If acetabular cartilage is viable, hemi replacement prosthesis is preferred.
- Total hip replacement if acetabular cartilage is not viable.

Osteoarthritis of the Hip (Secondary)

This is an inevitable outcome of the nonunion and avascular necrosis following neck femur fracture.

Clinical Features

Pain, early morning stiffness and restricted hip movements are the usual complaints.

Investigations

Radiograph shows reduction in joint space, sclerosis, osteophytes, etc. (Fig. 21.16).

Treatment

Conservative methods in mild cases and in advanced cases osteotomy or arthrodosis in younger patients and THR in elderly patients.

Remember

Fracture neck of femur at a glance:
- An unsolved problem
- Fracture of the elderly
- Majority due to trivial fall
- Garden's classification widely accepted
- It is an orthopedic emergency
- Speed is the watchword in management
- Early anatomical reduction, impaction, and rigid internal fixation are the aim of treatment
- DHS and multiple cannulated cancellous screws is the currently accepted method of fixation
- Nonunion and AVN are very common.

SUBTROCHANTERIC FRACTURE

Subtrochanteric region is defined as an area between the lesser trochanter and a point 5 cm distal to it (Fig. 21.16). Subtrochanteric fracture is a difficult fracture due to problems like malunion, delayed union, nonunion, shortening, angular deformity, rotational malalignment.

Mechanism of injury: It is usually due to direct trauma due to high velocity RTA or fall and is common in young individuals.

Clinical Features

The patient presents with pain, swelling, shortening, complete external rotation deformity and other usual features of fractures.

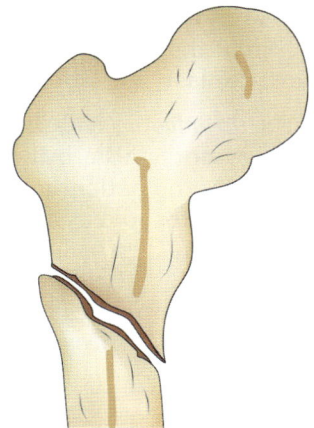

Fig. 21.16: Subtrochanteric fracture

Classification: Seinsheiner has described five varieties of subtrochanteric fracture and it ranges from undisplaced to comminuted varieties.

Radiology: Radiograph helps to study the level and pattern of fracture and thereby helps plan the treatment (Figs 21.17A and B)

Treatment

Conservative methods are advocated if the patient is young. In severely comminuted fractures, modified cast brace with pelvic band is used.

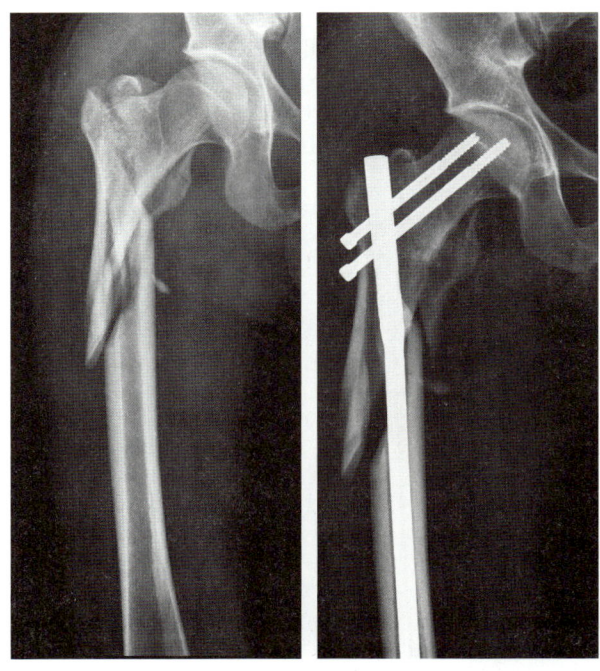

Figs 21.17A and B: (A) Subtrochanteric fracture with trochanteric extension, (B) Fixed with long PFN

Surgery: This is the preferred method of treatment in adults and ORIF is chosen for those fractures, which can be made stable by closed or open reduction. The choice of internal fixation with implants at different levels of the fracture is between PFN interlocking nail, Zickel's nail, Gamma nail, etc. (Fig. 21.18).

INTERTROCHANTERIC FRACTURE

It is seen in elderly patients 10 to 12 years older than intracapsular neck femur fracture and is more common in females (2.8:1) due to osteoporosis.

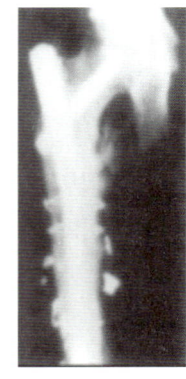

Fig. 21.18: Fixation with gamma nail

Mechanism

- *Direct trauma* as in RTA, fall, etc.
- *Indirect* due to violent muscle pull, etc.
- Axial loading due to high energy trauma as in young adults.

Clinical Features

The patient will have pain, marked shortening of the lower limb, complete external rotation deformity, swelling, ecchymosis and tenderness over the greater trochanter.

Classification: Boyd and Griffin (5 types) and Evan's (6 types) are the classification commonly followed.

Radiology: A true anteroposterior view in internal rotation and a lateral view helps to study the fracture pattern (Fig. 21.19).

Treatment

Conservative treatment: This is indicated in poor medical and surgical risk patients, terminally ill patients and very old patients. Methods commonly employed are:

- Skeletal traction is applied through distal femur or tibia for 10 to 12 weeks over a BB frame or a Thomas splint (See Fig. 10.2).
- Russell skin traction is the most widely recommended method of skin traction in this variety of fracture (See Fig. 5.4)

Surgical methods: Goal is to fix a stably reduced fracture either by closed or open methods internally and thus maintain a normal femoral neck shaft angle.

Once stable reduction has been obtained either anatomically or by any one of the non-anatomical means (e.g. by osteotomy), rigid internal fixation is done preferably by DHS screw and plates, PFN, etc. (Figs 21.20 and 21.21A and B).

Complications

Due to the cancellous nature of bone, these fractures unite well unlike neck femur fracture but malunion is quite common. Coxa vara, nonunion is less than 2 percent (rare) and traumatic osteoarthritis is seen. These fractures also carry a higher incidence of mortality (more than 10%). Avascular necrosis is very rare (0.8%).

21

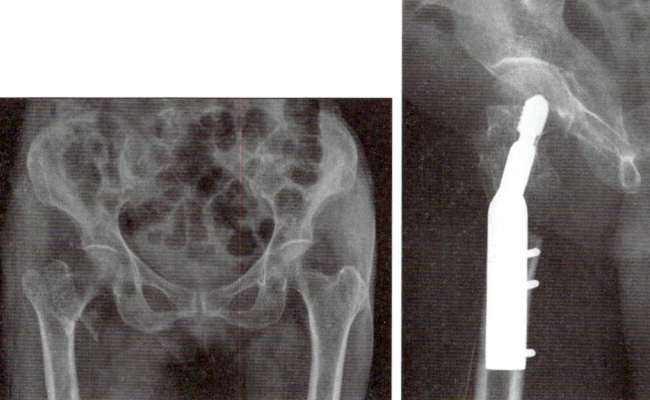

Fig. 21.20: Trochanteric fracture fixed with DHS

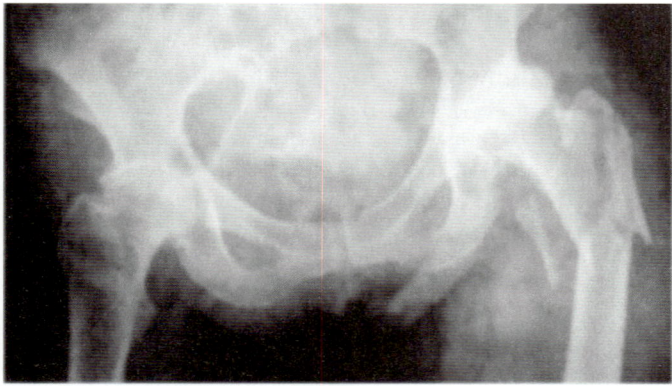

Fig. 21.19: Comminuted trochanteric femur fracture

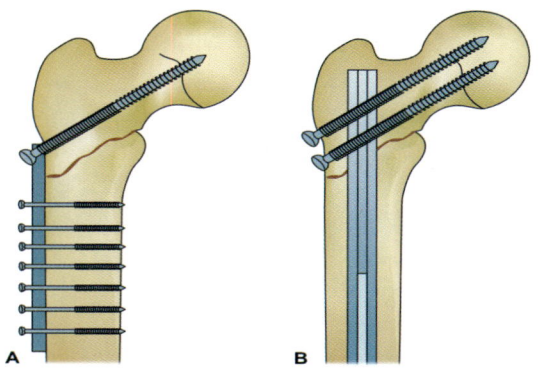

Figs 21.21A and B: (A) Trochanteric fracture, fixed with DHS, (B) Fixed with PFN nail

Comparison of neck femur fracture and trochanteric fracture		
Features	*Neck femur fracture*	*Trochanteric fracture*
1. Age	Elderly	More elderly
2. Incidence	Common	Four times more common
3. Blood loss	Less	More
4. Mechanism	Trivial fall	Major trauma
5. Signs:		
• Shortening	Minimum	Gross
• Deformity	Minimum external	Gross external rotation
• Site of trochanter	Anterior hip joint tenderness	Over greater line
6. Conservative treatment	Not successful	Successful
7. Surgery	Absolutely indicated	Indicated for early mobilization
8. Complications		
Nonunion	Very common	Rare (1%)
Malunion	Unheard	Very common

POSTERIOR DISLOCATION OF HIP JOINT

It is an interesting observation that if anterior dislocation is common in shoulder joint, it is the posterior dislocation, which is common in the hip joint. Incidence is around 70%.

Mechanism of Injury

It is usually due to a backward directed force along the line of femur in a flexed hip (dashboard injury). If the femur is more adducted at the time of impact, pure dislocation results and if the femur is slightly abducted fracture dislocation results (Fig. 21.22).

Clinical Features

There is usually history of trauma and the patient has a flexion, adduction and medial rotation deformity of the

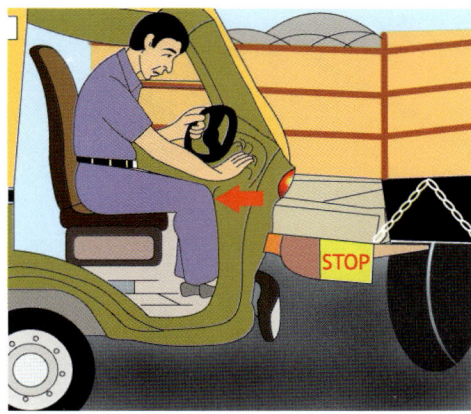

Fig. 21.22: A dashboard injury

affected limb (Figs 21.23A and B). There is marked shortening and gross restriction of all hip movements. Head of the femur is felt as a hard mass in the glutei region and it moves along with the femur. There could be features of sciatic nerve palsy. It may be difficult to feel the femoral pulse (Vascular sign of Narath is negative).

Investigations

Radiography: AP views of the pelvis showing both the hip joints are usually preferred. Lateral view and oblique views of the affected joint gives clue to the fractures of the posterior acetabular rim (Fig. 21.24).

CT scan and MRI: Study of the hip joint is more reliable in assessing the acetabular fractures.

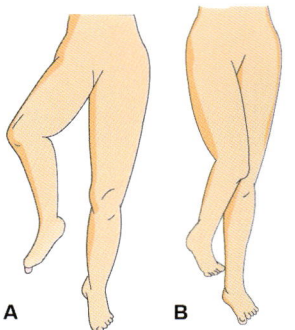
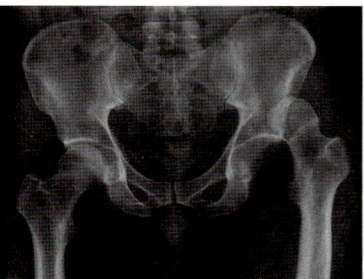

Figs 21.23A and B: Appearance of classical deformities in dislocation hip: (A) anterior, and (B) posterior

Fig. 21.24: Posterior dislocation of hip

Treatment

In order to prevent early onset of secondary osteoarthritis and to reduce pain, immediate reduction of the hip has to be carried out under general anesthesia.

Techniques of reduction: There are various methods of reduction of the hip joint but the most commonly employed method is the "classical method". In this method, the patient is supine and is on the floor under general anesthesia. The hip is flexed to 90° and with an assistant stabilizing the pelvis, a longitudinal traction is given in the line of femur. If reduction is achieved a loud click sound is heard. Immediately after the reduction, tests for the stability of hip joint is done by moving it around in all directions. In fracture dislocations, the hip joint redislocates again (Fig. 21.25). Bigelow's method of reduction can also be done (See Box).

Note: To clinically assess the stability after reduction, flex the hip to 90° and apply a posterior force. If the hip remains reduced, it is considered stable.

21

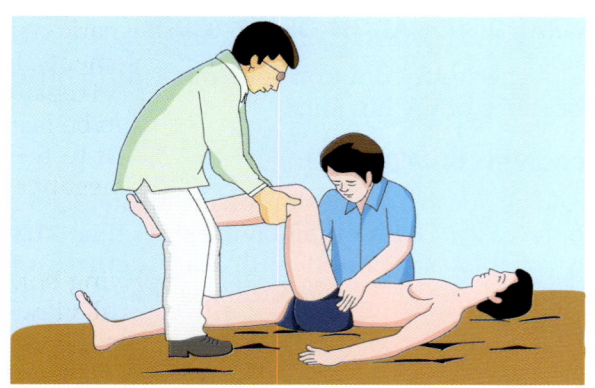

Fig. 21.25: Classical Watson Jones technique for reduction of hip dislocation

Allis method: Same as the classical method but along with the longitudinal traction, the affected limb is gently abducted, externally rotated and extended.

Stimson's gravity method: Here gravity aids in reduction. Here with the patient in the prone position, with the limb hanging over the edge of a table downward traction is applied along the long axis of the femur with the hip and knee flexed to 90° position.

After treatment: After reduction, the patient is put on skin traction or immobilized in a Thomas splint for 3 weeks. Full weight bearing is permitted after 6 weeks.

Indications for open reduction: The following are some of the important indications for open reduction.
- *Failure of close reduction:* This could be due to obstruction by bony fragments or by soft tissues like acetabular labrum and capsule or locking of fracture surfaces or due to buttonholing of femoral head through the capsule.
- Instability after reduction is usually due to large posterior chunk of acetabulum.
- Sciatic nerve palsy, etc.

Complications

Myositis ossificans (2%): It is seen with associated head injury and is unknown in simple posterior dislocation. It can be prevented by avoiding repeated manipulation and by immobilizing for 6 weeks in hip spica.

Sciatic nerve injury: Incidence of this injury is 10 to 13 percent. It is 3 times more common in fracture dislocation than simple dislocation. Usually a Neuropraxia recovers on its own.

Traumatic osteoarthritis due to avascular necrosis (35%): Incidence is about 10 percent and the treatment has already been discussed.

Recurrent dislocation: This is due to fracture acetabulum and sometimes due to rent in the capsule and gluteus minimus. This requires exploration and fixing of the acetabular fragments with screws.

Unreduced dislocation: This is common in Asian patients due to ignorance and illiteracy. Manipulative reduction is tried first. If it is unsuccessful, operative reduction is attempted.

Irreducible dislocation (31%): This may be due to bony (acetabular fragments, femoral head, etc.) or soft tissue (acetabular labrum, etc.) obstruction. It may also be due to coma, ipsilateral fracture femur or dislocation of opposite hip. It may require exploration and open reduction.

Remember

The story of a student who was smarter than his teacher was: Jacob Bigelow when working as a house surgeon in the casualty in one of the hospitals in UK encountered a case of posterior dislocation of hip. A call was officially sent to the professor. Meanwhile Bigelow carried out the reduction by his own technique. Expecting a congratulatory note from his professor, he was dismayed when he was severely reprimanded by his professor for having carried out the reduction before he could attend the case! Bigelow promptly redislocated the hip and sent the case back to his professor who could not reduce the dislocation in spite of several attempts! Bigelow was summoned and was asked to reduce the dislocation again which he promptly obliged! This time he received a bouquet and not brickbat from his professor. His technique consisted of creating the opposite movements of extension, abduction and external rotation for reducing post-dislocation of the hip and vice versa for anterior dislocation. However, his method is now replaced by a simpler classical Watson Jones method.

Note: Posterior dislocation of the hip should be reduced early to prevent post-traumatic osteonecrosis and relieve compression on the sciatic nerve.

ANTERIOR DISLOCATION OF THE HIP (ADH)

This is relatively less common than the posterior variety and accounts for 10–15% of the cases.

Mechanism of Injury

- Dashboard injury as in posterior dislocation but here the thigh is in abduction at the time of impact.
- Fall from heights, say a tree, when one of the legs is stuck in the branches and leaves the hip joint widely abducted.
- Blow to the back in a squatted position or in RTA (Fig. 21.26).
- While standing at the bank of a river, with one foot in the boat and the other on the shore. Now if the boat suddenly moves forwards, the resulting abduction force dislocates the hip anteriorly.

Clinical Features

Patient may complain of severe pain and restriction of the hip movements. The hip is in flexion, abduction and

21

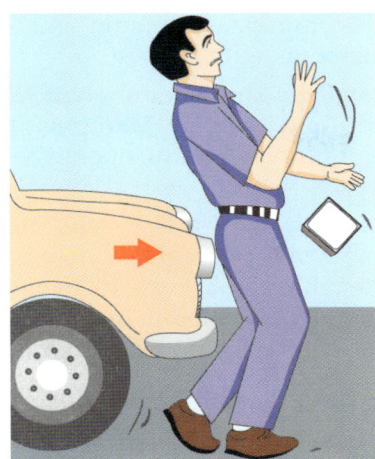

Fig. 21.26: Mechanism of injury in anterior dislocation of the hip

21

external rotation position. The head may be felt in the groin and the femoral pulse is readily felt (Vascular sign of Narath is positive).

Investigations

Radiography: AP views of the pelvis showing both the hip joints are usually preferred (Fig. 21.27).

CT scan and MRI: Study of the hip joint may be required in some situations.

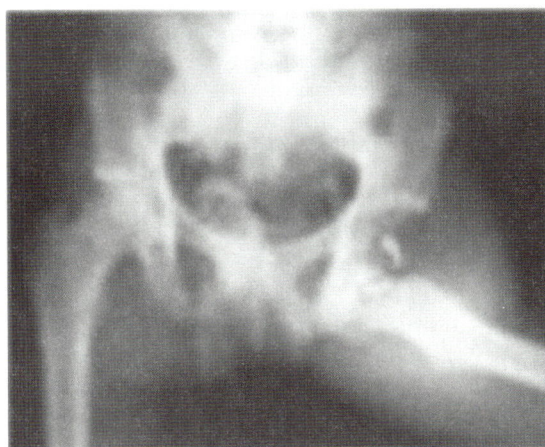

Fig. 21.27: Plain X-ray of the pelvis showing Anterior dislocation of the hip

Treatment

Consists of prompt closed reduction only and this is similar to the posterior dislocation of hip.

Complications: The femoral vessels and the nerves are more commonly injured. Rest of the complications is same as that of posterior dislocation of the hip.

CENTRAL DISLOCATION OF HIP (CDH)

This is the least common and most difficult of all dislocations of the hip joint.

Mechanism of Injury

It could be due to a direct blow on the greater trochanter as in the case of RTA or fall on the sides (Fig. 21.28). It is invariably associated with the fractures of the acetabulum and this is what makes it a very difficult problem to treat.

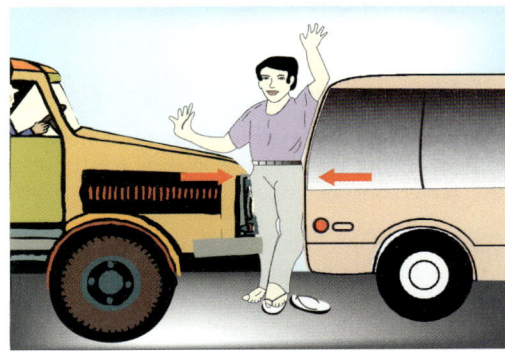

Fig. 21.28: Common mechanism of injury of central dislocation of the hip

Clinical Features

Interestingly none of the features as in ADH or PDH is seen. On the other hand, in CDH there is no limb shortening, no external rotation deformity, head is not externally palpable. The limb is in neutral position; there is pain, severe restriction of hip movements and a huge bruise over the greater trochanter. Head is felt easily by a per rectal examination typical of CDH.

Investigations

Routine plain X-rays (See Fig. 27.8C), CT scan (See Fig. 27.8D) are the recommended investigation procedures.

Treatment

Reduction is achieved through skeletal traction over the greater trochanter in line of the neck of femur. Open reduction is reserved for cases of failed closed reduction. The skeletal traction is maintained for 10–12 weeks if the acetabulum is reasonably reconstructed or else open reduction and surgical reconstruction of the acetabulum is recommended.

Complications

Post-traumatic osteoarthritis is an escapable complication of central dislocation. Other fearful complications include myositis, avascular necrosis of the femoral head and a stiff and disabling hip.

22 | Injuries of the Femur

Shaft femur fracture
Distal femur fracture
Supracondylar fracture

FRACTURE SHAFT FEMUR

Before discussing about fracture femur, it is in the fitness of things that an attempt is made to know certain relevant salient features about femur.

Remember

A must know facts about the salient features of femur (Fig. 22.1):
- It is the longest and the strongest bone in the body.
- It is the heaviest bone.
- A person's height is almost four times the length of femur.
- It has three parts: proximal end, distal end and shaft.
- The shaft extends from the level of the lesser trochanter to the flare of the condyles.
- The shaft is slightly bowed anteriorly and is narrowest at the midshaft.
- The cross-section is circular.
- Linea aspera is the thick ridge of bone situated mid posterior.
- Muscle forces acting on the femur at different sites causes displacements of the fracture fragments in different directions like:
  - Proximal third iliopsoas flex, abductors abduct and external rotators cause abduction and external rotation of proximal fragment, while, adductors adduct the distal fragment (Fig. 22.2).
  - Middle third there is shortening and adduction.
  - Distal third this is flexed due to the action of gastrocnemius muscle (Fig. 22.3).
- The blood supply to the femur shaft is rich and adequate and thus the fracture in this area usually unites well.
- It is a fracture common in the adults.
- Usually heavy force as in road traffic accidents is required to break the thighbone.
- Due to the heavy violence causing it, it may be associated with multiple fractures and multisystem injuries.
- Compound fractures are rare due to the heavy musculature.
- Due to the ball and socket variety of hip joint above, certain degree of malunion is concealed and hence acceptable.

Note: The above muscular forces should be taken into consideration while planning the treatment for shaft femur fracture.

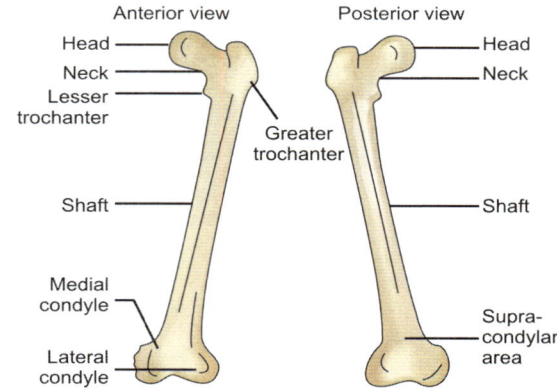

Fig. 22.1: Bony anatomy of femur

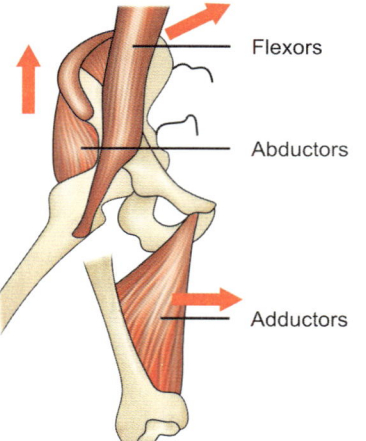

Fig. 22.2: Muscle forces acting across the shaft of femur

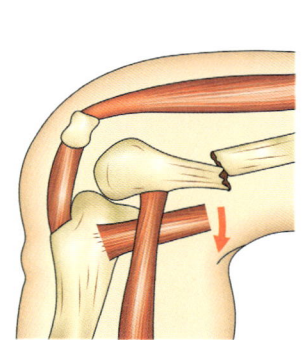

Fig. 22.3: In the distal third the gastrocnemius flexes the distal end of femur

Mechanism of Injury

Usually it is due to direct or indirect forces following a major violence as in RTA and is common in young adults because the strong metaphyseal areas transmit the forces to the shaft causing fracture (See Fig. 6.1). In old age, the metaphyseal areas are brittle and hence the shaft fracture is rare, but fracture of metaphyseal region is common.

Clinical Features

Apart from all the features of fractures there could be shortening of the lower limb and complete external

rotation deformity such that the lateral border of the foot touches the bed (Fig. 22.4). Since the fracture femur is usually due to major violence, the patient may also present with features of shock: (unconsciousness, pallor, cold nose, tachycardia, cold and clammy skin, hypotension, etc.).

Radiography: Routine anteroposterior and lateral views of the femur suffice but care should be taken to include the neighboring joints (hip and knee) to rule out the possibilities of injuries to these joints (Fig. 22.5).

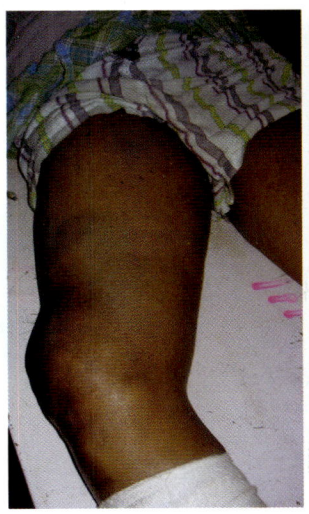 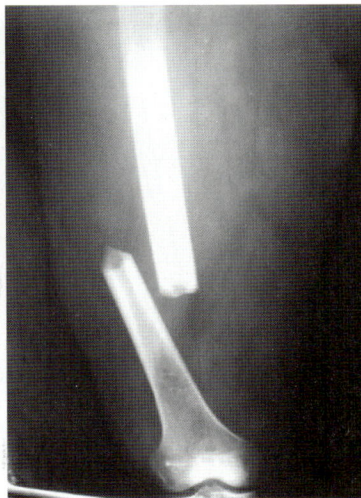

Fig. 22.4: Deformity in fracture femur **Fig. 22.5:** Shaft femur fracture

Management

Conservative Methods

Children: It is mainly conservative in children (Table 22.1). Nowadays older children beyond 8–10 years, are treated operatively by TENS nails (Fig. 22.7D) as this eliminates the need for plaster immobilization and helps in faster rehabilitation. Sometimes in adults it can be treated by skeletal traction and functional cast brace after 4–6 weeks once the fracture becomes sticky (See Fig. 9.5).

Surgery: The best method of managing a fracture shaft femur in adults is by open reduction and rigid internal fixation with the following implants:

Intramedullary (IM) nails: This is used for fractures from 2.5 cm below the lesser trochanter to that 8 to 10 cm above the knee joint. It can be used in simple or comminuted fractures. It can be done immediately following the trauma or delayed for a few days.

Note: Human position is 90° of flexion and 45° of external rotation at the hip.

Technique of open intramedullary nailing (Küntscher's nail): After anesthesia (preferably spinal), strong traction is

Table 22.1: Conservative methods in children	
0 to 2 years	– Plaster spica in human position or modified Bryant or Gallow's traction (See Fig. 11.3)
2 to 10 years	– Most femoral fractures are seen in this age group. Here split Russell traction is more useful (Fig. 22.6)
10 to 15 years	– 90 to 90° Femoral skeletal traction or hip spica or both (See Fig. 9.4)
More than 15 year	– Treatment is as in adults

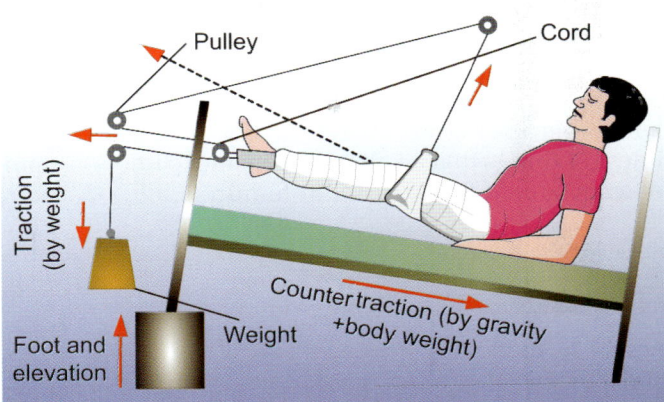

Fig. 22.6: Russell traction

exerted on the affected limb to reduce the fracture and the patient is firmly fastened to the operating table. The limb is painted and draped. Through a lateral or poster lateral approach the fracture is exposed. By using suitable sized medullary reamers, the proximal and distal fragments are reamed. Appropriate sized snugly fitting Küntscher's nail is chosen and driven in a retrograde fashion through the proximal fragment until it emerges into the subcutaneous tissue through the greater trochanter. The fracture is now reduced under direct vision and the nail is driven down into the distal fragment. The wound is closed in layers over a drain (Fig. 22.7C). However K-nailing is seldom done of late.

Note: Open method allows direct visualization of fracture site and hence fracture can be anatomically fixed. Nevertheless, the chances of infection are quite high with this technique.

DCP plate and screws: Earlier this was a very popular method of treating shaft femur fracture. Dynamic compression plating is used for proximal and distal one-third fractures where medullary canal is wide and intramedullary nailing is not suitable. However, it is less commonly used nowadays due to the availability of better methods of fixation like the interlocking nailing (Fig. 22.7B). MIPPO technique is gaining importane of late.

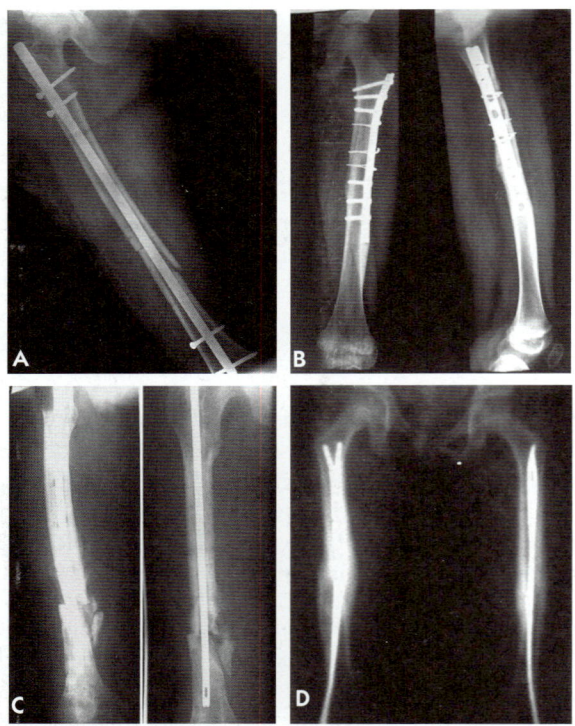

Figs 22.7A to D: Methods of internal fixation for shaft femur fracture: (A) Interlocking nail, (B) DCP plate and screws, (C) Kuntschner's intermedullary nails and (D) Titanium nail fracture femur in children

Interlocking nails of late, this is being regarded as the gold standard in the method of internal fixation of shaft femur fracture. These extend the indications of standard IM nail.

Interlocking nailing technique: In this, the patient is securely fixed to a fracture table. Under C-arm control, a suitable sized interlocking nail is passed through the trochanter into the proximal fragment over a guide wire and driven down into the distal fragment after reducing the fracture and reaming it. The interlocking nail has two holes in the upper and lower ends unlike the standard IM nails. Transverse screws are passed through the upper and lower holes and the nail is locked into position (Fig. 22.7A).

Note: This is the best method but technically difficult as it requires sophisticated equipment like C-arm, instrumentation and has a learning curve.

Flexible medullary nails: E.g. Ender's nail this is usually passed from below upwards through the distal femur.

Complications of Shaft Femur Fracture

Immediate complications: These are life-threatening and the common ones are shock, fat embolism neurovascular injury to the femoral artery, sciatic nerve, etc.

Delayed complications: These are more common and include:
- *Nerve injury:* Injury to the common peroneal nerve is more often seen in these fractures. However, it is not a very common occurrence.
- *Malunion:* This is one of the most common complication seen in fracture shaft femur and is due to the strong and variable muscular forces already described. It is more often seen following conservative treatment and traction than in operative treatment (Fig. 22.8).
- *Nonunion:* It is not that common, as fracture shaft femur is known to unite well (Fig. 22.9).

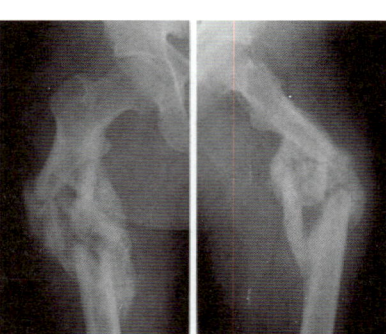 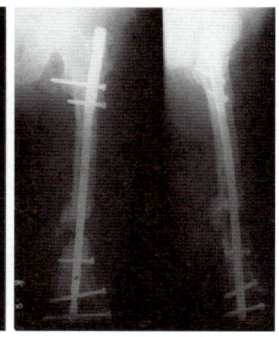

Fig. 22.8: Malunion femur shaft   **Fig. 22.9:** Nonunion femur shaft

- *Joint stiffness:* In fracture shaft femur knee joint may become stiff due to quadriceps atrophy following prolonged immobilization and due to intraarticular or extraarticular adhesions.
- *Infection:* It is rare and is seen in compound fractures of the femur and as a complication of internal fixation like plating, intramedullary nailing.

DISTAL FEMUR FRACTURE

The distal part of the femur encompasses the lower one-third. It varies between 7.6 cm and 15 cm of distal femur. The supracondylar area is a transition zone between the distal diaphysis and the femoral articular surface. The distal femur is subjected to the quadriceps force anteriorly and the flexion force of the gastrocnemius posteriorly. The fractures of the distal femur could be classified into supracondylar, intercondylar, unicondylar and comminuted fractures. The intercondylar fractures could be either T, Y or comminuted. The distal femur fracture accounts for 4.7 percent of all femoral fractures (Figs 22.10A to C).

Mechanism of Injury

These fractures are usually due to severe valgus or varus forces with axial loading and rotation due to RTA, fall, etc.

22

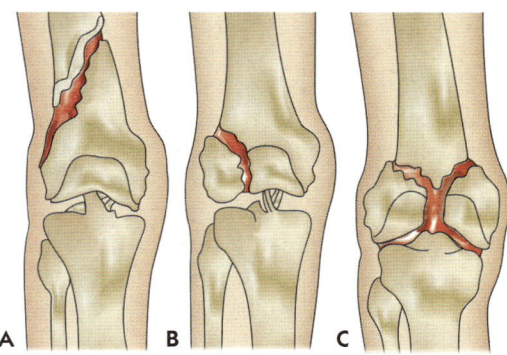

Figs 22.10A to C: Distal femur fracture: (A) Supracondylar fracture, (B) unicondylar fracture, (C) intercondylar fracture (Muller's types)

Clinical Features

It consists of the usual features of fractures but what is specific to this fracture is the flexion deformity caused by the pull of gastrocnemius. Hemarthrosis is commonly seen especially with fractures extending into the joint.

Radiography: Radiograph helps to study the fracture pattern more accurately (Fig. 22.11).

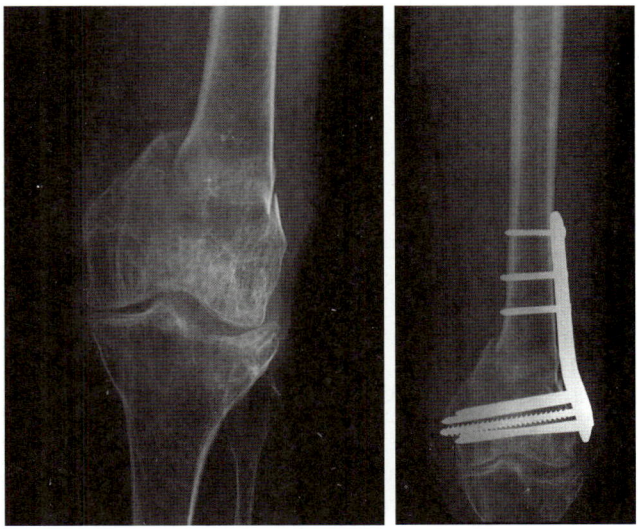

Fig. 22.11: Distal femur fracture and blade plate fixation

Treatment

The treatment usually consists of conservative methods, traction and operative methods.

Conservative methods: This has a limited role and is usually useful in impacted and undisplaced fractures. In the former, a long leg or spica cast is sufficient and in the latter a long above knee cast after an initial period of skin or skeletal traction is all that is required.

Traction methods: The choice is mainly skeletal traction through the upper tibia over the BB frame. This method of treatment is sparingly used is some instances of comminuted or compound fractures (See Fig. 10.2).

Note: The support is given at the fracture site and not the knee to prevent angulation.

Operative methods: This consists of ORIF and is preferred as the closed reduction is associated with troublesome complications like limited knee motion, residual varus and internal rotation deformities. The advantages of open reduction are early mobilization of the knee joint due to an accurate reduction and rigid fixation.

Fixation methods: The choice is between medullary fixation and blade plate fixation. Rush pins, Ender's nail, medullary nails, split nails, etc. are some of the commonly used medullary fixation methods (Figs 22.12A and B). While AO plates, Elliott or Jewett plates comprise the blade fixation methods (Fig. 22.11).

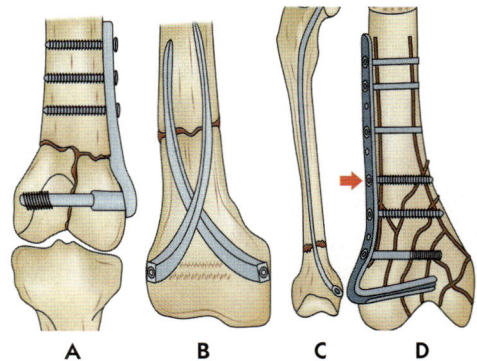

Figs 22.12A to D: Methods of fracture fixation of distal femur fracture: (A) DCS, (B) SC nails, (C) Ender's nail, (D) Angle blade plate

Complications

The complications commonly encountered in supracondylar fractures are delayed union, malunion, nonunion, injury to the popliteal vessels and common peroneal nerves, knee stiffness, deep vein thrombosis, infection, implant failure, etc.

23

Injuries of the Leg

Proximal tibial fracture
Tibia and fibula fracture
Open tibial fractures
Pylon fractures

PROXIMAL TIBIAL FRACTURE

Proximal tibia consists of the medial and lateral condyles along with the upper tibial articular surface and includes the proximal 10 to 12 cm of the tibia. These fractures are usually due to bumper injuries, are frequently intraarticular and unite well considering the cancellous nature of the bone.

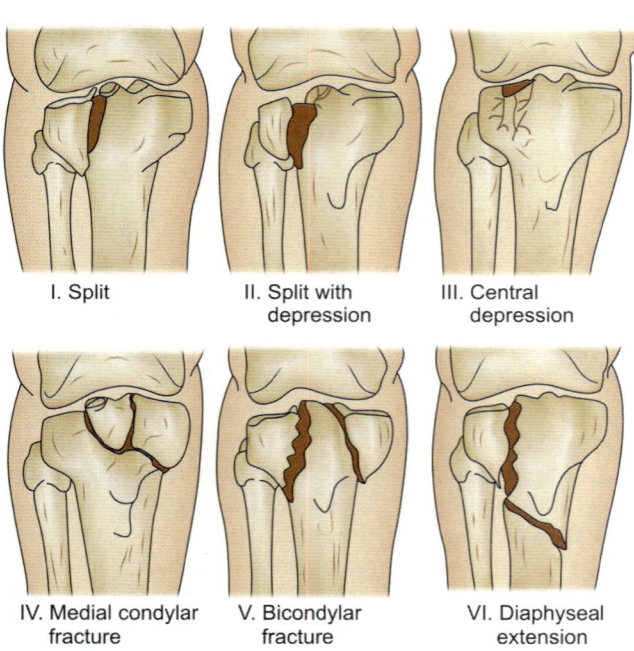

I. Split   II. Split with   III. Central
                depression   depression

IV. Medial condylar   V. Bicondylar   VI. Diaphyseal
fracture   fracture   extension

Fig. 23.1: Types of proximal tibial fractures

Classification: Schatzker's has classified proximal tibial fracture into six types (Fig. 23.1).

Clinical Features

The patient with proximal tibial fractures presents with pain, swelling, deformity, hemarthrosis, decreased movements of the knee and instability in valgus or varus.

Investigations

The routine AP and lateral radiographs of the knee helps to detect a majority of tibial condyle fractures (Figs 23.2A and B). Oblique view may be required to localize the fractures accurately. CT scan and MRI are preferable.

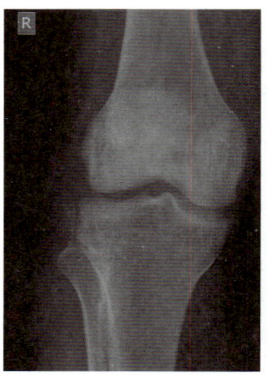 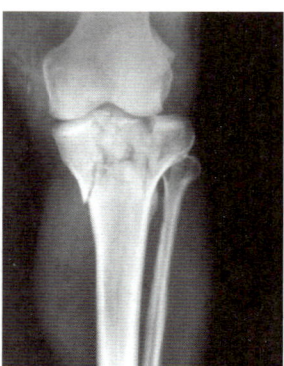

Fig. 23.2A: Type I Schatzker's fracture

Fig. 23.2B: Comminuted proximal tibial fracture

Treatment

Conservative treatment: It is indicated for fractures with < 4 mm depression or displacement and consists of a long cast for a period of 8–12 weeks.

Surgery: Open reduction and rigid internal fixation with cancellous screws, buttress plate, etc. for grossly displaced fractures. Of late, locked compression plates (LCP) are being preferred. MIPO (minimally invasive plate osteosynthesis) is another better alternative (Fig. 23.3).

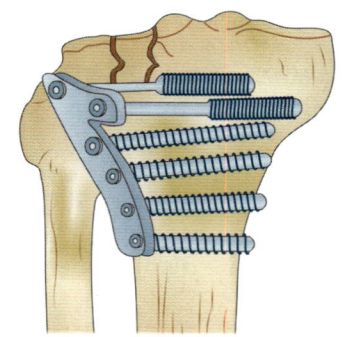 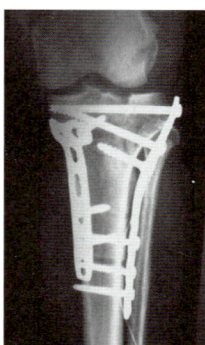

Fig. 23.3: Internal fixation of proximal tibial fracture with buttress plate and screws

Skeletal traction: This is reserved for grossly comminuted fractures.

Complications: These include compartment syndrome, peroneal nerve palsy, popliteal artery laceration, nonunion (rare), malunion and degenerative arthritis.

TIBIA AND FIBULA FRACTURE

Tibia and fibula like their upper limb counterparts, radius and ulna, are twin bones residing together and hence more often than not break together. But unlike in the forearm where both radius and ulna play stellar roles in the forearm function, in lower limbs tibia does bulk of the work while fibula is non-functional and is reduced to the role of providing attachment to the bulkier leg muscles. About 1/3 of tibia is subcutaneous.

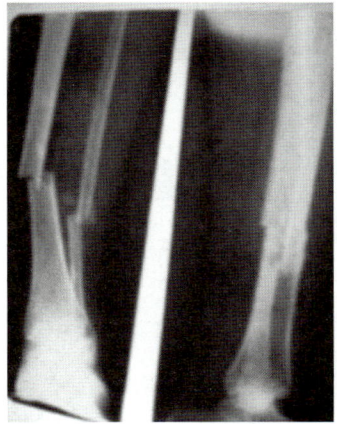

Fig. 23.4: Tibia and fibula fracture

Mechanism of Injury

Direct violence: Due to road traffic accident (most common mode of injury), fall, etc. Open fractures are common in this mode of injury (See Fig. 11.3).

Indirect violence: Due to falls, twisting force, usually cause spiral fractures.

The leg fractures could be simple or compound and more often, it is compound due to the subcutaneous location of the tibia. Tibia and fibula may be breaking in isolation or more commonly together.

Clinical Features

In these fractures, the common symptom is pain and the obvious sign is the deformity, apart from other features of fractures. Damage to the blood vessels and nerves is not that common but fibular neck fracture may injure the lateral popliteal nerve and if the posterior tibial vessels are injured, compartmental syndrome may develop.

Radiography: Radiograph for acute cases requires AP and lateral views. For delayed cases AP, lateral and oblique views may be required (Fig. 23.4).

Methods of Treatment

Conservative management: This consists of above knee cast for undisplaced fractures and for displaced closed reduction under general anesthesia and a long leg cast application is advised (Fig. 23.6).

Indications

• Most closed fractures.
• Undisplaced fractures.
• Fractures with minor or moderate displacements.

Methods of Reduction

There are two methods of closed reduction. In the first, patient is supine and is under general anesthesia. With

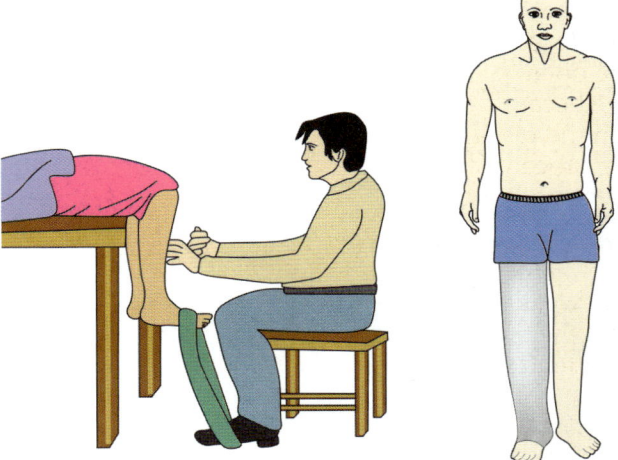

Fig. 23.5: Reduction technique of tibia fracture by the surgeon himself

Fig. 23.6: Tibia fracture treated with long leg cast

the limb held parallel to the table, the fracture is reduced by traction and countertraction method (by an assistant) and a long leg cast is applied. The disadvantage with this technique is due to the gravitational forces posterior angulation develops at the fracture site.

In the second and more commonly followed method, the patient is either sitting if no aneshtesia is required or is supine under anesthesia. Patient is brought to the edge of the table and both the legs are kept dangling. Through a halter, the clinician holds the leg of the patient and manipulates the fracture (Fig. 23.5). A long leg cast is then put with the knee in slight flexion and the ankle at 90°. The advantages of this method are:

• Traction and countertraction do not require the services of an assistant and can be given by the surgeon himself.
• Patient's own weight of the leg provides traction through the gravity.

- Easy to compare with the normal leg regarding the accuracy of closed reduction by looking at the control of rotation and angle.

Concept of wedge plaster correction: For post-reduction angulation of the fracture tibia, which is in a plaster cast, the technique of wedge correction of the plaster, will enable the surgeon to correct the residual angulation without removing the original plaster cast.

In a post-reduction radiograph, the direction of the angulation whether medial or lateral, anterior or posterior is noted. Then an attempt is made to correct the angulation by either opening a wedge or closing a wedge in the cast. In the open wedge plaster correction, the plaster is cut at the opposite end of the angulation and opened thereby correcting the angulation. In the closed wedge technique a wedge of plaster cast is removed at the apex of the angulation and the plaster cast is closed correcting the angulation (Fig. 23.7).

The open wedge technique is preferred over closed wedge because of the chances of the skin being caught within the plaster edges in the closed technique. After either procedure the plaster cast is completed and a check radiograph is taken to confirm the correction.

Sarmiento's total contact below knee cast: After reduction of the fracture and application of a long leg cast for several weeks, a total below knee cast which is molded around the tibial condyles and patella in the fashion of patellar tendon bearing prosthesis is applied (Fig. 23.8).

Advantages

- It allows knee movements.
- Sitting can be permitted early.
- Ease of ambulation for patients with bilateral fracture.
- It decreases the incidence of delayed union and nonunion.

Surgery

Open reduction and internal fixation (ORIF): As mentioned earlier only 5 percent of the cases require operative treatment in tibial fractures. After open reduction, the tibial fracture can be fixed internally either by a DCP plate (Fig. 23.9A), IM nail or interlocking nail. Luckily most of the times, fibula needs no fixation. Interlocking nail is the current gold standard internal fixation method (Fig. 23.9B). MIPPO (minimally invasive percutaneous plate osteosynthesis): This technique is increasingly being employed of late.

Closed interlocking nailing: In some specific instances like simple, comminuted or segmental fractures, closed reduction is followed by closed interlocking nailing

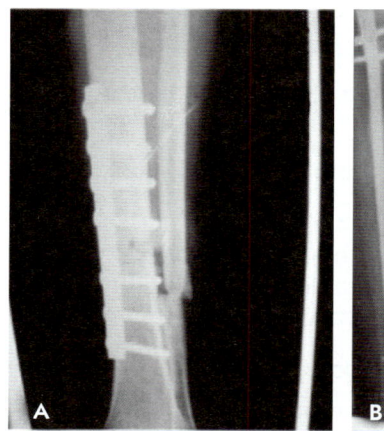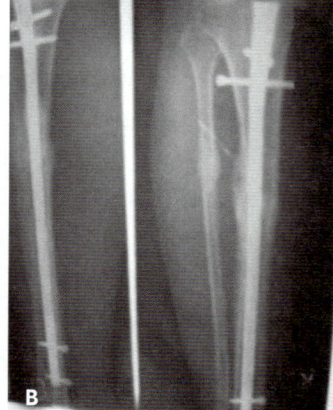

Figs 23.9A and B: Methods of internal fixation in tibial fracture: (A) DCP plate and screws, (B) interlocking nailing

Flow chart 23.1: Internal fixation methods

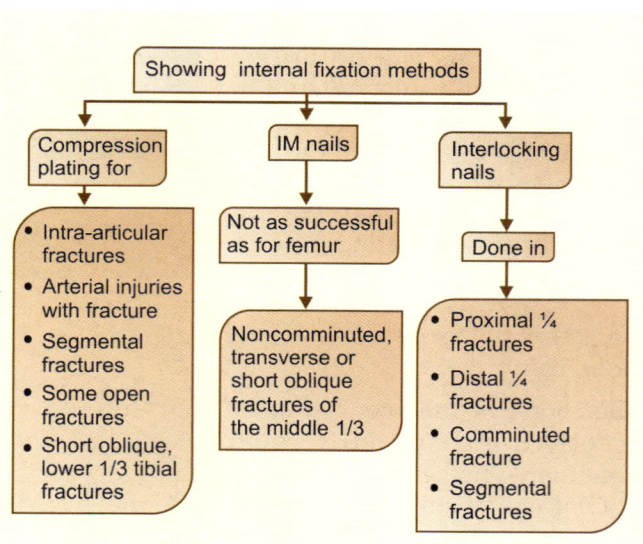

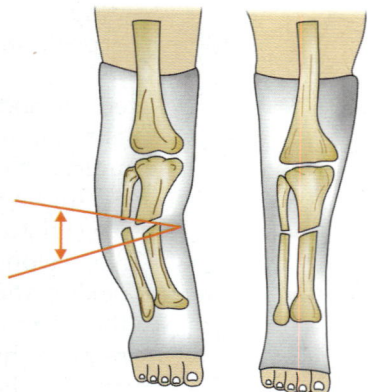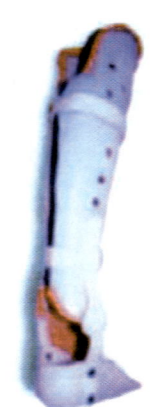

Fig. 23.7: Residual post-reduction angulation corrected by closed wedge plaster technique

Fig. 23.8: Sarmiento's total contact below knee cast

23

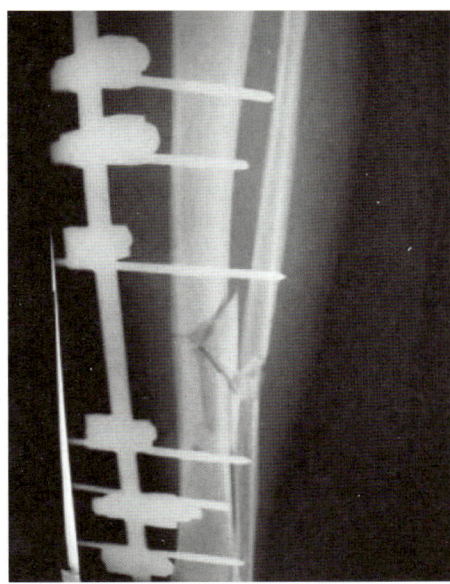

Fig. 23.10: External fixator treatment for compound tibia fracture

technique under C-arm control. The results are good in the hands of experts.

Role of external fixators: This is useful in compound fractures of the tibia as it enables to stabilize the fracture and helps to take care of the wound (Fig. 23.10).

Complications of Tibial Fractures

Delayed union This is a common complication and has an incidence of 1 to 17 percent. If there is no evidence of union of the fracture even after 20 weeks, delayed union is suspected and is treated with cancellous bone graft.

Nonunion: This is a notorious problem usually encountered in fractures at the junction of middle one-third and lower one-third. It can be treated by electric stimulation or rigid internal fixation with compression plating and cancellous bone grafting (Fig. 23.11).

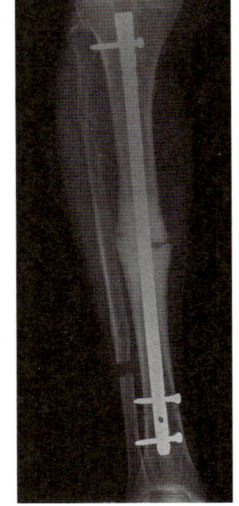

Fig. 23.11: Nonunion of tibia

Treatment of Delayed Union and Nonunion

The choice of treatment in cases of delayed or nonunion depends upon the status of the nonunion whether complete or partial.

- *Complete nonunion:* Here the fracture site is opened, the sclerotic ends are denuded and they are fixed rigidly either by compression plating or by nailing techniques.
- *Incomplete nonunion:* Here the fracture is partially united by a good fibrous tissue and there is acceptable alignment. In such cases, Phemister grafting is the recommended form of treatment. Without opening the nonunion site, cancellous bone grafts are placed posteriorly by raising an osteoperiosteal flap. This hastens the union.

Infected nonunion: It poses a tough challenge to the orthopedic surgeon and is best managed by Ilizarov's method of treatment.

Malunion: Because of the parallel hinge knee and ankle joints above and below, Malunion of tibia is an unacceptable problem as it may cause early degenerative arthritis. Corrective osteotomy is the treatment of choice (Figs 23.12A and B).

Shortening: This may be due to malunion or overlap of the fracture fragments and less than 2 cm shortening is acceptable and may be corrected by footwear adjustments while more than 2 cm shortening may require bone-lengthening procedures.

Infection: Due to the subcutaneous location of the bone, infection is a fairly common complication in these fractures due to a higher frequency of compound fractures following RTAs.

Other complications: Compartmental syndromes, joint stiffness, refractures, fat embolism and claw toes due to tethering of the long extensors over the callus are the other common complications.

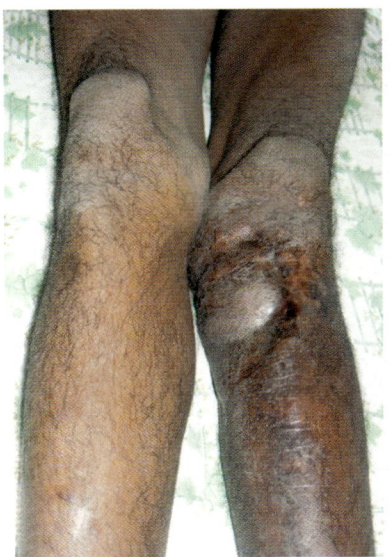

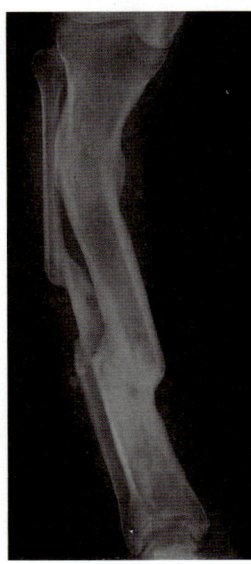

Fig. 23.12A: Deformity due to malunion of tibia

Fig. 23.12B: Malunion of tibia and fibula

Complications of tibial fracture
- Delayed union
- Nonunion
- Infected nonunion
- Malunion
- Shortening
- Infection
- Compartmental syndromes
- Joint stiffness
- Refracture
- Fat embolism
- Claw toes—due to tethering of long extensors over callus.

OPEN TIBIAL FRACTURES

As mentioned previously open fractures are frequently seen in tibial fractures due to its subcutaneous location. The principles of treatment, methods of treatment and complications are as discussed in chapter on open fractures.

PYLON FRACTURES

These are intraarticular fractures caused by the impaction of the talus on the distal tibial articular surface due to high-energy trauma and fall from a height. These fractures are frequently comminuted and are associated with extensive soft tissue injury. Plain

X-rays and CT scan help us to identify and classify the fractures (Figs 23.13 and 23.14). The treatment of choice is open reduction, limited internal fixation and autogenous bone grafting. External fixators are also being tried for fixation with good results (Fig. 23.15).

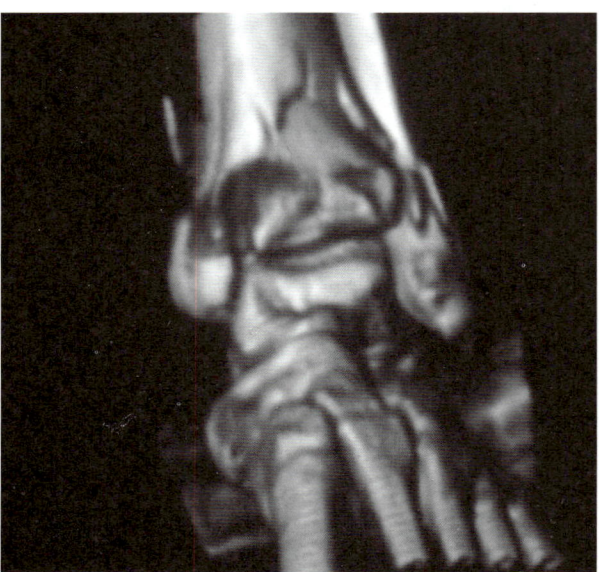

Fig. 23.14: CT of pilon fracture

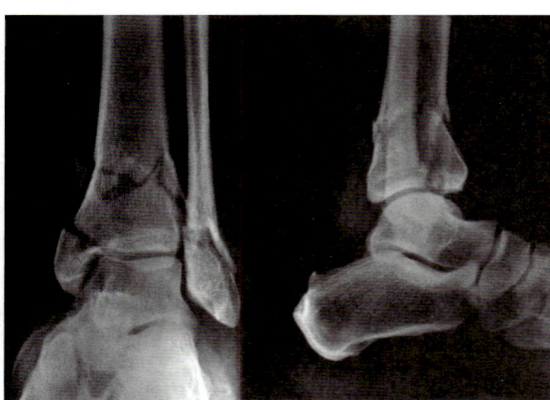

Fig. 23.13: Pilon fracture

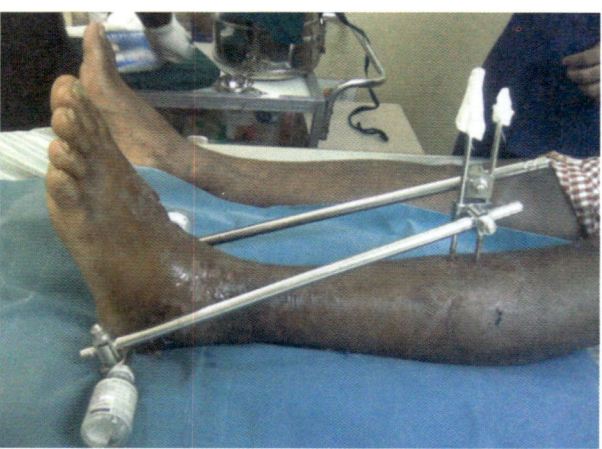

Fig. 23.15: Pilon fracture fixed by external fixation

24 | Injuries Around the Knee

BRIEF ANATOMY OF KNEE

Knee consists of a hinge joint between the lower end of femur and upper end of tibia and a saddle joint between the patella and the femur. Hence, it is rightly called a compound synovial joint. It is heavily dependent for stability on the following ligaments.

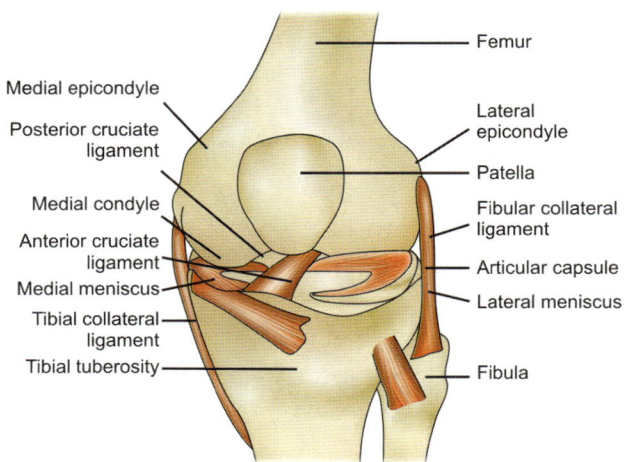

Fig. 24.1: Anatomy of knee joint

Medial side: In the anterior third it is supported by the anterior capsule and extensor retinaculum, in the middle third by the superficial and deep layers of tibial collateral ligament, in the posterior third the capsule is reinforced by posterior oblique ligament, expansions from semitendinosus, etc.

Lateral side: In the anterior third, capsule and the lateral extensor retinaculum; in the middle third, the iliotibial band; in the posterior third by the arcuate complex formed by fibular collateral ligament, and a slip from the popliteus, biceps femoris, etc.

Anteroposterior stability: This is provided by two cruciate ligaments: one anterior and the other posterior and are the primary stabilizers in the anteroposterior plane.

Menisci: These are two wonderful structures in the form of *menisci* whose structure and function are discussed in the section on Meniscal Injury.

Extensor apparatus: The structures, which form a part of the "Extensor Apparatus" whose primary function is to bring about knee extension, are:

- The quadriceps muscle
- The quadriceps tendon
- Patella and the ligamentum patellae
- Patella and their retinaculae
- Patellar tendon.

If any of these structures are injured or if they develop weakness following a period of inactivity or surgery, the extension will not be complete or weak leading to the development of a troublesome complication called the "Extensor Lag".

> **QUICK FACTS: KNEE STABILITY DEPENDS UPON**
> - Mechanical axes of the joint.
> - The bony contours.
> - Extraarticular stabilizers (synovium, capsules, collaterals, muscles and tendons).
> - Intraarticular stabilizers (menisci and cruciates).

KNEE LIGAMENT INJURIES

Etiology

- *Athletes:* Knee ligament injuries are very common in athletes who are involved both in contact and non-contact sports. The injury could be either direct due to the collision with another athlete or indirect due to rotation and twisting injuries (Fig. 24.2).

- *Road traffic accident* (RTA): Here the mechanism is usually direct and could be due to a dashboard injury.

- Fall from height with twisting forces.

COLLATERAL LIGAMENT INJURY

Collateral ligament injury is due to direct or indirect violence as described earlier. Medial collateral ligament injury is more common due to the valgus stress caused by striking the lateral aspect of the knee joint during collision in sports. The varus force on the medial side required to cause the lateral collateral ligament injury is less common because of the protection offered by the other leg.

MEDIAL COLLATERAL LIGAMENT TEAR

This is more common than the lateral collateral ligament injury for reasons mentioned earlier.

Mechanism of injury: Patient gives history of valgus and external rotation force in mild sprains (Fig. 24.2). In severe sprains, patient gives history of valgus stress force due to the direct blow on the lower thigh or upper leg seen commonly in contact sports like football, rugby, etc. It may be associated with ACL tear or meniscal injury.

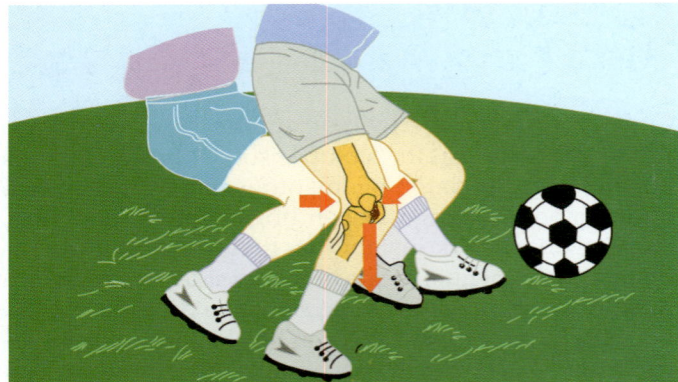

Fig. 24.2: Mechanism of injury of medial collateral ligament of the knee

Classification: The MCL injuries are graded from 1 to 3 depending on the degree of tear (Fig. 24.3).

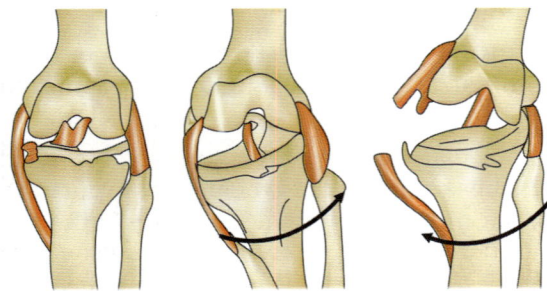

Fig. 24.3: Different grades of sprains of medial collateral ligament injuries of the knee

Clinical Features

A patient with medial collateral ligament injury may present with pain, swelling, hemarthrosis, painful and restricted knee movements, instability, etc. On examination, the point of local tenderness could be at the adductor tubercle, joint line or at the insertion of the tibial collateral ligament.

About 10 to 20 percent of patients have damage to the extensor mechanism of the knee.

Note: MCL more often than not tears at its insertion near the adductor tubercle.

Clinical tests: These are abduction stress test, which is positive at 30 degrees of flexion. Tests to rule out other knee structures like the Anterior Drawer test and Lachman's test should be done.

Investigations

- Stress radiographs at 15 to 20° of valgus.
- MRI helps to localize the MCL tear.
- Arthrograms and arthroscopy to evaluate and rule out meniscal and cruciate injuries.

Treatment

Fresh Injury

I°sprain: RICE Concept (rest, ice, compression with bandages, E-elevation of the limb to prevent edema) is the recommended form of treatment. Other symptomatic treatment methods include non-steroidal anti-inflammatory drugs (NSAIDs), etc. to relieve pain, spasm and swelling.

II°sprain: Long leg cast for 4 to 6 weeks with knee in 30 to 40° of flexion.

III°sprain: Surgical repair consists of direct repair of the collateral ligament injury using non-absorbable sutures.

Reinforcements: Here along with the repair, additional reinforcement using fascial or tendon graft is done. This is reserved for patients reporting for treatment after 2 or 3 weeks.

Old cases: Here it is mainly reconstruction. If TCL is intact but lax then distal transfer is done. If ligament is destroyed, reconstruction using hamstrings or semitendinosus is done.

LATERAL COLLATERAL LIGAMENT INJURY

Mercifully this is not as common as its medial counterpart thanks to the protection provided by the other leg which disallows the varus force, so essential to tear the fibular collateral ligament. Unlike the MCL tear, it more commonly tears at the insertion near the head of the fibula (Fig. 24.4).

24

24

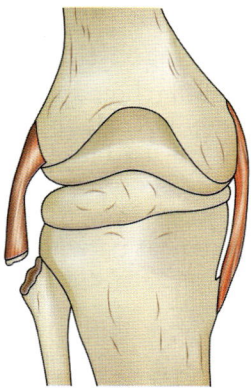

Fig. 24.4: Avulsion of lateral collateral ligament from the head of the fibula

Clinical Features

Patient may complain of pain and swelling on the lateral side of the knee. Varus stress test is positive at 30-degree flexion.

Investigations and treatment in fresh injuries proceeds on the similar lines as for the MCL injury.

In old cases, however, in fibular collateral ligament injury if the ligament is adequate and thick, distal transfer is recommended. If the ligament is torn badly and destroyed, then reconstruction using fascia lata, biceps tendon, etc. is done.

CRUCIATE LIGAMENT INJURIES

Anterior Cruciate Ligament (ACL) Tear

This is the most common knee ligament injury. Athletes and sportspersons are more prone and are due to the indirect forces like flexion, abduction, and internal rotation. It rarely tears in isolation and is associated with injuries to medial meniscus and medial collateral ligament (*Popularly known as the unhappy triad of O'donoghue*) (Fig. 24.5).

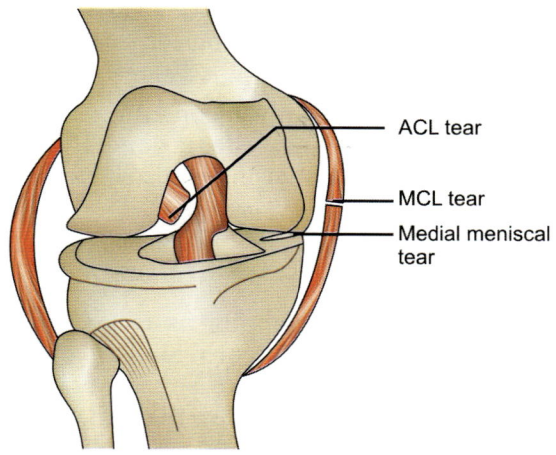

ACL tear

MCL tear

Medial meniscal tear

Fig. 24.5: Unhapply triad of O'donoghue

Mechanism of Injury

The most common mode of injury is external rotation with abduction of the flexed knee or hyperextension of knee in internal rotation.

Clinical Features

This is a disabling injury and the knee may immediately collapse and is painful. Popping sensation felt or heard at the time of injury signifies ligamentous injury (ACL tear). The patient also tells that the knee "gave away" or buckled at the time of injury. Swelling of the knee could develop immediately or over a period and could be due to either hemarthrosis or traumatic synovitis. The distended knee is held in partial flexion by the hamstrings (see box for differential diagnosis of hemarthrosis).

Remember

Differential diagnosis: Hemarthrosis
- Ligamentous tear (ACL, PCL, etc.)
- Osteochondral fracture
- Peripheral meniscal tear
- Capsular tear
- Patellar dislocation

Note: ACL tear is the most common cause of hemarthrosis.

Clinical examination: Always examine the normal knee first and form a basis for "comparison." Clinical findings depends on associated ligamentous injury or meniscal injury or bone damage. Depending on the combination, there will be specific instabilities that will allow anterior displacement of tibia on the involved side. Anterior subluxation of more than 5° suggests lax or disrupted ACL. Isolated injury is rare. This can be elicited by the anterior drawers test and the Lachman's test. See Section on clinical examination of the knee.

Investigations in ACL Tear

Radiograph of the knee: The views recommended are anteroposterior (AP) view, lateral view, intercondylar notch view, sunrise views, etc. Radiographs are usually normal in ACL tear. Avulsion fracture of tibial spine if present indicates ACL tear.

MRI: This is the best diagnostic tool. It is noninvasive and demonstrates the ACL tear with remarkable accuracy.

Arthroscopy: Diagnostic arthroscopy to detect ACL tear is remarkably accurate. It also helps to rule out damage to meniscus and other internal structures of the knee.

Treatment

Conservative treatment is indicated for minor ACL tears with no knee instability. Initially the treatment is as per

the RICE regime. In later stages treatment it is by rest, long leg casts for 4 to 6 weeks, NSAIDs, physiotherapy, etc.

Surgery is indicated in more severe tears and if the knee is unstable.

Fresh cases: Primary repair is indicated in young adults and athletes. Repair is successful if ACL is torn at its femoral or tibial attachments. It is not successful in mid-position tears. Failure rate is as high as 50 percent.

Old cases: Reinforcement of ACL tear should be augmented except when avulsion is with a fragment of bone, which is fixed with a screw. It could be either intraarticular or extraarticular or both by using iliotibial band, semitendinosus tendon, etc. Reconstruction in chronic ACL insufficiency could be either intraarticular or extraarticular replacement by using quadriceps, tendon, patellar tendon (central 1/3 BTB graft) semitendinosus and gracilis tendon (STG graft), etc.

POSTERIOR CRUCIATE LIGAMENT (PCL) TEAR

This is less common than ACL tear. It is ruptured due to severe rotational injury, dashboard injury or complete dislocation of the knee. Isolated PCL tear is rare and is accompanied with other ligament injuries.

Clinical presentation: Patient complains of pain, swelling and tenderness over the popliteal fossa. Clinically posterior drawer test and sag sign will be positive.

Investigations are similar to ACL injuries. See Section on Clinical examination of the knee.

Treatment

In fresh cases, the treatment is more or less similar to the ones described for fresh ACL tear. However, in old cases surgical reconstruction is the treatment method of choice. Reconstruction is done by using medial head of gastrocnemius, etc.

Rehabilitation: Knee rehabilitation is extremely important than the surgery. It consists of mobilization exercise, strengthening exercise, electrotherapy, CPM, etc.

MEDIAL MENISCUS INJURY

Medial meniscus is more commonly injured than the lateral and is usually associated with other ligament injuries of the knee.

Mechanism of Injury

Mechanism of injury is a rotational force when a flexed knee extends:
- In young, it can occur only when weight is being taken, knee is flexed and there is a twisting strain. Young active athletes are more prone.

- In middle life, fibrosis has decreased the mobility of meniscus and hence tear occurs with less force.

Predisposing factors: These could be abnormal meniscal shape, abnormal stress due to chronic ligament laxity, etc.

Smillie's classification: Medial meniscus injury is seen in over 71 percent of the cases. In 5 percent of cases, injury of medial meniscus is bilateral. Lateral meniscus is less commonly injured than the medial meniscus because it is smaller in diameter, thicker in periphery, wide, more mobile, attached to both cruciate ligaments and stabilized posteriorly to the femoral condyle by popliteus.

Types of Meniscal Tears (Figs 24.6A to F)

- *Longitudinal tears (35%):* In these peripheral attachments tear 10 percent, complete tear 23 percent (bucket handle tear), and segmental tear 2 percent anterior or posterior.
- *Horizontal tears (48%):* It could be posterior, middle, or anterior.
- Cystic degeneration (12%).
- Congenital abnormalities 5 percent.
- Regenerative lesions.

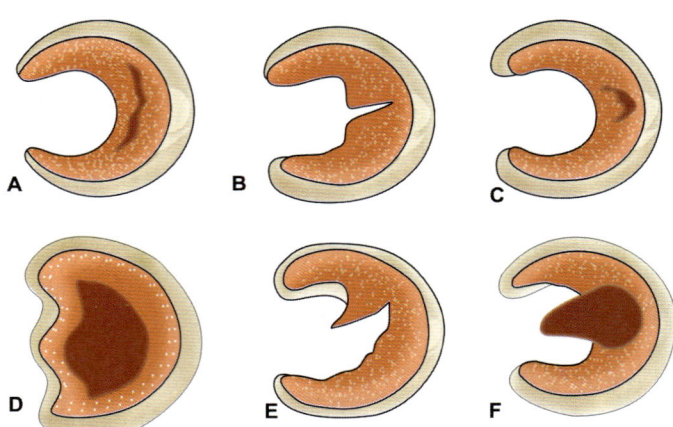

Figs 24.6A to F: Different types of meniscal injuries: (A) longitudinal tear, (B) radial tear, (C) horizontal tear, (D) bucket handle tear, (E) parrot beak tear, and (F) segmental tear

Note: Bucket handle tear is the most common variety of medial meniscus injury.

Clinical Features

A patient with medial meniscal injury complains of pain swelling and limp. There may or may not be history of giving way (this may also be seen in quadriceps insufficiency, loose bodies, chondromalacia, etc.). Joint line tenderness, McMurray's test, Apley's tests are

24

positive (See section on clinical examination of the knee). Patient may give history of locking in few instances (See Box) and is typically seen only in bucket handle tear.

Differential diagnosis of locking	
True locking	*Pseudo locking*
• Loose bodies	• Ligament injuries
• Recurrent dislocation of patella	• Chondromalacia patellar
• Tibial spine fracture	
• Meniscal injuries	

Investigations

- *Radiograph* is usually normal. The views recommended are anteroposterior, lateral, intercondylar notch and sunrise views of the patella.
- *Arthroscopy* helps to identify the torn meniscus more accurately (Fig. 24.7).
- *Arthrography* may reveal the tear. Double contrast arthrography is 95 percent accurate.
- *MRI* is expensive but useful in detecting the tears.

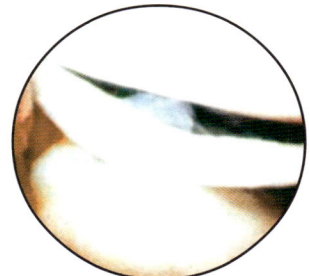

Fig. 24.7: Arthroscopic view of a bucket handle tear of medial meniscus injury

Treatment Methods

Conservative: This is indicated in patients soon after injury with no locking and with infrequent attacks of pain.

Measures

- Abstinence from weightbearing.
- Rest, Ice packs, Compressive bandage, elevation of the limb (RICE concept).
- Buck's extension skin traction.
- Joint aspiration.
- Quadriceps exercises.
- If symptom persists, a cylindrical cast may be considered.

Manipulations under anesthesia: If joint is locked due to the torn menisci, manipulation under anesthesia is recommended.

Surgery: It is indicated if joint cannot be unlocked and if symptoms are recurrent. Closed partial meniscectomy via an arthroscope is better than total removal of the menisci by open surgery. Complete removal of the menisci incapacitates the knee hence, the emphasis is on conservative surgery than radical removal. Suture of a peripheral tear by either open or arthroscopy is also tried is called meniscorrhaphy.

PATELLA FRACTURE

Patella is the largest sesamoid bone in the body. Incidence of fracture is around 1 percent.

Mechanism of Injury

Direct trauma: This is due to dashboard or bumper injuries or due to direct fall over the patella. They usually cause comminuted fractures (Stellate fracture and are the common causes of patella fracture (Fig. 24.8).

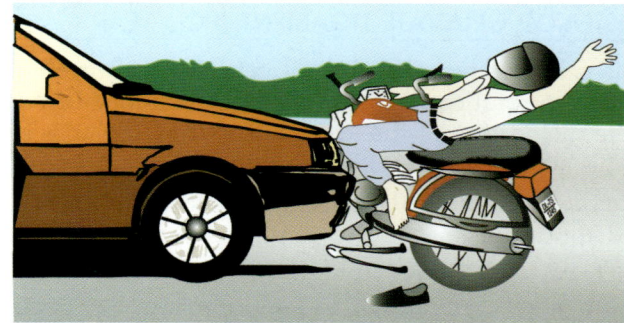

Fig. 24.8: Bumper injuries in RTA

Indirect trauma (quadriceps contraction) sudden forceful contraction of the quadriceps as in sportsperson and athletes can cause patellar fractures. Here the fracture is usually transverse and sometimes avulsion fractures of the proximal or distal poles may be seen.
Age: Common in the 40–50 age group.
Sex: Male:Female = 2:1

Classification: The following types (Figs 24.9A to D) are described:
- Undisplaced
- Displaced

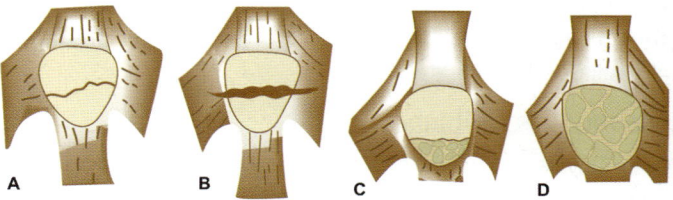

Figs 24.9A to D: Types of patellar fractures: (A) undisplaced fracture, (B) transverse fracture, (C) distal pole fracture, and (D) comminuted fracture

a. Transverse—involving upper or lower poles (50–85%).
b. Oblique fracture
c. Vertical fracture (12–27%).
d. Comminuted fracture (30–35%).

Clinical Features

Patient gives history of trauma following which there is pain and swelling at the knee joint. Patient is unable to extend the knee and both the active and passive movements are restricted. On examination, there could be a palpable gap, tenderness, signs of effusion and a positive patellar tap. Cross fluctuation test may be positive.

Radiology

Plain X-ray of the knee, AP and lateral views helps in identifying the type of fracture of the patella (Fig. 24.10).

Note: Bipartite patella and osteochondral fractures cause confusion in the diagnosis.

Management

Undisplaced fracture: Nonoperative treatment will produce good results in undisplaced fractures and if displacement is less than 1 to 2 mm and the methods include compression bandage, ice applications, aspiration of hemarthrosis, cylindrical cast early weight bearing and quadriceps exercises (See Fig. 9.2D).

Displaced fracture: In this variety surgery is the treatment of choice. Surgery is performed as early as possible preferably within 7 days.

Surgical Methods

Open reduction and internal fixation: This is indicated in transverse fractures of the patella. Internal fixation is done either by the circumferential wiring or by tension band wiring. Interfragmentary screws are also wide (Fig. 24.11).

Patellectomy: This could be either partial (for smaller distal or proximal pole fracture) or complete (for comminuted fractures). The emphasis is now on preserving as much patella as possible to prevent the disadvantages of patellectomy like extensive leg quadriceps atrophy, etc.

Complications

Postoperative complications: Early fracture dehiscence, postoperative infection, refracture (1–5%), avascular necrosis (25% incidence in proximal pole) are some of the common postoperative complications.

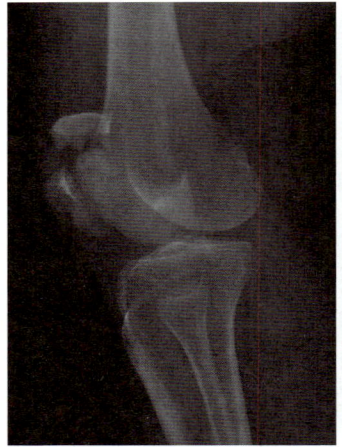 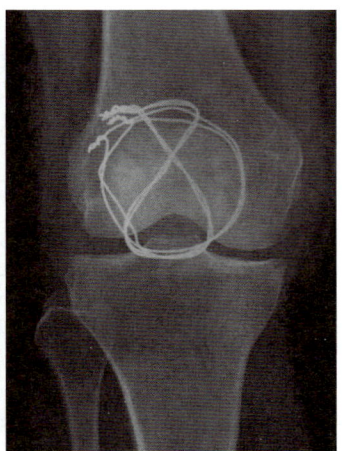

Fig. 24.10: Patella fracture— Lateral view   **Fig. 24.11:** Patella fracture wiring

Delayed complications: This is like knee stiffness, osteoarthritis of the patellofemoral and knee joint, extensor lag, etc. can occur.

Extensor lag: This is the inability of the patient to perform the last 5–10° of extension. About 80 percent of quadriceps strength is required to bring about the last 20° of extension. After patellectomy, due to the decreased lever arm, the efficiency of quadriceps is reduced and the patient will be unable to bring about the terminal extension of the knee. Thus an attempt is made to save as much of patella as possible, all of the patella or at least the proximal or distal half, if practical to preserve the quadriceps efficiency and prevent the extensor lag (Fig. 24.12).

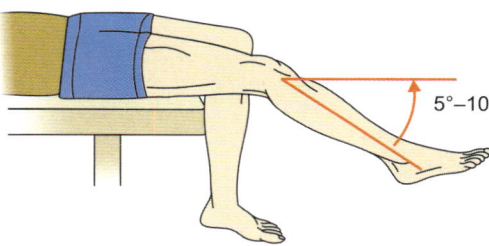

Fig. 24.12: Extensor lag following patellectomy

ACUTE DISLOCATION OF PATELLA

Lateral dislocation of patella are very common and are due to lateral force acting on a semi-flexed knee. Patient complains of severe pain, swelling and inability to bend the knee. Patella is seen and felt on the lateral side. Plain X-ray of the knee help in making the diagnosis.

24

Treatment

Closed reduction and above knee POP casting is done under GA. Immobilization in a long leg cast may be required for a period of 4–6 weeks.

ACUTE DISLOCATION OF KNEE

This is an uncommon injury and is due to severe violence as in RTA, fall, etc. (Fig. 24.13). It is usually associated with injuries to collaterals cruciates and meniscus. Patella may also be fractured or dislocated.

Treatment

Conservative: An attempt may be made for closed reduction under GA. An above knee POP cast is applied for 12 weeks.

Surgery: Open reduction may be required if the closed reduction fails or if there is extensive ligament injuries, repair, reconstruction, or both may be required. Knee is immobilized in an above knee POP cast for 12 weeks.

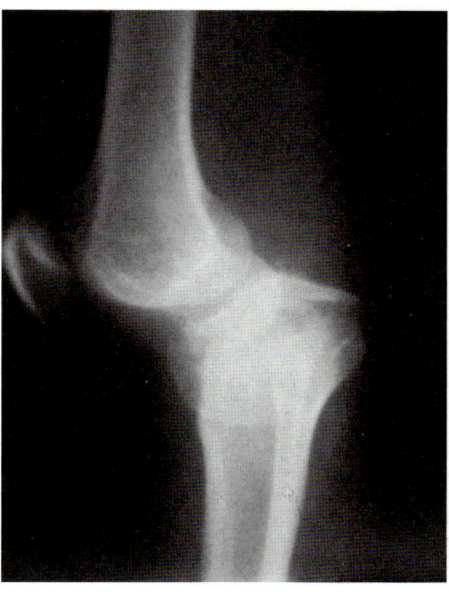

Fig. 24.13: Posterior dislocation of the knee

24

25

Injuries Around the Ankle

BRIEF ANATOMY OF THE ANKLE JOINT

It is a complex joint made up of distal ends of tibia, fibula and dome of the talus. The tibiofibular joint functions as a uniplanar hinge joint and in which about 25° of dorsiflexion and 35° of plantar flexion takes place. It is fully congruous in all positions. The stability is provided by the configuration of the ankle mortice and the ligaments which are arranged in the following three groups (Figs 25.1A and B).

Medial collateral ligament: It consists of deltoid ligament with a superficial and deep part.

Lateral collateral ligament: It is formed by anterior and posterior talofibular ligaments and calcaneofibular ligament.

Syndesmotic ligament: These are formed by the anterior tibiofibular ligament, the posterior tibiofibular ligament, the inferior transverse ligament and the interosseous ligament.

The posterior malleoli is the third malleolus other than the medial and lateral malleoli. It is formed by the posterior distal tibial articular surface.

ANKLE INJURIES

The ankle mortice is formed by the distal articular surface of the tibia, fibula, the intervening tibiofibular ligament and the inner articular surfaces of the medial and lateral malleoli. The strong ankle mortice and the ligaments make these dislocations a rarity. However, fracture dislocations do occur at a greater frequency. Pott described ankle injuries for the first time in 1768.

Mechanism of Injuries

- Twisting injury while walking, running, sports, athletes, etc. are the most common mode of ankle injuries (Figs 25.2A to C).
- *Fall from a height:* These are indirect injuries brought about by the displacing talus.

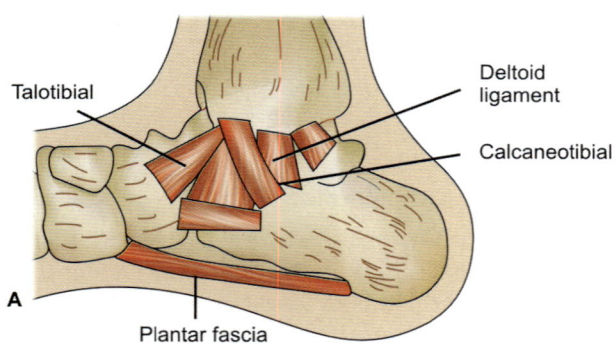

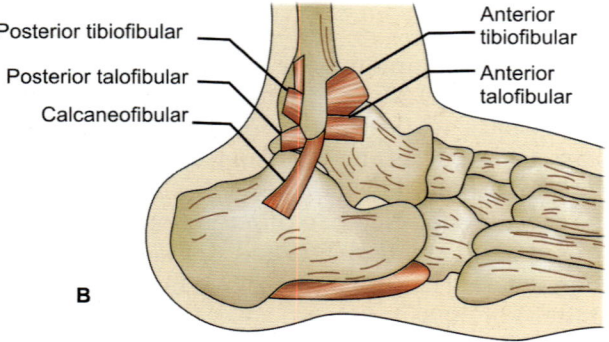

Figs 25.1A and B: Anatomy of ankle ligaments: (A) Medial side, (B) Lateral side

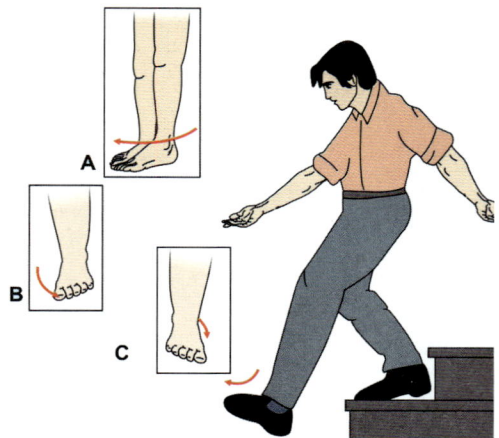

Figs 25.2A to C: Common mechanism of ankle injuries: (A) external rotation force, (B) abduction force, (C) adduction force

131

Classification

Ankle injuries are classified after the mechanism causing them. Hence it is of paramount importance to understand the movement of the ankle to comprehend the classification. What complicates the issue is the practice of using more than one term to describe the same motion.

There are six movements of the ankle and the hindfoot. *Plantar flexion* and *dorsiflexion* are the up and down movements of the foot. Movement causing the toes to point inwards is called *internal rotation* and movement causing the toes to point outwards is called *external rotation. Supination* is the movement which raises the medial aspect of the foot and the heel off the ground. In *pronation* the motion is to bring the lateral aspect of the foot and the heel from the ground. In *adduction,* the hindfoot is moves towards the midline and in *abduction* it moves laterally (Fig. 25.3). Pure vertical loading position as in landing, jumping, falling, etc. will cause pylon fracture by the driving of the talus into the tibia (see Fig. 26.1).

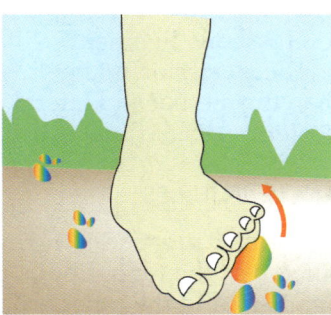

Fig. 25.3: Mechanism of eversion injuries

Lauge Hansen's Classification (Table 25.1)

Four major types are described (Fig. 25.4). The mechanism of injury could be adduction force, abduction force or supination and pronation force. First word refers to the position of the foot at the time of injury and the second to the direction of injuring force.

Note: About 75 percent of the cases fall into the first two groups.

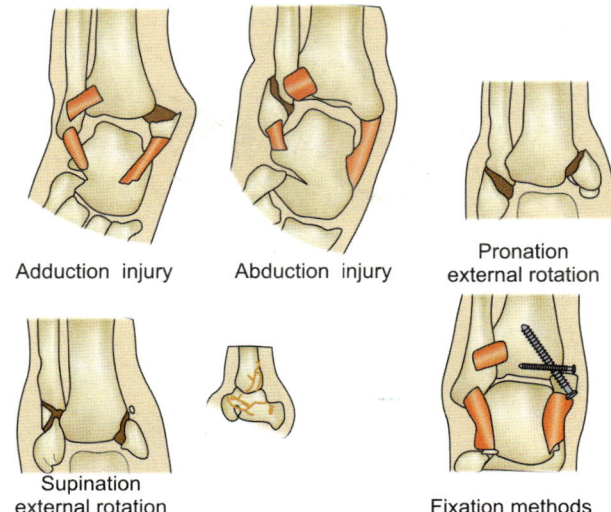

Adduction injury   Abduction injury   Pronation external rotation

Supination external rotation   Fixation methods

Fig. 25.4: Lauge Hansen's classification of ankle injuries

Table 25.1: Lauge Hansen's classification	
Supination adduction (Adduction injuries)	
Stage I	Transverse fracture of lateral malleolus or tear of lateral collateral ligament
Stage II	Stage I + fracture of medial malleolus
Pronation abduction (Abduction injuries)	
Stage I	Rupture of anterior inferior tibiofibular ligament
Stage II	Stage I + spiral oblique fracture of the lateral malleolus
Stage III	Stage II + posterior lip of fracture of tibia (posterior malleolar fracture)
Stage IV	Stage III + fracture medial malleolus or tear of deltoid ligament
Pronation external rotation	
Stage I	Fracture medial malleolus or tear of deltoid ligament
Stage II	Stage I + rupture of anteroinferior tibiofibular ligament and posterior inferior tibiofibular ligament with fracture posterior lip of tibia
Stage III	Stage II + oblique supramalleolar fracture of the fibula.
Supination external rotation	
Stage I	Fracture medial malleolus or tear of deltoid ligament
Stage II	Stage I + tear of anteroinferior tibiofibular and interosseous ligament
Stage III	Stage II + tear of interosseous membrane and spiral fracture of the fibula
Stage IV	Stage III + fracture of posterior lip of tibia due to ligamentous avulsion by posterior inferior and inferior and transverse tibiofibular ligament

Note: Pott's fracture refers to bimalleolar fracture; Cotton's fracture refers to trimalleolar fracture

Denis Weber Classification

This is the other classification proposed for ankle injuries and it is based on the *level of the fibular fracture,* while the Lauge Hansen's system is based on experimentally verified injury mechanism like adduction, abduction.

Adduction Injuries

This is the most common ankle injury. It happens when the ankle is forcefully adducted when you stumble upon an object while walking or getting down from the staircase. Athletes and sportsperson are more prone for such injuries (Fig. 25.2C).

The ankle is subjected two different forces, compression force on the medial side and distraction force on the lateral side. The sum of these two forces determine the pattern of injuries.

On the lateral side, there could be either a partial or a complete rupture of the lateral ligament and there could even be a low transverse fracture of the lateral

malleolus. These injuries could occur in isolation or in combination.

On the medial side, the scenario is different. An upwardly running oblique fracture of the medial malleolus starting at the angle of the ankle mortice is a distinct possibility.

Abduction Injuries

Here the pattern of injuries is opposite to that of the ones mentioned above (Fig. 25.2B). The medial side is subjected to distractive and the lateral side to compressive forces. Consequently, on the medial side, we get a partial or complete rupture of the deltoid ligament and sometimes if the force is more, there could be even an avulsion fracture of the medial malleoli. However, the compressive forces on the lateral side may result in oblique fractures of the lateral malleoli. If the forces are unkind then there could be comminution of the lateral cortex of the lateral malleolus (Fig. 25.6).

Pronation External Rotation Injuries

Here the talus rotates outwards on the vertical axis subjecting the medial structures to distractive forces and the lateral structures to compressive forces. In addition, there is a twisting element to both these forces which plays havoc with the ankle joint structures (Fig. 25.2A). Medially there could be a tear of the deltoid ligament or the transverse fracture of the medial malleolus. On the lateral side, the tibia fibular syndesmosis, may give way due to the rupture of the anterior tibiofibular ligament. If this happens the forces are free to break the fibula at its lower end or even as high as at the neck of the fibula (called the *Massionaive's fracture*). It is now obvious that the fibular fracture will be either spiral or oblique.

Dupuytren's Fracture

Here there is complete diastosis of inferior tibiofibular syndesmosis and comminuted fracture of the lower end of fibula.

Tillaux Fracture

This is an avulsion fracture of the anterior or posterior tip of the inferior fibular facet of the tibia.

Supination External Rotation Injuries

An externally rotating talus in a supinated foot presents a different scenario. A lax medial structure ensures that the catastrophe first strikes the lateral malleolus (causing a spiral fracture), then knocks off the posterior malleolus and if the forces continue unabated, it will cause transverse fracture of the medial malleolus. While all the three malleoli lies in ruins, the tibiofibular syndesmosis is still holding its fort. This trimalleolar fracture is known as "Cotton's fracture" (Fig. 25.6).

Axial or Vertically Compressive Forces

So far we have read about the misadventure of a tilting or a twisting talus. Now imagine the consequences if the talus decides to bull doze through the joint. Such an event is possible by a vertically compression force, so often a result of fall from the height and land on the feet phenomena. There could be comminuted fracture of the distal tibial articular surface (called the **Pylon fracture**) and fracture of the fibula. A less unkind force can just cause a marginal chip fracture of the anterior tibial margins of distal tibia.

Clinical Features

Patient usually gives history of inversion, eversion or rotational injury, following which there is pain, swelling, deformity of the ankle. Movements are decreased, Drawer's test, inversion and eversion stress tests may be positive.

Radiology: Anteroposterior, lateral and mortise views of the ankle are recommended in the radiographs. Radiology in ankle injuries speaks quite eloquently provided one sees it properly (Figs 25.5 and 25.6). Unlike in other fractures, radiology here helps you to study the fracture anatomy, enables you to guess the

25

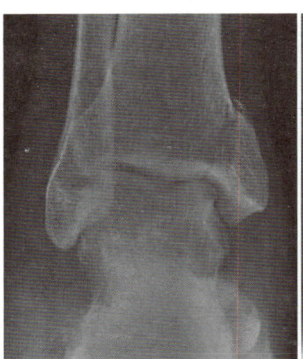 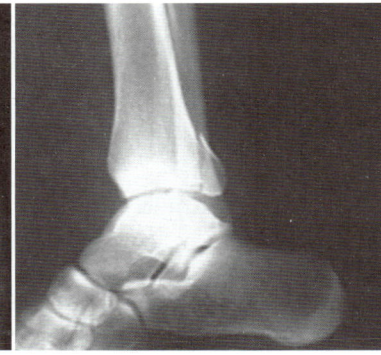

Fig. 25.5A: Medial malleolar fracture   **Fig. 25.5B:** Posterior malleolus fracture

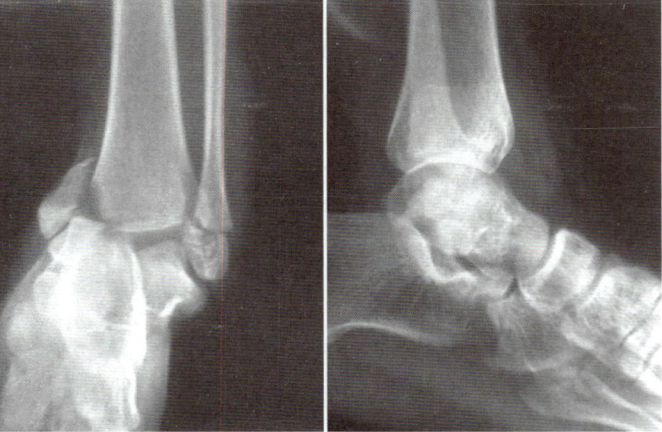

Figs 25.5C: Bimalleolar fracture

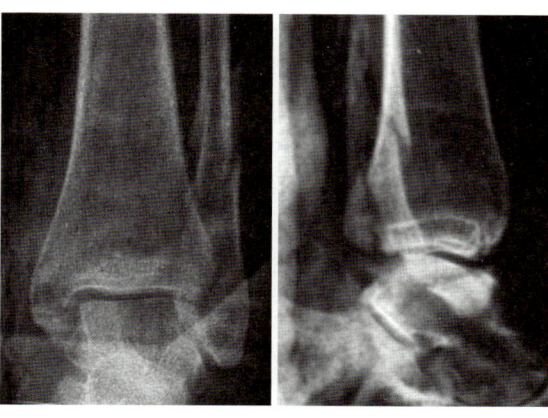

Fig. 25.6: Trimalleolar ankle fracture AP view and lateral view

nature of injury and plan the line of treatment. In fact it is hoping to tell you stories provided you have the eye to see it (Table 25.2).

Table 25.2: Radiological findings in ankle injury

Findings	Interpretation
• Transverse fracture	This is always the first to occur.
• Oblique/spiral fracture	This is the last to occur
• Inferior tibiofibular syndesmosis broke	Look for fibular fracture from lateral malleoli to the neck of the fibula
• Three malleoli fracture	Usually a supination, external rotation injury
• Huge soft tissue swelling	Suggests ligament sprain

Treatment of Ankle Injuries

Goals of the treatment: Whatever the ankle fractures, basic principles of treatment remain the same and consist of the following:

- Anatomical positioning of the talus and restoration of the ankle mortise.
- To obtain a joint line that is parallel to the ground and the knee joint.
- Smooth articular surface to be restored.

If these three things are not achieved, post-traumatic osteoarthritis results.

For stable injuries no reduction is required, immobilization with only plaster splints till the swelling decreases and then a below-knee plaster cast is applied with foot in neutral position (Fig. 25.7).

Unstable injuries require reduction and immobilization in plaster casts. The commonly encountered unstable injuries are:

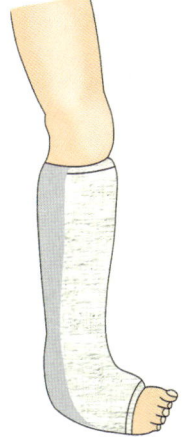

Fig. 25.7: A below knee plaster cast

a. *Fracture due to external rotation:* This is more common and can be managed both by conservative and operative methods.
Conservative method: This consists of reversal of the injuring forces by closed reduction (Fig. 25.8) and a below-knee plaster cast application. A walking cast is applied after a period of one month.
Surgical method: In these both the malleoli are fixed, first the lateral malleoli is fixed with pin or screws and later the medial malleolar fracture is fixed with a single screw perpendicular to the fracture line. Below knee splint is given initially and later a cast is applied.

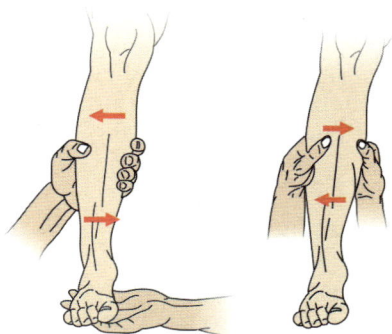

Fig. 25.8: Method of reduction of displaced ankle fractures

b. *Fracture primarily due to abduction:* These are less common than the fractures due to external rotation. Nevertheless, the principles of the treatment remain the same. Adduction force is required to bring about reduction and if closed reduction fails, open reduction is preferred. During the open reduction, both the malleoli are fixed (Figs 25.9A and B).

c. *Fracture primarily due to adduction:* Unlike external rotation and abduction, adduction violence is more frequently an isolated event. Wedging of small comminuted fragments into the fracture line often prevents closed reduction, so that open reduction and internal fixation (ORIF) is required more frequently. Medial malleolus is approached first, since it is more unstable, and the fracture is fixed with two screws one at a right angle to tibial cortex and another at right angle to the fracture line (Fig. 25.9). Lateral fibular fracture is stabilized with plate and screws (Fig. 25.9C).

d. *Fracture resulting from primarily vertical compression:* This may be isolated or associated with other forces described above. The anterior and posterior tibial plafond margins are fractured. Two types are described:
Posterior marginal fracture for undisplaced fracture below knee cast is sufficient. For more than 25 percent of articular surface involvement, ORIF with 2 screws is preferred.

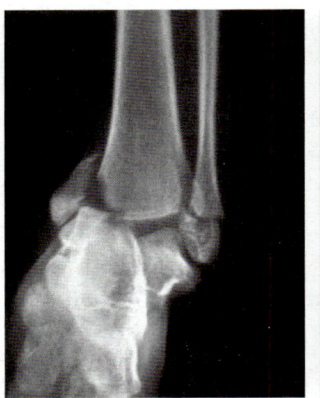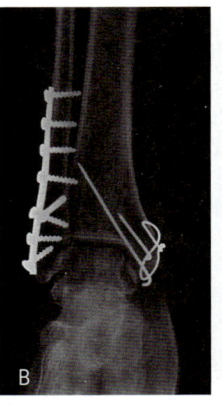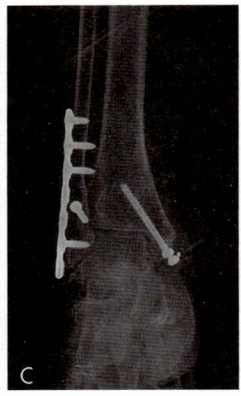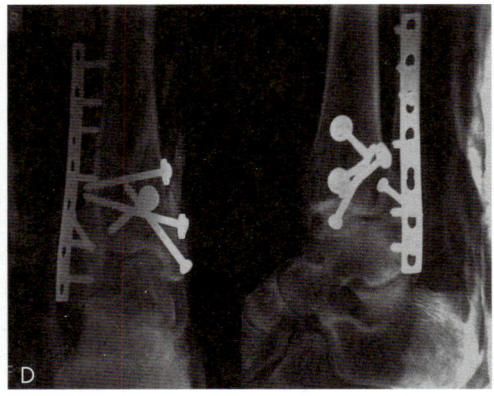

Figs. 25.9A to D: (A) bimalleolar fracture, (B) bimalleolar fracture fixation (plate and TBW), (C) bimalleolar fixation (plate and malleolar screw), (D) long plate and interfragmentary screw

Anterior marginal fracture (tibial plafond injury): It may include a crush of the anterior lip or it may include a major fragment. If crushed, calcaneal traction is given and if there is a large fragment, ORIF is required (Fig. 25.9D).

Complications of ankle fracture include post-traumatic arthritis, reflex sympathetic dystrophy, neurovascular injury (injury to posterior tibial vessels and nerve), nonunion (due to soft tissue interposition), malunion, etc.

ANKLE SPRAIN

These are common injury in sports. If improperly treated it may result in chronic laxity, pain or delayed recovery.

Lateral Ligament Sprain

This is the most common musculoskeletal injury with an incidence of 1/10,000/day. In 85 percent of cases it is due to inversion of supinated plantar flexed foot. The lateral ligament commonly injured is anterior talofibular ligament followed by calcaneofibular ligament (Fig. 25.10). The posterior talofibular ligament is rarely sprained.

Clinical Features

The patient complains of pain, swelling and tenderness over the affected ligament (Fig. 25.11). *Anterior drawer test* is positive and it is performed by stabilizing distal tibia with one hand, then grasps the posterior heel with the opposite hand and applies anterior force. If the displacement of talus is more than 8 mm anterior, it suggests laxity of the anterior talofibular ligament. Next, the talar tilt test is performed, if the tilt is more than 5°, it suggests laxity of anterior talofibular and calcaneofibular ligaments.

Radiograph of the ankle: Plain X-ray of the ankle joint AP, lateral and oblique views. If the talar tilt of the injured

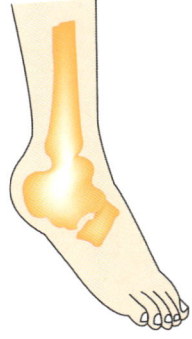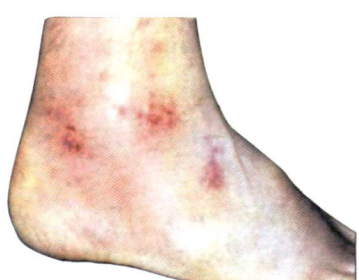

Fig. 25.10: Lateral ligament sprain (due to adduction injury)

Fig. 25.11: Clinical appearance of an ankle sprain

ankle is 10° greater than the uninjured ankle it is considered as significant.

Grading of Ankle Sprain

Grade I: Minimal pain, mild swelling and no laxity.
Grade II: Mild to moderate laxity, soft tissue swelling, anterior drawer and talar tilt is slightly positive.
Grade III: Severe swelling and pain, the anterior drawer and talar tilt tests are highly positive.

Treatment

Grade I sprain: Rest, Ice therapy, Compression bandage, foot Elevation, (RICE), Non-steroidal anti-inflammatory drugs (NSAIDs), crutch walking, etc. are the recommended treatment. Ankle straps help to maintain stability (Fig. 25.12).

Grade II sprain: Long leg cast, range of motion exercises, strengthening exercises, etc. are helpful.

Grade III sprain: Same lines as mentioned above and sometimes may rarely require surgical repair.

Medial Ligament Sprain

This is due to pronation eversion injury. In mild sprains, only the superficial part of the deltoid ligament is torn

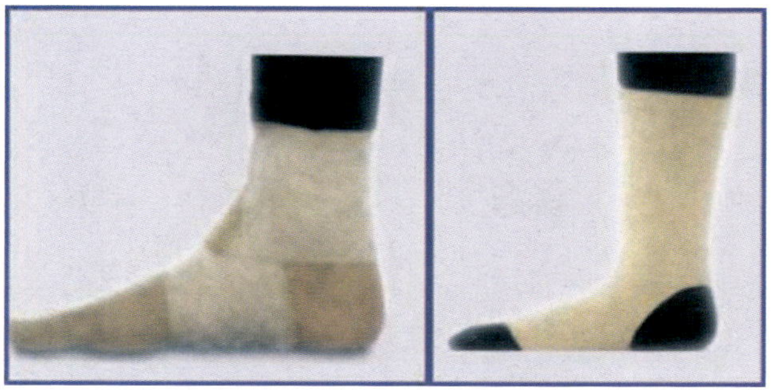

Fig. 25.12: Ankle strap

but in severe forms the deep part of the deltoid ligament is also torn resulting in a lateral talar tilt. If this exceeds more than 2 mm, significant alteration in the weightbearing mechanism takes place resulting in post-traumatic arthritis. For mild sprains, conservative treatment is sufficient and for severe sprains surgical reduction and repair are considered.

Remember

Know the concept of **RICE** in the treatment of ankle sprains: This is a simple and effective functional method of treatment of ankle sprains and consists of:
- R–rest to the ankle.
- I–ice therapy for 2 days.
- C–compression by Jones bandaging technique to decrease the swelling.
- E–elevation of the limb to drain the swelling.

25

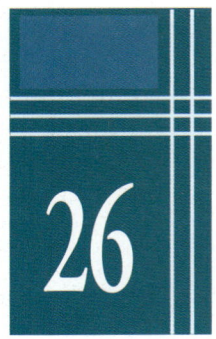

26 | Injuries of the Foot

- Calcaneum fracture
- Talus fracture
- Metatarsal fracture
- Jones fracture
- March fracture
- Phalangeal fracture
- Chopart's fracture
- Lisfranc's injury

CALCANEUM FRACTURE

Calcaneum is the most often fractured tarsal bone: No ideal method of treatment has been described yet.

> **INTERESTING FACTS**
> Calcaneum fractures are also known as Don-Juan or Lover's fracture

Anatomy

It is the heel bone and articulates above with the talus and with the cuboid in front. It is mostly cancellous in nature and has a thin cortical shell except at the posterior tuberosity. Two types of trabecular pattern are described (See Fig. 26.6).

1. *Traction trabeculae:* this radiates from the inferior cortex.
2. *Compression trabeculae:* Converge to support anterior and posterior facets.

The superior surface has three articular facets namely concave anterior and middle facets and convex posterior facet.

Mechanism of Injury

Twisting forces cause many of the extraarticular fractures. *Fall from height* and land on the feet phenomena causes a vast majority of intraarticular fractures (Fig. 26.1) and is due to axial loading and shearing forces. Look for associated fractures of pelvis, spine, etc. (See box).

> **Remember**
> *Vital facts*
> - Bilateral fracture is seen in 5 to 9 percent of cases.
> - Ten percent cases have compression fracture of dorsal or lumbar vertebral bodies.
> - Twenty-six percent are associated with other injuries of the lower limbs.

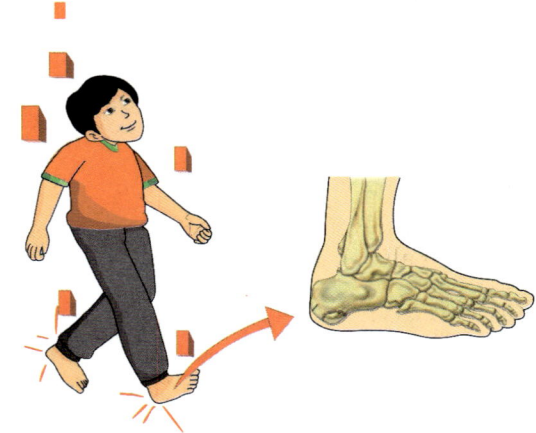

Fig. 26.1: Common mechanism of calcaneum fractures of fall and land on heels (Inset showing comminuted fracture of calcaneum)

Classification

Essex-Lopresti's classification is the most accepted classification for fracture calcaneum. It consists of extra-articular fractures (Figs 26.2A to D) (Less common accounting for only 25% of the cases) and intraarticular fractures, which is more common (Figs 26.3A to C).

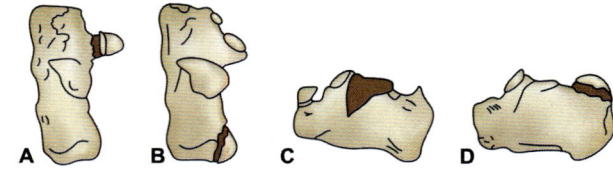

Figs 26.2A to D: Types of extra-articular fractures: (A) S. tali fracture, (B) medial process fracture, (C) anterior process fracture, and (D) tuberosity fracture

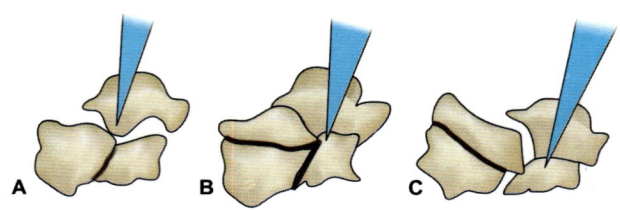

Figs 26.3A to C: Varieties of Intraarticular fractures: (A) undisplaced fracture, (B) tongue-shaped fracture, (C) comminuted fracture

137

Extraarticular (25–30%)	Intraarticular (70–75%)
1. Fracture anterior process	1. Undisplaced fracture
2. Fracture tuberosity	2. Tongue-shaped fractures
3. Medial process fracture	3. Joint depression
4. Fracture sustentaculum tali.	4. Comminuted fracture talus and body.

The other classifications are Sander's and Rowe's and is outside the scope of this book.

Extraarticular Fractures

1. Fracture of anterior process.
2. Fracture tuberosity.
3. Fracture medial calcaneal process.
4. Fracture sustentaculum tali.

Intraarticular Fractures

These account for 60 percent of all tarsal injuries and 75 percent of all calcaneal fractures.

Mechanism of Injury

Fall from height: Lateral process of the talus acts as a wedge and is forced through the Gissane's angle resulting in four fracture patterns:
• Undisplaced
• Tongue-shaped
• Joint depression
• Comminuted.

Clinical Features

After the fall, the patient may experience pain, swelling of the heel. Due to the compression, the heel may be broadened (Fig. 26.4). Patient may also complain of inability to bear weight on the heels. There may be ecchymosis around the heels after two days. Inversion and eversion of the foot may be affected but the ankle function remains unaltered. In undisplaced or incomplete fracture eliciting heel tenderness helps clinch the diagnosis (Fig. 26.5).

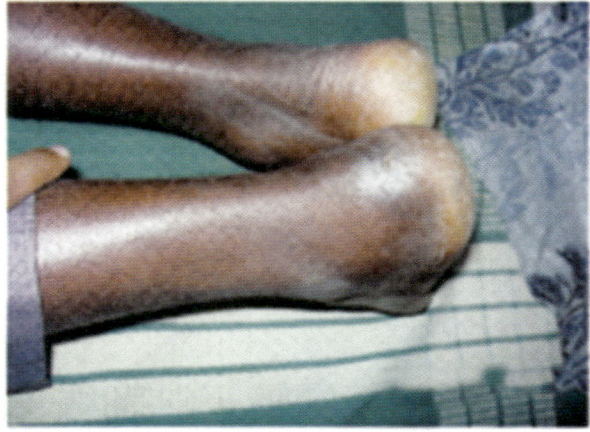

Fig. 26.4: Broadened heel in calcaneum fractures

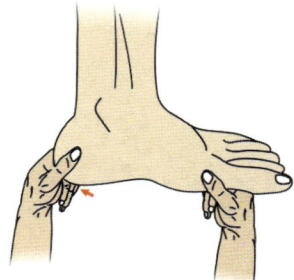

Fig. 26.5: Method of eliciting heel tenderness in calcaneum fractures

Radiograph

X-ray of the calcaneum especially the lateral view helps to make an accurate diagnosis (Fig. 26.6). Sometimes a special view like the axial view may be required. A careful study of the Bohler's and Gissane angle should be done before and after the reduction (Figs 26.7A and B). CT scan (3D scan) helps in making a better evaluation.

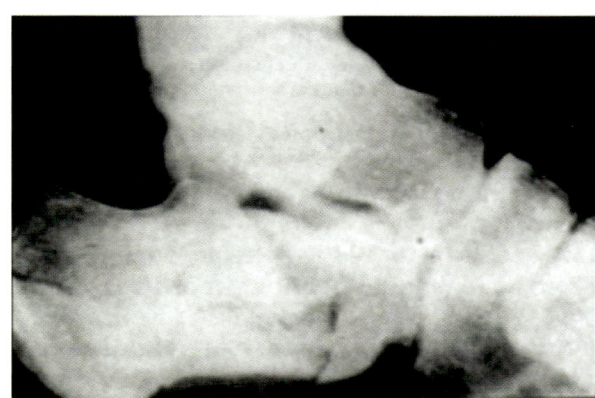

Fig. 26.6: Radiograph showing calcaneum fracture

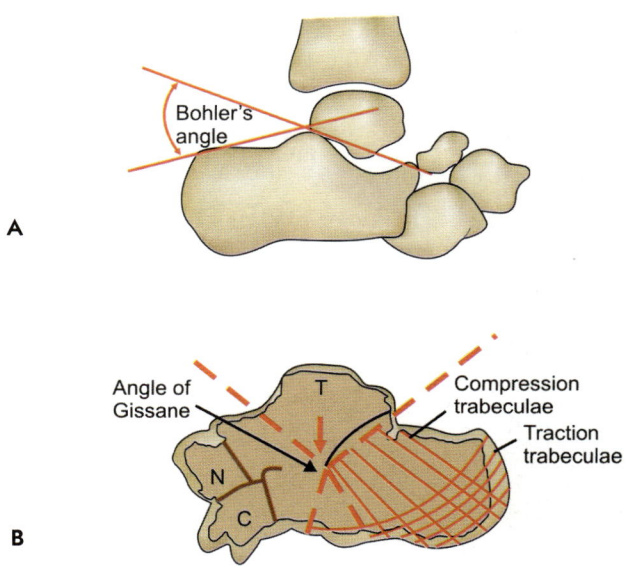

Figs 26.7A and B: (A) Bohler's angle (B) Angle of Gissane

Treatment

Aim of the treatment is to restore back both the radiological angles mentioned above. The following are the basic methods of treatment.

For undisplaced fractures: Obviously no reduction is required in these cases. A below knee cast for a period of 4–6 weeks usually helps.

For displaced fractures: Displaced calcaneum fracture needs closed reduction and fixation either by below knee calcaneum cast or by some internal fixation.

Calcaneum Cast

Here, after the reduction the leg and the foot are immobilized in a below-knee plaster cast for a period of 4–6 weeks (Fig. 26.8). After the removal of the plaster cast, compression bandage is applied for another 4–6 weeks and the foot is kept elevated during the above treatment. Weight bearing is permitted only at the end of 12 weeks.

Open Reduction

Open reduction and internal fixation with K-wires or small plate and screws with bone grafting is difficult and is rarely adopted (Figs 26.9A to C).

Complications

- Nonunion is rare due to the cancellous nature of the bone.
- Malunion is more common.
- Heel pain: The source of heel pain could be from:
  - Subtalar joint due to post-traumatic osteoarthritis.
  - Peroneal tendinitis due to stenosing tenovaginitis of the peroneal tendons.
  - Bone spurs due to malunion of fracture and disruption of fat pad of the heel.
  - Arthritis of calcaneocuboid joint is a major source.

FRACTURE TALUS

Anatomy: Talus peculiarly has no tendon or muscle attachments. It articular is with the tibia above, calcaneum below and navicular in front.

Highlights of Talus

- First discribed by Astley Cooper (1832)
- Also called Aviator's Astralgus (by Anderson in 1919).
- It takes part in weight transmission.
- It has a precarious blood supply.
- 3/5th of the bone is covered by articular cartilage.
- Sudden hyperextension of the forefoot causes fracture neck called "Aviators Astralgus".

Because of the precarious blood supply, AVN of the talus is more commonly seen in Talar neck and body fractures.

Blood Supply of Talus (Fig. 26.10)

- Sixty percent is covered by articular surface, only limited surface is available for vascular perforation.
- No muscle originates or inserts into talus.
- All the three major arteries of the foot supply talus. (Posterior tibial artery, anterior tibial artery, peroneal artery, artery of the tarsal canal and Sinus tarsi). These vessels form a plexus near the posterior tubercle and sinus tarsi.
- There is important contribution from capsular and ligamentous vessels.

Injuries of the talus are as follows:
- Talar neck fracture (common)
- Talar body fracture (rare)
- Talar head fracture
- Subtalar dislocation
- Total talar dislocation.

We will discuss about talar neck fracture as this is most common.

26

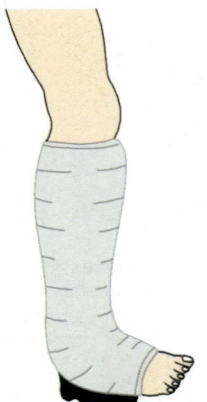

Fig. 26.8: Short leg POP cast with walking heel for calcaneum fracture

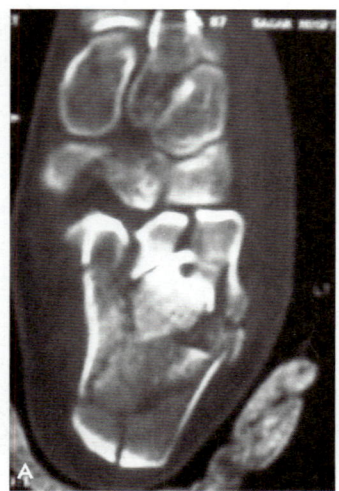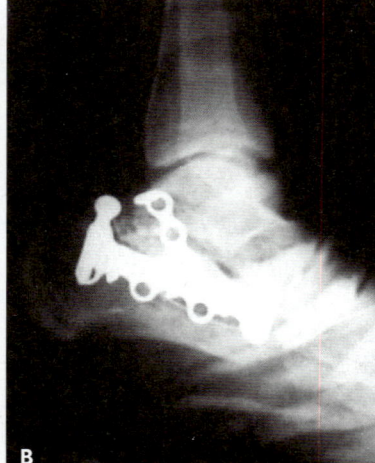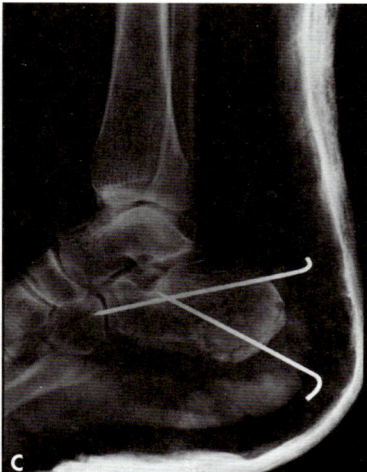

Figs 26.9A to C: (A) Comminuted calcaneum fracture, (B) Fixation with plate and screws, (C) K-wire fixation

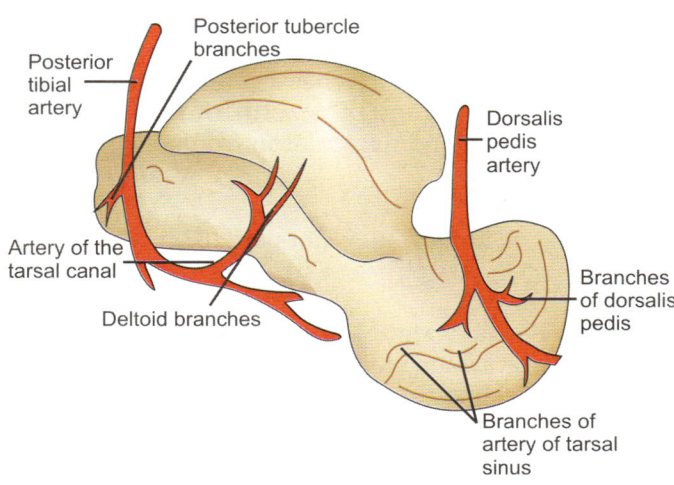

Fig. 26.10: Blood supply of talus bone

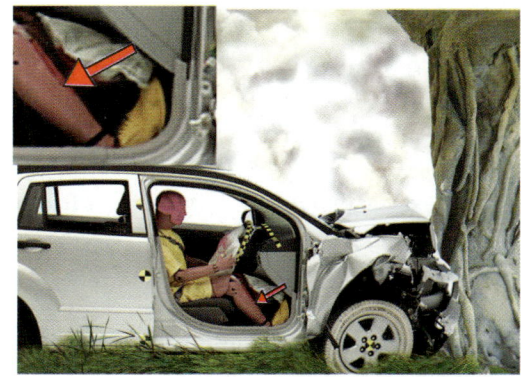

Fig. 26.11: Common mechanism of talus fracture

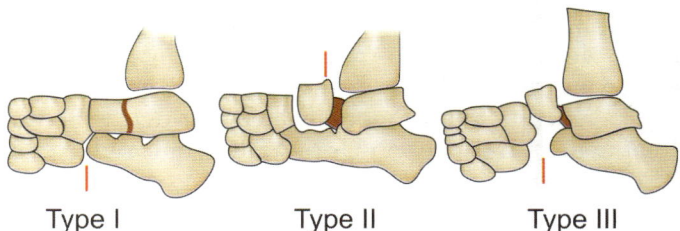

Type I   Type II   Type III

Fig. 26.12: Different types of neck of talus fractures (Hawkin's type)

Fracture Neck Talus

This is second in frequency to the chip and avulsion fracture of the talus.

Incidence is around 30 percent. Just as calcaneal fracture is common in people who are more prone for fall from heights, so is fracture neck of talus. It is more commonly seen in people who drive four wheelers and aircraft and get involved in a head on collision accidents.

Mechanism of Injury

The common mode of injury is hyperdorsiflexion of the foot on one leg. It may be associated with fracture of tarsal bones and fracture of the metatarsal bones.

The driver of any four-wheeler like car, bus, lorry etc. or of an aircraft, meets with an accident and has a head on collision with another vehicle, tree or any other object. If his foot is on the brake pedal at the time of impact, then it is forced into hyperdorsiflexion. In this position, the anterior rim of the tibia slices through the weak and unprotected neck of the talus breaking it. It was earlier popularly called the 'aviator's fracture' due to aircraft accidents. Now it is more commonly seen in automobile accidents (Fig. 26.11). Depending upon the severity of the forces, the fracture could be undisplaced or displaced.

Classification: Hawkin's has described three varieties of fractures (Fig. 26.12):
- Undisplaced fracture
- Displaced with subtalar joint involvement
- Displaced with both subtalar and ankle joint involvement.

Clinical features: There will be history of pain, swelling and in ability to bear weight. Movement of the ankle and subtalar joints are painfully restricted.

Radiography: The views recommended are AP view with foot in maximum equinus and 15° pronation, lateral and oblique views of the ankle joint (Fig. 26.13A).

Treatment

Undisplaced fractures: This is best treated by below-knee plaster cast for a period of 8–10 weeks.

Displaced fractures: In this, closed reduction is done by traction in plantar flexion and a plaster cast is put in equinus. If this fails, ORIF with lag screws is done. In these, approximately 25 percent are open fractures. Debridement is done first and closed reduction is attempted later. If unsuccessful, ORIF with K-wires or open reduction with lag screws is attempted (Fig. 26.13B).

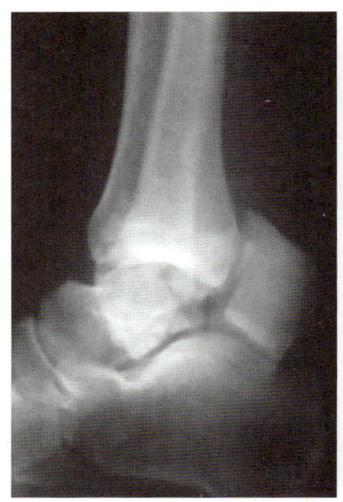

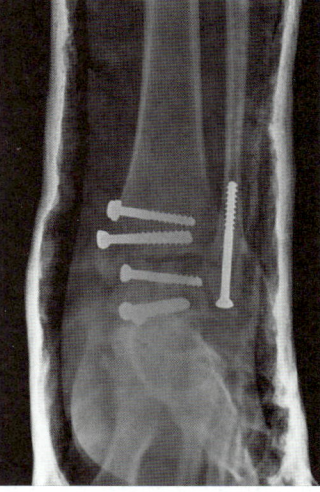

Fig. 26.13A: Plain X-ray showing fracture neck of talus

Fig. 26.13B: Talus fracture fixation

Other treatment method (4 As)

- **A**rthroscopy: To remove loose osteochondral fragments
- **A**rthroplasty: In AVN and Sec. OA
- **A**rthrodesis: In severely damaged joint due to Sec. OA
- **A**stragelectomy: As a salvage procedure.

Complications

Skin necrosis, infection, delayed union, nonunion, malunion, avascular necrosis (Fig. 26.14); post-traumatic arthritis, etc. are some of the well-known complications of fracture talus.

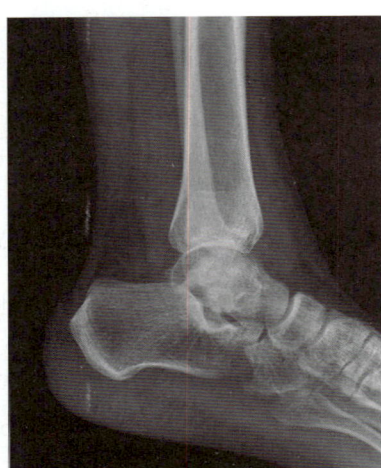

Fig. 26.14: AVN talus

METATARSAL FRACTURE

Common mechanism of injury is direct due to fall of a heavy object on the foot.

Clinical Features

Patient complains of pain, swelling and tenderness over the dorsum of the foot. There could be considerable soft tissue swelling. Limp is present. Pain in the foot increases with weight bearing.

Radiology

Plain X-ray with AP, lateral and oblique views help to make the diagnosis (Fig. 26.15).

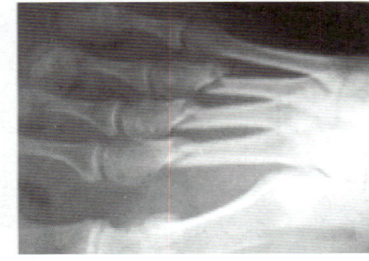

Fig. 26.15: Plain X-ray showing multiple metatarsal fractures

Treatment

Conservative treatment is by NWB below-knee plaster cast for 6 to 8 weeks for stable fractures with no loss of bone length.

Operative treatment is reserved for displaced and unstable fractures by closed reduction and percutaneous fixation with K-wires (Fig. 26.15), screws only or with plate and screws.

JONES FRACTURE

It is a fracture of the diaphysis of the fifth metatarsal bone approximately 1.5 to 3.0 cm above the tip of the tuberosity. This was first described by Sir Robert Jones in 1902.

Mechanism of Injury

This is due to indirect violence.

Clinical Features

Patient complains of pain, swelling and limp. On examination, tenderness can be elicited over the base of the fifth metatarsal bone.

Radiology: Radiograph of the foot helps to confirm the diagnosis (Fig. 26.16A).

Treatment

Treatment is essentially conservative and consists of the application of a below knee plaster for a period of 3 to 4 weeks. Surgical stabilization with a screw in may be considered in displaced fractures and in athletes (Fig. 26.16B).

Pseudo Jones-Fracture

This is also called as Tennis fracture. It is an avulsion fracture due to the pull of the peroneus brevis muscle.

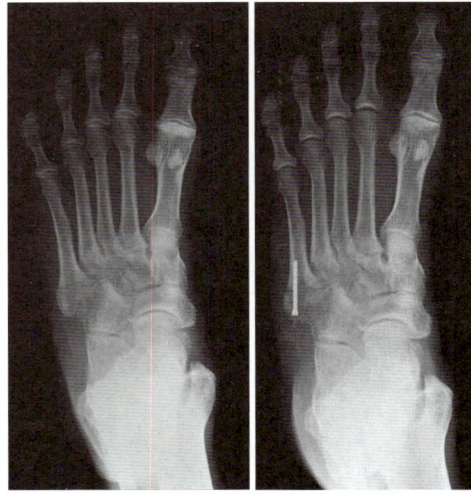

Figs 26.16A and B: (A) Jones fracture, (B) Jones fracture fixed with a screw

26

Treatment: This is mainly conservative and consists of compression bandage or a below knee walking cast for 3 weeks.

MARCH FRACTURE

This is a stress or fatigue fracture of the metatarsals particularly the second or third metatarsal bone. It is more often encountered in military personnel who indulge in frequent and prolonged marching and hence its name. It is also seen in police officers, dancers, nurses and surgeons who require to dance or stand for a long duration. Pain, tenderness and limp could be the usual complaints. Radiograph helps in the diagnosis (Fig. 26.17) and treatment is rest and symptomatic like NSAIDs, splints, elasto crepe bandage application, etc.

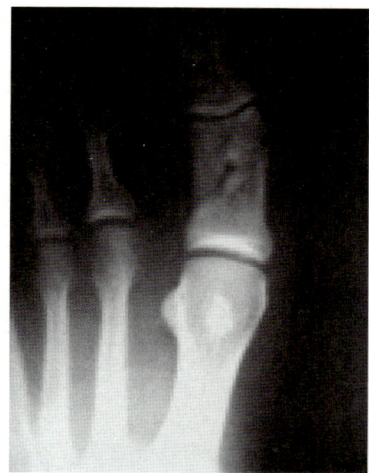

Fig. 26.18: Comminuted phalangeal fracture

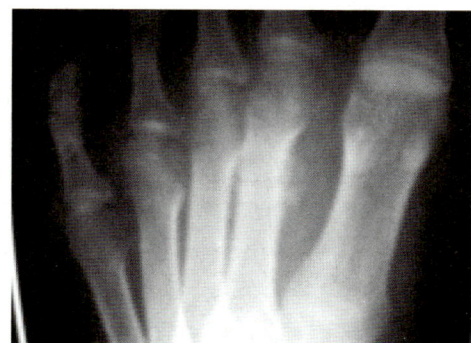

Fig. 26.17: Plain X-ray showing march fracture

PHALANGEAL FRACTURE

This is the most common injury of the foot. Proximal phalanx is more commonly injured than all other phalanx. Direct blow due to fall of a heavy object on the toes is the common mechanism of injury.

Clinical Features

The patient presents with pain, swelling, limp and difficulty to wear the footwear.

Radiology

Standard AP and lateral films of the forefoot help to make the diagnosis (Fig. 26.18).

Treatment

It consists of buddy taping for undisplaced and slightly displaced fractures. Operative treatment is indicated for grossly unstable intra-articular fractures. The treatment method of choice is closed reduction and percutaneous K-wire fixation or open reduction, K-wire or screw fixation.

Chopart's Fracture

It is a mid-foot fracture involving the talonavicular and calcaneocuboid joints and is commonly due to twisting force (80%) and rarely due to eversion force. Patient presents with pain swelling, limp, etc. There could be associated fractures of the calcaneum, talus and navicular bones.

Plain X-ray of the foot helps to make a diagnosis.

Treatment consists of conservative methods like plaster immobilization, etc. for mild cases and operative reduction and stabilization for more severe cases.

Lisfranc's Injury

This is a fracture or fracture dislocation of the tarometatarsal joints. The common mechanism of injury is severe plantar flexion of the foot.

If all the metatarsals are dislocated to the same side, it is called homolateral and if dislocated in different directions, it is divergent (more severe). These could be associated fractures of other tarsal and metatarsal bones.

Plain X-ray of the foot helps in making the diagnosis.

Treatment consists of conservative management like plasters for mild injury, for more severe injury closed reduction and pinning or open reduction and internal fixation is done.

26

4

Injuries of the Pelvis and Spine

27 Fractures of the Pelvis and Trunk

Brief anatomy
Pelvis fracture
Coccyx fractures
Ribs fractures

BRIEF ANATOMY

Pelvis is made up of two innominate bones, a portion of spine and sacrum. The innominate bone is formed by fusion of three separate bones, the ilium, ischium and pubis. The ilium forms the superior part, the ischium the posteroinferior part, the pubis the antero-inferior part. These three bones meet to form the acetabulum. Anteriorly it is connected by a strong minimally mobile fibrocartilaginous joint called the pubis symphysis. Posteriorly it articulates with the sacrum through the almost immobile sacroiliac joint. It derives its stability in the posterior aspect from the sacroiliac and the sacrospinous ligament complex, anteriorly by the pubic symphysis and inferiorly by the muscles and ligaments forming the pelvic floor and perineum. The main functions are:

- To transmit the forces from the spine to the lower limbs and vice versa.
- In the standing position it transmits the weight through the ilium and in the sitting position through the ischium.
- It gives attachment to the muscles helping in posture and locomotion.
- It protects the vital genitourinary system and lower abdominal viscera.

Fracture Pelvis: Stability Facts

Stability of the pelvis: It depends on both bony and ligamentous structures. Anterior portion of the pelvic ring neither participates in normal weight bearing nor is it essential for maintenance of pelvic stability. The posterior arch is formed by the sacrum, SI joints and iliac bone and is the weight-bearing portion of the pelvis. The posterosuperior SI ligaments provide most of the ligamentous stability of the SI joints.

Stable pelvic fracture: These fractures do not involve the pelvic ring and they are minimally displaced.
Unstable pelvic fracture: They involve the pelvic ring and are widely displaced. Pelvic fractures pose a problem

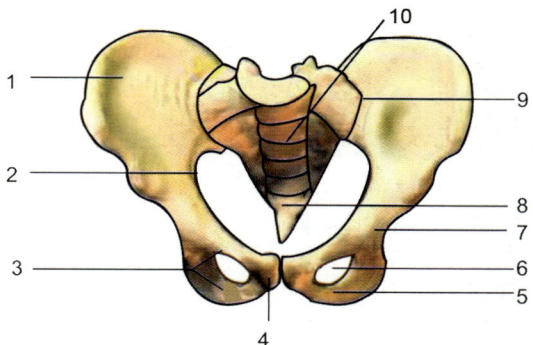

Fig. 27.1: Bony anatomy of pelvis (1) Ilium (2) Iliopentineal line (3) Pubic rami (4) Pubis symphysis (5) Ischium (6) Obturator foramen (7) Acetabulum (8) Coccyx (9) SI joint (10) Sacrum

different from others. Here the emphasis is on recognition of potential complications associated with these fractures, the notable ones being injuries to the major vessels and nerves of the pelvis and major viscera like intestines, bladder and urethra, severe intrapelvic hemorrhage from fracture of pelvic ring. Mortality from pelvic fracture varies from 10 to 50 percent. Proper fracture management decreases the blood loss and controls the hemorrhage. A to F management as proposed by MacMurthy in multiple trauma patients is important in management of the pelvic fractures.

VITAL PRACTICE POINTS
A to F management of MacMurthy
 A Airway management
 B Blood and fluid replacement
 C Central nervous system management
 D Digestive system management
 E Excretory system management
 F Fracture management

History: Pelvic fractures usually occur due to high-velocity trauma following a road traffic accident (RTA) or due to fall from a height. The relative incidences are as follows:

- RTA—80.7 percent
- Fall—16.1 percent
- Compression fracture—rest

Mechanism of Injury

There are four mechanisms by which pelvic ring fractures are produced:

144

in shear. At the affected level, one part of sacral canal has been displaced in the transverse plane.

Clinical Features

Patient gives history of trauma due to RTA or fall from height and complains of pain, posterior swelling, tenderness, palpable interspinous gap or a step may be felt. Neurological involvement may vary from paraplegia to individual nerve root involvement. Spinal shock is present for 24 hrs during which all the reflexes are lost. Cauda equina paralysis is present if the lesion is below L_1.

Investigations

Radiography of the affected spine: This is the preliminary investigation and all three views (AP, lateral and oblique) are taken (Fig. 28.23).

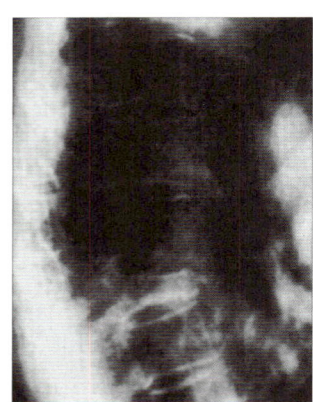

Fig. 28.23: Radiograph showing flexion anterior compression fracture of T_{12} vertebra

CT scan and MRI: Both CT scan and MRI have found to be more useful than radiographs in evaluation of spinal trauma. While CT scan helps in studying the bony elements, MRI helps in the study of both bone and soft tissue elements. The damage to the cord is detected fairly accurately and is now being considered as the "gold standard" in the investigation of spine injury (Fig. 28.24).

Management

This is discussed under two heads.

Management at the site of accident: This consists of careful handling of the patient suspected to have spine injury. Consider all patients with spine injury to have neurological damage and shift them to the hospital with utmost care and caution avoiding all unnecessary movements.

Definitive treatment at the hospital: This varies depending upon the nature of injury and the presence or absence of neurological damage.

• *Practice:* Caution in handling the neck.

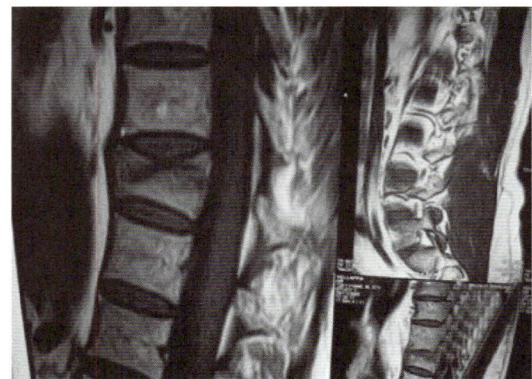

Fig. 28.24: MRI showing fracture to T_6 Vertebra

• *Examination:* The general condition and other systems like CNS/CVS/RS/PA/GI tract. Also, examine from head to toe, the presence of other fractures, head, chest injuries, blunt injury abdomen and pelvic fractures.
• *Evaluate:* The spine injury by gentle careful clinical examination. This has to be supplemented by proper investigations like X-ray, CT-scan, MRI.
• *Assess:* Carefully assess the level and extent of neurological damage by examining the dermatome, myotome and reflexes.
• *Plan:* After evaluating and assessing the damage, plan the line of treatment. The treatment options include nonoperative, traction and operative methods. Now let us carefully look into various treatment modalities:

Treatment Methods

a. *For stable fracture without neurological deficit:* Less than 30 percent anterior wedge, lateral, central compression fracture of the vertebral body is considered as stable fracture. In these injuries there is no fracture of the posterior cortex of the vertebral body, and there is no disruption of the neural arch.
Treatment: This is essentially conservative and consists of bed rest, NSAIDs and external spine supports like brace, corsets (Fig. 28.25). If the vertebral body compression is less than 30 percent,

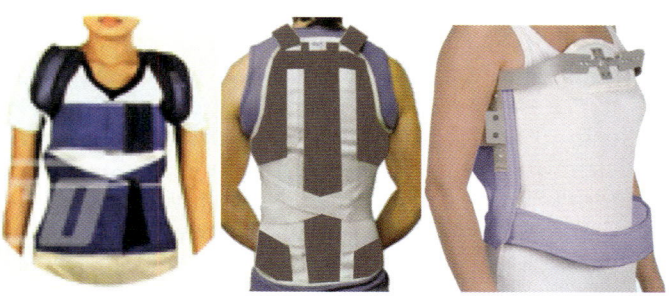

Fig. 28.25: Various spinal corsets

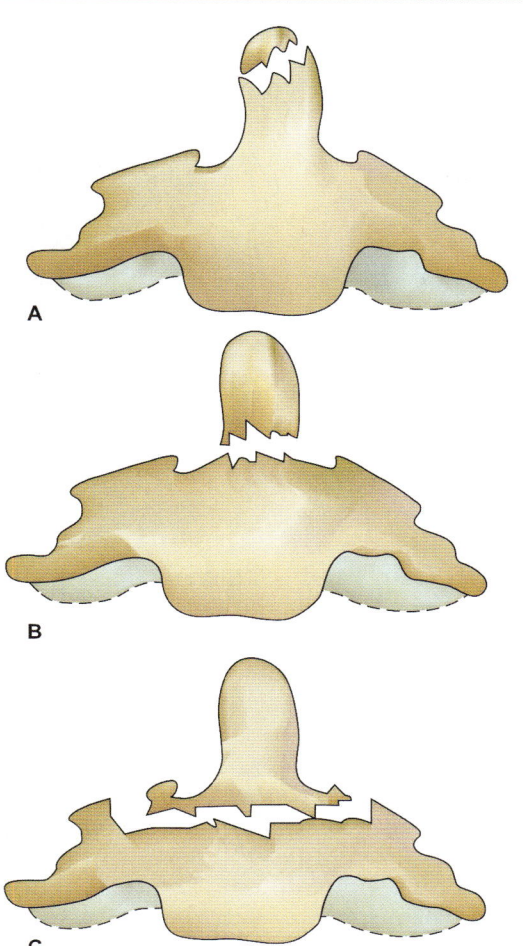

Figs 28.21A to C: Odontoid process fracture: (A) Type I, (B) Type II, and (C) Type III.

Investigations: Plain X-ray, CT scan, MRI, etc. are indicated.

Treatment: Heals with immobilization in cervical collar in 2–3 weeks. Sometimes there may be residual pain.

THORACIC AND LUMBOSACRAL SPINE INJURIES

Thoracolumbar spine is generally regarded as extending from tenth thoracic vertebrae to second lumbar vertebrae and is the transitional area between the kyphotic upper thoracic spines to the lordotic lumbar spine. The general anatomy of the vertebral column is more or less the same as in other areas of spine. The three-column concept has already been described. Anterior column is the load-bearing structure and the posterior column functions as motion limiters as well as load-bearing structures. Mercifully, the thoracolumbar injuries spare the upper limbs and vital functions. Though a lesser challenge than cervical injury nevertheless it poses problems, no less risky than the former.

Mechanism of Injury

- Fall from a height.
- RTAs: Seat belt injury (chance fracture).
- Other causes like gunshot injuries, assault.

McAfee's Classification (Figs 28.22A to D) **3-Column Classification Wedge compression:** Isolated failure of anterior column due to forward flexion. No neurological deficit.

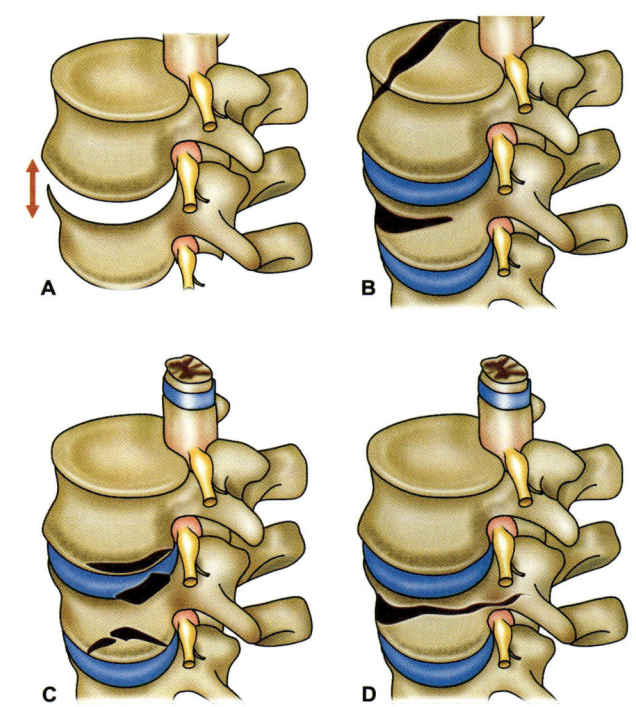

Figs 28.22A to D: Thoracolumbar fractures: (A) flexion compression fracture, (B) burst fracture, (C) flexion distraction fractures (seat belt fractures), (D) lateral compression fractures or jack knife fracture

Stable burst fractures: Anterior and middle columns fail. No loss of integrity of posterior elements.

Unstable burst fractures: Anterior and middle column fail in compression. Posterior column fail in compression, lateral flexion or rotation. Post-traumatic kyphosis and neural symptoms are present.

Chance fracture (Seat belt injury): Horizontal avulsion fracture of vertebral bodies caused by flexion about an axis anterior to the anterior longitudinal ligament. A strong tensile force pulls entire vertebrae apart.

Flexion distraction injury: Flexion axis is posterior to the anterior longitudinal ligament. Anterior column fails in compression. Middle and posterior column fail in tension. It is unstable because supraspinous, interspinous and ligamentum flavum fail.

Translational injuries: Malalignment of neural canal, which has been much disrupted. All three columns fail

28

If reduction is obtained, weight is reduced by 50 percent. If reduction is not obtained, open reduction is attempted.

Traction is given for 3 to 6 weeks and once satisfactory reduction is achieved, patient is mobilized with a collar, corset or jacket (Figs 28.18 and 28.19).

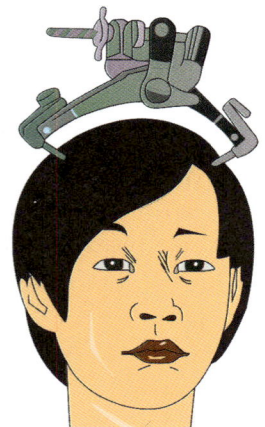

Fig. 28.18: Crutchfield tongs

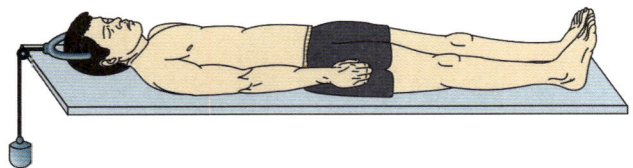

Fig. 28.19: Skeletal traction applied through Crutchfield tongs

Surgical Treatment

Indications: Unstable injury with or without neurologic damage require surgery.

Methods: In most patients early open reduction and internal fixation (ORIF) is indicated to obtain stability. Cervical spine is stabilized through an anterior or posterior approach. Usually a posterior approach is used with triple wire stabilization and fusion with iliac bone grafting. This allows rapid mobilization of patient in a cervical orthosis.

INDIVIDUAL CERVICAL FRACTURE OF INTEREST

Fracture of C_1 this is popularly known as Jefferson fracture. Here the patient usually presents with neck pain without neurological deficit. This can be radiologically diagnosed by open mouth odontoid view (Fig. 28.20).

Treatment

For stable fracture rigid cervicothoracic, brace for three months.

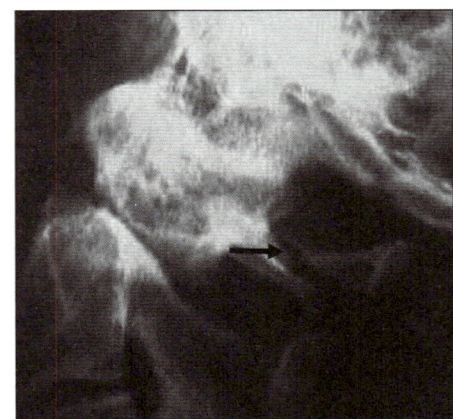

Fig. 28.20: Jefferson fracture

For unstable fractures: Skeletal, traction or halo cast for three months.

Rotary subluxation of C_1 or C_2: Here the patient presents with torticollis and neck pain and is diagnosed radiologically. Treatment is usually by reduction and skull traction.

Odontoid process fracture: Anderson and D'olonzo's classification (Figs 28.21A to C).

Type I Oblique fracture of the upper part of the odontoid process. It is uncommon and is treated by cervical cast.

Type II Junction of odontoid process and body. It is common and has a nonunion rate of 36 percent. Requires surgical wiring and fusion.

Type III fracture is through the upper part body of the body of vertebra. Cancellous area hence fracture unites well with a halo cast.

Hangman's Fracture

It is a fracture through pedicle of C_2 and is due to distraction extension force. There is no neurological deficit and patient needs rigid cervical support.

Clay Shoveler's Fracture

Laborers involved in Shovelling clay, mud, stone, etc. are prone to suffer from avulsion fracture of the spinous process of vertebra from C_6 to T_1. Conservative management is all that is required in these cases.

Whiplash Injury

It is an interesting injury that happen in the rear end collision in an RTA. The neck is thrown back violently and then jerked forwards (Fig. 28.6). Depending upon the force, it could be soft tissue injury only or injury to muscles, nerves, facets, discs, etc. in more violent force.

Presentation: Patient complains of pain, stiffness, restricted movements of the neck, hoarseness, difficulty in swallowing, headache, dizziness, pain in the back, paresthesia, etc.

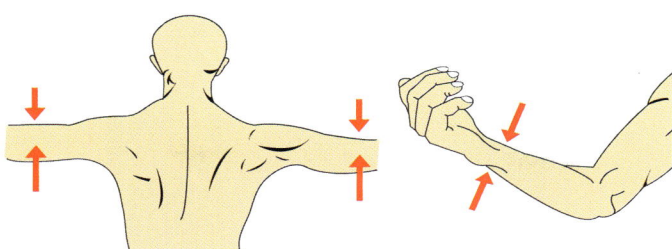

Fig. 28.10: Examination of C_5–C_6 roots (deltoid muscle)

Fig. 28.11: Examination of C_5–C_6 roots (biceps muscle)

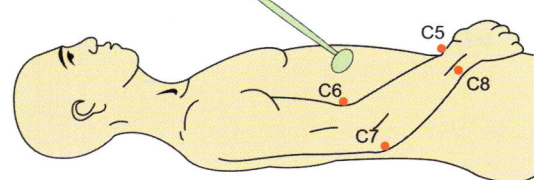

Fig. 28.12: Examination of upper limb reflexes

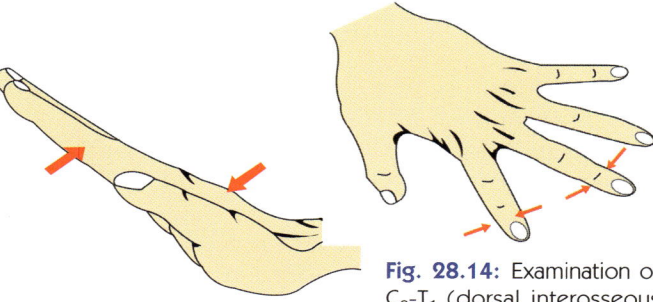

Fig. 28.13: Examination of C_7–C_8 (wrist extensors)

Fig. 28.14: Examination of C_8-T_1 (dorsal interosseous muscle)

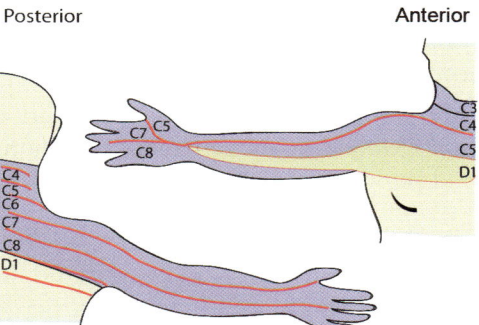

Fig. 28.15: Dermatomal pattern of cervical nerve roots

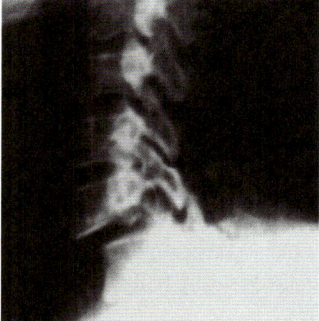

Fig. 28.16: Cervical fracture dislocation

- Obtain and maintain spinal stability
- Aim at early functional recovery

Treatment Methods

At the accident site: Resuscitation and transport is important. *If a person is lying still without using his neck after an RTA, a cervical spine injury is always suspected until proved otherwise.* The patient is transported with utmost care over a stretcher to the hospital. All unnecessary neck movements should be totally avoided. If patient needs resuscitation it has to be carried out with a lot of care.

At the hospital: When the patient reaches the hospital, in the causality the patient is stabilized and the definitive management is done as follows:

Nonoperative treatment: Most cases can be treated nonoperatively by halo vest, Minerva jacket, cervical collars, etc. (Figs 28.17A to C).

28

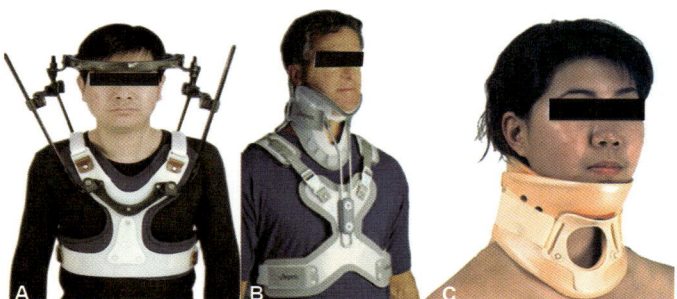

Figs 28.17A to C: Methods of cervical immobilization: (A) Halo vest traction, (B) Four post-cervical collar, (C) Cervical collar

Indications: Stable cervical spine fractures with no neurological injury. A rigid cervical brace or halo for 8 to 12 weeks is usually sufficient.

Skeletal traction: Reduction with traction is done for unstable fracture. Urgency of reduction is based on neurological loss (Flow chart 28.1).

Flow chart 28.1: Skeletal traction	
Neurologic loss ↓	*No neurologic loss* ↓
Urgent skeletal Traction through ↓	No urgency Only maintenance of reduction of skeletal traction
Crutchfield tongs or Gardner-Wells tongs ↓	
10 lb weight for head, 5 lb weight for each vertebra to a maximum of 40 lb.	

Table 28.1		
Roots sensory system		*Motor system*
C_2	Sensation decreased over back of the scalp	C_2–C_4 root involvement Survival of patient is rare
C_3	↓ Sensation over anterior aspect of the neck	-do-
C_4	↓ Sensation over lateral aspect of neck and inferiorly over clavicles down to the rib space	-do-
C_5	↓ Sensation over the lateral	↓ voluntary activity deltoid of deltoid and biceps
C_6	↓ Sensation over the radial aspect of the forearm, thumb, index and middle finger activity	↓ ECRL, ECRB
C_7	↓ Sensation over the ulnar border of ring and small fingers	↓ triceps, finger extensors, pronator teres, and FCR activity
C_8	↓ Sensation over ulnar border of hand and forearm	↓ FDS or profundus activity
T_1	↓ Sensation over the medial aspect of the upper arm	
T_2	↓ Over the anterior chest wall above the nipple	Intrinsic function of the hand is intact

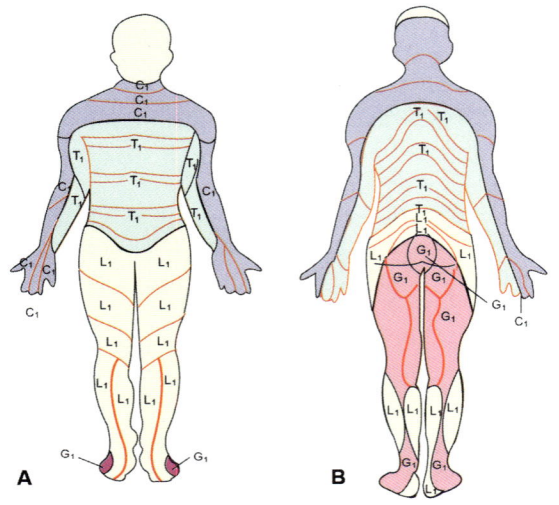

Figs 28.8A and B: Dermatomal levels: (A) anterior, and (B) posterior

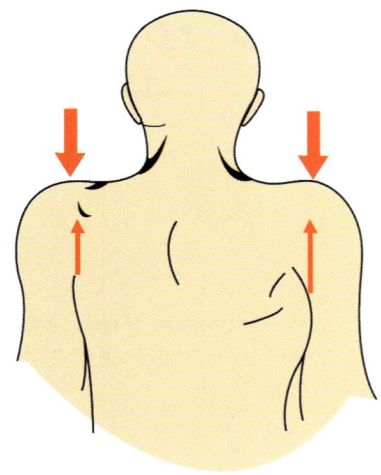

Fig. 28.9: Examination of C_3–C_4 (trapezius muscle)

finger. *Bulbocavernosus reflex* involves S_1, S_2 and S_3 nerve roots. Squeeze the glans penis, anal sphincter contracts around the gloved finger.

> **Remember**
>
> Features suggestive of spine injuries:
> - Kyphosis/scoliosis
> - Loss of vertebral height or fracture vertebral body
> - Displacement of spine anteroposterior or lateral
> - Fracture of posterior neural arches.
>
> Features suggestive of unstable spine injuries:
> - Vertebral body compression >50%
> - Fracture of posterior neural arches
> - Fracture dislocation
> - Rotation of vertebra

Radiography: Lateral view is important (Fig. 28.16). If an adequate lateral radiography reveals no fracture or dislocation, then a complete radiographic examination including anteroposterior, open mouth and oblique projections are performed.

Pitfalls: In "Whiplash injury", sometimes the X-ray may appear normally leading to errors in diagnosis.

Myelography is of value in incomplete lesion who fails to show progressive improvement.

CT scan makes an accurate diagnosis of hidden fracture. It is not helpful in assessing the soft tissue injury.

MRI evaluates cord injuries better. MRI is found to be very reliable and helpful in assessing the bony, soft tissue damages and injury to the cord very accurately.

General laboratory investigations like Hb percentage, blood group, bleeding time, clotting time, electrolyte states, etc. are done.

Treatment Facts

Goals of treatment of cervical spine injury

- Realign the spine
- Prevent further neurological damage
- Aid neurological recovery

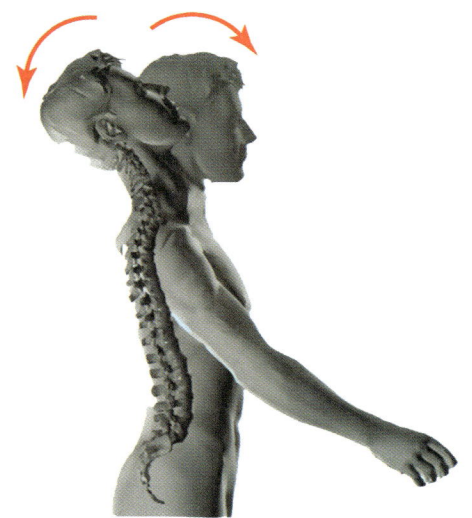

Fig. 28.6: Whiplash injury: Due to sudden deceleration, forceful hyperextension is followed by flexion of the neck

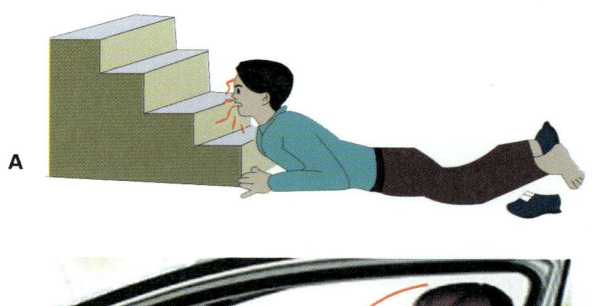

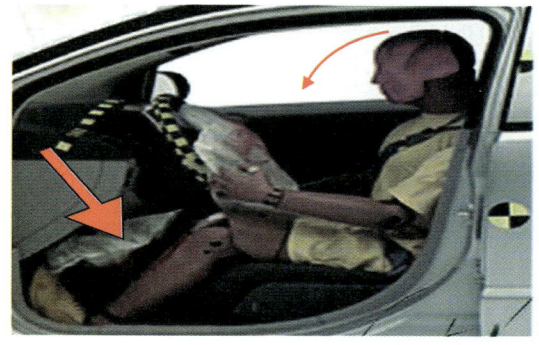

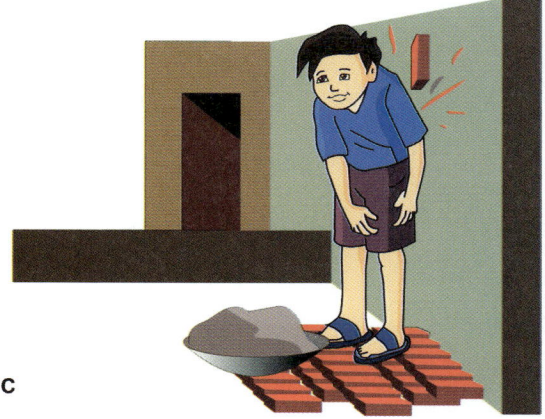

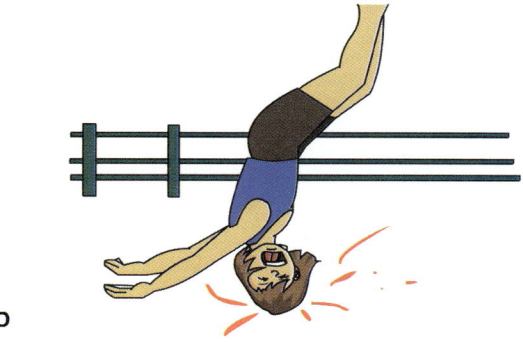

Mechanism of Injury

Pure flexion force: Compression fracture of vertebral body from C_5–C_7, e.g. fall from height. *Flexion rotation force* e.g. fall on one side of shoulder or head, disruption of facet joint and capsule is seen in C_5–C_7. *Axial compression*, e.g. fall of an object on the head results in load compression, e.g. explosive comminuted fracture of C_5 body (burst fracture i.e. from C_5–C_6). *Extension force*, e.g. avulsion fracture of superior margin of vertebral body, e.g. whiplash injury. *Lateral flexion*, e.g. fracture pedicle, fracture transverse process and facet joints, etc. *Direct injuries*, e.g. fracture spinous process and body due to assault, gunshot injury, etc. (Figs 28.7A to D).

Clinical Features

Patient usually gives history of trauma following which there will be pain, swelling and inability to move the neck. There will be tenderness over the involved spinous process and there could be a palpable gap. There may be signs of neurological involvement and is examined the following way. After examining the sensory system (Fig. 28.8), the lowermost functioning muscle is documented and a functional level is established (Table 28.1). This is followed by the examination of the Motor functions of the upper limb muscles its power and reflexes (Figs 28.9 to 28.14). Next, the sacrally innervated skin is examined. Perianal, anal, scrotal, labia and plantar surface of the toes are examined. *Perianal sensation may be the only sign to indicate an incomplete lesion* (Figs 28.8A and B).

Note: FCR—flexor carpi radialis, ECRL—extensor carpi radialis longus, ECRB—extensor carpi radialis brevis, FDS—flexor digitorum superficialis.

Figs 28.7A to D: Common mechanism of spine injuries: (A) hyperextension injury, (B) flexion extension injury, (C) flexion rotation injury, (D) flexion injury

Other Examinations

Rectal sensation—loss of sensation around the anus
Rectal motor—sphincter contracts, over the gloved

along with the posterior surface of the body. In this canal lies all the important spinal cord (Fig. 28.3).

While ligamentum flavum binds the laminae together, the interspinous ligament binds the spinous processes, and the supraspinous ligament binds the tip of the spinous process. All the structures mentioned so far help in providing the much needed stability.

Spine: Unstable vs Stable When We Call Spine as Stable

A spine, which after the initial injury refuses to be displaced further due to its intact posterior element, is called stable. Conversely, an unstable spine is one, which displaces further due to serious disruptions of the structures jeopardizing the spinal cord.

The *three-column concept* is the latest description of the spine stability. The *anterior column* consists of anterior half of the vertebral body, anterior part of the disc and anterior longitudinal ligament. The *middle column* consists of posterior half of the body and the disc the posterior longitudinal ligament. The *posterior column* consists of the posterior vertebral arch consisting of transverse process, spinous process and the accompanying ligaments. One-column injury is stable, two-column injury is unstable and three-columns injury are invariably unstable. Unstable spine is a dangerous spine for it may injure the spinal cord (Fig. 28.4).

QUICK FACTS: SPINE

- It is the principal load bearing structure of the head and torso.
- Each portion of the spine has specific functions:
  Cervical spine provides head with limited mobility and protects proximal part of spinal cord.

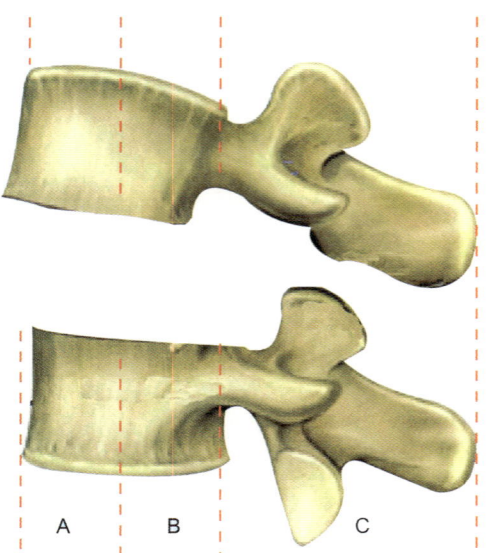

Fig. 28.4: Three-column concept of spine: (A) anterior column, (B) middle column, and (C) posterior column

Thoracic spine provides mobility to the upper torso and rib cage and protects the cord.
  Lumbar spine provides the lower torso, its mobility and protects the cord.
- Like the skull which protects the brain, spinal column protects the cord.
- Spine should be flexible yet strong.
- Spinal cord injury could result, quadriplegia, paraplegia or in death.

INJURIES OF THE CERVICAL SPINE

Injuries of the cervical spine are dangerous and if associated with neurological damage the results can be devastating (Fig. 28.5). Though diagnostic and treatment methods have vastly improved over years, still injuries of the cervical spine pose the greatest challenge to the skill and acumen of orthopedic and neurosurgeons. Jefferson pointed two areas commonly involved in cervical spine injuries, C1-2 and C5-7. According to Meyer C2 and C5 are commonly involved. Neurological damage is seen in 40 percent of cases. In 10 percent of cases, radiographs are normal.

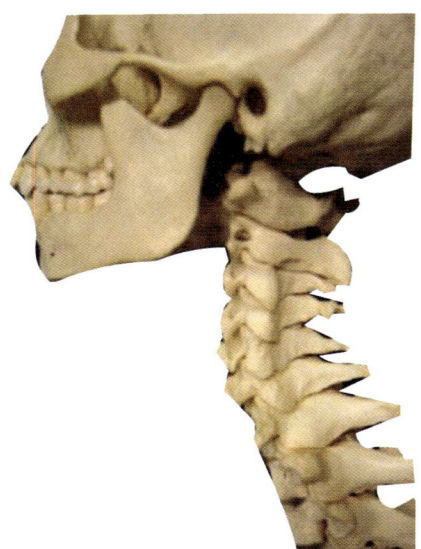

Fig. 28.5: Cervical vertebrae

Causes

- Fall from height—it is the most common cause in developing countries.
- Diving injuries—diving into water with insufficient depth or in an inebriated condition (Fig. 28.7D).
- Road traffic accidents (RTAs)—common cause in developed countries, e.g. Whiplash injury (Fig. 28.6).
- Gunshot injuries, etc. these injure the cervical spine and the cord directly.

28

Injuries of the Spine

BRIEF ANATOMY

Spine is a family of 33 bones running from the skull to the pelvis and has 4 spinal curvatures (Fig. 28.1). It has been assigned the twin responsibility of carrying the load of the body and head, thanks to the two-legged posture human beings enjoy and the still more important responsibility of protecting the vital spinal cord.

The neck bones are called *cervical vertebrae*, bones of upper back and in line with the chest are called *thoracic vertebrae* and the bones of the lower back are called *lumbar vertebrae*. Each vertebra rest on the vertebra above and below. At these points they articulate with each other through the *facet* joint which keeps all the vertebrae in their correct position and in alignment with each other. There is a spinal shock absorber called the *disc* which separates each vertebra from the next.

Each vertebra has an *anterior body* and a *posterior neural arch*. The body has a tough outer cortex and a cancellous middle portion. It is supported in front and back by anterior longitudinal ligament and posterior longitudinal ligament respectively (Fig. 28.2). The posterior neural arch consists of two pedicles, two transverse processes, a posterior spinous process and a pair of lamina which together form the spinal canal

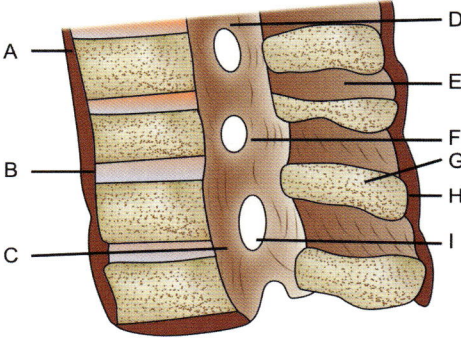

Fig. 28.2: Bony anatomy of spine: (A) anterolongitudinal ligament, (B) intervertebral disc, (C) posterior longitudinal ligament, (D) facet joint, (E) interspinous ligament, (F) ligamentum flavum, (G) spinous process, (H) supraspinous ligament, (I) intervertebral foramen

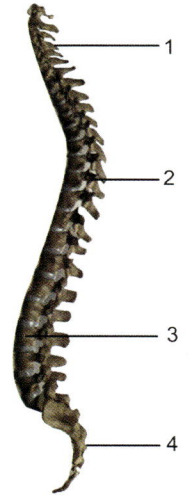

Fig. 28.1: Normal spinal curves: (1) cervical lordosis, (2) thoracic kyphosis, (3) lumbar lordosis, and (4) sacral kyphosis

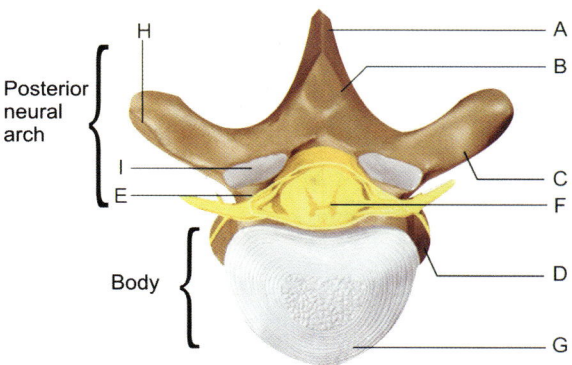

Fig. 28.3: Anatomy of a vertebra: (A) spinous process, (B) lamina, (C) transverse process, (D) superior articular facet, (E) pedicle, (F) spinal canal, (G) body, (H) transverse costal facet, (I) inferior articular facet

151

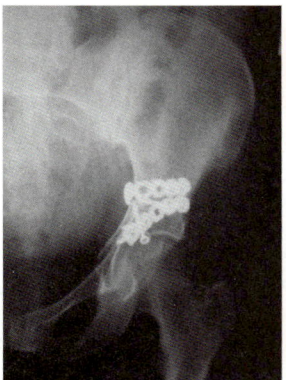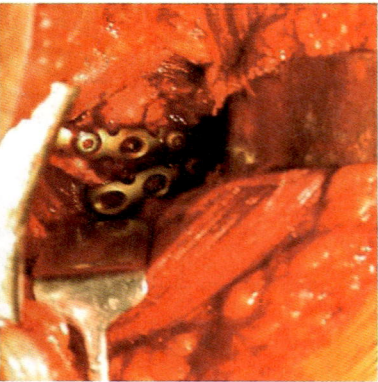

Fig. 27.12: Internal fixation methods

Other indications for surgery:
• SI joint dislocation
• Unstable sacral fractures
• SI joint dislocations
• Hemi pelvis displaed posterior or vertical > 1 cm.

Complications of Pelvic Fracture

Pelvic fracture is a dreaded injury as it is associated with a plethora of complications. The following are some of them.

Hemorrhage: It is usually intraabdominal and the incidence is around 20 percent. Patient usually presents with features of shock. If the pulse is greater than 100/min it suggests 20 percent blood volume deficit, if the blood pressure is less than 100 mm systolic it suggests 30 percent volume deficit. Diagnostic peritoneal lavage and open paracentesis has an accuracy rate of 98 percent in intraabdominal injuries. CT scan is also sensitive and specific. Treatment is by laparotomy and is indicated if there is continuing blood loss, visceral perforation, expanding palpable suprapubic hematoma.

Injuries of lower urinary tract: Rupture of urethra and rupture of urinary bladder are the common lower urinary tract injuries frequently seen in separation of pubic symphysis and fracture pubic rami. It has an average incidence of 13 percent. The dictum is "All pelvic fractures must be assumed to have urinary tract injuries until proved otherwise."

Presence of hematuria is not pathognomonic but its presence calls for three radiographic studies like retrograde urethrogram, cystogram and IVP. Rupture of anterior urethra is seen in straddle fractures and is not very common. Rupture of posterior urethra is relatively more common and is limited to male. Suprapubic cystostomy, direct repair, rail road repair, urethroplasties are some of the treatment methods.

Bladder injuries are seen in 4 percent of the cases and are associated with symphysis pubis injuries and rami fracture. Eighty percent injuries are extra-

peritoneal and calls for direct surgical intervention as quickly as possible.

Other injuries: Testicular injuries and vaginal lacerations, bowel and rectal injuries and urethral injuries are all common and require immediate surgical intervention.

Other complications: Loss of reduction, sepsis, thrombophlebitis, delayed union, nonunion, post-traumatic arthritis, fat embolism, major arterial injuries, abdominal wall injury, neurological injuries usually L_5, S_1 roots due to sacral fracture are the other common complications.

Remember

Pelvic fractures
• A fracture feared for its complications.
• RTA accounts for 80% of cases.
• Fracture broadly classified into not affecting and affecting integrity of the pelvic ring.
• Fracture pubic rami, usually single, is the commonest pelvic fracture (69%).
• Usual presentation is hypovolemic shock.
• Correction of hypovolemia and other general measures takes precedence over fracture management.
• Conservative treatment is the mainstay.
• External and internal fixation is done for specific indications
• Intraabdominal and genitourinary injuries are common possibilities and need early recognition and prompt treatment.
• Mortality is 10–30%.

Note: Mortality in closed pelvic fractures is 10 to 30 percent and open fractures are 40 to 50 percent.

QUICK FACTS: INTERESTING PELVIC FRACTURES

a. *Straddle fracture:* Double vertical fractures of pubic rami.
b. *Malgaigne's fracture:* Ipsilateral pubic rami fracture and SI joint dislocation.
c. *Bucket handle fracture:* pubic rami fracture with contra-lateral SI joint dislocation.
d. *Open back fractures:* Disruption of the pubic symphysis or rami fracture and external rotation of the hemi pelvis over an intact posterior SI joints.

COCCYX FRACTURES

Coccyx in human beings represents the extinct tail. It is formed by the fusion of five vertebral bones. Injury to the coccyx is relatively the common.

Mechanism: It is commonly due to direct fall on the buttocks (Figs 27.13A and B).

Clinical Features

Patient usually complains of chronic pain in between the buttocks, difficulty in sitting, etc.

27

Radiology: X-ray of the pelvis helps in the diagnosis and AP and lateral views are recommended (Figs 27.13A and B).

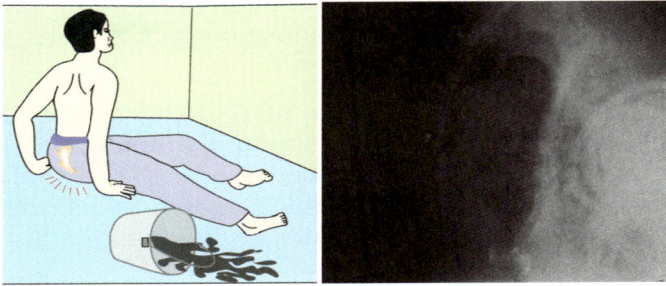

Figs 27.13A and B: (A) Mechanism of injury in coccyx fractures, (B) coccyx fractures

Conservative Management

- The treatment is essentially conservative in nature with periods of bed-rest and symptomatic treatment for pain and inflammation.
- To relieve pain, thermotherapy like ultrasound and TENS.
- To relieve prolonged pressure on the buttocks, sitting on a ring cushion and sitting on alternate buttocks is advised.
- Isometric exercises to the glutei maximus muscle in sitting, lying and prone positions are advisable.
- *Seitz bath helps to relieve pain (See Box).

Remember About Coccyx Fracture

Note: These injuries are difficult to tackle.
Reasons:
- Due to the position of coccyx which is deep and covered by thick muscles on either side.
- Due to the pressure from sitting. Hence long sitting posture needs to be controlled.
- *Note:* *Seitz bath—this consists of sitting in a shallow tub of warm water. Commonly advocated in Piles patients after surgery.

RIB FRACTURES

These are relatively rare injuries and are usually due to direct trauma. The rib usually breaks at the angle which is a point of maximum convexity (Fig. 27.14).

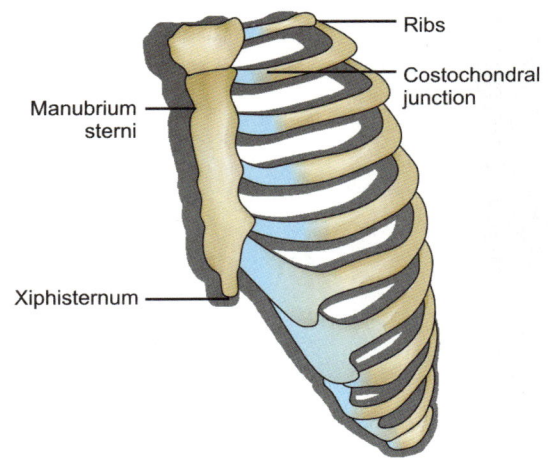

Fig. 27.14: Anatomical features of ribs

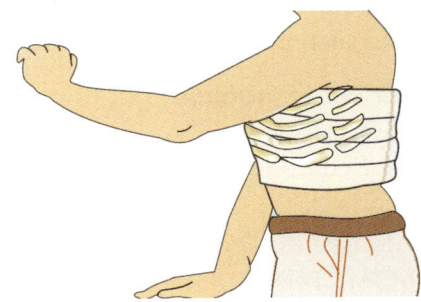

Fig. 27.15: Strapping method for treatment of fracture ribs

Intercostal muscles provide natural immobilization to the fractured ribs and hence no aggressive management is required. Strapping (Fig. 27.15). Ultrasound or TENS, etc. are effective in reducing the pain. Occasionally a local infiltration of hydrocortisone helps.

Very rarely the fracture fragments may pierce the pleura causing pneumothorax, hemothorax, etc. These are dangerous injuries and need to be managed aggressively.

Rehabilitation: This essentially consists of deep breathing exercises, which are progressively made more vigorous to improve the mobility of the thorax.

28

Injuries of the Spine

BRIEF ANATOMY

Spine is a family of 33 bones running from the skull to the pelvis and has 4 spinal curvatures (Fig. 28.1). It has been assigned the twin responsibility of carrying the load of the body and head, thanks to the two-legged posture human beings enjoy and the still more important responsibility of protecting the vital spinal cord.

The neck bones are called *cervical vertebrae,* bones of upper back and in line with the chest are called *thoracic vertebrae* and the bones of the lower back are called *lumbar vertebrae.* Each vertebra rest on the vertebra above and below. At these points they articulate with each other through the *facet* joint which keeps all the vertebrae in their correct position and in alignment with each other. There is a spinal shock absorber called the *disc* which separates each vertebra from the next.

Each vertebra has an *anterior body* and a *posterior neural arch.* The body has a tough outer cortex and a cancellous middle portion. It is supported in front and back by anterior longitudinal ligament and posterior longitudinal ligament respectively (Fig. 28.2). The posterior neural arch consists of two pedicles, two transverse processes, a posterior spinous process and a pair of lamina which together form the spinal canal

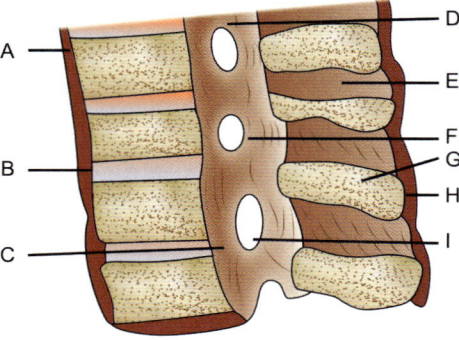

Fig. 28.2: Bony anatomy of spine: (A) anterolongitudinal ligament, (B) intervertebral disc, (C) posterior longitudinal ligament, (D) facet joint, (E) interspinous ligament, (F) ligamentum flavum, (G) spinous process, (H) supraspinous ligament, (I) intervertebral foramen

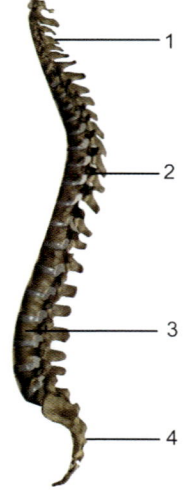

Fig. 28.1: Normal spinal curves: (1) cervical lordosis, (2) thoracic kyphosis, (3) lumbar lordosis, and (4) sacral kyphosis

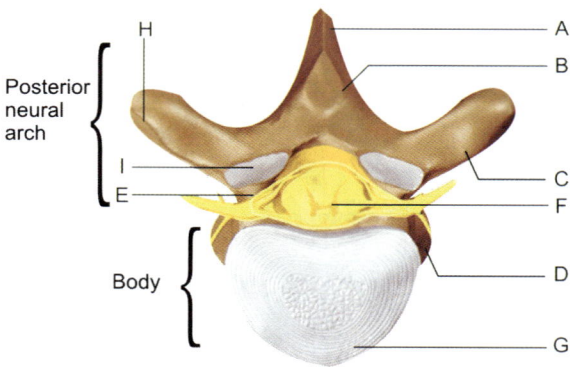

Fig. 28.3: Anatomy of a vertebra: (A) spinous process, (B) lamina, (C) transverse process, (D) superior articular facet, (E) pedicle, (F) spinal canal, (G) body, (H) transverse costal facet, (I) inferior articular facet

along with the posterior surface of the body. In this canal lies all the important spinal cord (Fig. 28.3).

While ligamentum flavum binds the laminae together, the interspinous ligament binds the spinous processes, and the supraspinous ligament binds the tip of the spinous process. All the structures mentioned so far help in providing the much needed stability.

Spine: Unstable vs Stable When We Call Spine as Stable

A spine, which after the initial injury refuses to be displaced further due to its intact posterior element, is called stable. Conversely, an unstable spine is one, which displaces further due to serious disruptions of the structures jeopardizing the spinal cord.

The *three-column concept* is the latest description of the spine stability. The *anterior column* consists of anterior half of the vertebral body, anterior part of the disc and anterior longitudinal ligament. The *middle column* consists of posterior half of the body and the disc the posterior longitudinal ligament. The *posterior column* consists of the posterior vertebral arch consisting of transverse process, spinous process and the accompanying ligaments. One-column injury is stable, two-column injury is unstable and three-columns injury are invariably unstable. Unstable spine is a dangerous spine for it may injure the spinal cord (Fig. 28.4).

> QUICK FACTS: SPINE
>
> - It is the principal load bearing structure of the head and torso.
> - Each portion of the spine has specific functions:
>   **Cervical spine** provides head with limited mobility and protects proximal part of spinal cord.

Thoracic spine provides mobility to the upper torso and rib cage and protects the cord.
Lumbar spine provides the lower torso, its mobility and protects the cord.
- Like the skull which protects the brain, spinal column protects the cord.
- Spine should be flexible yet strong.
- Spinal cord injury could result, quadriplegia, paraplegia or in death.

INJURIES OF THE CERVICAL SPINE

Injuries of the cervical spine are dangerous and if associated with neurological damage the results can be devastating (Fig. 28.5). Though diagnostic and treatment methods have vastly improved over years, still injuries of the cervical spine pose the greatest challenge to the skill and acumen of orthopedic and neurosurgeons. Jefferson pointed two areas commonly involved in cervical spine injuries, C1-2 and C5-7. According to Meyer C2 and C5 are commonly involved. Neurological damage is seen in 40 percent of cases. In 10 percent of cases, radiographs are normal.

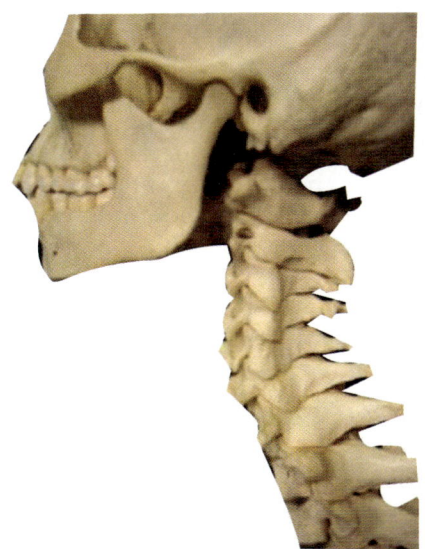

Fig. 28.5: Cervical vertebrae

Causes

- Fall from height—it is the most common cause in developing countries.
- Diving injuries—diving into water with insufficient depth or in an inebriated condition (Fig. 28.7D).
- Road traffic accidents (RTAs)—common cause in developed countries, e.g. Whiplash injury (Fig. 28.6).
- Gunshot injuries, etc. these injure the cervical spine and the cord directly.

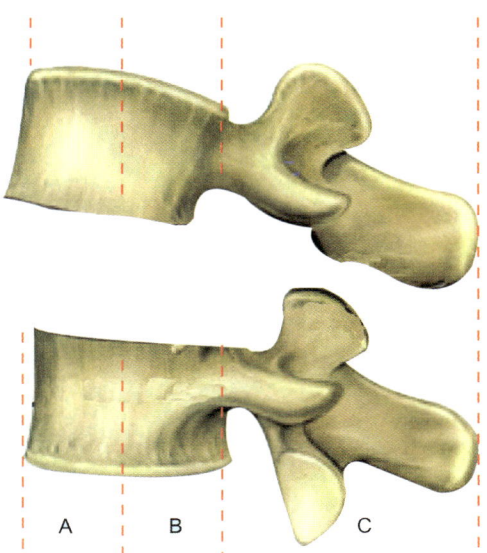

Fig. 28.4: Three-column concept of spine: (A) anterior column, (B) middle column, and (C) posterior column

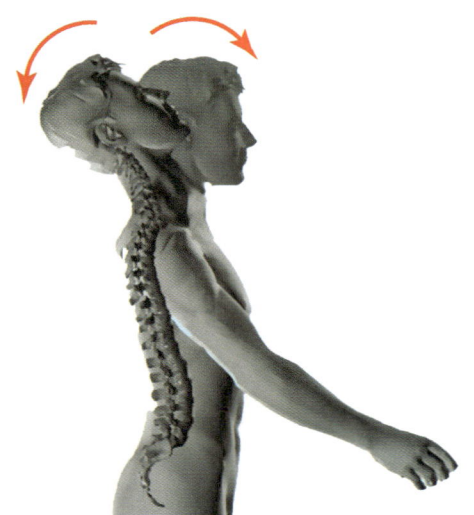

Fig. 28.6: Whiplash injury: Due to sudden deceleration, forceful hyperextension is followed by flexion of the neck

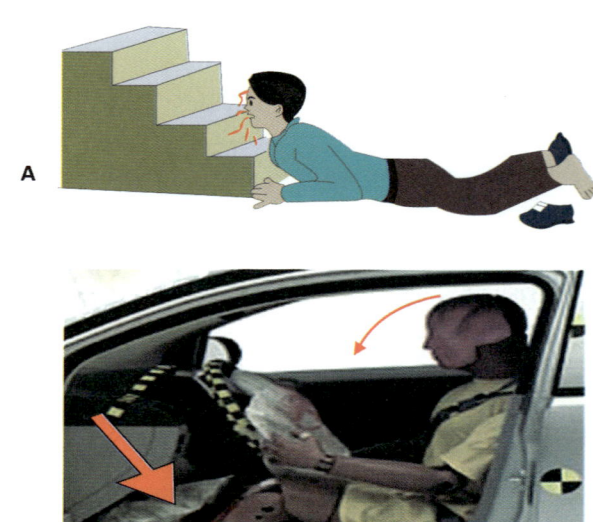

Mechanism of Injury

Pure flexion force: Compression fracture of vertebral body from C_5–C_7, e.g. fall from height. *Flexion rotation force* e.g. fall on one side of shoulder or head, disruption of facet joint and capsule is seen in C_5–C_7. *Axial compression*, e.g. fall of an object on the head results in load compression, e.g. explosive comminuted fracture of C_5 body (burst fracture i.e. from C_5–C_6). *Extension force*, e.g. avulsion fracture of superior margin of vertebral body, e.g. whiplash injury. *Lateral flexion*, e.g. fracture pedicle, fracture transverse process and facet joints, etc. *Direct injuries*, e.g. fracture spinous process and body due to assault, gunshot injury, etc. (Figs 28.7A to D).

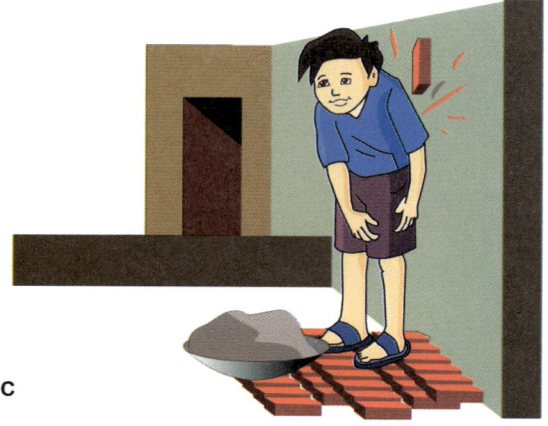

Clinical Features

Patient usually gives history of trauma following which there will be pain, swelling and inability to move the neck. There will be tenderness over the involved spinous process and there could be a palpable gap. There may be signs of neurological involvement and is examined the following way. After examining the sensory system (Fig. 28.8), the lowermost functioning muscle is documented and a functional level is established (Table 28.1). This is followed by the examination of the Motor functions of the upper limb muscles its power and reflexes (Figs 28.9 to 28.14). Next, the sacrally innervated skin is examined. Perianal, anal, scrotal, labia and plantar surface of the toes are examined. *Perianal sensation may be the only sign to indicate an incomplete lesion* (Figs 28.8A and B).

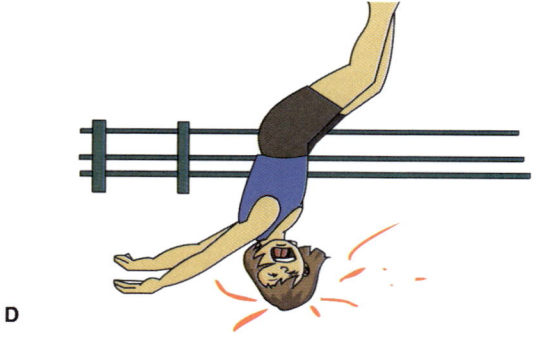

Figs 28.7A to D: Common mechanism of spine injuries: (A) hyperextension injury, (B) flexion extension injury, (C) flexion rotation injury, (D) flexion injury

Note: FCR—flexor carpi radialis, ECRL—extensor carpi radialis longus, ECRB—extensor carpi radialis brevis, FDS—flexor digitorum superficialis.

Other Examinations

Rectal sensation—loss of sensation around the anus
Rectal motor—sphincter contracts, over the gloved

Table 28.1		
Roots sensory system		*Motor system*
C_2	Sensation decreased over back of the scalp	C_2–C_4 root involvement Survival of patient is rare
C_3	↓ Sensation over anterior aspect of the neck	-do-
C_4	↓ Sensation over lateral aspect of neck and inferiorly over clavicles down to the rib space	-do-
C_5	↓ Sensation over the lateral	↓ voluntary activity deltoid of deltoid and biceps
C_6	↓ Sensation over the radial aspect of the forearm, thumb, index and middle finger activity	↓ ECRL, ECRB
C_7	↓ Sensation over the ulnar border of ring and small fingers	↓ triceps, finger extensors, pronator teres, and FCR activity
C_8	↓ Sensation over ulnar border of hand and forearm	↓ FDS or profundus activity
T_1	↓ Sensation over the medial aspect of the upper arm	
T_2	↓ Over the anterior chest wall above the nipple	Intrinsic function of the hand is intact

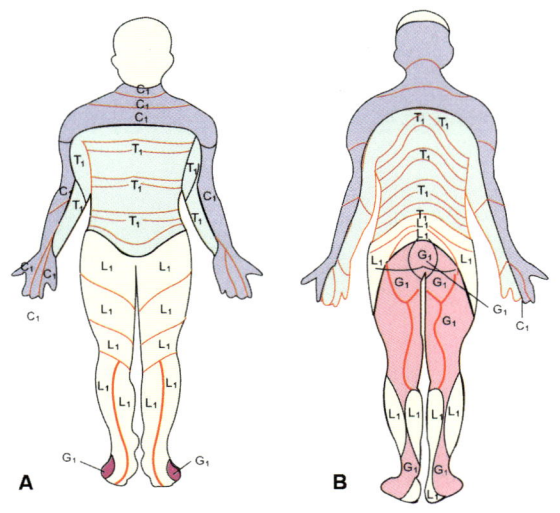

Figs 28.8A and B: Dermatomal levels: (A) anterior, and (B) posterior

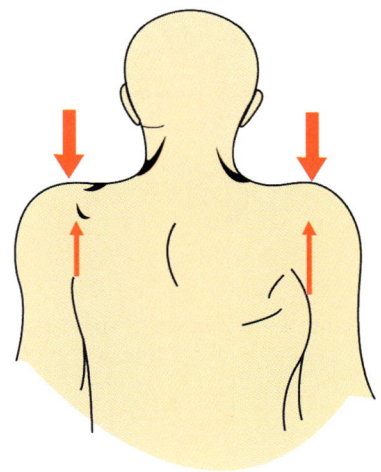

Fig. 28.9: Examination of C_3–C_4 (trapezius muscle)

finger. *Bulbocavernosus reflex* involves S_1, S_2 and S_3 nerve roots. Squeeze the glans penis, anal sphincter contracts around the gloved finger.

Remember

Features suggestive of spine injuries:
- Kyphosis/scoliosis
- Loss of vertebral height or fracture vertebral body
- Displacement of spine anteroposterior or lateral
- Fracture of posterior neural arches.

Features suggestive of unstable spine injuries:
- Vertebral body compression >50%
- Fracture of posterior neural arches
- Fracture dislocation
- Rotation of vertebra

Radiography: Lateral view is important (Fig. 28.16). If an adequate lateral radiography reveals no fracture or dislocation, then a complete radiographic examination including anteroposterior, open mouth and oblique projections are performed.

Pitfalls: In "Whiplash injury", sometimes the X-ray may appear normally leading to errors in diagnosis.

Myelography is of value in incomplete lesion who fails to show progressive improvement.

CT scan makes an accurate diagnosis of hidden fracture. It is not helpful in assessing the soft tissue injury.

MRI evaluates cord injuries better. MRI is found to be very reliable and helpful in assessing the bony, soft tissue damages and injury to the cord very accurately.

General laboratory investigations like Hb percentage, blood group, bleeding time, clotting time, electrolyte states, etc. are done.

Treatment Facts

Goals of treatment of cervical spine injury

- Realign the spine
- Prevent further neurological damage
- Aid neurological recovery

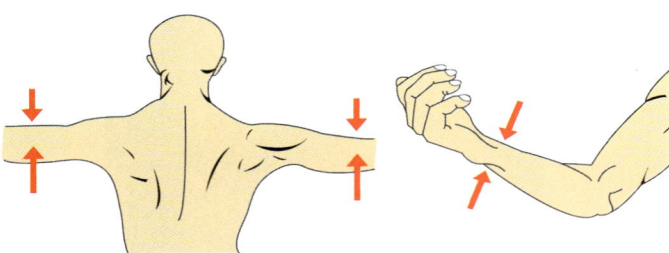

Fig. 28.10: Examination of C₅–C₆ roots (deltoid muscle)

Fig. 28.11: Examination of C₅–C₆ roots (biceps muscle)

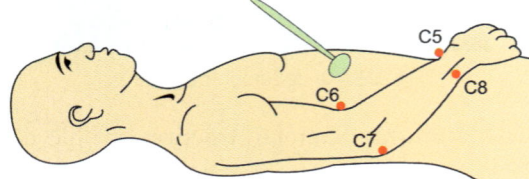

Fig. 28.12: Examination of upper limb reflexes

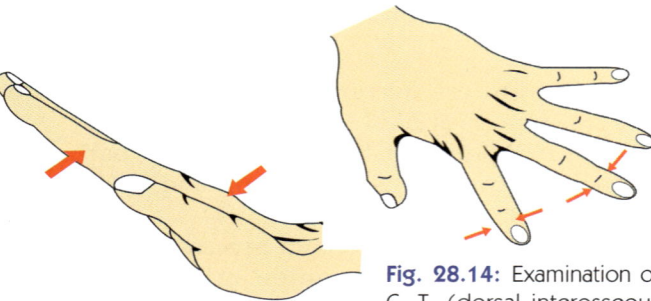

Fig. 28.14: Examination of C₈-T₁ (dorsal interosseous muscle)

Fig. 28.13: Examination of C₇–C₈ (wrist extensors)

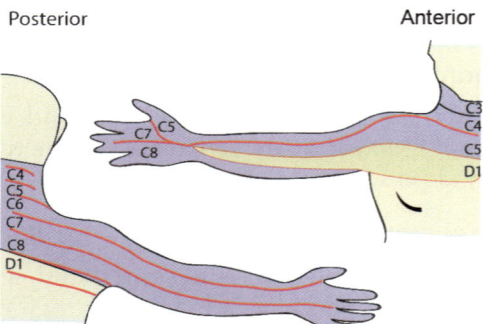

Fig. 28.15: Dermatomal pattern of cervical nerve roots

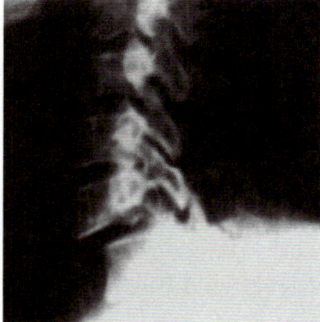

Fig. 28.16: Cervical fracture dislocation

- Obtain and maintain spinal stability
- Aim at early functional recovery

Treatment Methods

At the accident site: Resuscitation and transport is important. *If a person is lying still without using his neck after an RTA, a cervical spine injury is always suspected until proved otherwise.* The patient is transported with utmost care over a stretcher to the hospital. All unnecessary neck movements should be totally avoided. If patient needs resuscitation it has to be carried out with a lot of care.

At the hospital: When the patient reaches the hospital, in the causality the patient is stabilized and the definitive management is done as follows:

Nonoperative treatment: Most cases can be treated nonoperatively by halo vest, Minerva jacket, cervical collars, etc. (Figs 28.17A to C).

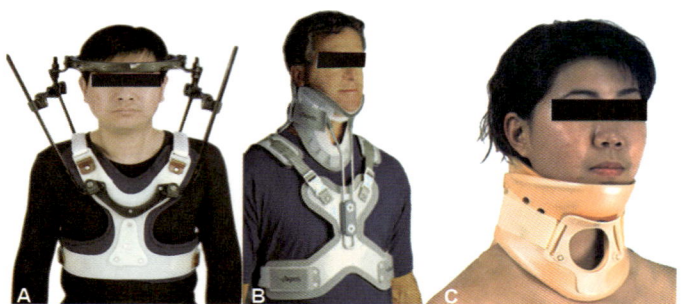

Figs 28.17A to C: Methods of cervical immobilization: (A) Halo vest traction, (B) Four post-cervical collar, (C) Cervical collar

Indications: Stable cervical spine fractures with no neurological injury. A rigid cervical brace or halo for 8 to 12 weeks is usually sufficient.

Skeletal traction: Reduction with traction is done for unstable fracture. Urgency of reduction is based on neurological loss (Flow chart 28.1).

Flow chart 28.1: Skeletal traction	
Neurologic loss	*No neurologic loss*
↓	↓
Urgent skeletal Traction through	No urgency Only maintenance of
↓	reduction of skeletal traction
Crutchfield tongs or Gardner-Wells tongs	
↓	
10 lb weight for head, 5 lb weight for each vertebra to a maximum of 40 lb.	

28

If reduction is obtained, weight is reduced by 50 percent. If reduction is not obtained, open reduction is attempted.

Traction is given for 3 to 6 weeks and once satisfactory reduction is achieved, patient is mobilized with a collar, corset or jacket (Figs 28.18 and 28.19).

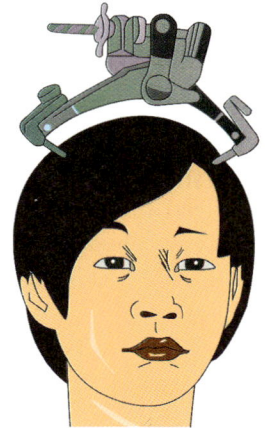

Fig. 28.18: Crutchfield tongs

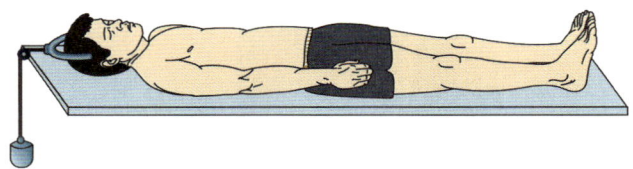

Fig. 28.19: Skeletal traction applied through Crutchfield tongs

Surgical Treatment

Indications: Unstable injury with or without neurologic damage require surgery.

Methods: In most patients early open reduction and internal fixation (ORIF) is indicated to obtain stability. Cervical spine is stabilized through an anterior or posterior approach. Usually a posterior approach is used with triple wire stabilization and fusion with iliac bone grafting. This allows rapid mobilization of patient in a cervical orthosis.

INDIVIDUAL CERVICAL FRACTURE OF INTEREST

Fracture of C_1 this is popularly known as Jefferson fracture. Here the patient usually presents with neck pain without neurological deficit. This can be radiologically diagnosed by open mouth odontoid view (Fig. 28.20).

Treatment

For stable fracture rigid cervicothoracic, brace for three months.

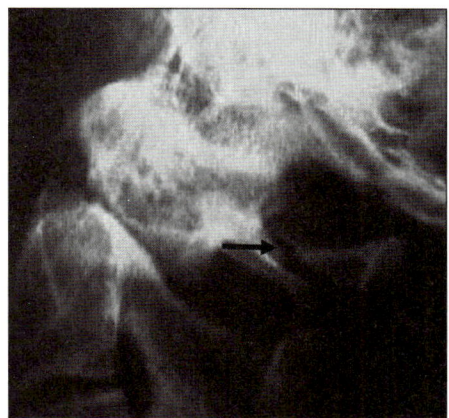

Fig. 28.20: Jefferson fracture

For unstable fractures: Skeletal, traction or halo cast for three months.

Rotary subluxation of C_1 or C_2: Here the patient presents with torticollis and neck pain and is diagnosed radiologically. Treatment is usually by reduction and skull traction.

Odontoid process fracture: Anderson and D'olonzo's classification (Figs 28.21A to C).

Type I Oblique fracture of the upper part of the odontoid process. It is uncommon and is treated by cervical cast.

Type II Junction of odontoid process and body. It is common and has a nonunion rate of 36 percent. Requires surgical wiring and fusion.

Type III fracture is through the upper part body of the body of vertebra. Cancellous area hence fracture unites well with a halo cast.

Hangman's Fracture

It is a fracture through pedicle of C_2 and is due to distraction extension force. There is no neurological deficit and patient needs rigid cervical support.

Clay Shoveler's Fracture

Laborers involved in Shovelling clay, mud, stone, etc. are prone to suffer from avulsion fracture of the spinous process of vertebra from C_6 to T_1. Conservative management is all that is required in these cases.

Whiplash Injury

It is an interesting injury that happen in the rear end collision in an RTA. The neck is thrown back violently and then jerked forwards (Fig. 28.6). Depending upon the force, it could be soft tissue injury only or injury to muscles, nerves, facets, discs, etc. in more violent force.

Presentation: Patient complains of pain, stiffness, restricted movements of the neck, hoarseness, difficulty in swallowing, headache, dizziness, pain in the back, paresthesia, etc.

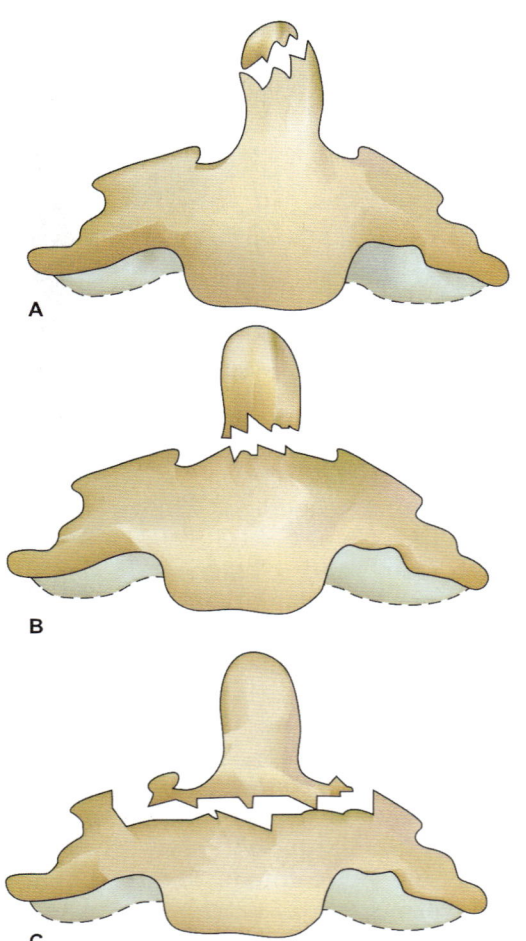

Figs 28.21A to C: Odontoid process fracture: (A) Type I, (B) Type II, and (C) Type III.

Investigations: Plain X-ray, CT scan, MRI, etc. are indicated.

Treatment: Heals with immobilization in cervical collar in 2–3 weeks. Sometimes there may be residual pain.

THORACIC AND LUMBOSACRAL SPINE INJURIES

Thoracolumbar spine is generally regarded as extending from tenth thoracic vertebrae to second lumbar vertebrae and is the transitional area between the kyphotic upper thoracic spines to the lordotic lumbar spine. The general anatomy of the vertebral column is more or less the same as in other areas of spine. The three-column concept has already been described. Anterior column is the load-bearing structure and the posterior column functions as motion limiters as well as load-bearing structures. Mercifully, the thoracolumbar injuries spare the upper limbs and vital functions. Though a lesser challenge than cervical injury nevertheless it poses problems, no less risky than the former.

Mechanism of Injury

- Fall from a height.
- RTAs: Seat belt injury (chance fracture).
- Other causes like gunshot injuries, assault.

McAfee's Classification (Figs 28.22A to D) **3-Column Classification Wedge compression:** Isolated failure of anterior column due to forward flexion. No neurological deficit.

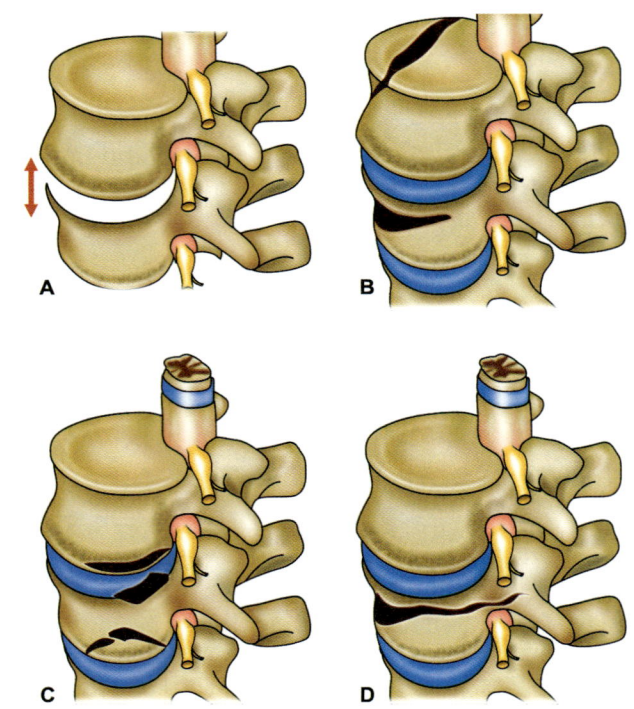

Figs 28.22A to D: Thoracolumbar fractures: (A) flexion compression fracture, (B) burst fracture, (C) flexion distraction fractures (seat belt fractures), (D) lateral compression fractures or jack knife fracture

Stable burst fractures: Anterior and middle columns fail. No loss of integrity of posterior elements.

Unstable burst fractures: Anterior and middle column fail in compression. Posterior column fail in compression, lateral flexion or rotation. Post-traumatic kyphosis and neural symptoms are present.

Chance fracture (Seat belt injury): Horizontal avulsion fracture of vertebral bodies caused by flexion about an axis anterior to the anterior longitudinal ligament. A strong tensile force pulls entire vertebrae apart.

Flexion distraction injury: Flexion axis is posterior to the anterior longitudinal ligament. Anterior column fails in compression. Middle and posterior column fail in tension. It is unstable because supraspinous, interspinous and ligamentum flavum fail.

Translational injuries: Malalignment of neural canal, which has been much disrupted. All three columns fail

28

in shear. At the affected level, one part of sacral canal has been displaced in the transverse plane.

Clinical Features

Patient gives history of trauma due to RTA or fall from height and complains of pain, posterior swelling, tenderness, palpable interspinous gap or a step may be felt. Neurological involvement may vary from paraplegia to individual nerve root involvement. Spinal shock is present for 24 hrs during which all the reflexes are lost. Cauda equina paralysis is present if the lesion is below L_1.

Investigations

Radiography of the affected spine: This is the preliminary investigation and all three views (AP, lateral and oblique) are taken (Fig. 28.23).

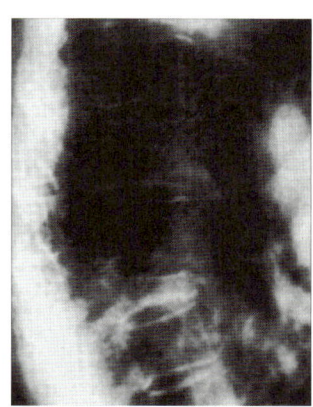

Fig. 28.23: Radiograph showing flexion anterior compression fracture of T_{12} vertebra

CT scan and MRI: Both CT scan and MRI have found to be more useful than radiographs in evaluation of spinal trauma. While CT scan helps in studying the bony elements, MRI helps in the study of both bone and soft tissue elements. The damage to the cord is detected fairly accurately and is now being considered as the "gold standard" in the investigation of spine injury (Fig. 28.24).

Management

This is discussed under two heads.

Management at the site of accident: This consists of careful handling of the patient suspected to have spine injury. Consider all patients with spine injury to have neurological damage and shift them to the hospital with utmost care and caution avoiding all unnecessary movements.

Definitive treatment at the hospital: This varies depending upon the nature of injury and the presence or absence of neurological damage.
- *Practice:* Caution in handling the neck.

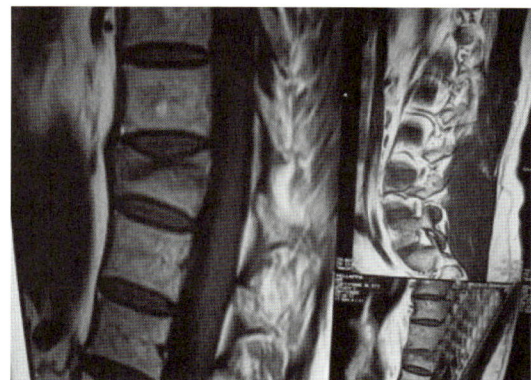

Fig. 28.24: MRI showing fracture to T_6 Vertebra

- *Examination:* The general condition and other systems like CNS/CVS/RS/PA/GI tract. Also, examine from head to toe, the presence of other fractures, head, chest injuries, blunt injury abdomen and pelvic fractures.
- *Evaluate:* The spine injury by gentle careful clinical examination. This has to be supplemented by proper investigations like X-ray, CT-scan, MRI.
- *Assess:* Carefully assess the level and extent of neurological damage by examining the dermatome, myotome and reflexes.
- *Plan:* After evaluating and assessing the damage, plan the line of treatment. The treatment options include nonoperative, traction and operative methods. Now let us carefully look into various treatment modalities:

Treatment Methods

a. *For stable fracture without neurological deficit:* Less than 30 percent anterior wedge, lateral, central compression fracture of the vertebral body is considered as stable fracture. In these injuries there is no fracture of the posterior cortex of the vertebral body, and there is no disruption of the neural arch.
   Treatment: This is essentially conservative and consists of bed rest, NSAIDs and external spine supports like brace, corsets (Fig. 28.25). If the vertebral body compression is less than 30 percent,

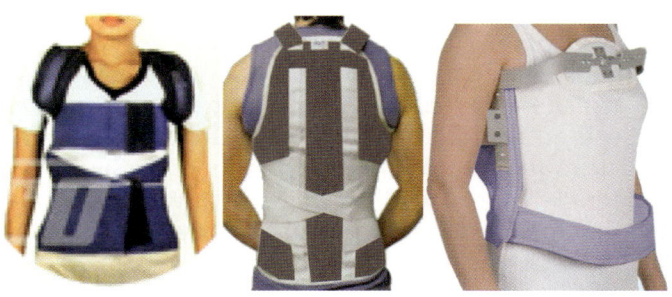

Fig. 28.25: Various spinal corsets

only corset is used and if the compression is more than 30 percent but less than 50 percent a plaster jacket along with a corset is preferred.

b. *For stable fracture with neural deficit:* It has to be first determined whether the neurological deficit is complete (loss of motor power, sensory loss and absent reflexes) or incomplete (only cord or only spinal nerve roots).

If neurological damage is incomplete, IV steroids are given for 4 days later anterior decompression and anterior interbody fusion in the first stage is done. Posterior segmental spinal stabilization by pedicle screws, Hartshill rectangle frame, Luque instrumentation, etc. can be done one week later. Laminectomy has fewer roles as it makes the spine less stable.

c. *Unstable fracture without neurological deficit:* This is best treated by early open reduction, internal fixation, fusion and is done preferably within 12 to 24 hours. It is done with spinal cord monitoring. Internal fixation is either by VSP plates, Hartshill frame, Harrington instrumentation, etc. (Fig. 28.26).

d. *Unstable fracture with neurological deficit:* Systemic Decadron 4 to 6 mg/every 6 hrs IV for 3 days is given. Early open reduction and internal fixation and fusion are done in incomplete neurological deficit cases. This is also desirable in complete neurological deficit to permit early-uninhibited rehabilitation. Segmental

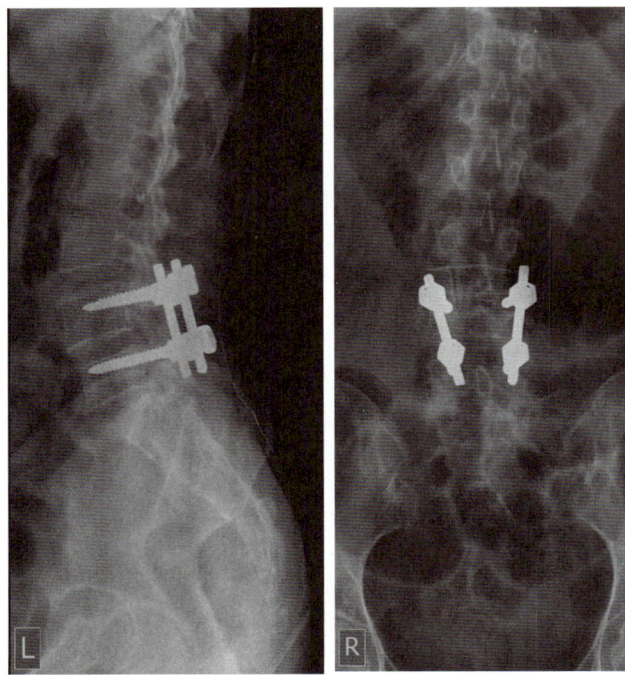

Fig. 28.26: Posterior spinal stabilization

spinal stabilization with Luque or Hartshill frame is recommended.

28

29 Spinal Cord Injuries

Spinal cord could be damaged due to injuries of spine extending from cervical vertebrae to the thoracolumbar junction. Below this the cord ends and the cauda equina begins (Fig. 29.1).

PATHOLOGY

The pathology may vary from extradural hemorrhage to cord concussion, laceration to cord crushing. Lesion has longitudinal, sagittal and coronal dimensions. Amount of neural damage has no relationship to radiographic appearance.

Cord Concussion

This is a state of spinal shock and there will be sensory loss, flaccid paralysis, visceral paralysis, reflexes are in abeyance and anal reflex is absent. By 8 hours, concussion is known to regress and by 8–10 days, there is complete recovery.

Fig. 29.1

Spinal Shock

Immediately following a cord injury there is flaccid motor paralysis as the cord is in a state of spinal shock. After some time the cord recovers and acts independently without the control from the higher centers. Sligh test voluntary movement and sensation below the level of cord lesion indicate cord continuity with better prognosis.

Return of reflex activity (e.g. anal reflex, bulbocavernosus reflex and plantar response) if paralysis is complete even after 8 hrs and if there is symmetrical returning of reflexes and priapism in male, it indicates an unfavorable prognosis as it indicates complete cord transection. Return of reflex activity below the lesion indicates that the spinal shock has passed off and remaining paralysis and anesthesia may be due to

injury to the long tracts of cauda equina. Total sensory and motor paralysis after 8 hrs with return of reflex activity indicates that distal part of spinal cord has been separated from the cerebral control.

Cord transection: This could be:
Complete: This can lead to quadriplegia or quadriparesis at the cervical level, paraparesis and paraplegia at the thoracic or thoracolumbar level.
Incomplete: Here the central cord, lateral cord, anterior or posterior cord could be involved.

Nerve root involvement: Individual nerve roots could be affected at their respective intervertebral foramen. All the features of peripheral nerve injury with LMN type of lesion are seen. The myotome and the dermatome should be assessed to know the root involvement.

> **QUICK FACTS:** Signs of bad prognosis in spinal shock
> - Complete cord transection.
> - Anal reflex (anal wink): Anal sphincter reflexly contracts when stimulated with a sharp pin (Fig. 29.2)
> - If the anesthesia persists it indicates complete cord injury. If there is descrimination between dullness and sharpness it indicates incomplete injury
> - Bulbo cavernous reflex contraction of the anal sphincter squeezing of glans penis will cause contraction (Fig. 29.3)
> - Explanation: In spinal shock there is flaccid paralysis and these reflexes are absent. Return of these reflexes with 24 hours to 7 days indicates passing off spinal shock and return of these cord mediated reflexes of S_1, S_2 and S_3. This is an indicator of grave prognosis

> **Remember**
>
> Cord concussion
> A state of "spinal shock", i.e. temporary electrical dysfunction
> **Features**
> - Sensory loss.
> - Flaccid paralysis.
> - Visceral paralysis.
> - Reflexes are in abeyance.
> - Anal reflex lost (anal wink lost).
> **Usually**
> - 8 hr later concussion regresses.
> - 7–10 days later complete recovery. If the reflexes appear and the motor paralysis does not return within 24 hrs to 10 days a diagnosis of complete cord transection is made.

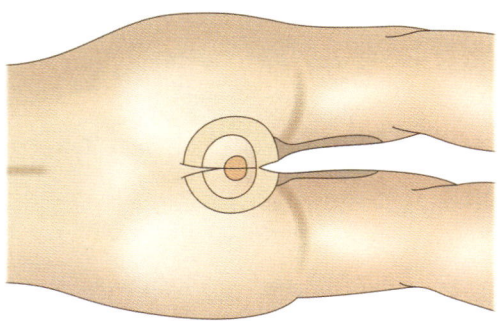

Fig. 29.2: Anal wink indicator of the status of spinal shock

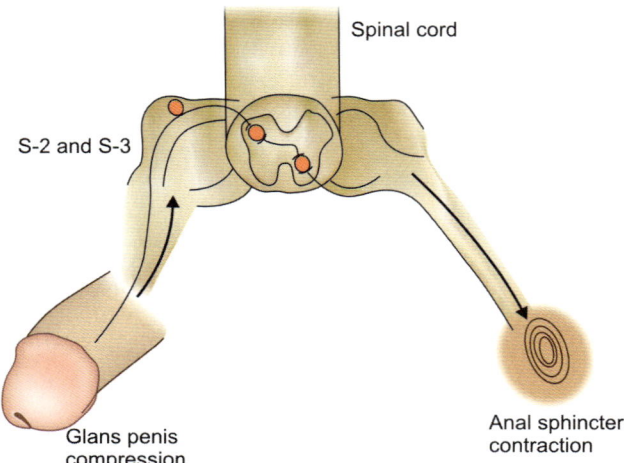

Fig. 29.3: Bulbocavernous reflex

Clinical Assessment

General examination: This consists of examination of the head, chest, pelvis and other systems for incidence of injuries and recording the vital statistics.

Neurological examination: Examine the level of the vertebral injury and find out the level of the corresponding cord injury (See box). Next, examine the individual muscle group and dermatome.

a. *Cervical level*: Each muscle group and dermatome has to be checked. In cases of cervical cord injury survival is impossible if the cord is injured above C_4 level due to paralysis of the diaphragm and respiratory muscles. In injuries below C_4 and above C_7, the level of lesion can easily be detected by examining the respective myotome, dermatome and reflexes (ref p. 155 and 156).

b. *Thoracic level (T_1–T_{10}):* This could result in paraplegia and paralysis of the trunk muscles.

c. *Thoracolumbar level (T_{11}–L_1):* Due to injuries at the thoracolumbar junction, three things can occur:
   - Complete cord division and nerves intact
   - Complete cord division and partial nerve division
   - Complete cord division and complete nerve division.

The most common spinal injury causing paraplegia is the flexion rotation injury at the thoracolumbar junction. Alternatively a mixed picture of both cord and root lesion may emerge and there could be a UMN and LMN features in the lower limbs.

d. *Lumbar level:* Injury below L_1 causes cauda equina paralysis due to nerve root transection only. It is easy to identify the injured nerve root by a careful examination of myotome, dermatome and reflexes of the lower limb.

Remember

Nerve-wracking points remember the neurological facts
- Cervical spine level as mentioned previously.
- Between T_1 and T_{10}: Paralysis of trunk and lower limb muscles.
- At T_{10}: Paraplegia and the corresponding cord damage are at L_1.
- Between D_{11} and L_1: Paraplegia and here the lumbar and sacral sections of the spinal cord are damaged along with their nerve roots.
- Below L_1: No cord damage, only root damage leading to cauda equina paralysis.
- So to arrive at the proper level of spinal cord damage, remember this rule:

Do you know how to find out the level of cord injury by looking at the level of vertebral injury?

Bone segment	Cord segment
C_1 to C_7	Add 1 to vertebral level
T_1 to T_4	Add 2 to vertebral level
T_4 to T_{10}	Add 3 to vertebral level
T_{10}	Dorsal segments complete
T_{12}	Lumbar segments complete
L_1	Sacral segments complete
Below L_1	Cauda equina paralysis

Investigations: This consists of plain radiograph of the affected part and all three views antero-posterior, lateral and oblique views are done. MRI and CT scan are also done and their role has already been stressed.

TREATMENT

First aid and management of vertebral fracture and dislocations in individual injuries has already been discussed in the previous chapter. Good nursing care is essential for the management of the bowel, bladder and back due to spinal injuries and is done as follows.

Bedsore Management

Preventing bedsores: *Nursing goals:* Education of the patients and relatives.

Only sure method of preventing pressure ulcers is strict nursing care and gradual shifting of responsibility of the skin care to the patient's family.

Spinal beds, mattresses and pads are not reliable to prevent pressure sores.

29

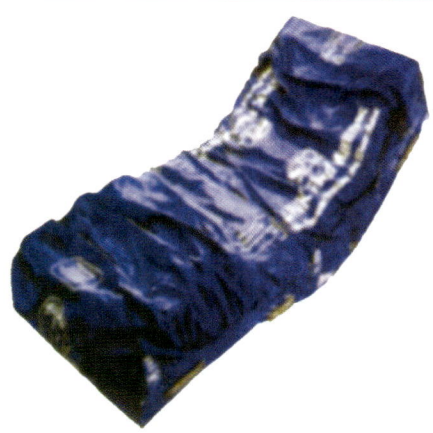

Fig. 29.4: Waterbed, a boon for prevention of bedsores

Using waterbed also helps prevent bedsores (Fig. 29.4).

Sleeping in prone position with a pillow bridging the bony prominences is the most reliable method of preventing bedsores (Fig. 29.5).

Managing bedsores: While prevention is the best mantra, the following measures are recommended once a bedsore develops:

- Keep the back dry
- Apply a dry powder to the back
- Turn the patient every 2 hours
- Use water or air beds
- Do period dressings taking all aseptic precautions.

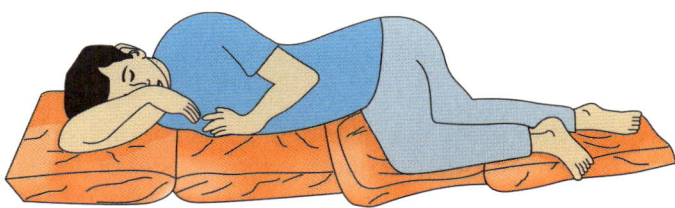

Fig. 29.5: Bed posture (side lying) to prevent formation of bedsores

Paralyzed Bladder

Bladder injuries could be either UMN type or LMN type (Table 29.1).

UMN type (automatic bladder): This is seen in injury above S2 due to complete transection of the cord. Here the bladder is distended and there is no real sensation of vesical filling and the bladder is controlled by the reflex centers. There is automatic involuntary emptying and no residual urine is left.

LMN type (autonomous bladder): This occurs in injuries at or below S2. The bladder reflex center is destroyed. It now depends on the intrinsic plexus in the musculature of the bladder wall (detrusor ganglion). Here

Table 29.1: Characteristic features of UMN and LMN bladder injuries		
Bladder	*Automatic*	*Autonomous*
1. Type	UMN	LMN
2. Level	Above S2	S2 and below
3. Reflex center of bladder	Takes over	Lost
4. Controlled by	Reflex centre	Intrinsic plexus of bladder
5. Emptying by	Involuntary	Voluntary
6. Residual urine	Minimal	Large > 200–300 cc

emptying is to be done by manual pressure or by trained contraction of abdominal musculature. There is a large amount of residual urine in this condition.

Crede's maneuver: Here the patient himself applies pressure over the suprapubic area and empties the bladder himself (Fig. 29.6).

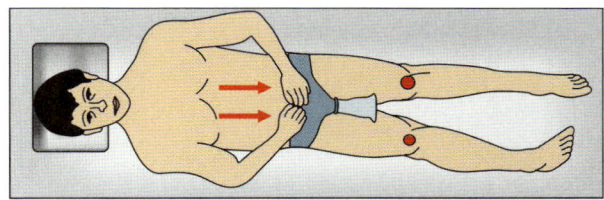

Fig. 29.6: Crede's maneuver

Note: Goal in either case is to attain an automatic reflex emptying of the bladder

Treatment: In either condition mentioned above, the treatment method aims at obtaining automatic reflex emptying. This is done as follows.

- Urinary retention catheter is placed in the bladder for 24 to 48 hours.
- After 48 hours, intermittent catheterization is started, to develop the automatic reflex emptying of the bladder.
- Persons with traumatic quadriplegia have a UMN bladder controlled by reflexes through conus medullaris.
- If intermittent catheterization is not available, bladder range of motion exercises are performed by clamping the catheter tube for 50 minutes and opening for 10 minutes every hour to allow the bladder to develop a reflex pattern of emptying.
- If reflex emptying with residual bladder urine volume of less than 100 cc does not occur within 6 to 9 months, urological procedures like external sphincterotomy or bladder neck resection is done to achieve a balanced bladder.
- Urinary diversion through ileal loops, etc. is not superior to reflex emptying of the bladder and hence is not recommended.

All possible attempts should be made to remove the catheter and have a catheter-free reflex emptying of the bladder.

Bowel Program: *Reflex emptying of the bowel with suppository stimulation is the goal of bowel training* every second or third day bowel reflex is stimulated by insertion of glycerin or Dulcolax suppository with digital stimulation. Enemas should not be given as this destroys the bowel reflex. Stool softeners and mild laxatives may be necessary.

Beds: A conventional hospital bed and pillow is preferred. Side-to-side rotating bed is used during the first week. Proper positioning of the patient with supportive pillows, frequent turning in the bed and care towards personal hygiene is very much needed.

Rehabilitation: Rehabilitation programs in neurological injury following spinal fractures are as shown in Table 29.2.

The Table shows the level of spinal injuries, their corresponding disabilities and the measures to be followed

Family education: The family members of the victim are trained to take care of the victim's bowel, back, bladder and bed. They are also encouraged to give all the necessary moral support which is so essentially required to rehabilitate the patient back to normalcy.

Physical therapy: This consists of putting joints through all the range of movements by passive stretching and exercises. Parallel bar walking, walking with the help of walkers or crutches is encouraged (Figs 29.7A to C). Wheelchair transfer activities are encouraged for injuries from C_6 level onwards (Fig. 29.8).

Occupational therapy: If possible patient is allowed to return to his original work with minor adjustments if necessary. But however if the patient is unable to return to his original work, an alternative employment depending upon his present status of health is suggested.

Social therapy: The attitude of the people towards these patients should not be of sympathy, but of support and encouragement. The right attitude of the

Table 29.2: Rehabilitative measures for neurological injury

Level	Disabilities	Measures
$S_{2,4}$	Only bowel and bladder injured	Bladder and bowel programme
L_4–S_1	Bladder, bowel and prolonged sitting impaired	Short leg braces
$L_{1,2,3}$	Bladder, bowel and walking impaired	Walking with long leg brace
T_{7-12}	UMN bladder	Long leg brace and wheelchair
T_2-T_6	Bowel, bladder, walking, sitting impaired	Wheelchair is necessary
C_7-T_1	Up to the level patient can become independent in all activities of daily living	Wheelchair is a must
C_5	Assistance to all activities of daily living required	Electrical chair is required
Above C_5	Total dependence + impaired breathing	

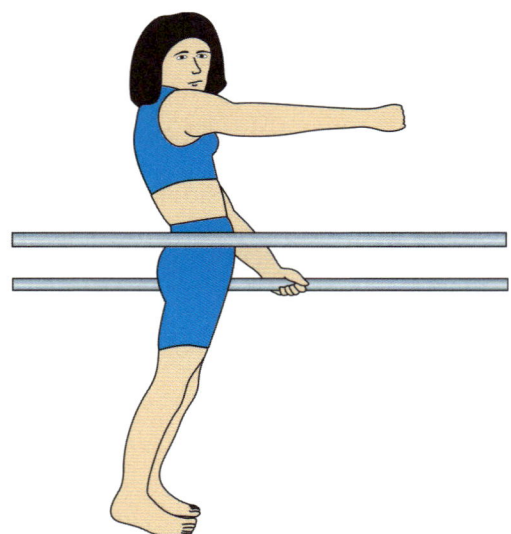

Fig. 29.8: A paraplegic patient learning to balance and walk within a parallel bar

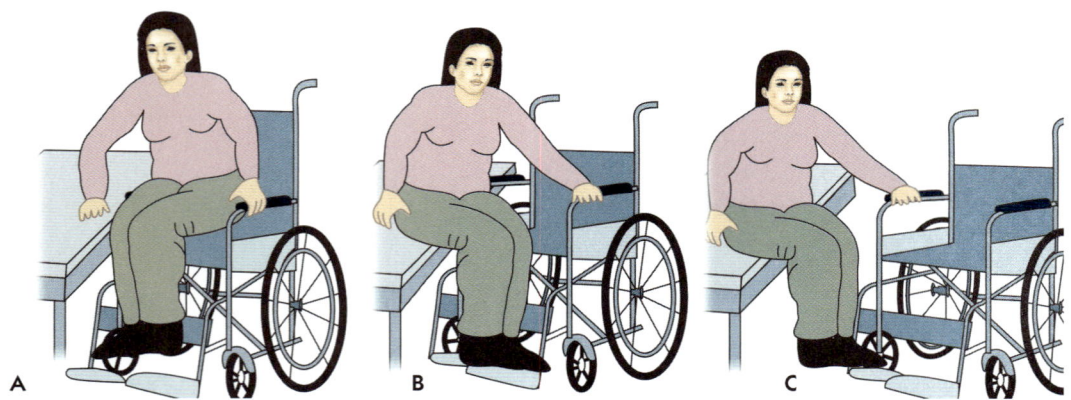

Figs 29.7A to C: Method of self-transfer by a paraplegic patient from wheelchair to the bed (A, B, C) and from bed to wheelchair (C, B, A).

society towards these unfortunate victims will go a long way in rehabilitating them back to normal.

CAUDA EQUINA SYNDROME

Cauda equina syndrome is seen in injuries below the level of first lumbar vertebra.
It is essentially injury to the nerve roots below:

Causes

- Tumors of the spine.
- Pott's disease.
- Protrusion of disc—large midline disc prolapse at 4–5 levels.
- Fracture dislocation of the thoracolumbar spine.

Clinical Features

Patient complains of back pain, perineal pain, difficulty in micturition, impotence in male, etc.

Sensory signs: Most salient feature of a cauda equina lesion is an area of saddle-shaped hyperesthesia and later anesthesia (involving buttocks, anus and perineum) (Fig. 29.9).

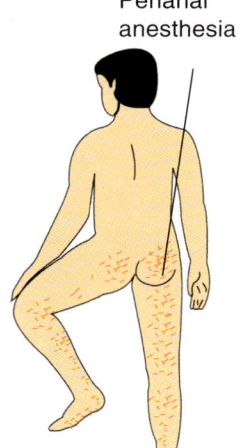

Perianal anesthesia

Fig. 29.9: Cauda equina lesion

Motor signs: Flaccid paralysis below the knee.

Reflexes: Ankle jerk is lost and the knee jerk is increased due to the weakness of the opposing hamstrings.

Bladder symptoms: Common problems are retention of urine with overflow. Even after a severe cauda equina lesion, reflex micturition is established later, reflex being mediated through the vesical plexus.

Anal sphincter: Relaxation

Treatment

Prompt surgical intervention is the treatment of choice. This consists of operative stabilization of the fractures, bowel, back and bladder care and other rehabilitating measures that have already been described above.

QUICK FACTS

Common site	Level	Result
Cervical spine	C_5–C_6	Quadriperesis/Quadriplegia
Thoraco-lumbar spine	D_{12}–L_1	Paraparesis/Paraplegia
Below L_1	Cauda equina paralysis	

WHAT IS NEW?

Stem cell therapy for permanently damaged spinal cord injury is offering a ray of hope. About 2 million stem cells are injected within 14 days after the injury helps develop new oligodendrocyte progenitor cells that can lead to development of new myelin cells. Truly a remarkable development and offers hope to millions of people with spinal cord injury.

29

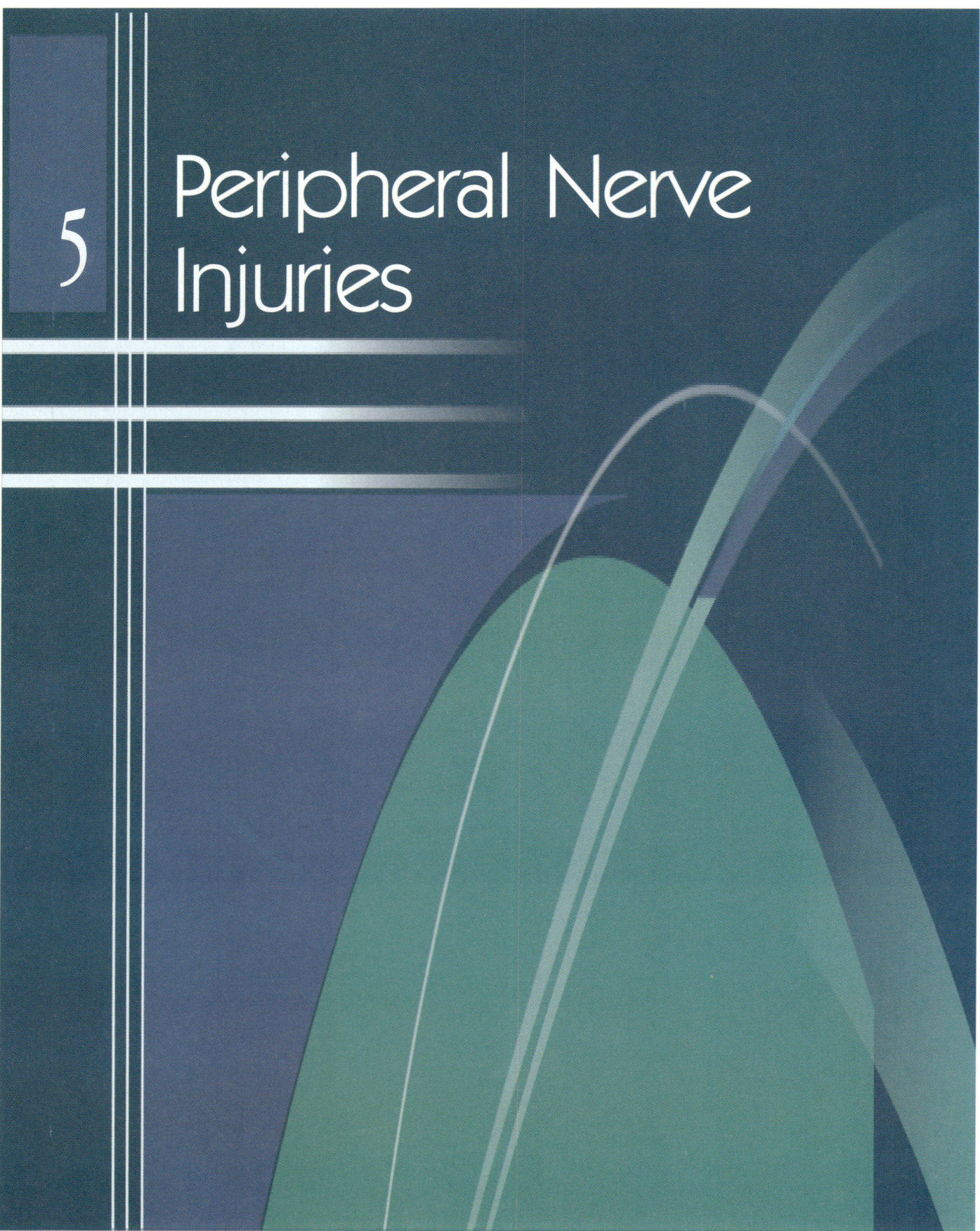

5

Peripheral Nerve Injuries

Peripheral Nerve Injuries I

BRIEF ANATOMY

The dorsal and ventral nerve roots arising from the spinal cord join at the intervertebral foramen to form a spinal nerve. In the thoracic segments, these mixed spinal nerves retain their autonomy and supply one intercostal segment both dermatome and myotomal. In virtually all other segments spinal nerves join with others to form a plexus. There are 31 pairs of spinal nerves consisting of 8 cervical, 12 thoracic, 5 lumbar, 5 sacral and 1 coccygeal.

A spinal nerve has got three components: motor, sensory and sympathetic (Fig. 30.1). The sympathetic components of all 31 mixed spinal nerves leave along the 14 motor roots (12 thoracic and 2 lumbar roots). Each spinal nerve now divides into *anterior and posterior rami*. The anterior rami of the upper four cervical nerves forms the *cervical plexus* and the lower four cervical together with upper thoracic nerves form the *brachial plexus*. The anterior rami of the first three lumbar nerves and part of the fourth lumbar nerve form the *lumbar plexus*. The sacral anterior rami along with the anterior rami of the fifth lumbar and part of fourth lumbar form the *lumbosacral plexus*.

The posterior rami supply the para spinal muscles and the skin of the back. They are smaller than anterior rami except for upper three cervical posterior rami. The spinal nerves are then distributed to the limb buds through several peripheral nerves. *So basically a peripheral nerve is also a mixed nerve like the spinal nerve.* Cross section of the nerve shows epineurium as the outermost covering, perineurium which encloses the nerve bundle, endoneurium enclosing the individual axons and mesoneurium the connective tissue that holds all these structures together (Fig. 30.2).

Note
- *Dermatome* is an area of skin supplied by a single spinal root.
- *Myotome* represents a muscle unit supplied by a single spinal root.

PATHOLOGY

Nerve degeneration: Any part of the neuron detached from its nucleus degenerates and is destroyed by phagocytosis. This process of degeneration distal to a point of injury is called *secondary or wallerian degeneration*. Reaction in proximal end is called as *primary or retrograde degeneration* (Fig. 30.3).

Nerve regeneration: Axonal sprouting starts from 24 hour after the injury. Unmyelinated initially but later on it gets myelinated. Now if the endoneurium is intact sprouts will readily pass along their former courses and after regeneration may innervate their previous end organs. If the endoneurium is interrupted, then the sprouting axons may migrate aimlessly throughout the

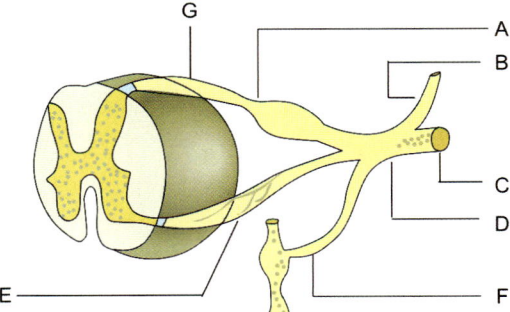

Fig. 30.1: Components of a mixed spinal nerve: (A) dorsal root ganglion on the sensory root, (B) posterior rami, (C) anterior rami, (D) mixed spinal nerve, (E) grey ramus communicans from the sympathetic ganglion, and (F) motor root

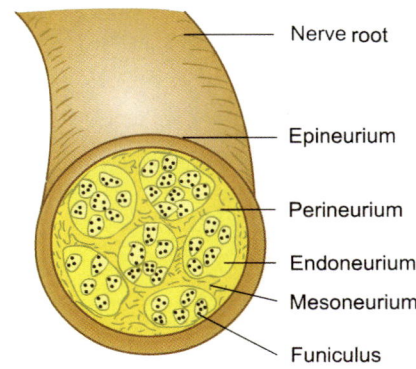

Fig. 30.2: Cross-section of the nerve root

damaged area into the epineurial, perineurial regions forming a *stump neuroma or neuroma in continuity* or they may enter into the other empty endoneural tubes or newly formed endoneural tubes only to terminate in myotomal or dermatomal areas of their own. Hence, recovery is difficult if entire axon is transected and filled with scar tissue.

> *Note:*
> The rate of axonal regeneration is 1 mm/day.
> The regenerating nerve reinervates the muscles from proximal to distal, phenomena called motor march.

Classification of Nerve Injuries

Seddon's (1943) classification (Table 30.1): Seddon identified three types of nerve injuries: the first one is a mere contusion, second is the transection of axons only, and third complete transection of the nerve. This classification is less accepted clinically.

Table 30.1: Seddon's classification

Neuropraxia	Axonotmesis	Neurotmesis
• Minor contusion of the peripheral nerve	• Axon breakdown	• Complete anatomic section
• Axis cylinder is preserved	• Endoneurium is intact	• No recovery
• Spontaneous	• Spontaneous recovery is expected	
• Temporary		
• Recovery is complete		

Sunderland's classification: *Accepted clinically* Arranged in ascending order of severity from 1 to 5. Various degrees represent injury to myelin, axon, endoneurium, perineurium and entire trunk (Table 30.2).

Etiology

General causes: Metabolic diseases, collagen diseases, malignancies, endogenous or exogenous toxins; thermal, chemical or mechanical trauma, etc. can cause injury to the peripheral nerves.

Local causes: Forty percent of bone and joint injuries are associated with peripheral nerve lesions.

Types

Primary: This is due to injury of a peripheral nerve resulting from the same trauma that has injured a bone or joint.

Secondary: This is due to involvement of the nerve in infection, scar, callus, etc. following a trauma.

Incidence of Peripheral Nerve Injuries

- Radial nerve is commonly injured
- Ulnar nerve 30 percent
- Median nerve 15 percent
- Peroneal nerve
- Lumbosacral plexus 3 percent
- Tibial nerve

30

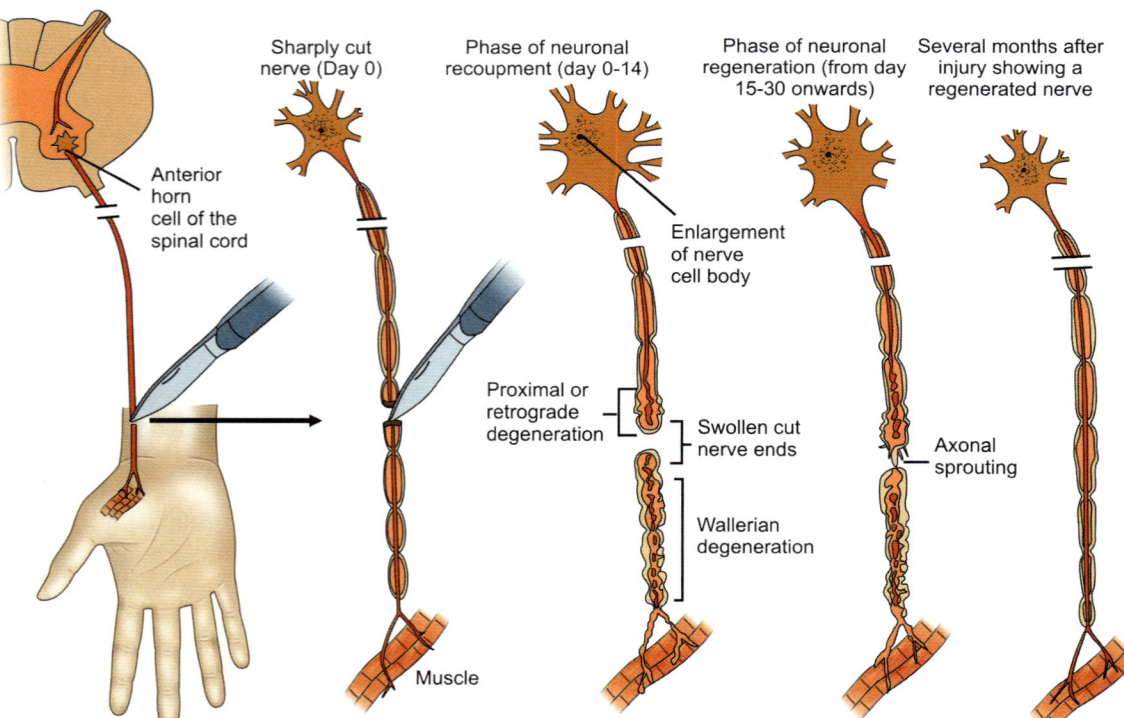

Fig. 30.3: Different types of response of the nerve to injuries

Table 30.2: Sunderland's classification of nerve injuries

Degrees	I°	II°	III°	IV°	V°
• Axon	Contusion	Disrupted	Disrupted	Disrupted	Disrupted
• Endoneurium	Intact	Intact	Disrupted	Disrupted	Disrupted
• Perineurium	Intact	Intact	Intact	Few fibers preserved	Disrupted
• Entire nerve	Intact	Intact	Intact	Intact	Disrupted
• Myelin	Intact	Intact	Intact	Intact	Disrupted
*Motor march: Recovery of the motor innervation in a progressive manner from proximal to distal	• No motor march • No Tinel's sign • Complete 3 restoration of function	• Motor march present • Tinel's sign present • Good reccovery	• Motor march present • Tinel's sign present • Incompete reccovery	• No Tinel's sign or present • No recovery	• No recovery • Grade VI° is mixture of the above injuries from 1° to V°

Clinical Diagnosis

The diagnostic approach towards a peripheral nerve injury should essentially consist of the following steps:

• *Listen:* Carefully listen to what the patient has got to tell you about the history of the injury. Many a time mere listening can help you clinch the diagnosis. Here are some samples:

Remember

History	Nerves affected
1. I am suffering from leprosy	Ulnar, median and sciatic nerves
2. I took an injection in the Arm or buttocks	Arm—Deltoid nerve. Buttocks—Sciatic nerve
3. I traveled in a bus overnight	Sciatic nerve compression neuropathy
4. I cut my wrist by a glass piece.	Medial nerve injury
5. I suffered from an arm bone fracture	Radial nerve injury
6. I broke my elbow in a fall	Radial nerve injury Median/ulnar injury
7. I have suffered a hip dislocation due to dashboard injury.	Sciatic nerve injury

QUICK FACTS: It is difficult to evaluate a nerve injury immediately after a severe trauma. However, typical attitudes and simple screening test help clinch the diagnosis with reasonable accuracy.

TYPICAL DEFORMITIES
• Wrist drop → Radial nerve injury
• Claw hand → Ulnar nerve injury
• Foot drop → Lateral popliteal nerve injury
• Ape thumb → Median nerve injury
• Winging of scapula → Thoracodorsal nerve injury
• Pointing index → Median nerve injury
• Policeman tip → Brachial plexus injury (Erb's palsy).

SIMPLE SCREENING TESTS
• In ulnar nerve injury, loss of pain at tip of the little finger.
• In median nerve injury, loss of pain on the tip of index finger.
• In radial nerve injury, inability to extend the thumb (Hitchhiker's sign)

• *Look:* This is the second step in the diagnosis of PNI. After listening to the story, look for the typical tell tale evidences. Each nerve injury is associated with a particular attitude. Look for those (See Box).
• *Feel and touch:* This helps you to detect damage to the sensory component of a nerve. The affected skin could be cold or clammy. Patient may not be able to feel the temperature, touch, vibrations, and pressure in the affected areas. Loss of sweating is an omnious sign. Do sensory grading (See Box).

QUICK FACTS: Sensory vs motor grading

	Sensory grading	Motor grading
Grade 0	No sensation (So)	No movement
Grade 1	Pain prevent	filicker
Grade 2	Presence of pain and some touch	Movement with gravity eliminated
Grade 3	Pain touch with no over reaction	Movement against gravity
Grade 4	Pain touch 2 point discrimination	Movement against partial resistance
Grade 5	Normal sensation	Normal powr

• *Move:* Instruct the patient to move the limb and joints distal to the site of injury. Inability to do so totally reveal complete nerve damage, slight movements possible suggests less than complete damage to the nerve. Do motor grading as shown above.
  Beware of the trick movements a patient may resort to overcome the loss of a particular muscle function. This is a diagnostic "pitfall" one should carefully avoid.
• *Knock:* Using a knee hammer, 'knock' over the knee, ankle, elbow, etc. to elicit the appropriate reflexes. They are normally absent in peripheral nerve injuries.
• *Measure:* With a measuring tape, measure the muscle girth of the limbs for wasting.
• *Investigate:* After following the various clinical steps, certain investigations need to be done to confirm the diagnosis and plan the appropriate line of treatment.

30

Investigations (Diagnostic tests)

Electromyography (EMG): Electromyography helps to record the electrical activity of a muscle at rest and during activity graphically.

Intact muscle: There is no electrical activity in an intact muscle at rest. During a weak contraction, the electrodes record a single action potential. In powerful muscle contractions, these motor action potentials superimpose to give an interference pattern.

Injured or denervated muscle: These muscles show denervation potentials, which are spontaneous electrical activity at rest. These are primitive responses, which is normally suppressed by the stronger nerve action potentials. These denervation potentials normally appear by 1 to 2 weeks after injury. If they do not appear by 15 to 20 days after muscle denervation, it indicates a good prognostic sign.

> **Quick facts: EMG**
> - Normal insertional activity immediately after section.
> - Positive waves seen after 5 to 14 days.
> - Denervation fibrillation after 14 days.
> - Spontaneous fibrillation after 15 to 30 days of interruption.

Uses of EMG: Electromyography helps to detect the presence or absence of nerve injury, if present whether it is complete or incomplete and whether any regeneration is taking place or not. EMG does not give the level of injury or the degree of injury accurately.

Limitations of EMG: It merely indicates whether the muscle is innervated or not. It gives no specific indications as to the level of injury or degree of injury.

Strength duration curve: A muscle usually responds to an electric stimulus. However, greater strength of current is required to excite a denervated muscle than normal muscle. Minimum current required to elicit a muscle contraction is called the "rheobase" and is

expressed in milliamperes. The "chronaxie" is the duration of current required to excite a muscle with a current strength of double the rheobase. This is expressed in milliseconds.

To know the excitability of a muscle in relation to the current strength and its duration, the muscle is stimulated by decreasing the duration of the current from 300 milliseconds to 1 millisecond and a consequent increase in the strength of the current required is detected and plotted on a graph as the strength duration curve.

Utility of Strength Duration Curve (SDC)

Normal muscle: A normal muscle responds to stimuli from duration of 300 milliseconds to 1 second without any increase in the strength of the current. However if it is less than one millisecond, increase in the strength of the current is required. This curve is called the *nerve curve.*

Completely denervated muscle: Records a muscle curve and here either more strength or longer duration stimulation is required to produce a contraction.

Partially denervated muscle: The curve here lies in between the two curves mentioned above. However, there is an upward kink, which denotes the super-imposition of the two basic types of curves.

Nerve conduction studies: Stimulation of a peripheral nerve by an electrode placed on the skin overlying the nerve will readily evoke a response from the muscle innervated by that nerve. Immediately after section, stimulation distal to the point of injury will elicit an essentially normal response for 18 to 72 hrs after injury until Wallerian degeneration sets in. This failure of response after about 3 days excludes "neuropraxia". Slowed conduction at a specific point indicates "compression neuropathy".

Tinel's sign: This is an important sign, which helps in recording the rate of regeneration of the nerve clinically.

Procedure: Gentle percussion is done along the course of injured nerve. The patient in the distribution of injured nerve rather than the area-percussed experiences tingling sensation, and the sensation should persist for several seconds following the stimulation. Positive Tinel's sign indicates regenerating axonal sprouts have not obtained complete myelinization. Response fades as myelinization takes place. Distal progression of the response and the rate of the progression have been used by some to establish prognosis (rate of recovery should be 3 cm per month). Presence of this sign is encouraging. Even a few regenerating sensory fibers can result in positive Tinel's sign. Thus, its presence cannot be taken as an absolute evidence of recovery.

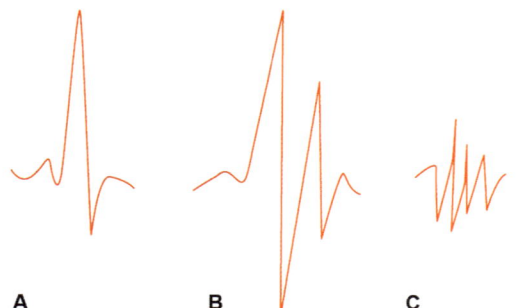

A   B   C

Figs 30.4A to C: Pattern of electromyography curves: (A) normal insertional activity, (B) positive waves (5–14 days), and (C) denervation fibrillation after (15–30 days)

30

Sweat test (Starch test): Presence of sweating within *autonomous zone suggests that complete interruption of the nerve has not occurred.

Skin resistance test: It is another method of evaluating autonomic interruption by using Richter's thermometer.

> *Note:*
> **Small area of complete anesthesia after section of a peripheral nerve or root*

Electrical Stimulation

Faradic stimulation: It is of little value (because even normally innervated muscles may fail to respond).

Galvanic stimulation: Recording of chronaxie and strength duration curve by galvanic stimulation is more helpful in evaluating nerve injuries.

Management

General principles resuscitation is carried out first, if the patient is in shock. General condition is improved by the emergency management measures. A thorough debridement of the wound is carried out, and if the wound is clean direct suturing of the perineurium or epineurium or epiperineurium of both the cut ends carries out primary repair of the nerve. If the wound is contaminated nerve is repaired after 3 to 6 weeks. In closed fractures with peripheral nerve injuries, conservative management is the treatment of choice. Careful assessment of the recovery is made and early surgical exploration is done if the recovery is not satisfactory.

Conservative management: This consists of the following essential steps.
a. *Splinting of the limbs* different splints are required to immobilize the limbs in functional positions in various nerve injuries to prevent contractures from developing.
  1. *Upper limb*
     Brachial plexus injury—aeroplane splint
     Axillary nerve injury—shoulder abduction splint
     Radial nerve injury—cock-up splint.
  2. *Lower limb:* Common peroneal nerve injury—foot drop splint
b. *Passive movements* of all joints are done to prevent contractures.
c. *Physiotherapy* measures include massage, exercise, stimulation, etc.
d. *Care of the skin.*

Operative management: This consists of various types of nerve repair, tendon transfers, arthrodesis, etc. (Figs 30.5A to D)

Types of Nerve Repair

• Primary repair is done within 6 to 8 hours after injury and if the wound is clean cut.

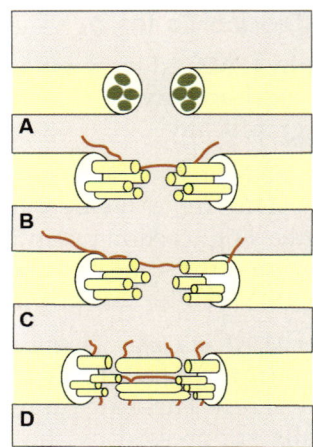

Figs 30.5A to D: Types of nerve repair: (A) epineural neurorrhaphy, (B) perineural neurorrhaphy, (C) epiperineural neurorrhaphy, and (D) interfascicular nerve grafting

• Delayed primary repair is done between 7 and 18 days after injury and if the wound is contaminated.
• Secondary repair is carried out 18 days after injury, if the injury is seen late, failure of conservative treatment, incomplete injury, etc.

Techniques

• *Endoneurolysis:* It is freeing of the nerve entrapped either within the scar tissue external scar (external neurolysis) or within nerve (internal neurolysis).
• *Partial neurorrhaphy:* This is advisable if one-half of a large nerve is disrupted, e.g. sciatic nerve injury.
• Neurorrhaphy and nerve grafting if there is a gap after injury.
• Methods of closing the gaps between the nerve ends if the nerves cannot be approximated end to end
  – Mobilization of the nerves by sectioning its cutaneous branches and freeing it from the fibrous tissue around.
  – Positioning of the extremities in functional position.
  – Transposition of the nerves, e.g. ulnar nerve transposition.
  – Bone resection.
  – Nerve grafting by using sural nerve.
  – Nerve crossing.

By these above methods, the cut ends of the nerves can be brought together and sutured by any one of the techniques mentioned above.

Other Surgeries

• Tendon transfers are contemplated after 18 months of injury when there is no recovery after various nerve repair techniques or if the patient presents late.
• Arthrodesis is considered if no tendons are available for transfers and if there is no hope of recovery.
• Amputation may be required in an anesthetic limb.

Remember

Quick summary
- Peripheral nerve is a mixed nerve
- Sunderland's classification is clinically accepted
- Forty percent of bone and joint injuries are associated with peripheral nerve lesions
- Radial nerve is the most common peripheral nerve to be injured
- Screening test helps in quick diagnosis
- In closed injuries conservative management is the treatment of choice
- In open injuries, primary nerve repair if the wound is clean and if the wound is contaminated delayed primary nerve repair or secondary repair is done

Methods of nerve suture
- Epineural repair
- Epiperineural repair
- Perineural repair
- Fascicular repair

30

31 | Peripheral Nerve Injuries II

Ulnar nerve injury
Median nerve injury
Radial nerve injury
Erb's palsy (upper brachial plexus)
Klumpke's palsy (lower brachial plexus)
Axillary nerve injury
Sciatic nerve injury

ULNAR NERVE INJURY

Brief Anatomy

It is the largest branch of the medial cord of the brachial plexus with a root value of C_8–T_1. It arises at the level of pectoralis minor muscle, run through the axilla and lie in the medial compartment of the arm. It pierces the medial intermuscular septum at the level of coraco-brachialis and lie in the posterior compartment of the arm. It passes over the posterior aspect of the medial epicondyle and enter the forearm through the two heads of flexor carpi ulnaris via the elbow. It lies beneath the flexor carpi ulnaris muscle within the forearm. At the junction of middle and lower one-third of forearm. It gives a dorsal sensory branch, which winds round the forearm and passes dorsally to supply the dorsum of the ulnar border of the hand, the little finger and medial half of ring finger. Later it passes through the Guyon's canal at the wrist formed by the pisohamate ligament and the hook of the hamate. On the exit from the canal, it splits into a superficial and deep branch. It supplies the following muscles during the course.

- In the arm—Nil.
- In the forearm—Flexor carpi ulnaris and medial half of flexor digitorum profundus it supplies both these muscles at the proximal third. As already mentioned it gives off a dorsal sensory branch at the distal third.
- In the hand—superficial branch supply palmaris brevis and digital branches to volar aspect of little finger and medial half of ring finger. Through the deep branch, it supply the hypothenar, the dorsal and the palmar interossei, two medial lumbricals and the adductor pollicis muscles.

In short, it supplies ulnar flexors of the wrist, deep finger flexors of the little and ring fingers and mainly it supplies the intrinsic muscles of the hand comprising hypothenar, lumbricals and interossei muscles (Fig. 31.1).

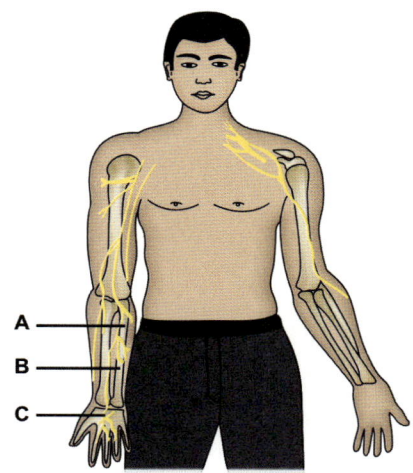

Fig. 31.1: Ulnar nerve course and supply: (A) flexor carpi ulnaris, (B) flexor digitorum profundus, and (C) intrinsic muscles of the hand

> **Remember**
>
> *Role of lumbricals:* Mainly flexes the metacarpo-phalangeal joints and extends the proximal interphalangeal joint. Role of interossei Palmar interossei adducts the fingers and dorsal abducts the fingers. Through the dorsal digital expansion they aid the action of lumbricals.
>
> *Role of hypothenar:* Abducts and helps in the movement of apposition of little finger.

Causes of Ulnar Nerve Injury

General causes are as described in the general principles of peripheral nerve injury.

Local causes are more important and could be in the following areas:

Causes in the axilla:
- Crutch pressure.
- Aneurysm of the axillary vessels.

Causes in the arm:
- Fracture shaft of humerus.
- Gunshot and penetrating injuries.

Causes at the elbow:
- Compression by the accessory muscle (anserina epitrochlearis).
- Fracture lateral epicondyle of humerus.
- Repeated occupational strains.
- Recurrent subluxation of the nerve.

- Compression by the osteophytes as in rheumatoid and osteoarthritis.
- Cubitus valgus deformity due to various causes results in repeated friction of the nerve giving rise to tardy (late) ulnar nerve palsy.

Causes in the forearm:
- Fracture both bones forearm.
- Incised wounds, gunshot wounds and penetrating injuries of the forearm.

Causes at the wrist:
- Compression by osteophytes.
- Fracture hook of the hamate.
- Compression by ganglion.

Wrist injuries
Causes in the hand:
- Blunt trauma
- Penetrating injuries
- Occupational—people operating high-speed drills in rock mining, etc.
- Associated ulnar artery aneurysm.

Ulnar nerve injuries give rise to *clawhand* deformity either true type or ulnar clawhand. It is a deformity with hyperextension of the metacarpophalangeal joints and flexion of the interphalangeal joints of the fingers.

Types: Two varieties are described: one is a true claw hand involving both median and ulnar nerves and the second an ulnar clawhand or claw-like hand due to ulnar nerve injury.

Clinical Features

These include the classical deformity, loss of sensation along the ulnar nerve distribution and wasting of the hypothenar muscles, intrinsic muscles of the hand leading to hollow intermetacarpal spaces on the dorsum of the hand (Figs 31.2A to D). A test for loss of sensation along the distribution (Fig. 31.3) of the ulnar nerve in the hand and fingers is carried out. However, the clinical features vary depending upon the level of lesion (Table 31.1).

Clinical Tests

For ulnar nerve injury:
Froment's sign: This is a reliable clinical test for ulnar nerve injury. Three muscles (first palmar interossei,

Table 31.1: Levels of lesion

High above the level of elbow entire nerve function is lost

Low

1. Below the elbow at the junction of middle and lower third of forearm	Spared: Function of FDP and FCU	
	Lost: Motor-HTM, Its, Lum, PB.	• Sensory—dorsal aspect of hand (medial border) and one and a half fingers
2. Proximal to Guyon's canal	Spared: FDP, FCU and dorsal sensation. Lost: Same as above + loss of volar sensation.	
3. Distal to Guyon's canal	Spared FDP, FCU, HTM, PB dorsal and volar Lost: Interossei and lumbricals.	• Sensations

FCU—flexor carpi ulnaris, FDP—flexor digitorum profundus, HTM—hypothenar muscles, PB—palmaris brevis, Lum—lumbricals, Its—interossei.

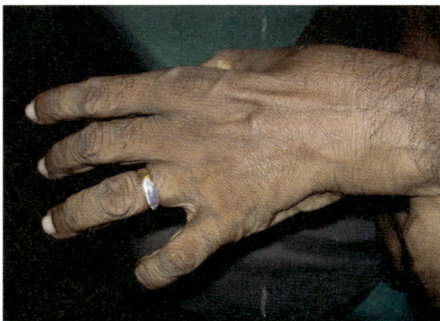

Fig. 31.2B: Wasting of intermetacarpal spaces

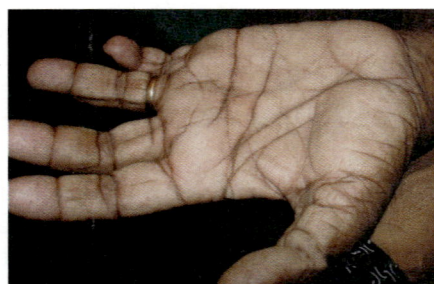

Fig. 31.2A: Clawhand deformity with hypothenar muscle wasting

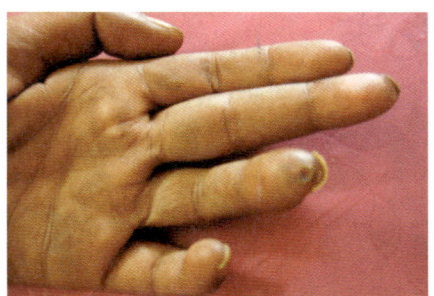

Fig. 31.2C: Trophic ulcer at the tips of fingers

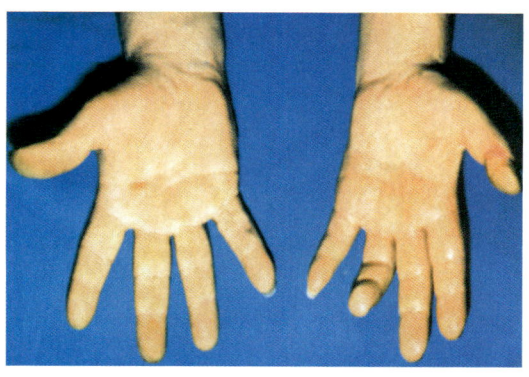

Fig. 31.2D: Bilateral clawing generally seen in diseases like leprosy

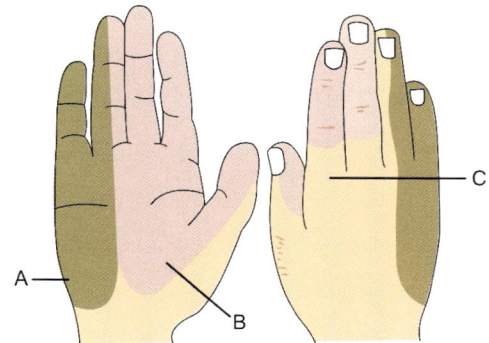

Fig. 31.3: Sensory distribution of the hand: (A) ulnar nerve distribution, (B) median nerve distribution, and (C) radial nerve distribution

adductor pollicis and flexor pollicis longus) are required to hold a book between the thumb and other fingers. In ulnar nerve injury, the first two muscles are paralyzed and now to hold the book, patient has to depend only on flexor pollicis longus, which flexes the thumb prominently. This is the positive Froment's sign (Figs 31.4A and B).

Card test: Inability to hold a card or paper in between fingers due to loss of adduction by the palmar interossei (Fig. 31.5).

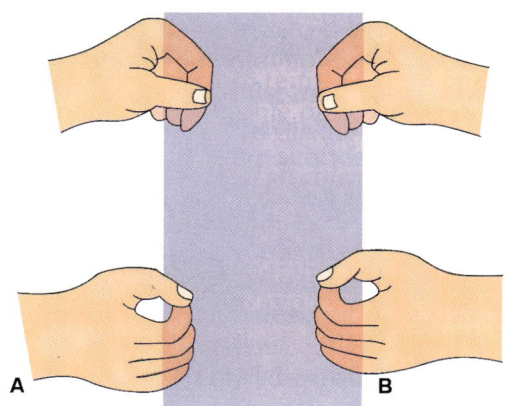

Figs 31.4A and B: Froment's sign: (A) normal, and (B) ulnar nerve injury

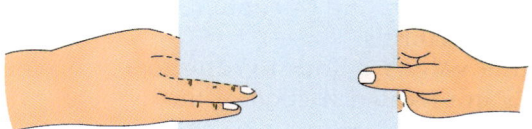

Fig. 31.5: Card test

Egawa test: With palm flat on the table the patient is asked to move the middle finger sideways. This is a test for the dorsal interossei of middle finger (Fig. 31.6).

MEDIAN NERVE INJURY

In total clawing median nerve is also injured. Following tests will help to detect the median nerve injuries.

Pen test: Patient is unable to touch the pen due to the loss of action of abductor pollicis brevis (Fig. 31.7).

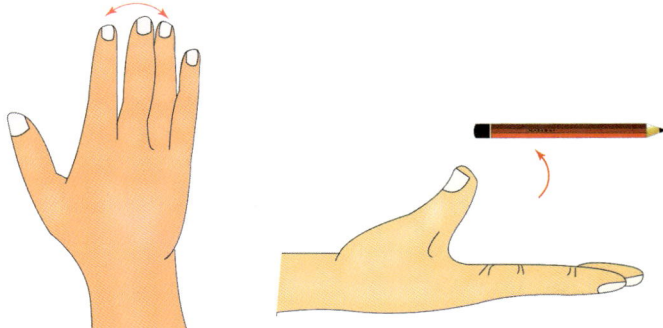

Fig. 31.6: Egawa test   **Fig. 31.7:** Pen test

Pointing index or Oschner's clasp test: When both the hands are clasped together, index and middle fingers, fail to flex due to the loss of action of long finger flexors of the index and middle fingers, which are supplied by the median nerve (Fig. 31.8).

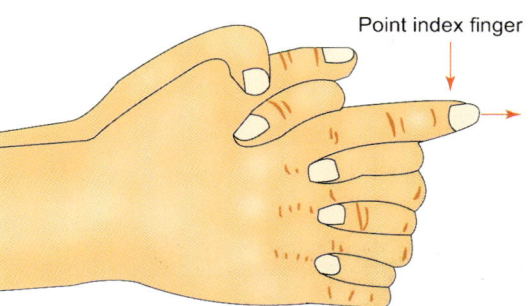

Point index finger

Fig. 31.8: Oschner's clasp test for median nerve—Pointing index finger

Benediction test: For the same reason mentioned above patient is unable to flex the index and middle finger on lifting the hand (this is the position a clergyman uses to bless the couple during marriage. Hence, called Benediction test) (Fig. 31.9).

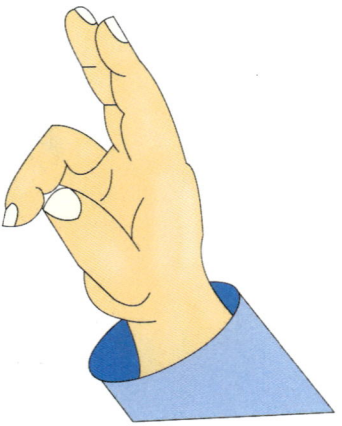

Fig. 31.9: Benediction test

Treatment

In acute injuries the treatment is as discussed in the general principles.

For Claw Hand Deformity

Principles of treatment: All the treatment measures aim at blocking the hyperextension at the metacarpophalangeal joint. Once this joint is stabilized, the long extensors will bring about the extension of IP joints. The long finger flexors will help in flexion of the MP joints along with their action of finger and wrist flexion.

> *Note:* Median nerve supplies the following muscles
> - *In the forearm* Pronator teres, flexor carpi radialis, palmaris longus, flexor digitorum superficialis, flexor digitorum profundus, flexor pollicis longus and pronator quadratus.
> - *In the hand* Abductor and flexor pollicis brevis, opponens pollicis middle and index lumbricals.

> **Remember**
> **What is ulnar paradox?**
> The higher the lesion of the median and ulnar nerve injury, the less prominent is the deformity and vice versa. This is because in higher lesions the long finger flexors are paralyzed. The loss of finger flexion makes the deformity look less obvious.

Methods of stabilization of MP joints: This can be done by the active method, which involves tendon transfer, or by passive method, which involves arthrodesis, capsulodesis or tenodesis.

Tendon transfers: Choice of surgery.

Modified S. Bunnell's operation: Flexor digitorum superficialis of the ring finger is transferred through the lumbrical canal into the dorsal digital expansion.

Riordan's operation: The flexor carpi radialis muscle is removed and transferred with a free tendon graft.

> **Remember**
> ***At a glance: ulnar nerve injury***
> - Ulnar nerve root value is C_8T_1.
> - Injury causes ulnar clawing.
> - Total clawing when median nerve is also affected.
> - Froment's sign is a reliable test.
> - For quick clinical evaluation after injury, the tip of the little finger is tested for sensation.
> - Ulnar paradox—higher the lesion less is the deformity and vice versa.
> ***Correction is by tendon transfers if all criteria are met.***
> - If no tendons are available for transfer, MP joint is stabilized by capsulodesis, tenodesis or arthrodesis.
> - All surgeries aim at correcting the hyperextension at MP joint.

Brand's operation: The extensor carpi radialis longus or brevis is transferred by a free tendon graft.

Fowler's operation: The extensor digitorum longus tendon of the index and little fingers are transferred.

When no muscle is available for transfer and if the joints are supple, capsulodesis of MP joint or tenodesis is done. If the joints are not supple, arthrodesis in functional position is done.

RADIAL NERVE INJURY

Brief Anatomy

It is the continuation of the posterior cord of the brachial plexus and its largest branch. The root value is C5-8 T1. In the axilla, it lies behind the axillary artery, pass posterior to the humerus beneath the teres major, and enter in the interval between the long and medial head of triceps. It winds round the spiral groove, pierces the lateral intermuscular septum at the junction of the distal third and the middle third, and come to lie in the anterior compartment of the arm. Here it lies between the brachoradialis and extensor carpi radialis longus and at the level of the lateral epicondyle, it splits into superficial branch and posterior interosseous nerve. Superficial branch is the direct continuation, which runs distally in the forearm under cover of brachioradialis and about two inches above the wrist it pierces the deep fascia turns dorsally and laterally and reaches the dorsum of the hand supplying three and a half fingers until the level of middle phalanges. The posterior interosseous branch penetrates the supinator muscle through the arcade of Frohse, runs distally in the forearm, and lies on the interosseous membrane. It ends as a pseudoganglion over the wrist joint. It supplies the following muscles during its course (Fig. 31.10).
- **Above the spiral groove:** All the three heads of triceps and anconeus.
- **In the spiral groove:** It gives off three cutaneous branches, posterior cutaneous nerve of the arm,

31

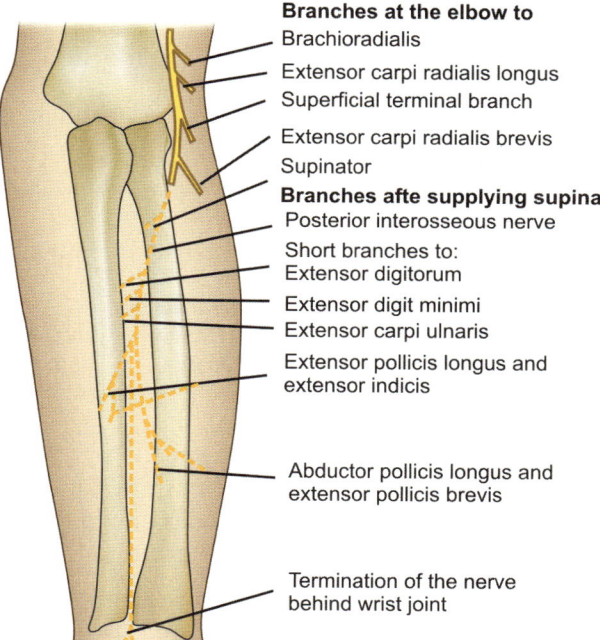

Branches at the elbow to
Brachioradialis
Extensor carpi radialis longus
Superficial terminal branch
Extensor carpi radialis brevis
Supinator
Branches afte supplying supinator
Posterior interosseous nerve
Short branches to:
Extensor digitorum
Extensor digit minimi
Extensor carpi ulnaris
Extensor pollicis longus and
extensor indicis
Abductor pollicis longus and
extensor pollicis brevis
Termination of the nerve
behind wrist joint

Fig. 31.10: Distribution of the radial nerve in the elbow and the forearm

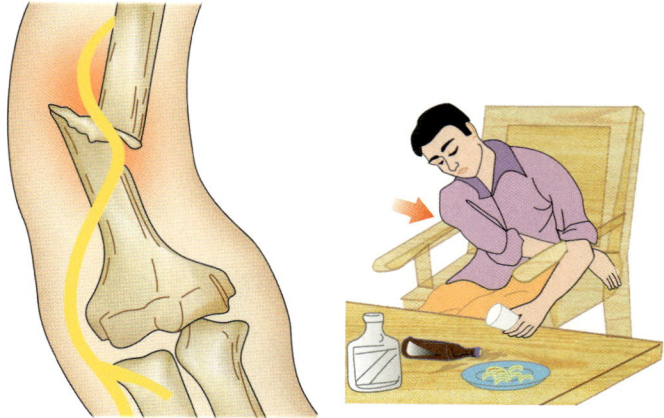

Fig. 31.11: Radial nerve injury in fracture shaft of humerus

Fig. 31.12: Saturday night palsy.

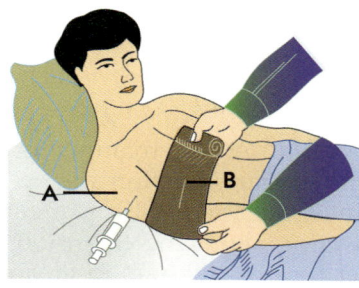

Fig. 31.13: Causes of RNP (A) syringe palsy, (B) tourniquet palsy

posterior cutaneous nerve of the forearm and lower lateral cutaneous nerve of the arm.

- **Between the spiral groove and lateral epicondyle:** It supplies the brachialis, brachioradialis and extensor carpi radialis longus muscle.
- **Before piercing the supinator** it supplies extensor carpi radialis brevis and part of supinator.
- In the supinator it supplies the rest of it. After emerging out of the supinator, it supplies all the remaining extensor muscles of the forearm and abductor pollicis longus.

Thus, you can say that it supply all the muscles on the lateral and dorsal aspects of the forearm, except the brachioradialis and extensor carpi radialis longus, through the posterior interosseous branch.

Causes for Radial Nerve Injury

General causes already discussed *(ref. p. 175)*
Local causes

In the axilla
- Aneurysm of the axillary vessels
- Crutch palsy

In the shoulder
- Proximal humeral fractures
- Shoulder dislocation

In the spiral groove **5 S**s
- **S**haft fracture (Fig. 31.11)
- **S**aturday night palsy (Fig. 31.12)
- **S**yringe palsy (Fig. 31.13A)
- **S**urgical positions (Trendelenburg)
- **'S'**march's (Esmarch) tourniquet palsy (Fig. 31.13B)

Between spiral groove and lateral epicondyle
- Fracture shaft humerus
- Supracondylar fracture humerus
- Lateral epicondyle fracture of the humerus
- Penetrating and gunshot injuries
- Cubitus valgus deformity

At the elbow
- Posterior dislocation of the elbow
- Fracture head of radius
- Monteggia's fractures

Causes in the forearm
- Fracture both bones forearm
- Penetrating and gunshot injuries.

Clinical Features

If the lesion is high patient will present with wrist drop, thumb drop and finger drop (Fig. 31.14). He will be unable to extend the elbow. If the lesion is low, the elbow extension is spared but the wrist, thumb and the finger extensions are lost but *the patient can extend the IP joints of the fingers because of the action of the intrinsic muscles of the hand.* Sensation along the posterior surface of the arm and forearm is lost in high lesions and in low lesions the above sensations are spared, but there is loss of sensation over the first dorsal web space.

Levels of lesion	Features
High Above spiral groove Low: Type I	Total palsy
Between the spiral groove and the lateral epicondyle	Spared: Elbow extensor Lost: Motor • Wrist extensor • Thumb extensor • Finger extensors Sensory: Dorsum of first web space.
Low: Type II Below the elbow	Spared • Elbow extensor • Wrist extensor Lost: Motor • Thumb extensor • Finger extensor Sensation first web space

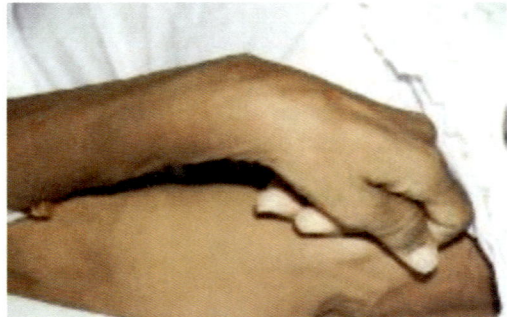

Fig. 31.14: Wrist drop

In acute injuries, it is difficult to evaluate the injury to the radial nerve. In such situations, the Hitchhiker's sign (inability to extend the thumb) is used as the screening test.

Investigations: Radiograph of the injured part and all other investigations mentioned in the general principles are carried out.

Treatment

Early cases: As mentioned in the general principles for closed fractures conservative treatment is adopted. Patient is put on a cock-up splint or dynamic splint. This is followed by active and passive physiotherapy. In failed conservative treatment, operative treatment is considered after a period of 12 to 18 months (Figs 31.15A and B).

In open fractures, surgery is the treatment of choice. If the wound is clean, primary nerve repair is done and if the wound is contaminated delayed primary or secondary nerve repair is resorted to.

Late cases (> 1 yr): Broad Principles are as follows:

Active treatment: If neighboring tendons are intact and if all the criteria for tendon transfers are met, then

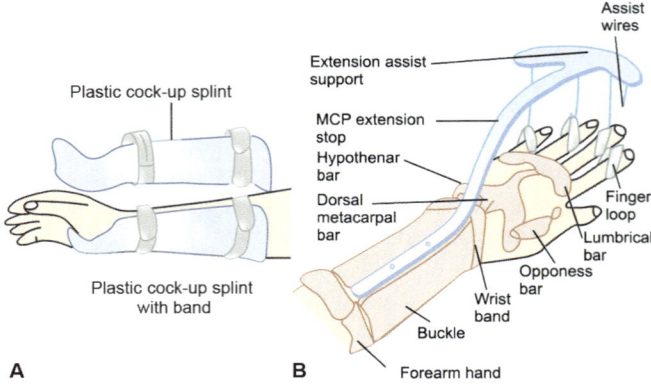

Figs 31.15A and B: Wrist drop splints: (A) static or cock-up splint, (B) dynamic splint

tendon transfer is the treatment of choice. The tendons commonly used for the transfers are pronetor teres, flexor carpi ulnaris and palmaris longus muscles (Robert Jones operation).

Passive method: If no tendons are available for transfer then tenodesis or wrist arthrodesis in functional position is preferred.

Remember
Radial nerve injury at a glance
- Continuation of posterior cord of the brachial plexus.
- Most common peripheral nerve to be injured.
- Most common site of injury is the distal end of humerus.
- Thumb extension test (Hitchhiker's sign) is the screening test.
- In radial nerve injury extension at finger IP joint is still possible.
- For early cases in closed fractures conservative treatment.
- For open fractures operative treatment and repair.
- For late cases, tendon transfers if neighboring tendons are available and if all the criteria are met.
- If no tendons are available wrist arthrodesis is done in functional position.

ERB'S PALSY

This is due to injury to the C_5 nerve root and rarely the C_6 nerve root. It occurs either very early in life due to birth trauma (obstetric palsy, due to faulty application of forceps) or in young adults due to bike trauma.

The Effects of the Injury

At the shoulder here, there is paralysis of the deltoid, rhomboids, supra and infraspinatus and teres minor muscles. This results in the loss of shoulder abduction and external rotation.

At the elbow, biceps and brachialis muscles are paralyzed. This results in loss of flexion of the elbow joint.

At the forearm supinator, muscles are paralyzed resulting in loss of supination of the forearm.

The combined effect of the injury is an arm hanging loosely by the side of the trunk. The shoulder is internally rotated, the elbow is in extension, the forearm is pronated and the wrist is in flexion. This characteristic posture is popularly known as *"Policeman or Waiter's tip"* (Fig. 31.16).

Apart from this, there may be sensory loss on the outer aspects of the arm and forearm both in the front and back.

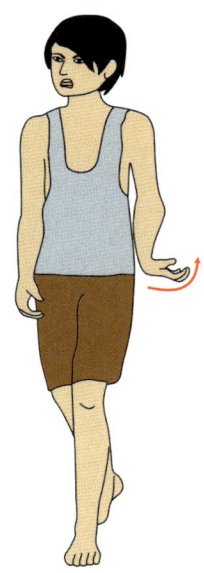

Fig. 31.16: Waiter or Porter's tip position in Erb's palsy

Management

Splinting: This is done by using an abduction or aeroplane splint. The shoulder is maintained in abduction and external rotation, elbow in 90° of flexion, forearm in supination and wrist in extension.

Measures to prevent contractures: A full range of passive movements to the affected joints helps prevent the contractures. This is a home treatment program and should be taught to the mother.

Electrical: Stimulation of the affected muscles by using bilaterally symmetrical PNF stimulus helps to activate them.

Surgery: This is rarely indicated as most of the cases recover spontaneously with the above treatment. Some of the recommended surgical measures are
a. Exploration and repair of the nerve roots
b. Tendon transfers to improve abduction and external rotation of the shoulder
c. Release of soft tissue contractures
d. Derotation osteotomy for the rotational deformity.

KLUMPKE'S PARALYSIS

This is also due to either a birth trauma or a bike trauma.

The C_8T_1 nerve roots are involved and there will be paralysis of the wrist flexors, finger flexors and intrinsic muscles of the hand. This results in a clawhand deformity (Fig. 31.17). The clinical features and management are discussed in the section on ulnar and median nerve injuries (see page 220).

AXILLARY NERVE INJURY

It takes origin from the posterior cord of the brachial plexus and winds round the lower border of the subscapularis. It goes through the quadrangular space and lies medial to the surgical neck of the humerus and divides into anterior and posterior branches. The anterior branch winds around the surgical neck of the humerus and supplies the deltoid muscle except the

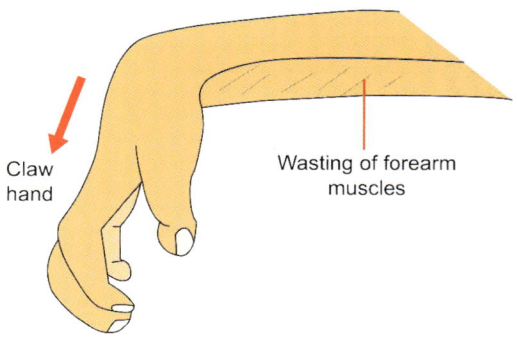

Claw hand

Wasting of forearm muscles

Fig. 31.17: Klumpke's paralysis

lower half. Posterior branch supplies the teres minor, lower half of the deltoid and ends as a cutaneous nerve that supplies the lower half of the deltoid region.

Wasting of the deltoid muscle, regiment badge anesthesia (Fig. 31.18), inability of the patient to abduct the shoulder are some of the classical features.

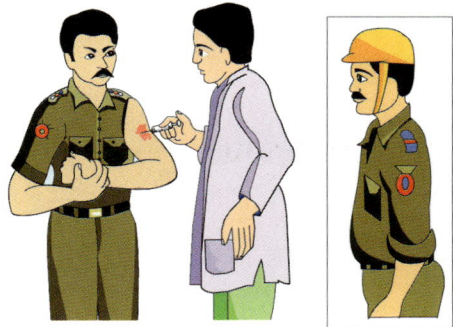

Fig. 31.18: Regiment badge anesthesia in axillary nerve injury

FOOT-DROP

Sciatic Nerve Brief Anatomy

It is the thickest nerve in the body with a root value of L_{4-5} S_{1-3}. It enters the glutei region through the greater sciatic notch and passes between the greater trochanter of femur and ischial tuberosity. From here, it enters the thigh and in the middle, it divides into *common peroneal and the tibial part*. Before doing so it supplies biceps, semitendinosus, semimebranosus and adductor magnus. The *common peroneal part* is the smaller of the two terminal divisions. This runs along the medial border of biceps, leaves the popliteal fossa at the lateral angle, passes behind the head of the fibula, winds round the neck and divides into *superficial (musculocutaneous nerve) and deep peroneal nerve*. The superficial nerve descends in the substance of peroneus longus and supplies the peroneal muscles, skin over the lower part of front of the leg, whole of the dorsum of the foot except the first web space and most of the toes. The deep peroneal nerve supplies all the four muscles of the anterior compartment and divides into *medial*

terminal branch and lateral terminal branch. The former supplies the first web space and the latter *ends as a ganglion* after supplying extensor digitorum brevis and second dorsal interosseous. The medial terminal branch also supplies the first dorsal interossei (Fig. 31.19).

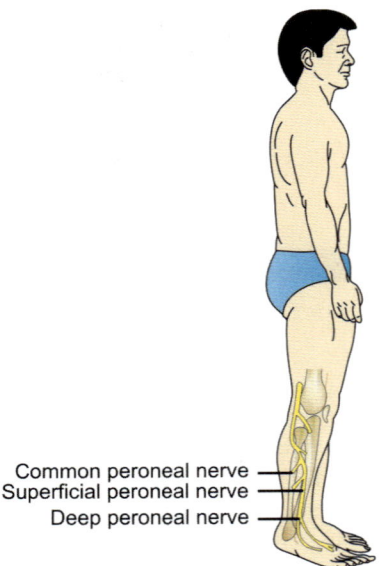

Fig. 31.19: Course and supply of common peroneal nerve

Common peroneal nerve
Superficial peroneal nerve
Deep peroneal nerve

The tibial component supplies muscles of the posterior compartment of the leg and provides cutaneous distribution to the entire sole of the foot. (Fig. 31.20).

Causes of Foot-Drop

General causes have been already mentioned, the important one being leprosy as a cause of foot-drop. *Local causes* are seen along the course of the nerve

At the spine
• Spina bifida
• Tumors
• Disc prolapse, etc.

At the hip
• Posterior dislocation of the hip (Fig. 31.21).

• Fractures around the hip
• Fracture acetabulum

At the gluteal region
• Deep intramuscular injections

At the thigh
• Fracture shaft femur
• Penetrating injury and gunshot injury

At the knee (common causes)
• Forcible inversion of the knee
• Dislocation of knee
• Fracture lateral condyle of tibia
• Lateral meniscal cysts and tumors
• Dislocation of superior tibiofibular joint
• Tight plaster casts around the knee
• Poor padding during traction
• Surgical damage during application of skeletal traction.
• *Direct injuries*—gunshot injuries, incised and penetrating injuries, etc.

31

Levels of Lesion

• *High lesion* (Above knee) Both tibial nerve and common peroneal nerve is paralyzed.
• *Low lesion* (Below knee) Spared: Peroneus longus and brevis.

Type I
Anterior tibial nerve injury

Lost: Tibialis anterior, extensor hallucis longus, extensor digitorum longus and peroneus tertius.
Sensation: Over first web, space is lost.

Type II
Musculo-cutaneous nerve injury

Spared: All the above muscles innervated by anterior tibial nerve.
Lost: Peroneus longus and brevis.
Sensation: Over outer leg and foot.

Clinical Features

The resulting deformity following injury to the above nerves is *foot-drop* (Fig. 31.22). This could be either *complete* (in sciatic nerve or lateral popliteal nerve

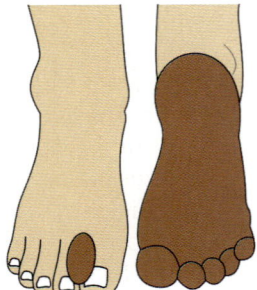
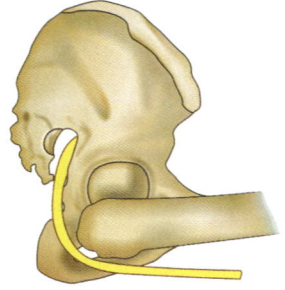

Fig. 31.20: Dorsal web space is supplied by anterior tibial nerve. Sole of the foot is by posterior tibial nerve

Fig. 31.21: Injury to sciatic nerve due to posterior dislocation of hip joint

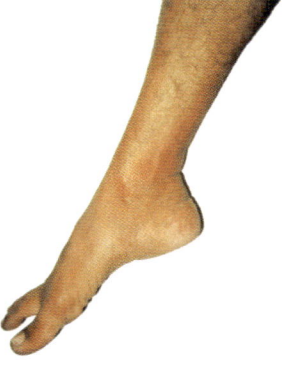

Fig. 31.22: Wasting of the leg muscles, foot-drop and trophic changes in the heel and foot

injury) or *incomplete* (injury to either superficial or deep peroneal nerve).

In high lesions, it is a total foot-drop and in low lesions, the foot-drop is usually incomplete. In low type I patient cannot dorsiflex and invert the foot but eversion is possible, front of the leg is wasted. In low type II, patient cannot evert but can dorsiflex and invert the foot. There is wasting of the outer half of the leg and there could be trophic changes in the heel and foot (Fig. 31.23). In type I injury, sensation over the dorsal web space is lost and in type II injury, it is lost over outer leg and foot. The gait typical of foot-drop is a *high stepping gait.*

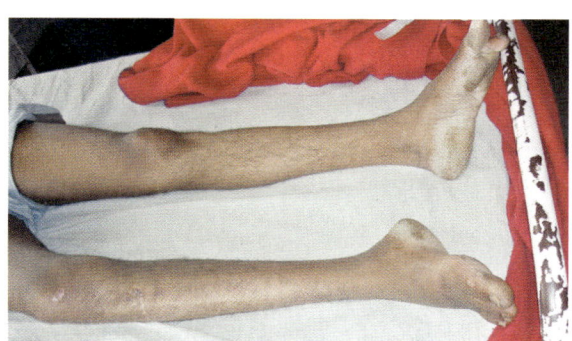

Fig. 31.23: Wasting of the leg muscles, foot-drop and trophic changes in the heel and foot

Treatment of early foot-drop: The lesions show a high incidence of recovery. Hence, conservative treatment with a view to encourage recovery (at least for 1 year) should be carried out.

Splintage of knee in 20° of flexion and ankle in 90° for night time. In daytime, walking is allowed by using a "Foot-drop appliance".

Foot-drop appliances are of two varieties:
Static—backstop shoe (Fig. 31.24).
Dynamic—spring shoe (Fig. 31.25)

Along with the splintage, general treatment to correct the underlying etiology is undertaken. Steroids are also known to help.

Treatment of late foot drop: In these cases surgery is the treatment of choice and the following procedures are described:

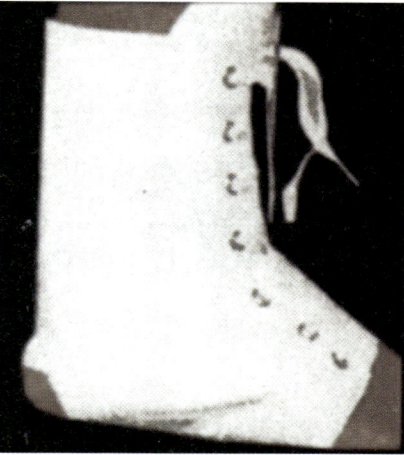 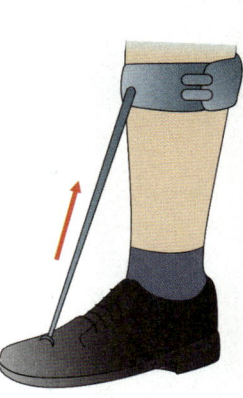

Fig. 31.24: Foot-drop splint (Static type)   **Fig. 31.25:** Dynamic foot drop splint

Surgery: *Choice of surgery*
- *Common peroneal nerve stripping* is done in leprosy. It is done in a thickened, tender nerve in a tuberculoid case with history of recent paralysis.
- Tendon transfers for mobile foot-drop, and the popular choice is posterior tibialis tendon transfer.
  Ober's technique: Here tibials posterior is transferred to base of the III metatarsal and III Geneiform.
  Barr's technique: Tibials posterior is inserted to III cuneiform.
- Tendo-Achilles lengthening—in fixed equinus.
- Subtalar stabilizing procedure—for fixed varus.
- Triple arthrodesis—for fixed varus at the subtalar joint.

Remember

At a glance: About sciatic nerve injury
- Sciatic nerve is the thickest nerve in the body.
- Common peroneal nerve also called as lateral popliteal nerve is commonly injured at the fibular neck.
- Leprosy is the commonest general cause.
- Foot-drop could be complete or incomplete.
- High stepping gait is characteristic.
- Dynamic foot-drop splint is the mainstay of conservative treatment.
- Conservative treatment is indicated up to one year.
- Tendon transfer for mobile foot-drop is contemplated after 1 year.

Regional Orthopedic Disorders: General Principles

32 General Principles of Orthopedic Disorders

History
Examination
Investigations

APPROACH TO ORTHOPEDIC DISORDERS

As in other branches of medicine, the diagnosis of orthopedic disorders revolves around the following fundamentals (Fig. 32.1). So we will try to discuss in brief the three steps of diagnosis in orthopedics.

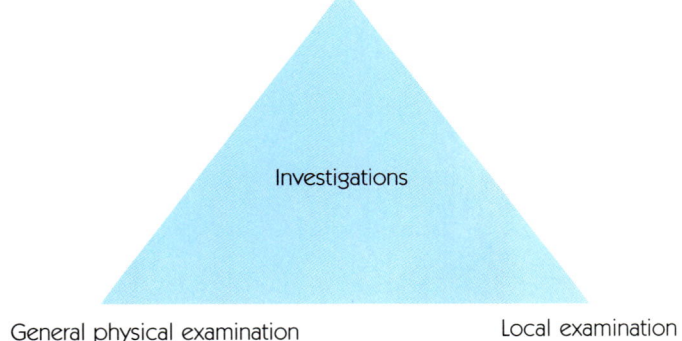

Fig. 32.1: Fundamentals of diagnosing orthopedic disorders

HISTORY

History is "His-Story", as told by the patient. History taking is an art. Caution has to be exercised in the story "told" and the story "untold." Everything told should be taken with a pinch of salt lest the examiner is misled.

Certain Points of Importance in the History

Age

Certain diseases have predilection for certain age groups, e.g. Perthes' disease and acute osteomyelitis are common in children. Avascular necrosis and degenerative disorders are common in the elderly. Some diseases may be seen in all the age groups, e.g. tuberculosis of bone and joints.

QUICK FACTS: AGE VS ORTHOPEDIC DISEASE

< 1 year	Congenital dislocation of hip and cerebral palsy
1–2 years	Nutritional rickets
	Poliomyelitis
	Ewing's tumor
5–10 years	Tuberculosis of hip
	Perthes' disease
15–20 years	Slipped capital epiphysis
<15 years	Osteomyelitis
10–20 years	Bone malignancies
30–40 years	Rheumatoid arthritis
> 40 years	Degenerative disorders
	Prolapsed intervertebral disc (PIVD)
	Multiple myeloma, etc.

Sex

Congenital dislocation of hip (CDH) is common in females. Congenital talipes equinovarus (CTEV) is more common in males.

QUICK FACTS—SEX VS ORTHOPEDIC DISEASE

- Males: Perthes, slipped epiphysis, traumatic disorders, multiple myeloma, etc.
- Females: Rheumatoid arthritis, CDH, osteoporosis, etc.

Onset

It may be sudden (Trauma infection, etc.) or gradual (diseases).

Trauma

It could be a predisposing factor (TB, osteomyelitis, etc.) or the causative factor (fractures or dislocations).

TRAUMATIC POINTS

Role of trauma vs orthopedic disorders—trauma as a causative factor
- Fracture
- Dislocation
- Sprain
- Strain
- Subluxation

Trauma as a predisposing factor
- TB hip
- Perthes' disease
- Slipped capital epiphysis
- Osteogenic sarcoma
- Acute osteomyelitis, etc.

Fever

It may be high as in acute osteomyelitis or low grade as in tuberculosis.

Pain

This could be continuous or intermittent, low or high grade. One should be on guard about the radiating pains as these often misleads the examiner.

QUICK FACTS: ABOUT RADIATING PAINS

Region	Radiation sites
• Cervical spine	Shoulder, arm, forearm, and fingertips
• Upper limbs	
a. shoulder	Arm and elbow
b. elbow	Forearm
• Thoracic spine	Girdle pains
• Lumbar spine	Groin, buttocks, posterior thigh, legs and foot
• Hip	Knee

Any constitutional problems: Like weight loss, anorexia, etc. if present is a pointer towards neoplasm, tuberculosis, etc.

Seasonal variation: If present, it is suggestive of rheumatoid disorders. Apart from these points, relevant past history, socioeconomic status and personal history should be taken into account.

An attempt should be now made to place the problem into one of the following categories at the end of history taking (See box).

DIAGNOSTIC FACTS

• Present since birth	Congenital
• During the development process	Developmental
• History of fever, chills, rigors	Infective
• Nutrition, socioeconomic status	Metabolic
• Other evidences of hormonal imbalance	Endocrinal
• Seasonal variation, multiple joint involvement, etc.	Inflammatory
• History of RTA, fall, assault	Traumatic
• Features of either benign or malignant	Neoplastic
• Advancing age, etc.	Degenerative
• If no obvious complaints	Idiopathic

If it cannot be categorised into any of the above, then it could be *idiopathic.* Having made a tentative diagnosis at the end of history taking , next important step is resorted to.

EXAMINATION

A good systematic clinical examination will help to clinch the diagnosis with certainty. *No sophisticated technology can replace the value of a good clinical examination.* A good clinician will make the diagnosis clinically and will make use of the investigation armamentarium judiciously. *A clinician should command the investigation and not vice versa.*

Examination of the locomotor system involves four steps.

STEP I

Examination of Gait

It is a term used to describe the style of walking. An examination of the gait is extremely important as it gives vital clues regarding the diagnosis. This is dependent not only on normal muscles and joints but also upon an intact central nervous system (CNS), peripheral nervous system and normal labyrinthine function.

STEP II

General Physical Examination

A good general physical examination (GPE) from head to toe gives vital clues in the diagnosis of most of the orthopedic disorders, particularly generalized disorders of the skeleton (see chapter).

STEP III

Clinical Examination

Symptoms

The following are the usual presenting symptoms in a patient with orthopedic disorder.

1. *Pain:* This is the first and the most common complaint. It is a highly subjective complaint and can be classified as mild, moderate or severe. The must-ask questions regarding the pain are: How did it start? Is it related to trauma? Site of pain? Does it radiate? What are the aggravating and relieving factors? Does it interfere with sleep? etc.
2. *Swelling:* It may precede or follow pain. Relevant questions to be asked are: Site of the swelling, painful or painless? Is it rapidly growing (e.g. malignancy) or slow growing (benign growth)? Is it associated with fever, chills, etc. (e.g. infective origin), single or multiple (e.g. neurofibromas)?
3. *Deformity:* Sudden onset of deformity is usually seen in fresh fractures and dislocations. Long-standing deformities are usually seen in old fractures and other non-traumatic disorders like congenital, developmental, and metabolic conditions. The patient may complain of cosmetic and functional impairment due to the deformity.
4. *Limitations of joint movements:* In the initial stages, it may be due to muscle spasm; and in the later stages, it may be due to intraarticular adhesions (e.g. TB, septic arthritis, rheumatoid arthritis) or extra-articular contractures (like postburn contractures, Volkmann's ischaemic contracture).
5. *Limp:* This could be painful (e.g. arthritis of hip, trauma) or painless (e.g. CDH, coxa vara).The patient may complain of difficulty or alteration in various

32

day-to-day activities like walking, squatting, running, working.

6. *Limb weakness:* This may be due to disuse atrophy, motor problems like polio, motor neuron disease, etc., muscle problems like muscular dystrophies, etc. or due to peripheral or diabetic neuropathies.

Signs

General: Look for the signs of anemia, fever, weight loss, etc.

Local

1. *Deformity:* It may be due to an abnormality of bone or joint. If a joint is out of its anatomical position, a deformity is said to exist. And in case of bone, deviation from its normal anatomy is deformity. In cases of old fractures and dislocations, the deformity may be fixed.

32

> **Remember**
> - A fixed deformity is the angle between the neutral position of the normal joint and the position the deformed joint will reach.

2. *Temperature:* This is always compared with the normal side. Check with dorsum of the hand as this is the most sensitive part.

3. *Tenderness:* This is elicited by examining from the normal to the affected area and is graded I to IV (Fig. 32.2).

4. *Swelling:* The following things are noted in the examination of a swelling.
   - Decide the anatomical plane. Also, examine the level of the swelling and identify whether it is epiphyseal, metaphyseal or diaphyseal (Figs 32.3A to D).
   - Describe the shape as globular, oval or round, etc.
   - Grade the consistency (*see* below).
   - Decide whether it is congenital, neoplastic, etc.
   - Look for slipping sign, sign of emptying, indentation sign and expansile impulse.

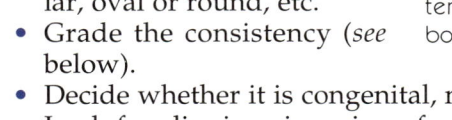

Fig. 32.2: Method of eliciting joint line tenderness (A) and bony tenderness (B)

> **Remember**
>
> Grading of consistency
> - Grade I   :   Very soft (like jelly)
> - Grade II   :   Soft (as relaxed muscle)
> - Grade III   :   Firm (like a contracted muscle)
> - Grade IV   :   Hard (as a contracted biceps)
> - Grade V   :   Stony and bone hard

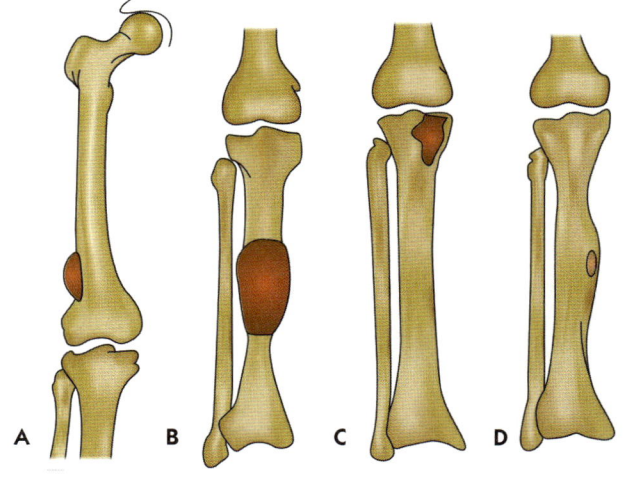

Figs 32.3A to D: Different levels of bony swelling (A) metaphyseal, (B and D) diaphyseal, (C) epiphyseal

5. *Movements of joint*
   Active movement: the patient himself moves the joint in one direction and later in the other. The extent of active movement is noted. Both the joints should be tested.
   Passive movement of the joint is tested by the examiner without causing pain. The extent of passive movement is noted.

> **Remember**
> - Limitation of all movements of a joint indicates arthritis.
> - Limitation of certain movements of a joint indicates an extraarticular lesion or mechanical block.
> - If passive movements exceed active movements, paralysis of muscle is likely.

6. *Measurements:* Accurate limb length measurements give vital clues regarding the diagnosis. Measurement should be taken for two purposes.

To know the limb length: For this, measurement is taken between two fixed bony points and is always compared with the normal.

Upper limbs
- *Arm length:* From the angle of acromion to the lateral epicondyle of humerus (Fig. 32.4).
- *Forearm length:* From the lateral epicondyle of humerus to the radial styloid process.

Lower limbs
- *Thigh length:* From anterior superior iliac spine to the medial knee joint line.
- *Leg length:* From the medial knee joint line to the medial malleolus.

   To know the apparent length of the lower limbs measurement is taken from the xiphisternum to the medial malleolus (Fig. 32.5).

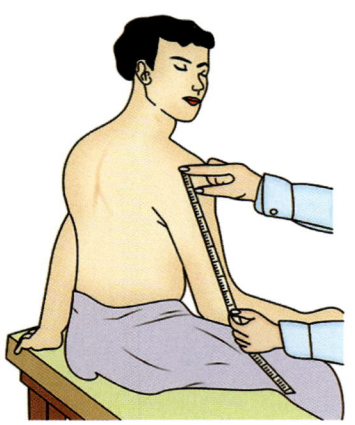

Fig. 32.4: Method of upper arm length measurement

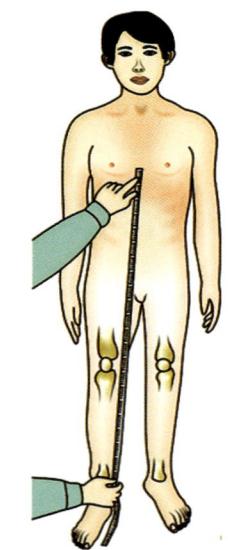

Fig. 32.5: Method of measuring apparent lower limb length

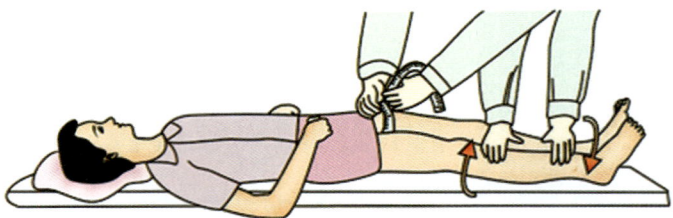

Fig. 32.6: Method of measuring the girth of a limb and checking the movements

INVESTIGATIONS

These help to confirm the diagnosis and in some cases help to make the diagnosis (e.g. crack fracture, etc. can be diagnosed only by X-ray). One has to choose carefully from the following vast armamentarium:

• *Laboratory investigation:* This consists of blood investigations like routine hemogram, urine examination, ECG, chest X-ray.

• *Special investigations:*
Radiography: At least two views of the affected part should be taken, oblique views and some special views are required in some cases.
CT scan to study the cross section of the limb anatomy and bones.
MRI: This is the recent gold standard in the investigative armamentarium of bone disorders. It helps to study the bone, soft tissues, medullary spread, etc. with greater accuracy. The only problem is its prohibitive cost.
Angiography and *biopsy* help in tumor diagnosis.

Thus, a reasonably accurate diagnosis can be made by following the guidelines discussed above.

To know the girth of the limb: To detect wasting of muscles, the circumference of the limb is measured at fixed points on both sides, e.g. 18 cm above joint line in the thigh (Fig. 32.6).

7. *Irregular thickening of bone and persistent discharging sinus:* If this is present along with scars fixed to bone, it indicates chronic osteomyelitis (see box for causes of persistent sinus) (See Fig. 51.17A).

Peripheral, vascular and nervous system examination should be done next. This is discussed in appropriate sections.

QUICK FACTS—SINUS TRACTS

Causes of persistent discharging sinus:
• Unobliterated cavities
• Unabsorbed sequestra
• Epithelialization of sinus tract
• Presence of foreign body
• Secondary infection
• Diabetes, steroid therapy, etc.
• Malignant change in the sinus

STEPS IN THE PROCESS OF DIAGNOSIS	
At the end of investigation	Final
At the end of examination	Provisional
At the end of history	Guess

Management

The general principles of the management of orthopedic disorders and related deformities are discussed in the next chapter. Detailed discussion on individual orthopedic disorders are dealt in relevant sections.

32

33 | Management of Orthopedic Disorders and Deformities

Introduction
Types of deformities
Causes: Bones, joints and soft tissues
Treatment options

INTRODUCTION

Any deviation from the normal anatomy of a bone and joint is called a deformity.

Congenital deformities are present since birth and are due to some genetic abnormalities or environmental variations or both. They may be obvious at birth or may be seen few years later. Incidence is around 2 to 3 per cent. They may be so severe that the child is stillborn or may be so minor that it is not noticeable.

Important Congenital Deformities

- *Neck* wry neck
- *Upper limbs* congenital radio-ulnar synostosis.
- *Lower limbs* CDH and CTEV.

    (See section on congenital deformities for details).

Acquired Deformities

These could be due to problems in the bone, joint or soft tissues.

Bone Causes

The following causes are responsible for deformities in the bone:

a. *Growth disturbances:* Tumor, infections or trauma near the growth epiphysis can cause unequal stimulus, suppression or stimulation of growth. This results in bending, shortening or lengthening of a bone respectively, e.g. osteomyelitis, epiphyseal injuries, tumor.
b. *Bone disorders:* Endocrine disorders, metabolic disorders, developmental disorders are some of the examples with bone deformities.
c. *Fractures:* This is by far the most important cause for a bone deformity. All displaced and fresh fractures cause temporary deformity while malunion or nonunion of fractures lead to deformities at a later date.

Joint Causes

The causes for the deformities due to joint problems are varied.

a. *Dislocation or subluxation:* This is usually due to trauma. It may also be seen due to pathological conditions of the hip, e.g. TB hip.
b. *Muscle imbalance:* Muscles balancing the joint on either side, if they are either over active (e.g. cerebral palsy) or under active, e.g. polio, deformity of the joint results.
c. *Tethering of muscles and tendons:* This can take place due to growth of fibrous tissue following infections or due to callus following fractures. Tethering restricts the joint movements and if held for some time deformity results, e.g. VIC, tenosynovitis of finger flexors.
d. *Arthritis:* Any joint may give rise to muscle spasm in the initial stages and fibrous or bony ankylosis in later stages giving rise to deformities, e.g. TB knee, rheumatoid hand, TB hip.
e. *Postural:* This is due to improper postural habits like hallux valgus in women due to tight and rigid shoes.
f. *Idiopathic:* There is no apparent cause for the joint deformities, e.g. Idiopathic scoliosis.

Soft Tissue Contractural Deformities

Soft tissue contractures (skin and deep fascia) other than the muscle contractures can also cause joint deformities, e.g. Dupuytren's contractures, post-burn contractures (Fig. 33.1).

Investigations: A good quality radiograph in all planes of the deformities need to be studied before zeroing in on the right choice of treatment.

Preventive Measures

Judicious and proper management of fractures and dislocations, use of proper splints like Mermaid splints in rickets during the growing phase in children can prevent most of the acquired deformity. Educating parents like avoiding smoking, alcohol, drugs, etc. during early pregnancy also helps prevent deformities.

Treatment Options

Masterly inactivity: Deformities do not need active intervention in the following situations:

a. Mild deformities, with no significant cosmetic or functional impairments (e.g. Clavicle fractures).
b. In very old and infirm patients.
c. Certain gross deformities that are beyond corrections, however, effort should be made to minimize the problem to the best possible extent.

Conservative measures: These include manipulative correction under anesthesia and retention by splints or casts, gradual correction by traction or splints, e.g. turn buckle splints. Correction by plaster wedging is hazardous.

Surgical measures: There are various surgical options available:

- *Ilizarov:* It is the gold standard for deformity correction in recent times.
- Soft tissue release.

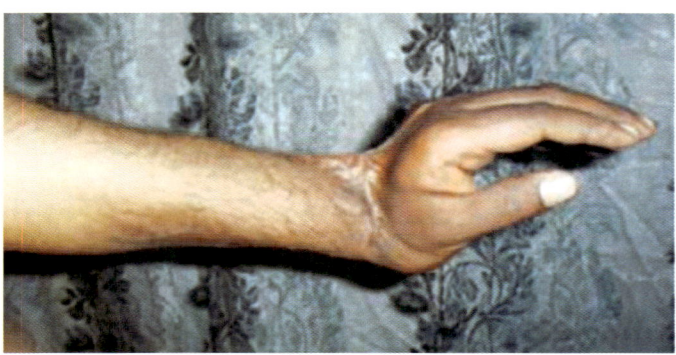

Fig. 33.1: Extensor contractures (post-burn)

- Tenolysis, tendon lengthening or tendon transfers are successfully employed in polio, cerebral palsy, etc.
- *Arthroplasty:* It can be crude as a salvage procedure (e.g. girdle stone excision in TB hip) or sophisticated as in total hip replacement or total knee replacement in rheumatoid and other disorders.
- *Corrective osteotomy:* This is a simple effective procedure to correct joint deformities, e.g. French osteotomy in cubitus varus deformity.
- *Arthrodesis:* The fusion of joints in functional positions in badly damaged joints, e.g. TB knee, rheumatoid arthritis.
- *Epiphyseal growth arrests:* When potential for growth is still left, stapling of the epiphysis can be attempted on one side to correct the bending deformity, e.g. in genu varum or valgum.

33

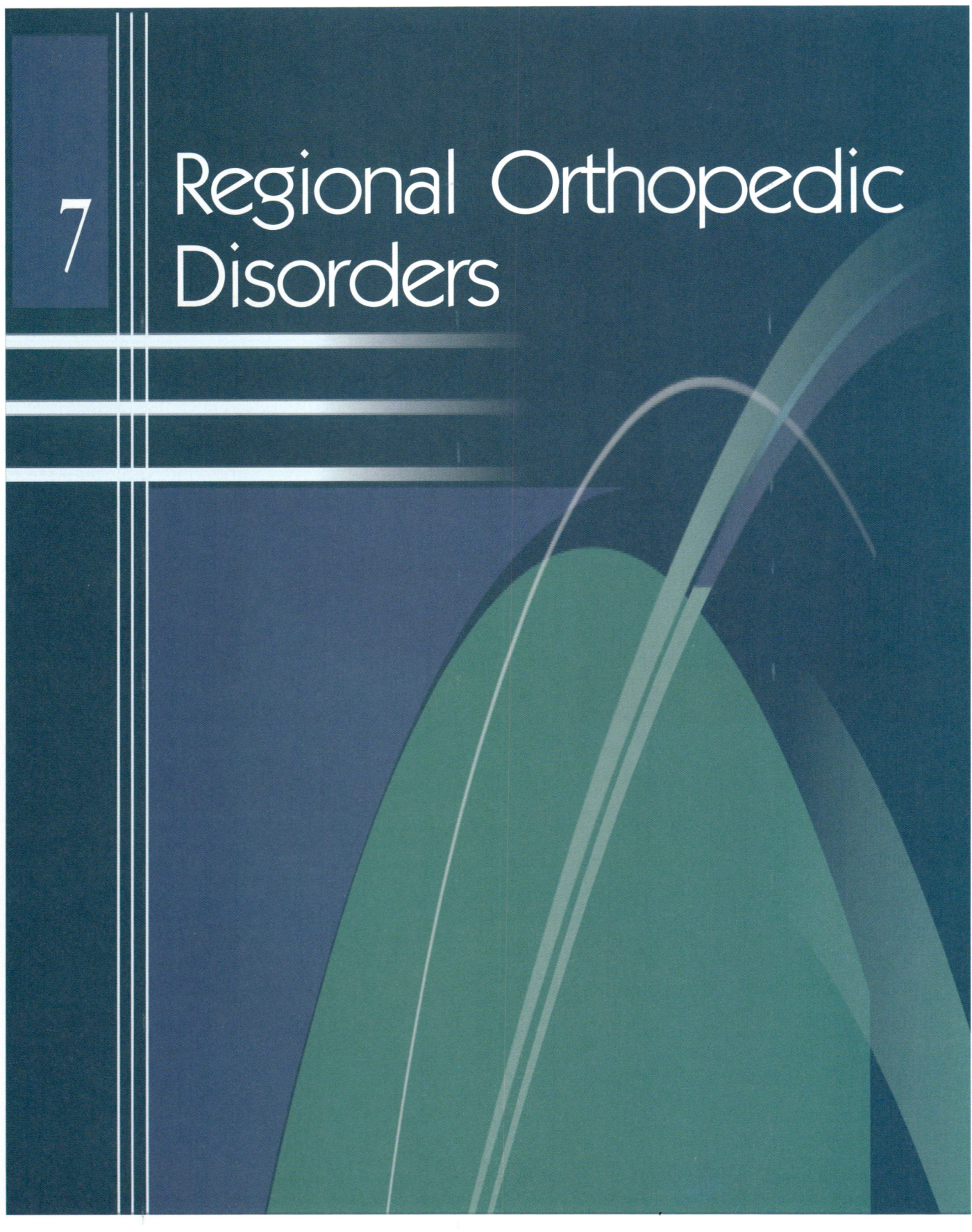

7 Regional Orthopedic Disorders

34 Regional Orthopedic Conditions of the Neck

Torticollis
Thoracic outlet syndromes
Cervical rib
Cervical disc syndromes

TORTICOLLIS (WRY NECK)

Torticollis is defined as the rotational deformity of cervical spine that causes turning and tilting deformity of the head and neck (Fig. 34.1).

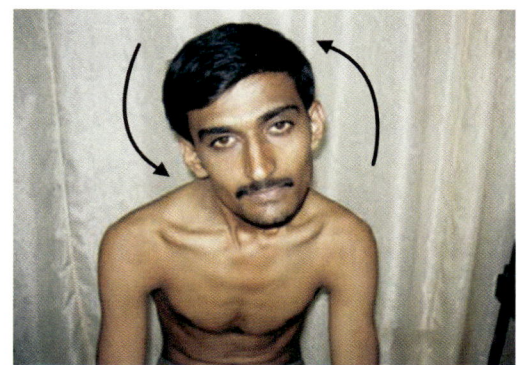

Fig. 34.1: Wry neck

Causes

- *Congenital* (see the Chapter on Congenital Disorder for description).
- *Infective* Tuberculosis of cervical spine, acute respiratory tract infection, etc.
- *Traumatic* Sprain, dislocation and fracture of the cervical spine.
- *Myositis or fibromyositis* of sternocleidomastoid, exposure to cold causes myositis.
- *Spasmodic* painful, persistent or intermittent sternomastoid muscle contraction.
- *Unilateral muscle paralysis,* e.g. polio
- *Neuritis* of spinal accessory nerve.
- *Ocular disturbances* child turns head to one side to compensate for defective vision.

Clinical Features

Head of the patient is tilted towards the affected side while the chin points to the other side. Sternocleidomastoid muscle is prominently seen. In the later stages,

the patient may develop facial asymmetry and macular disturbances in the eye. Among the acquired causes of torticollis, spasmodic muscle contraction of the sternocleidomastoid is the most common cause.

Plain X-ray of the neck AP and lateral views are recommended.

Management

Conservative: Initially conservative line of treatment is observed. This consists of non-steroidal anti-inflammatory drugs (NSAIDs), muscle relaxants drugs, etc. Physiotherapy like ultrasound, heat, massage is advocated. In acute pain, patient is encouraged to wear a collar. Gradual neck strengthening exercises are advised once the acute symptoms subside.
Surgical: Management is advised after the failure of conservative treatment. It consists of release of sternomastoid muscle from its clavicular attachment as in congenital torticollis and intradural section of both spinal accessory and three cervical roots in cases of torticollis due to spasmodic or neural causes.

THORACIC OUTLET SYNDROME

The space at the thoracic outlet or inlet when it is less than adequate, subjects the neurovascular structures seeking to gain entry into the upper limbs via this space, to undue pressure. The blame for the neurovascular complaints should be placed at the doorstep of the decreased space and not at the structures producing the problems (Fig. 34.2).

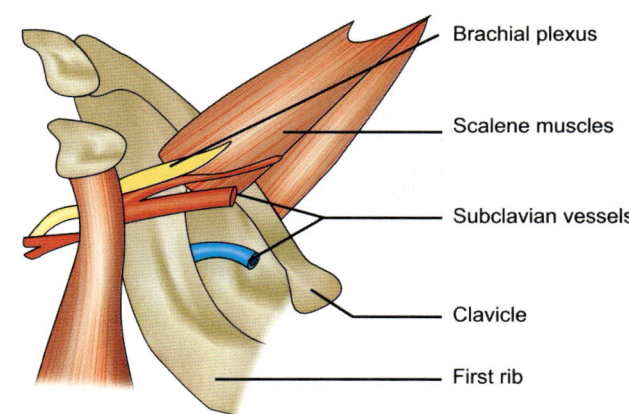

Fig. 34.2: Anatomy of the thoracic outlet causing compression

This syndrome results from the compression of neurovascular bundle comprising of subclavian artery and vein, axillary artery and vein and brachial plexus at the thoracic outlet. Thoracic outlet is a space between the first rib, clavicle and the scalene muscles. The above structures are liable to be compressed when this space gets narrowed either due to hypertrophy of the existing muscles or due to any other cause like congenital, trauma (Fig. 34.3).

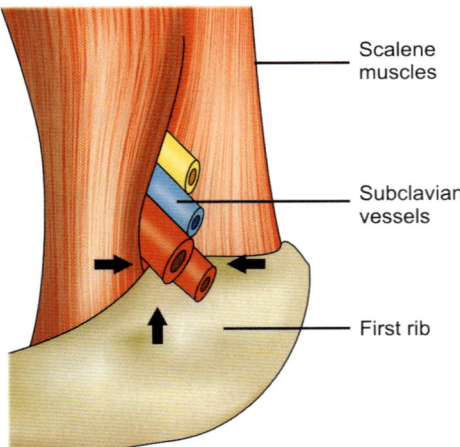

Fig. 34.3: Abnormal scalene muscle insertion causing compression

Clinical Features

Obviously this syndrome poses two major problems. The first one relates to the compression of the major vessels and secondly to the compression of the nerves.

Vascular problems: Patient complains of numbness of the whole arm, cold, cyanosis, pallor and Raynaud's phenomenon. Venous compression leaves the limb swollen and discoloured after exercises which disappears slowly with rest.

Neurogenic problems: This involves $C_8 T_1$ segment (Klumpke's paralysis). Patient complains of paraesthesia along the medial aspect of the arm, hand, little and ring fingers. There is weakness of the hand also.

Tests

Intermittent claudication test: The arm is abducted and elevated and fingers are exercised. The inference:
- If pain develops after 1 min; it is negative (normal)
- If pain develops before 1 min; the test is positive.

Other tests are costoclavicular manoeuvres, Adson's test (provocative tests) and Wright's test (Fig. 34.4).

Complications: Subclavian artery compression → results in poststenotic dilatation → stasis favours thrombosis → the thrombi break and migrate distally causing embolization → this results in the distal artery blockade causing ischemia and gangrene of the upper limbs.

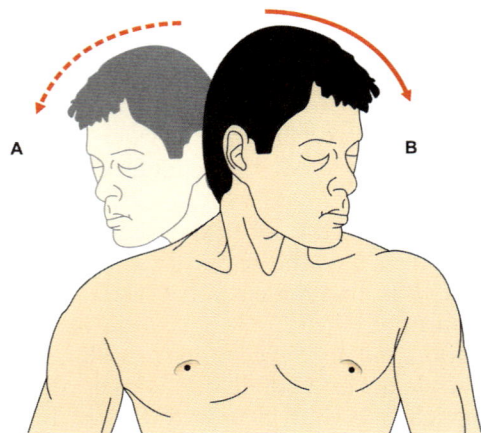

Fig. 34.4: Methods of performing (A) Wright's test, (B) Adson's test

Investigations

X-ray neck to rule out intrinsic causes like cervical spondylosis, cervical rib.
Nerve conduction studies: Difficult to determine the nerve conduction velocity through the thoracic outlet, but its biggest value is to rule out problems like entrapment, e.g. ulnar nerve at elbow, wrist.

Treatment

- *Conservative treatment* consists of rest, physiotherapy, exercises, etc.
- *Surgical treatment*

  Indications: Gangrene and poststenotic dilatation.

Methods

- *Removal of the first thoracic rib:* This is the most efffective treatment as it deals with both supraclavicular and infraclavicular etiological factors in this syndrome.
- *Removal of cervical rib:* If this is the cause of compression.
- *Scalenotomy:* It is indicated in scalenus anticus syndrome.

QUICK FACTS
- Sites of compression—could be supra-, sub-, or infra-clavicular.
- Clinical manifestation—could be neural, vascular, or both.
- Diagnosis is usually by exclusion and the screening test helps.
- Excision of the first thoracic rib is the most effective surgical procedure.

CERVICAL RIB

Cervical rib problem is akin to the story of the "Return of the Prodigal Son". But unlike the chastened prodigal son, cervical rib returns to torment the unfortunate victim! It is a rib arising from the 7th cervical vertebra, rarely 6th and 5th cervical vertebra.

34

Incidence: It is 0.46 percent. Nearly 50 percent of those are unilateral.

Side: It is more frequent on the right side.

Types: Four Varieties are Described

1. *Complete*: The cervical rib reaches up to the first thoracic rib.
2. *Bulbous end:* In this the cervical rib has a bulbous end.
3. *Tapering end*: In this the cervical rib tapers.
4. *Fibrous band:* In this the rib is represented by a thick fibrous band.

Pathological anatomy: The neurovascular structures, the brachial plexus and subclavial vessels are hung up by the cervical rib that is inserted into the scalene tubercle of 1st rib space. Pronounced drooping of the shoulder in women after middle age, trauma, unusual lifting operations, acute illness make the muscles weak, pulling the plexus and artery distally giving rise to symptoms.

Clinical Features

Cervical rib though largely asymptomatic, when symptomatic may present in the following manners:

Cervical rib with local symptoms: Show presence of a lump and tenderness in the supraclavicular fossa (Fig. 34.5).

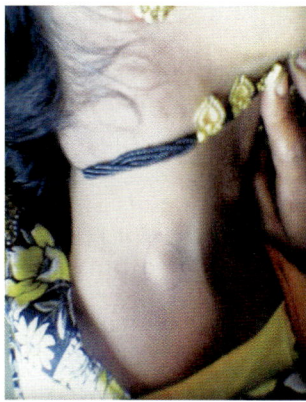

Fig. 34.5: A clinical photograph of the cervical rib

Cervical rib with vascular symptoms: This gives rise to pain in the upper limbs, temperature and colour changes, radial pulse is feeble or absent and a feeling of numbness is present.

Cervical rib with nerve pressure symptoms: The nerve pressure symptoms are due to the angulation of the first thoracic nerve root. The patient complains of paresthesia along the medial aspect of the arm, hand and little fingers. There is weakness of the hand muscles also.

Radiology

Plain X-ray AP view of the neck may show an extra rib from the C_7 vertebra on one or both sides (Fig. 34.6).

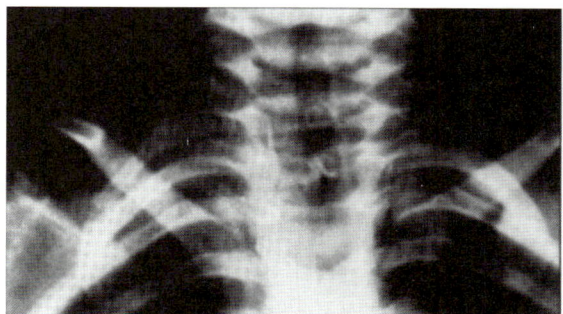

Fig. 34.6: Radiograph of the unilateral cervical rib

However in the fibrosis type X-rays of the neck may be normal. CT scan and MRI is a better alternative.

Treatment

In mild cases, shoulder shrugging exercises, avoiding carrying heavy weights, etc. and sling exercises often help. In more severe cases, scalenotomy (resection of scalenus anterior muscle) may be required and is successful in 70 percent of the cases. In troublesome cases removal of the cervical rib or the first rib surgically with its periosteum to prevent its regeneration is advocated. Weight lifting activities with affected extremities should be avoided.

> **INTERESTING CERVICAL RIB FACTS**
> - In 90% of cases cervical rib remains obscure and is accidentally detected radiologically.
> - In the remaining, symptoms usually begins after 30–40 years, when due to aging the shoulder sags.

CERVICAL DISC SYNDROMES

The cervical region consists of seven cervical vertebrae with their intervening discs. The disc is made up of central nucleus pulposus and annulus fibrosus at the periphery. The disc functions as an effective shock absorber and also gives the cervial spine more mobility. If the disc material herniates because of trauma or old age it gives rise to the cervical disc syndrome (Fig. 34.7).

More than 90 percent of the disc lesions in the cervical spine occur at the C_5 and C_6 levels as these are the most mobile segments.

Pathogenesis

Advancing age, improper neck postures, neck misadventures we indulge day in and day out (e.g. our habit of using thick pillows) takes its toll on the neck structures particulars the intervertebral discs. Over the years disc degenerates, disc space narrows, facet joints degenerates, muscles and ligaments stiffen causing pain in the neck. Consequent to all this unfortunate developments, extra bone growths called osteophytes develop herading the onset of nerve root compression. A tragic saga called cervical spondylosis thus unfolds.

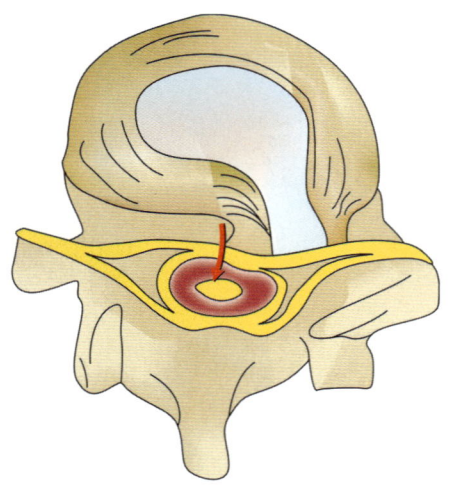

Fig. 34.7: Cervical disc herniation compressing the nerve root

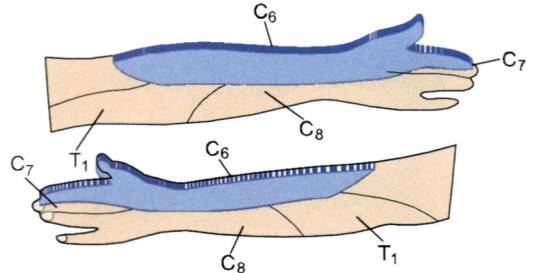

Fig. 34.10: Dermatomal pattern of upper limb

Catastrophe sets in when osteophytes compress the nerve roots or cord.

Clinical Features

Symptoms: Patient complains of pain in the neck which is gradual or acute in onset. The pain could radiate to the shoulder upper arm, forearm and fingers (Fig. 34.8). There is history of morning stiffness. Extension of the neck increases the pain. Tingling and numbness develops if the nerve root is compressed but it does not follow the dermatomal pattern.

Signs: Thee could be neck deformity (Fig. 34.9). Movements of the neck are decreased due to pain. Pain increases on hyperextension. There is localised tenderness over the spinous process. Trigger point tenderness at the scapular region is present. Pressure against the top of the head increases pain. If the nerve root is compressed by the disc herniation sensory, motor and reflex changes occur and follow the dermatomal pattern (Table 34.1 and Fig. 34.10). Cord compression could lead to features of UMN lesion.

Table 34.1: Dermatomal and myotomal pattern in cervical spondylosis			
Root	*Motor*	*Reflex*	*Sensation*
C$_5$ (C$_{4-5}$ lesion)	Deltoid↓	Biceps reflex↓	Numbness in the deltoid region
C$_6$ (C$_{5-6}$ lesion)	Wrist extension↓	Brachioradialis reflex↓	Dorsolateral aspect of the thumb and index finger
C$_7$ (C$_{5-6}$ lesion)	Wrist flexion↓	Triceps reflex↓	Index, middle and dorsum of the hand
C$_8$	Finger flexion↓	None	Ring, little finger, medial border of forearm

Investigations

X-ray: Normal in soft lesions but in hard lesions it shows, narrowing of disc space, anterior and posterior osteophyte formation, and narrowing of IV foramen (Figs 34.11A and B).

Myelography: It helps in localizing the lesion but is invasive.

MRI: This is useful, as it is non-invasive, and helps localize the lesion, but its high cost is prohibitive (Fig. 34.12).

CT scan: It is more useful in evaluating traumatic conditions of the neck than degenerative conditions.

EMG discography, thermography are occasionally used.

Treatment

Conservative treatment: It is the more accepted form of treatment in cervical disc syndrome. It consists of rest which is the cornerstone of the treatment as it allows soft parts to heal by reducing the inflammation. Cervical traction could be continuous or intermittent depending on the severity of the symptoms. Traction helps by reducing the muscle spasm, increasing the disc space and reducing the tension on the nerve roots. Wearing

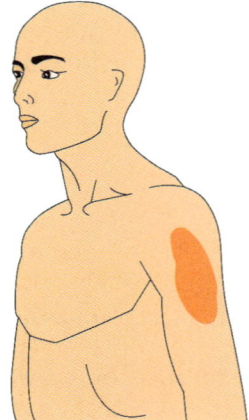

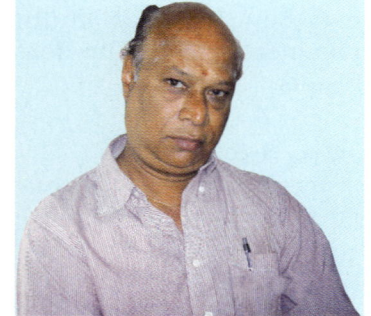

Fig. 34.8: Distribution of radiation pain in cervical spondylosis

Fig. 34.9: A clinical photograph of the cervical spondylosis

34

34

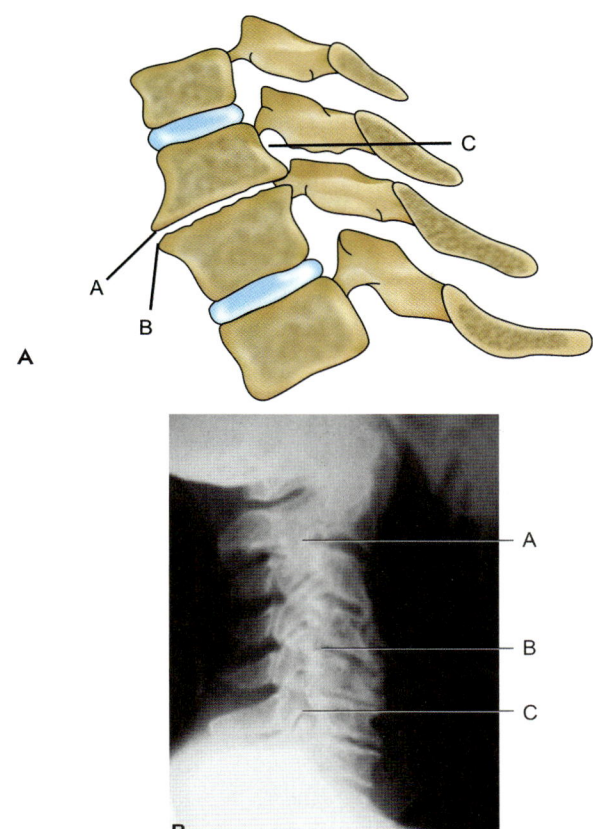

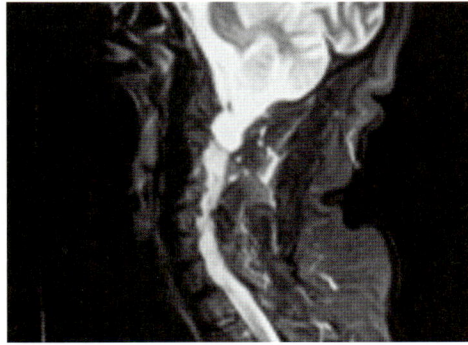

Figs 34.11A and B: (A) Diagramatic representation of radiograph in findings in cervical disc syndrome: (A) disc space narrowing, (B) osteophyte formation, and (C) narrowing of intervertebral foramina Plain X-ray of the neck

Fig. 34.12: MRI showing features of cervical spondylosis

cervical collars helps to relieve pain and muscle spasm due to acute exacerbation of chronic spondylosis (Fig. 28.17C). Physiotherapy like short wave diathermy, ultrasound, infrared rays are useful. NSAIDs once a day are usually preferred. After the pain decreases, patient is encouraged to perform gradual graded isometric neck exercises (Figs 34. 13A to E).

IMPORTANT PREVENTIVE MEASURES
- Practicing proper neck postures
- Avoiding thick pillows and using proper sized pillows (2")

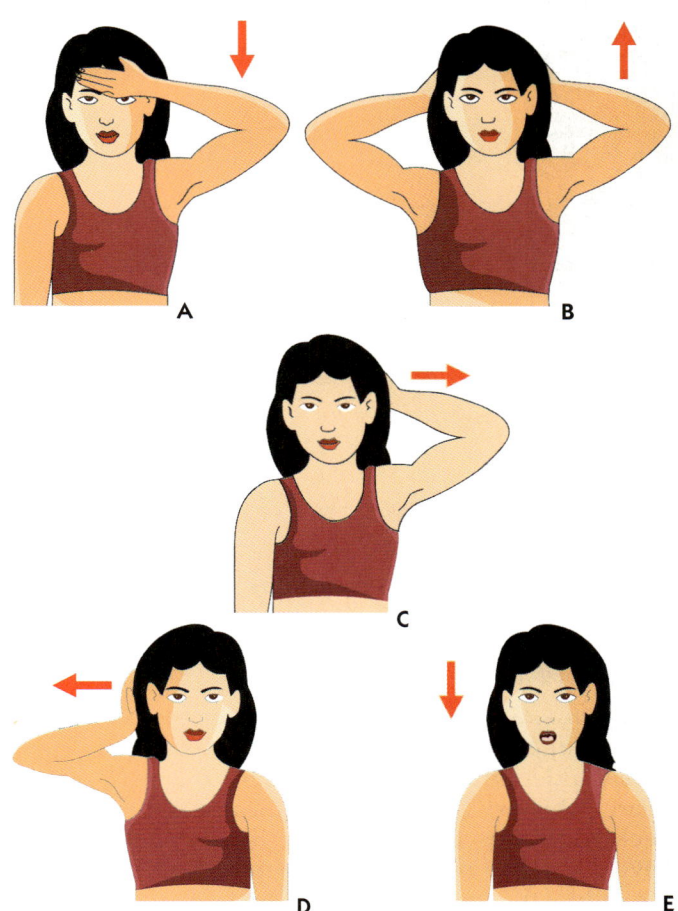

Figs 34.13A to E: Different self-resistive isometric neck exercises (A) neck flexion, (B) neck extension, (C) lateral flexion, (D) neck rotation, (E) for neck flexion

Surgical treatment: Less than 5 percent of the cases of cervical spondylosis require surgery and is usually indicated in cases of chronic pain, failed conservative treatment and neurological deficits due to root or cord compressions. The surgical procedure usually consists of removal of the cervical disc through an anterior approach and cervical interbody fusion by placing an autologous iliac bone graft. Excision of large osteophytes can also be done through this route. Excision of one or two cervical bodies (corpectomy) may be justified in multiple level disc pathology. Laminectomy usually does not produce the desired results.

QUICK FACTS
Surgical treatment of cervical spondylosis:
- Anterior cervical discectomy with interbody fusion for single or two level disc involvement.
- Corpectomy and strut graft for multiple level disc involvement.
- Laminectomy has a doubtful role.
- Surgery is required in less than 5 percent of cases.

35 Regional Orthopedic Conditions of the Shoulder

Frozen shoulder
Rotator cuff lesions

FROZEN SHOULDER
(Syn: Periarthritis, Adhesive Capsulitis)

It is defined as a clinical syndrome characterized by *painful restriction of both active and passive shoulder movements* due to causes within the shoulder joint or remote (other parts of the body) (Fig. 35.1).

History

Dupley first described it in 1872 and called it as *humeroscapular periarthritis.* In 1934 **Codman** coined the term *'frozen shoulder'*, and in 1945 **Neviaser** gave the name *'adhesive capsulitis.'*

Causes

Shoulder causes: Problems directly related to shoulder joint which can give rise to frozen shoulder are tendinitis of rotator cuff, bicipital tendinitis, fractures and dislocations around the shoulder, etc.

Nonshoulder causes: Problems not related to shoulder joint like:
- Diabetes (more common and severe in diabetics)
- Cardiovascular diseases with referred pain to the shoulder which keeps the joint immobile.
- Reflex sympathetic dystrophy, frozen hand shoulder syndrome, a complication of Colles' fracture can all lead to frozen shoulder.

The reason in all the cases mentioned above could be prolonged immobilization of the shoulder joint due to voluntary immobilization of the shoulder, referred pain, etc. In-Frozen shoulder, the patient will not be able to carry out day-to-day routine care activities like buttening a blouse (Fig. 35.1) combing the hair, carrying weights and will have difficulty in trying to sleep on the affected side.

Pathology

During abduction, and repeated overhead activities of the shoulder, long head of biceps, and rotator cuff undergo repeated strain. This results in inflammation, fibrosis and consequent thickening of the shoulder capsule which results in loss of movements (Figs 35.2A and B).

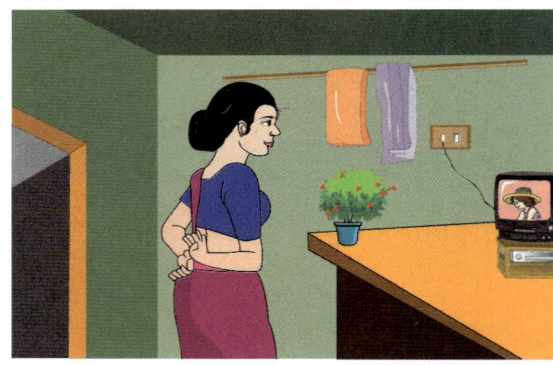

Fig. 35.1: Activities like these are not possible in frozen shoulder

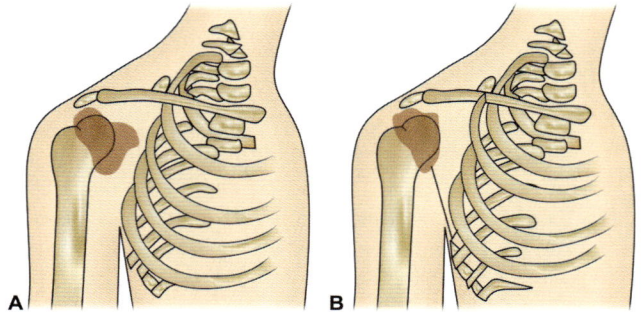

Figs 35.2A and B: (A) Normal capsular pattern, (B) contracted capsule in frozen shoulder

Clinical Features

Patient complains of pain, stiffness, inability to sleep on the affected side, etc. The following are the stages of the disease:

There are three classical stages in frozen shoulder:

Stage I (Stage of pain): Patient complains of acute pain, decreased movements (both active and passive movements are restricted Figs 35.3A and B), internal rotation greatest followed by loss of abduction and then forward flexion. *External rotation is less affected* (Figs 35.5A and B). This stage lasts for 10 to 36 weeks. Pain due to frozen shoulder will not radiate below the elbow unlike in cervical spondylosis (Fig. 35.4).

Stage II (Stage of stiffness): In this stage pain gradually decreases and the patient complains of stiff shoulder. Slight movements are present.

35

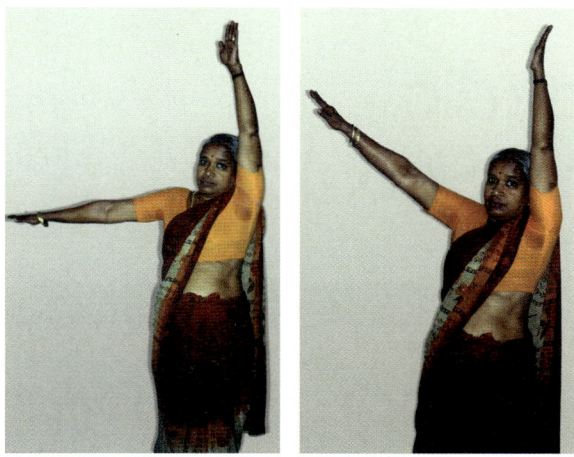

Figs 35.3A and B: (A) Active abduction restricted, (B) passive abduction restricted

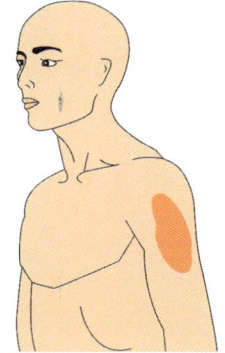

Fig. 35.4: Region of distribution of pain in frozen shoulder

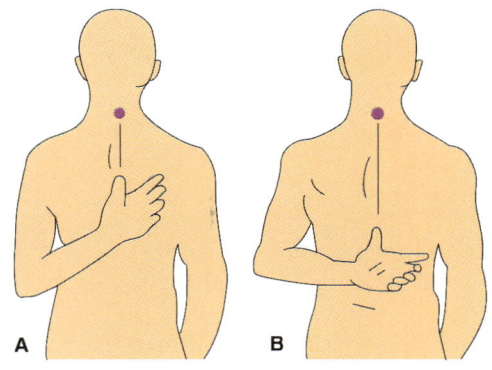

Figs 35.5A and B: Degrees of internal rotation: (A) normal, (B) frozen

Stage III *(Stage of recovery):* Patient will have no pain and movements will have recovered but will never be regained to normal. It lasts for 6 months to 2 years.

Investigations

Laboratory reports are normal, so is the plain X-ray of the shoulder. However sometimes a dense sclerotic line

may be seen on the outer aspect of the head of the humerus. If this is present it is quite pathognomonic and is called the "Golding's sign" (Fig. 35.6). Arthrography of the shoulder reveals decreased joint space and is quite reliable (Fig. 35.7).

Treatment

Stage I: In this stage long-acting once a day NSAIDs are usually preferred as this condition usually runs a long course (10–36 weeks). Intraarticular steroids may help.

Stage II: In this stage since the pain will have reduced considerably, exercises both active and passive are gradually begun followed by physiotherapy, ultrasound, heat and shoulder wheel exercises. The role of manipulation of the shoulder is controversial but can be attempted under general anesthesia in this stage.

Stage III: In this stage active and passive exercises, physiotherapy consisting of short wave diathermy, ultrasound, etc. are continued.

Mercifully frozen shoulder is a self-limiting disease and abates after 6–9 months of agonising experience to the patient. Some stiffness may remain as sequelae.

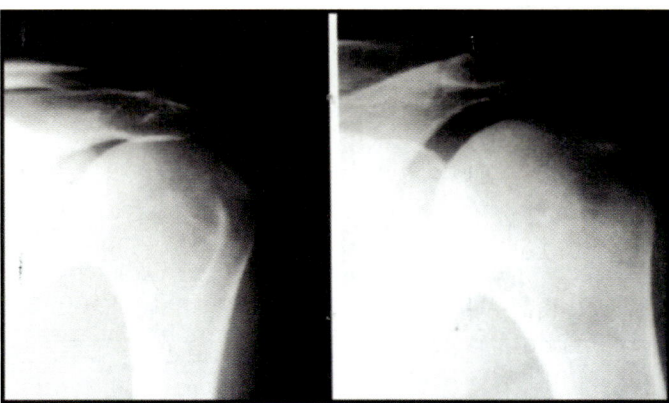

Fig. 35.6: Plain X-ray showing the Golding's sign

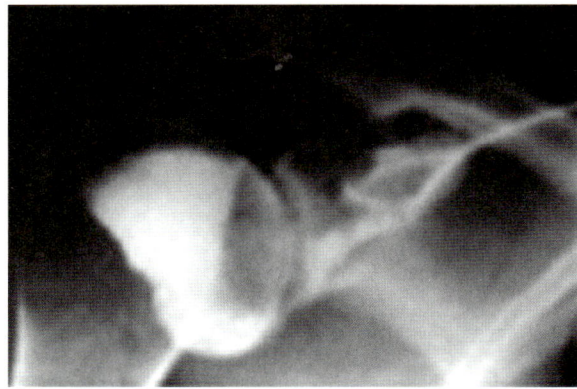

Fig. 35.7: Arthrography for frozen shoulder

PAINFUL ARC SYNDROMES

This is an interesting condition peculiar to the shoulder. Here patient complains of pain in the mid-range of abduction (60–120° range). A plethora of conditions (see box) are known to cause this intriguing problem but the most common cause seems to be rotator cuff lesions.

ROTATOR CUFF LESIONS

Fine adjustments of the humeral head within the glenoid is achieved by coordinated activity of four inter-related muscles arising from the scapula and is called the *rotator cuff.*

Note: Rotator cuff comprises supraspinatus, infraspinatus, subscapularis and teres minor (Fig. 35.8).

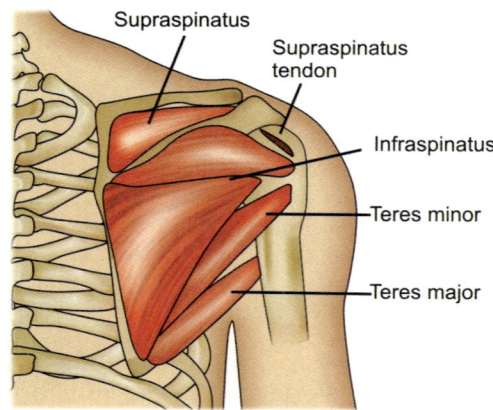

Fig. 35.8: Rotator cuff muscles

Rotator cuff lesion is a problem which is commonly associated with supraspinatus tendon. Other causes like bicipital tendinitis, etc. may give rise to rotator cuff problems but they are not that common. Rotator cuff tears are more frequently seen in the elderly due to the vulnerability of the rotators following degenerative changes.

Remember

Causes of painful syndrome
- Supraspinatus tendinitis
- Calcific deposits
- Subacromial bursitis
- Subdeltoid bursitis
- Bicipital tenosynovitis
- Fracture greater tuberosity.

Clinical Features

All patients with painful are syndrome have similar clinical features like pain, swelling, limitation of shoulder movements, muscle atrophy (supraspinatus and infraspinatus), tenderness over the greater tuberosity. Painful arc could be seen (Fig. 35.9).

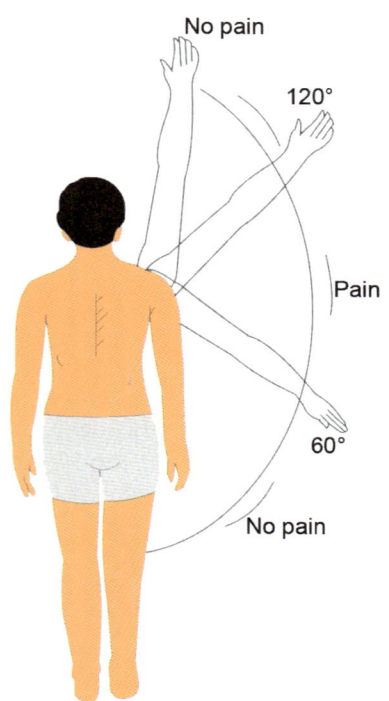

Fig. 35.9: Pain occurs in the impingement syndrome between 60 and 120° of shoulder abduction as it is in this position that the supraspinatus tendon is impinged against the undersurface of the acromion and head of the humerus. Rest of the movements are painless (painful arc syndrome)

Management

Conservative treatment: It consists of heat, massage, NSAIDs, local infiltration of hydrocortisone, subacromial steroid injections, exercises both active and passive, temporary immobilization, etc. *Ninety percent will recover with these measures.* Rarely manipulation of the shoulder under general anesthesia is required.

Surgical Treatment

Indications: Failure of conservative treatment for three months, if the patients are young and active, and if there is increasing loss of shoulder function, surgery is indicated.

Methods: Depending upon the etiological factors the following surgical techniques are described: excision of adhesions and manipulation of shoulder, excision of calcium deposits, repair of incomplete tear, acromioplasty, acromionectomy, etc.

35

36 Regional Orthopedic Conditions of the Elbow

- Tennis elbow
- Golfer's elbow
- Olecranon bursitis

TENNIS ELBOW

I am sure every one is fascinated by tennis. We may not get a place under the sun with Williams Sisters, Sania Mirza, Nadal and others but certainly, we may get an appointment with an orthopedic surgeon for a problem common in them, that too without playing tennis! Yes, the obvious reference is towards *tennis elbow.*

History

It was first described from the Writer's cramps by Range in 1873. It was Madrid who called it as "tennis elbow" shortly thereafter.

Tennis elbow syndrome encompasses lateral, medial and posterior elbow symptoms (Flow chart 36.1). The one commonly encountered is the lateral tennis elbow which is known as the classical tennis elbow and is the pain and tenderness on the lateral side of the elbow, some well defined and some vague that results from repetitive stress.

Flow chart 36.1

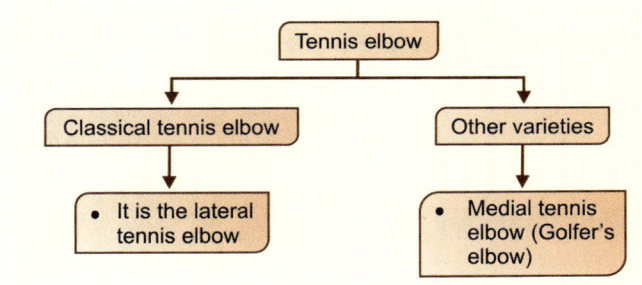

Remember

Location of pain in tennis elbow
- Lateral epicondyle (75%)
- Lateral muscle mass (17%)
- Medial epicondyle (10%)
- Posterior (8%)

LATERAL TENNIS ELBOW

It is a lesion affecting the tendinous origin of common wrist extensors from the lateral epicondyle arising from the humerus.

Causes: A number of pathological conditions in and around the elbow joint can lead to these conditions. However, the most common incriminating cause is single or multiple tears in the extensor carpi radialis brevis tendon.

SEEN IN

- All levels of tennis players.
- In world class players "SERVE" appears to be the cause.
- In less than world class players "backhand stroke".
- Seen in other sports also.
- Maybe occupational, carpenters, miners, etc.

Etiology

Problems in tennis players: More than one-third tennis players all over the world are affected with this problem over 35 years of age are obviously due to faulty playing techniques (Fig. 36.1).

Non-tennis players: Ironically tennis elbow is more common in non-tennis players. This unfortunate group is comprised of homemakers, carpenters, miners, drill workers, etc. India's Cricketing Legend Sachin

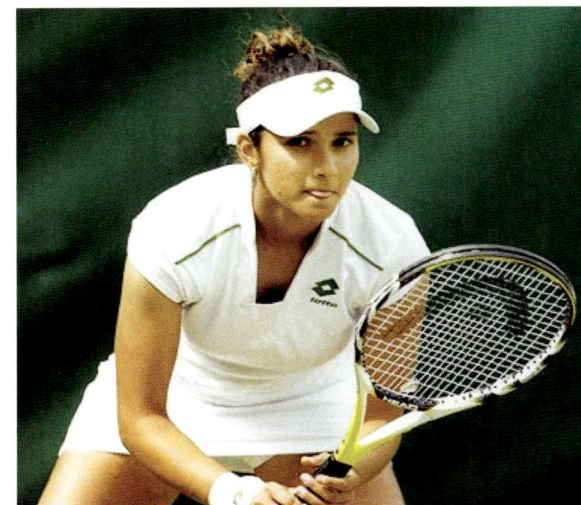

Fig. 36.1: Repetitive stress at common extensor origin in tennis players

Tendulkar has made Tennis Elbow very popular across the country and the world.

Indian housewives: This is the third largest group suffering from this condition. The household chores like washing, brooming, cooking, etc. require repeated extension of the elbow leading to the development of this condition (Fig. 36.2).

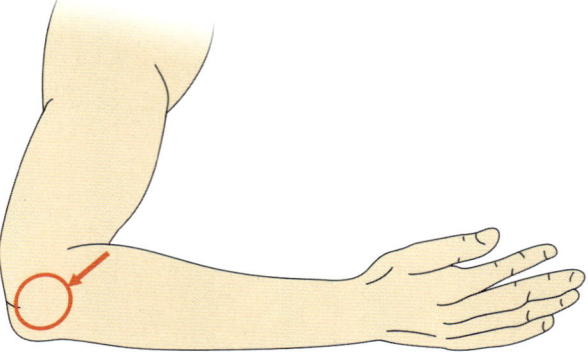

Fig. 36.3: Arrow showing site of tenderness in tennis elbow

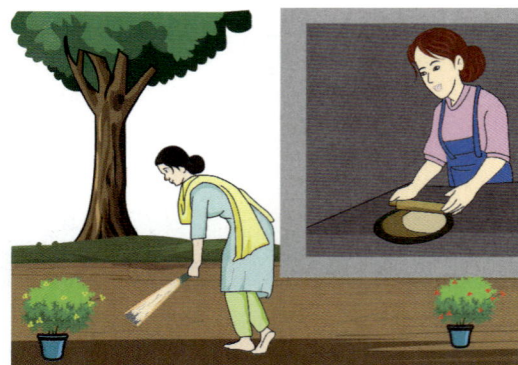

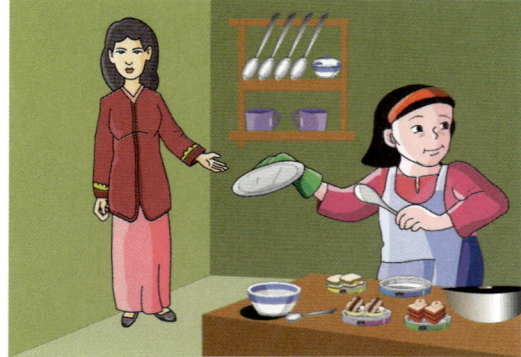

Fig. 36.2: Indian housewives are common victim of tennis elbow

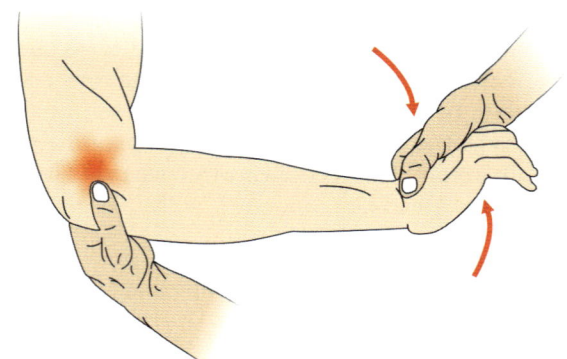

Fig. 36.4: Cozen's test

cases sclerosis may be seen in the vicinity of the lateral epicondyle.

Treatment

Conservative management: It consists of rest and physiotherapy. In tennis players exercises, light racket, smaller grip, elbow strap, etc. are helpful (Fig. 36.5). Injection of local anesthetic and steroid are useful in 40 percent of cases.

Surgical management: This is reserved for intractable cases that are unresponsive for the routine conservative regimen.

Surgical Methods

Percutaneous release of epicondylar muscles. Bosworth technique of excision of the proximal portion of the annular ligament, release of the origin of the extensor muscles, excision of the bursa and excision of synovial fringes.

Computer-related injuries: This is emerging as the recent epidemic among computer professionals across the globe due to repetitive stress while using laptops, mouse, etc.

Clinical Features

Patient complains of pain on the outer aspect of the elbow and has difficulty in gripping objects and lifting them. Sportspersons will have difficulty in extending the elbow. The following are some of the useful clinical tests:

- Local tenderness on the outside of the elbow at the common extensor origin with aching pain in the back of the forearm (Fig. 36.3).
- *Cozen's test:* Painful resisted extension of the wrist with elbow in full extension elicits pain at the lateral elbow (Fig. 36.4).

  Investigations: Routine AP and lateral views of the elbow radiographs are usually normal. However, in few

GOLFER'S ELBOW
(Syn: Epitrochleitis, Medial tennis elbow)

It is a tendinopathy of the insertion of the epitrochlear muscles (flexors of the fingers of the hand and pronators). Epitrochleitis is very similar to lateral epicondylitis (tennis elbow) but occurs on the medial

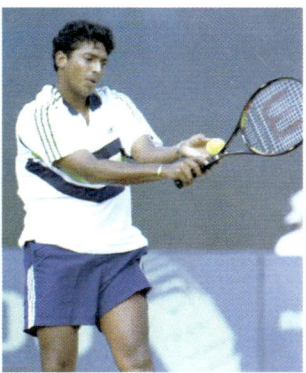

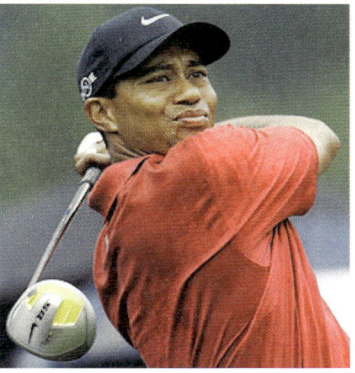

Fig. 36.5: Elbow supports to be used in tennis elbow

Fig. 36.6: Golf players are victims of medial epitrochleitis

Clinical Features

It usually manifests as a painless swelling over the tip of the Olecranon. There may be pain, if there is inflammation (Fig. 36.8). In extreme cases there could be ulceration.

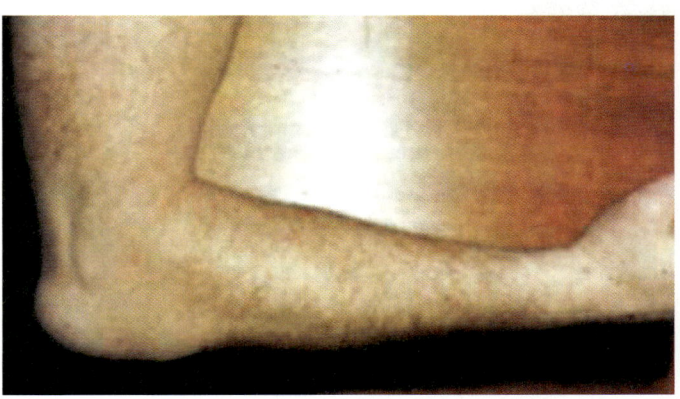

Fig. 36.8: Clinical photograph of student's elbow

side of the elbow, where the pronator teres and the flexors of the wrist and fingers originate and more so in Golf players (Fig. 36.6). Tensing of these muscles by resisted wrist and finger flexion in pronation will provoke the pain. Tenderness is often less well localized than in tennis elbow.

> **DID YOU KNOW?**
> Tennis elbow is nine times more common than Golfer's elbow.

Treatment: It is the same as for tennis elbow but the treatment is even less satisfactory.

OLECRANON BURSITIS (STUDENT'S ELBOW)

This is a chronic inflammation of the olecranon bursa. It may be the result of repetitive minor injuries, irritation, microcrystalline deposition, etc. Infection occurs due to chronic friction as in students who tend to keep their elbows repeatedly over the table, bench, etc. over long periods during writing, reading, etc. (Fig. 36.7).

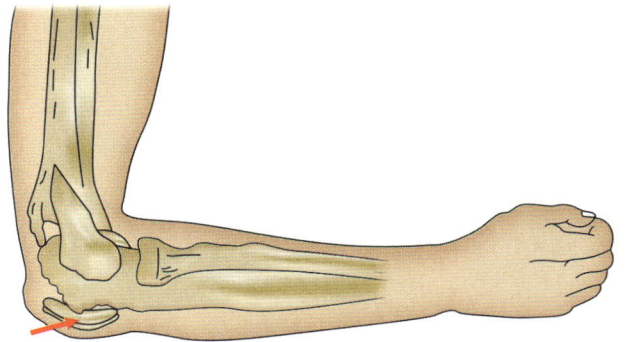

Fig. 36.9: Olecranon bursitis

Investigations

Aspiration and culture of the bursal fluid is necessary in order to exclude the possibility of an infectious etiology.

Treatment

This is essentially conservative and consists of NSAIDs, local steroids, etc. Surgical excision is done in chronic cases. Microcrystalline-induced bursitis has a good prognosis and the symptoms usually resolve after a few days, whether treated or not. Nevertheless, bursitis due to repeated minor irritation is more difficult to treat.

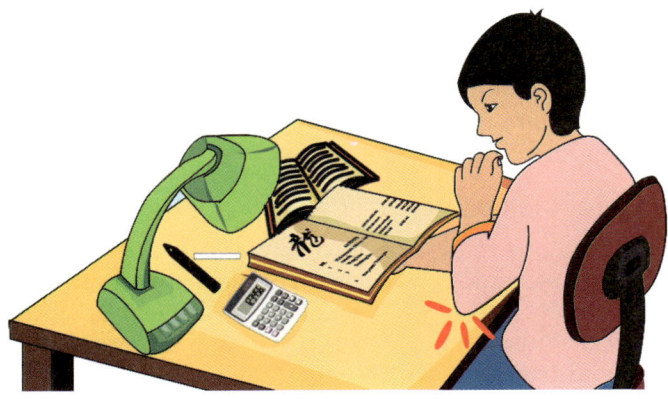

Fig. 36.7: Mechanism of students elbow

Regional Orthopedic Conditions of the Wrist

| deQuervain's disease |
| Ganglion |
| Carpal tunnel syndrome |

deQuervain'S DISEASE

Etiology: Exact cause is not known. deQuervain's disease is commonly seen in women and may be due to repeated overuse of the wrist. In this condition the common sheath of abductor pollicis longus, and extensor pollicis brevis tendons at the wrist are involved (Fig. 37.1).

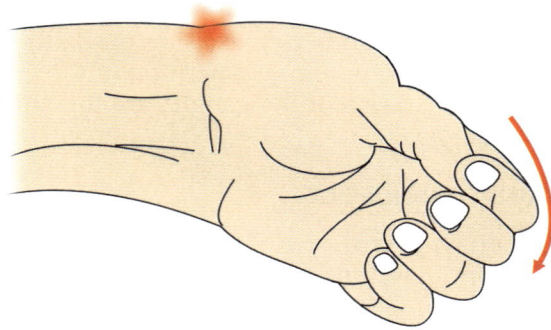

Fig. 37.2: Arrow showing the point of tenderness by sudden forceful ulnar deviation of the flexed hand. This is called Finkelstein's test.

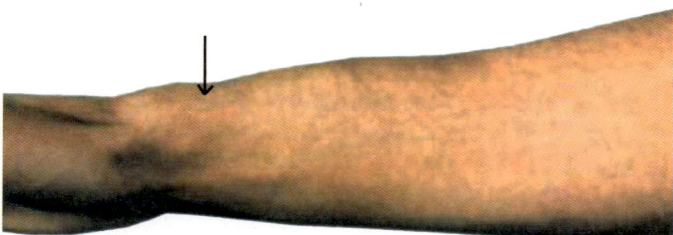

Fig. 37.1: deQuervain's disease: Arrow showing the site of tenovaginitis of the common sheath of abductor pollicis longus and extensor pollicis brevis

Note: It is popularly called as washerwoman's sprain

Clinical Features

Pain, swelling over the radial styloid process and limitation of the movements of the involved tendons are the presenting features. Tenderness can be elicited by sudden ulnar deviation of the flexed hand (This is known as the Finkelstein's test—Fig. 37.2) with the thumb adducted and held inside the palm.

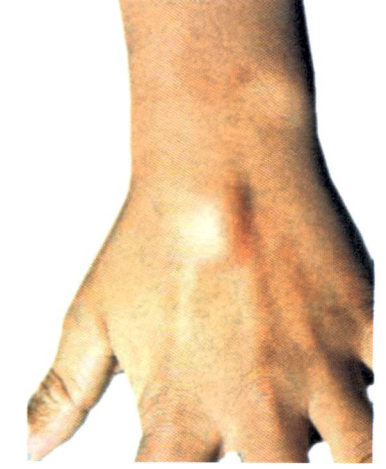

Fig. 37.3: Clinical photograph showing a ganglion

Treatment

Conservative treatment of this condition consists of rest, NSAIDs, local infiltration of hydrocortisone, etc.
Surgery: Division of the appropriate retinaculum and excision of a part of the tendon is considered if the above measures fail.

GANGLIA

It is a localized, tense, painless, cystic, swelling, containing clear gelatinous fluid (Fig. 37.3).

Remember
- Dorsal wrist ganglia accounts for 60 to 70% of all hand ganglia. It arises from scapholunate ligament
- Volar ganglion—18 to 20%
- Sheath at A pulley—10 to 12%
- Ganglion at the flexor tendon
- *Predisposing factors:* Chronic repetitive stress and sometimes injury.

Origin: The clear gelatinous fluid may be due to mucoid degeneration of the tendon sheath or capsule and leakage or subsequent fibrous encapsulation of synovial fluid through the capsule of a joint or a tendon sheath.

Sites: It is commonly seen over dorsum of the wrist, flexor aspects of the fingers and dorsum of the foot.

Clinical Features

Most of the times a cystic swelling over the dorsum of the wrist is the only complaint. Patient may complain of mild pain, discomfort in the wrist. Occasionally the ganglia may grow big and tense and may rupture causing enormous pain.

Treatment

It may resolve spontaneously or excision needs to be done if it is causing symptoms. Aspiration of the cyst and arthroscopic excision of the ganglia are the other treatment methods.

CARPAL TUNNEL SYNDROME

Carpal tunnel syndrome was first described by Sir James Paget in 1854, but the term was coined by Moerisch.

Anatomy: Bones bind the carpal tunnel on three sides and a ligament on one side. The floor is an osseous arch formed by the carpal bones and the transverse carpal ligament forms the roof (Fig. 37.4).

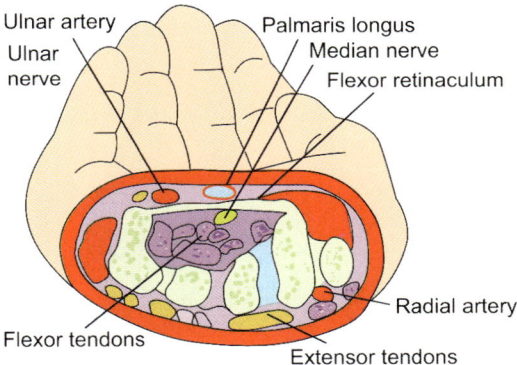

Fig. 37.4: Anatomy of the carpal tunnel

Contents: There are ten structures within the carpal tunnel and consists of tendons of flexor digitorum superficialis and profundus (four each) in a common sheath, tendon of flexor pollicis longus in an independent sheath and the median nerve. Synovitis of the above tendons can generate pressure on the nerve.

Causes

General
- Inflammatory—e.g. rheumatoid arthritis.
- Endocrine—hypothyroidism, diabetes mellitus, menopause, pregnancy, etc. are some of the important endocrine causes.
- Metabolic cause—gout.

- Idiopathic variety—this is the commonest type and the cause is unknown.

Local: These cause crowding of the space locally. Malunited Colles' fracture, ganglion in the carpal region, osteoarthritis of the carpal bones, wrist contusion, hematoma, etc. are some of the important local causes.

> **Remember**
>
> Mnemonic: **PRAGMTIC** for causes of carpal tunnel syndrome [**P**regnancy, **R**heumatoid arthritis, **A**rthritis degenerative, **G**rowth hormone abnormalities (acromegaly), **M**etabolic (gout, diabetes myxedema, etc.), **T**umors, **I**diopathic, **C**onnective tissue disorders (e.g. amyloidosis)]

Clinical Features

There will be symptoms of mild swelling tingling and numbness, pain, paraesthesia, etc. localized to the areas supplied by the median nerve. The patient may also complain of clumsiness in the hand and impairment of digital function, loss of sensation, etc. (Fig. 37.5). (See section on peripheral 'nerve' injury for examination of median nerve.)

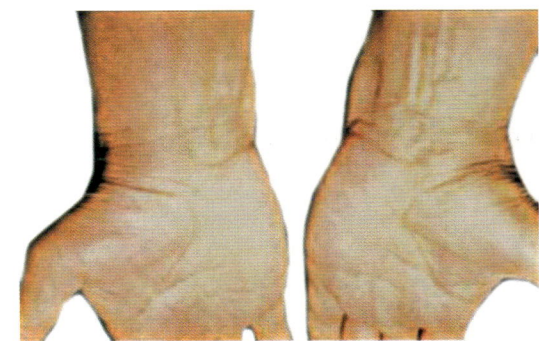

Fig. 37.5: The carpal tunnel

Clinical tests: These are provocative tests and act as important screening methods and as an adjunct to the electrophysiological testing.

Wrist flexion (Phalen's test): The patient is asked to actively place the wrist in complete but unforced flexion. If tingling and numbness are produced in the median nerve distribution of the hand within 60 secs, the test is positive. It is the most sensitive provocative test (Fig. 37.6). It has a specificity of 80 percent.

Tourniquet test: A pneumatic blood pressure cuff is applied proximal to the elbow and inflated higher than the patient's systolic blood pressure. The test is positive if there is paraesthesia or numbness in the region of median nerve distribution of the hand. It is less reliable and is specific in 65 percent of cases only.

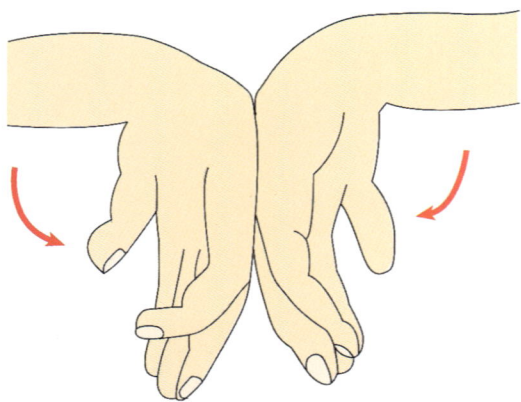

Fig. 37.6: Phalen's test

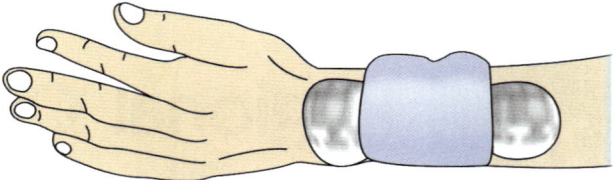

Fig. 37.7: Carpal tunnel splint

Two-point discrimination test: This test is positive in about one-third cases.

Electro diagnostic tests: These are not very infallible with 10 percent individuals having normal values. New conduction study indicates delayed conduction across the wrist.

Treatment

Nonoperative methods: In the initial stages non-steroidal anti-inflammatory drugs (NSAIDs) are given. If it is unsuccessful steroids like prednisolone for 8 days starting with 40 mg for 2 days and tapering by 10 mg every 2 days are tried. Use of carpal tunnel splint is also advocated (Fig. 37.7).

Injection treatment: This is indicated in patients with intermittent symptoms, duration of complaints less than one year and if there is no sensory deficits, no marked thenar wasting, etc. In the injection therapy a

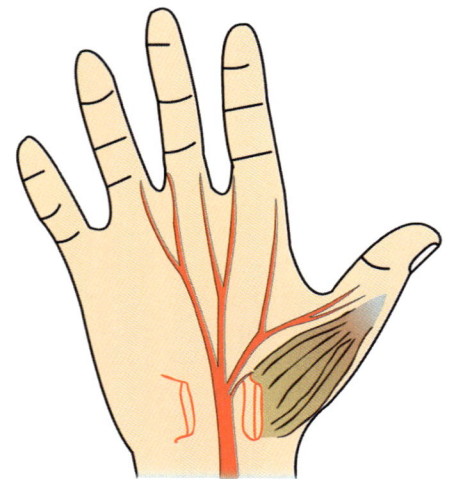

Fig. 37.8: Surgical division of transverse carpal ligament

single infusion of cortisone with splinting for 3 weeks is tried.

Surgery: This consists of division of flexor retinaculum and transverse carpal ligament (Fig. 37.8) and is indicated in failed nonoperative treatment, thenar atrophy, sensory loss, etc.

37

Regional Orthopedic Conditions of the Hand

38

Dupuytren's contracture
Compound palmar ganglion
Trigger finger

DUPUYTREN'S CONTRACTURE

Dupuytren's contracture is defined as proliferative fibroplasias of the subcutaneous palmar tissue, forming nodules of cords along its ulnar border. This fibroplasia results in finger contractures, thinning of subcutaneous fat, adhesions of skin to the lesion, pitting of skin, and knuckle pads on the dorsum of proximal interphalangeal (PIP) joints.

The following lesions may be associated with Dupuytren's namely lesions in medial plantar fascia in 5 percent, plastic indurations of penis in 3 percent (Peyronie's disease).

Causes

Exact cause is not known but it may be due to:
- Heredity
- Trauma of chronic repetitive nature.
- Occupational, seen in people employed in rock drilling due to the vibrations of the machine.
- Males—10 times more common in males.
- Whites are affected more than Blacks.
- Frequent and severe in epileptics and alcoholics (42%).
- Onset is usually less than 40 years of age.

Pathogenesis: Nodules and cords develop due to fibroplasias and hypertrophy of already existing fibers of palmar fascia on its ulnar border. This gradually contracts and pills the finger into flexion.

Clinical Features

Usually begins with ring finger at the distal palmar crease and later involves little finger. Flexion of MCP and PIP joints occur (Fig. 38.1). Discomfort is rare, itching or occasional pain over the nodules may be present.

Treatment

Observation consists of no treatment with observation being done at every three months interval.

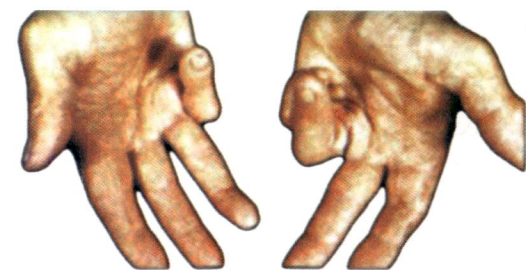

Fig. 38.1: Contractures of MCP and PIP joints of ring and little finger in Dupuytren's disease

Radiotherapy is given only during early fibroblastic phase.

Surgery is the best known treatment and is usually delayed.

Procedures chosen depend upon the degree of contractures, age, occupation, status of the palmar skin, presence or absence of arthritis of the finger joints, etc. More severe the involvement, more extensive is the surgery. The commonly done procedure is partial selective fasciectomy.

COMPOUND PALMAR GANGLION

This is a condition which affects the flexor tendons of the fingers mainly the ulnar bursa. It is usually due to tuberculosis though rheumatoid arthritis may also be a cause. The term *compound* is derived from a swelling one above and below the flexor retinaculum (Fig. 38.2).

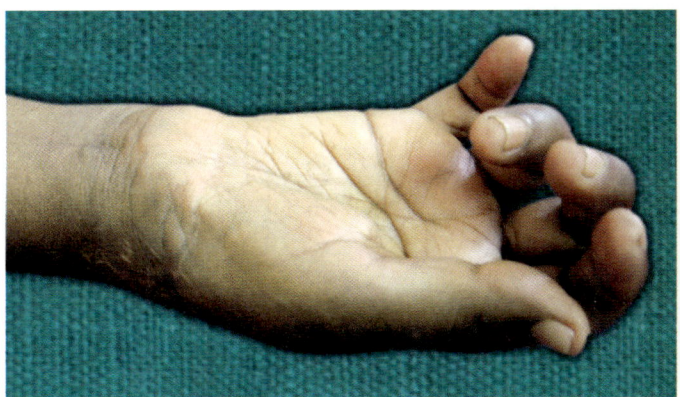

Fig. 38.2: Compound palmar ganglion

Here the endothelial lining of the sheath is substituted by granulation tissue containing miliary tubercles. The presence of *melon seed* bodies is a hallmark of this condition. Effusion may be seen and in the late stages the tendons may rupture.

QUICK FACTS: ABOUT MELON SEED BODIES
- Hallmark of compound palmar ganglion.
- Resemble grains of boiled sago.
- Give rise to soft, coarse crepitations.
- Made up of fibrin, cellular debris and occasional TB bacilli.

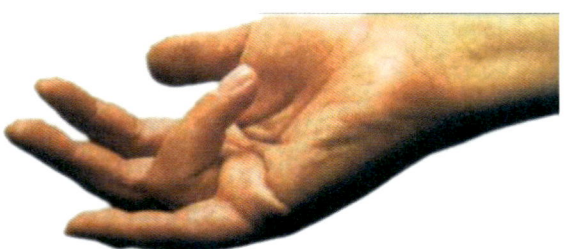

Fig. 38.3: Clinical photograph of trigger finger

Clinical Features

Those affected with this condition are usually less than 40 years and pain is not a feature. An hourglass swelling with cross-fluctuation may be noticed. There may be features of median nerve compression but there is definite evidence of wasting of the hand and forearm muscles.

Treatment

Antitubercular treatment, splinting of the forearm and exercises in the late stages, if it is due to tuberculosis. Complete excision forms the treatment in rheumatoid.

TRIGGER FINGER

The retinacula of the flexor tendons of the fingers and the thumb in the palm progressively thicken and constrict obstructing the fine glide of the flexor tenders. In the palm the flexor muscles are sufficiently strong to continue forcing the tendon through the diminished gap in the flexor retinaculum. The flexor tendon as a consequence gradually develops a constriction under the retinaculum and a bulge distal to it. Finally the flexor muscles may force the bulge through the retinaculum but the extensor muscles may be insufficiently powerful to extend the finger hereafter. The finger now snaps as it passes through the constriction and finally locks in a position of flexion from which attempts to passively extend the fingers are painful (Fig. 38.3). These are common in women. Congenital trigger fingers are seen in 25 percent of cases and may present as late as 2 years of age.

Note: Locking of the finger can be overcome by passive stretching or by a strong sustained active effort.

Treatment

Treatment of both the conditions is almost similar and consists of rest, NSAIDs, local infiltration of hydrocortisone, etc.

Surgery of the appropriate retinaculum if the above measures fail.

38

Regional Orthopedic Conditions of the Hip

Coxa vara
Legg-Calvé-Perthes disease
Slipped capital femoral epiphysis

COXA VARA

It is an abnormality of the proximal end of femur, which is characterized by decreased neck shaft angle (Figs 39.1A and B). Normal coxa vara is due to differential growth pattern of capital femoral and greater trochanteric epiphysis.

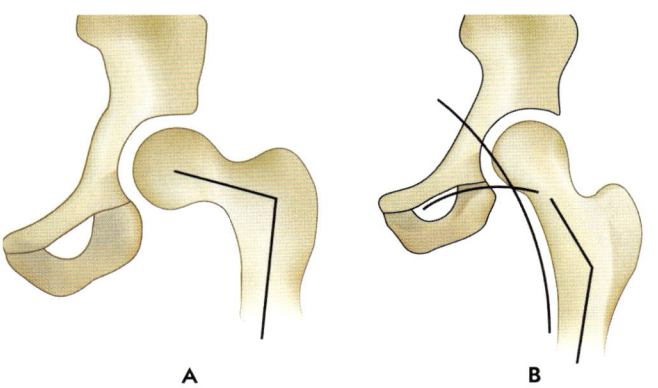

Figs 39.1A and B: (A) Coxa vara (< 125°), (B) coxa valga (> 135°)

Causes

It could be congenital or due to the effects of diseases like Perthes, slipped femoral epiphysis, rickets, septic arthritis, fibrous dysplasias, malunited trochanteric fractures.

Clinical Features

Small stature, limp, waddling gait, upward shift of greater trochanter, decreased rotation and abduction of hip, pain, stiffness and flexion contractures are some of the important clinical features of coxa vara.

Radiography

Radiographic features are neck shaft angle less than 90°, length of the neck is decreased, head is unusually translucent, and triangular fragment of bone is seen occupying lower part of the head close to the neck (called the Fairbank's triangle).

Treatment

It consists of corrective osteotomy at the intertrochanteric level. Usually a lateral wedge osteotomy is preferred. Macewen and Shands' corrective osteotomy corrects both coxa vara and retroversion of the femoral neck.

LEGG-CALVÉ-PERTHES DISEASE (Syn: Osteochondritis Deformans Juvenilis and Coxa Plana)

It is a disorder affecting the capital femoral epiphysis. It is the most common form of osteochondroses, characterized by avascular necrosis (AVN) and disordered enchondral ossification of the primary and secondary centers of ossification. It is associated with potential long-term morbidity.

Etiology

The etiology remains unknown, but it is currently accepted that the disorder is caused by an interruption of the blood supply to the capital femoral epiphysis causing avascular necrosis. Important predisposing factors are genetic (M:F > 5:1), trauma, low socio-economic group, smoking, etc.

Clinical Features

It is usually common in boys between 4 and 8 years (mean age 7 years) but can also occur less than 2 years and more than 12 years. If the child is older than 12 years, it is not true Perthes' disease but rather adolescent avascular necrosis.

Symptoms

Painless limp (classical presentation), mild pain in the hip or anterior thigh or knee, history of trauma may be present or absent, onset of pain may be acute or insidious.

Signs

Antalgic gait, muscle spasm (detected by roll test), proximal thigh atrophy (by 2–3 cm) limitation of abduction and internal rotation, short stature, etc. are some of the important clinical signs.

Clinical Tests

Thomas test reveals typically 15° fixed flexion deformity (FFD) of the hip (Fig. 39.2).

Internal rotation test (Figs 39.4A and B) for the hip shows decreased internal rotation.

Trendelenburg test is positive.

Abduction test abduction of the hip is limited on the affected side (Fig. 39.5).

Roll test (Fig. 39.3B) passive rotation of the lower limb is done to detect the muscle spasm. If this maneuver elicits pain the test is positive.

Mild wasting of the proximal thigh muscles could be seen (Fig. 39.3A).

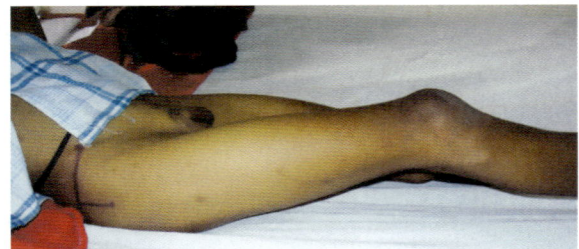

Fig. 39.2: A typical 15° FFD of hip

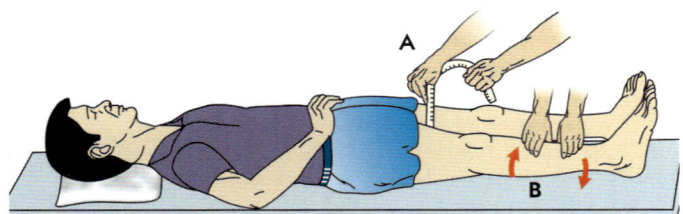

Figs 39.3A and B: Measurement of thigh muscle wasting (A) which is minimal in perthes and the roll test (B)

Stages

The disease passes, through three ill-defined stages of synovitis, necrosis and healing.

Classification

Catterall in 1971 proposed a four-group classification system for Perthes' disease based on the extent of involvement of head (radiographic appearance of the femoral head). This classification has been extremely useful in retrospective analysis of the results of treatment and has a very limited prognostic value. Salter and Thompson's classification is based on the extent of involvement of the capital femoral epiphysis. It has prognostic value.

Pathological and Radiological Staging

There are 4 stages described.

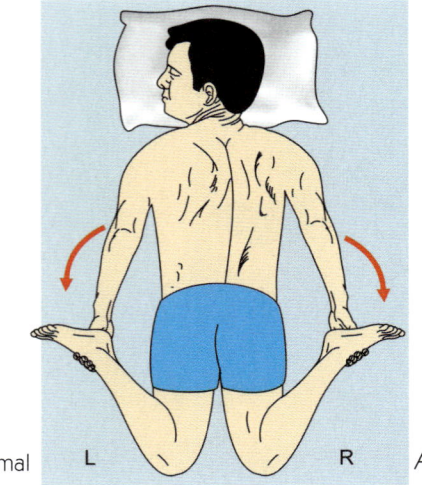

Normal   L   R   Affected

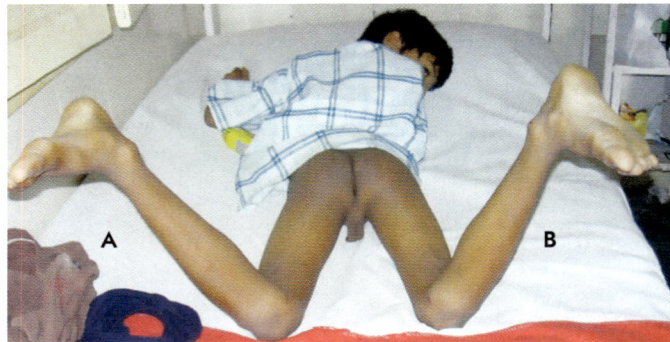

Figs 39.4A and B: (A) Internal rotation of the hip, (B) normal limited in Perthes

- *Stage of synovitis:* X-ray show increased sclerosis of the head.
- *Stage of AVN:* Fragmentation stage showing shrinkage of epiphysis.
- *Stage of revascularization:* New bone formation is seen.
- *Stage of healing:* Necrotic bone replaced with new bone.

Assessment

X-ray of the hip shows sclerosis and collapse of the femoral head in various stages (Fig. 39.6). Radiographic assessment is necessary to determine the progress of the disease, sphericity of the femoral head, epiphyseal extrusion or collapse and response to the treatment. Plain radiographs are usually adequate but rarely arthrography, MRI may be required.

Management

Perthes' disease is a local, self-healing disorder of the femoral head. Prevention of the femoral head deformity and secondary degenerative osteoarthritis is the only justification for treatment. This can be achieved by keeping the head of the femur in the acetabular cavity

39

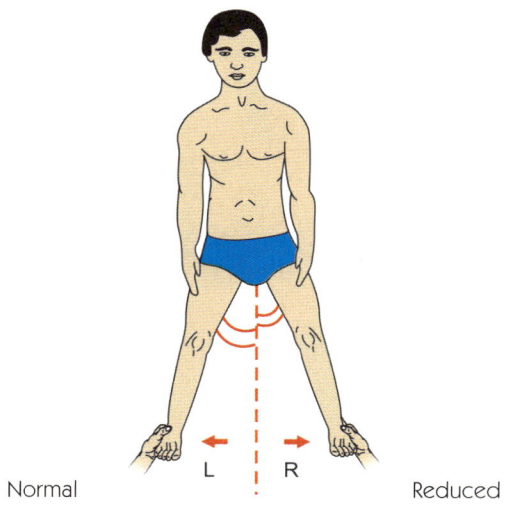

Normal   L   R   Reduced

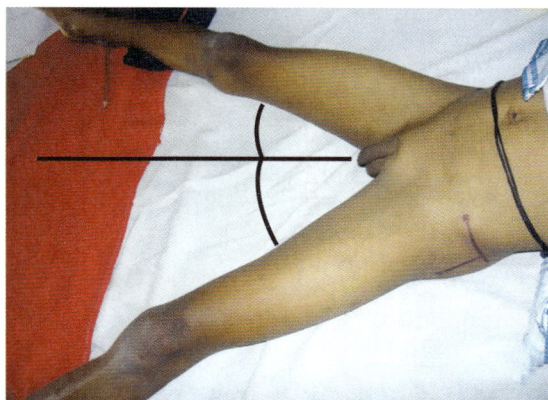

Fig. 39.5: Limitation of right hip abduction in Perthes

either by conservative or by surgical methods. Nonsurgical containment methods consist of abduction casts (Fig. 39.7), brace or Salter stirrup. Surgical containment is by in (Salter's type) nominate or femoral osteotomy (Varus derotation osteotomy).

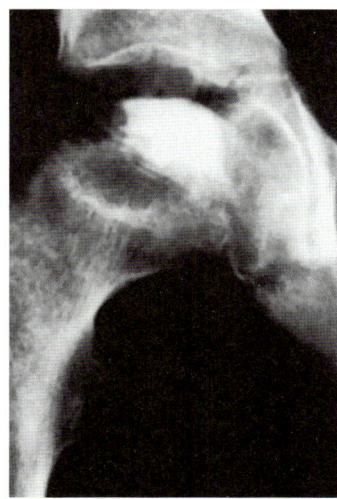

Fig. 39.6: Radiological features of Perthes

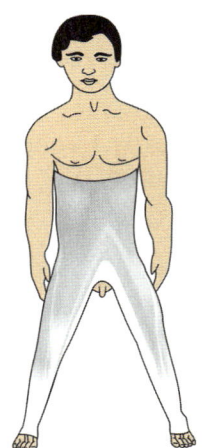

Fig. 39.7: Abduction cast in Perthes is a nonsurgical containment method

HEAD AT RISK SIGNS

Clinical	Radiological
• Overweight child	• Radiolucent V-shaped defect on the lateral epiphysis (Gage's sign)
• Elderly child	• Lateral subluxation
• Flexion and adduction deformities	• Calcification lateral to epiphysis
• Adduction contracture	• Horizontal growth plate
• Loss of movements	

QUICK FACTS: PERTHES' DISEASE

- Commonest osteochondroses.
- 80 percent affected are males between the age group 4 and 8 years.
- Two episodes of infarction
- First episode cause is not known
- Second episode is due to subchondral fracture
- Subchondral fracture heralds onset of true Perthes
- Painless limp is the characteristic symptom
- Decreased abduction, external rotation is present
- Catterall's grading helps plan the treatment
- Salter and Thompson's grading has prognostic value
- It is a local self-healing disorder
- The main goal of treatment is to attain a spherical femoral head either by non-surgical or surgical methods

Do you know the other famous osteochondritis in orthopedics?

Name	Site involved
Lower limbs	
• Perthes' disease	Head of the femur
• Osgood-Schlatter disease	Tibial tubercle
• Sever's disease	Calcaneal epiphysis
• Köhler's disease	Navicular bone
• Freiberg's disease	Metatarsal head
Spine	
• Scheuermann's disease	Ring epiphysis of the vertebrae
• Calve's disease	Central nucleus of the vertebra
Upper limbs	
• Panner's disease	Capitulum
• Keinbock's disease	Lunate

SLIPPED CAPITAL FEMORAL EPIPHYSIS (Syn: Epiphyseal Coxa Vara; Adolescent Coxa Vara)

Slipped capital femoral epiphysis occurs during adolescent rapid growth period when epiphyseal plate is weak and the capital epiphysis is displaced down and back. It was first described by **Muller** in 1889.

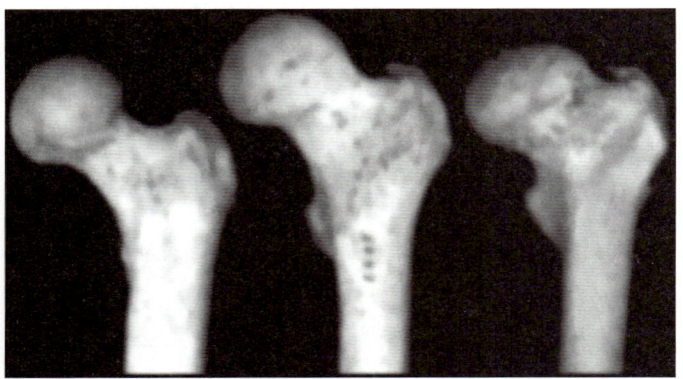

Fig. 39.8: Skeletal specimen of SCFE

Etiology

Predisposing factors

Age: It is common in 10–17 years of age

Sex: Males: Females is 5:2 ratio

Body type: Female—slender long built, and male—obesity type (hormonal type)

Location: Left hip is involved in 58 percent of cases

Trauma: Trivial or none at all.

Pathology

The slip mainly happens in the zone of hypertrophic cartilage and rarely in the zone of provisional calcification (Fig. 39.8).

Clinical Features

The presenting complaints and the clinical signs vary depending upon the stages of the disease. In the initial stages, the common presenting complaint is pain in the groin radiating to the thigh and the knee. In the later stages, there could be shortening, minimal thigh wasting, restricted abduction and internal rotation and increased adduction and external rotation. On flexion, the knee points towards the axilla on the same side.

Stages

The slip could be acute or chronic or it could be mild, moderate and severe.

X-ray of the Hip

The routine AP, lateral and frog leg views of the hip show the following radiological changes (Fig. 39.9).

Early Changes

- Marginal blurring of the proximal metaphysis.
- Lower margin of metaphysis is included within the acetabulum normally but excluded in the early epiphyseal slip (Fig. 39.9).

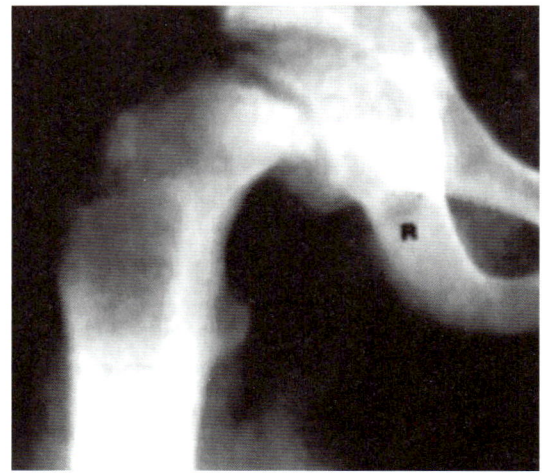

Fig. 39.9: Slipped capital femoral epiphysis

- *Trethovan's line:* Line drawn along the superior margin of the neck, transects the epiphysis normally, but will be above it in slip (Figs 39.10A and B).
- Depth of epiphysis is reduced.
- There is a step between the metaphysis and the epiphysis.

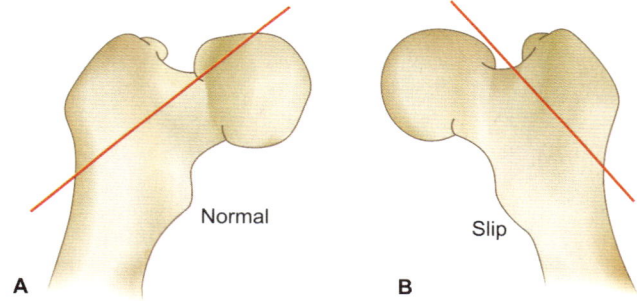

Figs 39.10A and B: Trethovan's sign

RADIOLOGICAL GRADING OF THE SLIP
- Type I slip: < 33% displacement
- Type II slip: < 33–50% slip
- Type III slip: > 50% slip

Late Changes

- Trethovan's sign is present.
- Head is atrophic.

- Neck shaft angle is less than 90°.
- New bone formation is seen at the anterior superior part of the neck.
- Joint space is usually clear.
- Shenton's line is broken.

CT scan: This is very useful in assessing the degree of slips and other changes more clearly than plain X-rays.

Treatment

Aim:
- To prevent further slip.
- To achieve premature closure
- To reduce risk of chondrolysis and AVN.

Acute major slip: Emergency reduction is done under (GA) or reduction is obtained by traction and fixed with pins.

Irreducible displacement: This is treated by open reduction and cervical osteotomy.

Old fixed displacement: This is treated by a corrective osteotomy at intertrochanteric or subtrochanteric level.

Gradual slip: If slip is less than one-third of the femoral neck *in situ* internal fixation is done. If more than one-third, corrective osteotomy is done at the inter-trochanteric region.

Complications: Chondrolysis, avascular necrosis, Sec. OA, etc.

39

40

Regional Orthopedic Conditions of the Knee

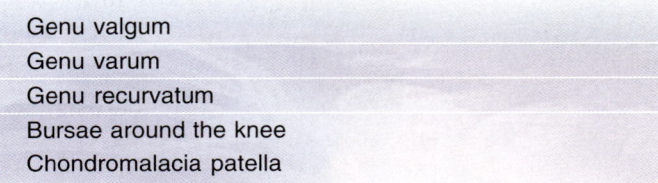

Genu valgum
Genu varum
Genu recurvatum
Bursae around the knee
Chondromalacia patella

Deformities around the knee joint could be in two planes. In the coronal plane we may encounter genu valgum and genu varum deformities and in the sagittal plane antevertum and recurvatum deformities (Figs 40.1A to C).

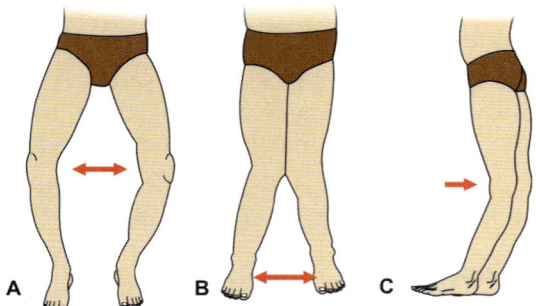

Figs 40.1A to C: Principal knee deformities: (A) genu varum, (B) genu valgum, (C) genu recurvatum

GENU VALGUM (KNOCK KNEE)

It is an outward deviation of the longitudinal axis of both tibia and femur. Apex of the curve or angulation of the knee is medial (Fig. 40.2).

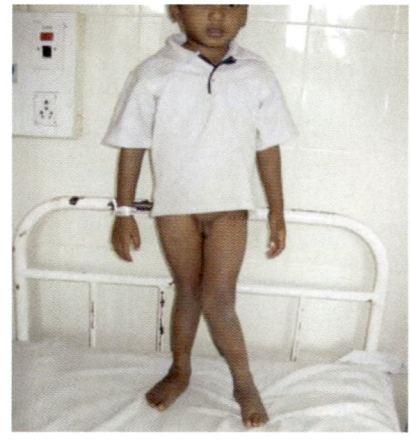

Fig. 40.2: Genu valgum or knock-knee deformity

Incidence

Seventy-five percent children have genu valgum up to 4 years of age. This is called physiological genu valgum, which usually disappears by 7 years.

Types

It is broadly classified into physiological and pathological, the latter could be unilateral or bilateral (Table 40.1).

Table 40.1: Causes of genu valgum	
Unilateral	*Bilateral*
• Trauma	• Physiological (disappears by 4 yrs)
• Osteomyelitis	• Pathological
• Tumors	• Congenital disorders
	• Idiopathic (most common)
	• Developmental disorders (e.g. epiphyseal dysplasia)
	• Endocrine disorders (e.g. thyroid disorders)
	• Metabolic disorders (e.g. rickets)
	• Paralytic disorders
	• Traumatic disorders
	• Infective disorders
	• Degenerative disorders
	• Inflammatory disorders (e.g. rheumatoid arthritis)

Clinical Features

The primary deformity in a genu valgum is a medial angulation of the knee. In response to this, secondary deformities develop in the femur, tibia and foot.

Assessment of genu valgum deformity: Clinical assessment of the severity of the deformity is measured by noting the intermalleolar distance and studying the plumb line. The methods are described in the section on clinical examination of the knee.

Plain X-ray of the knee is useful in evaluating the changes (Fig. 40.3).

Treatment of Genu Valgum

• *Mild cases:* Child is seen at intervals of 3 months and the progress is recorded. These cases usually require

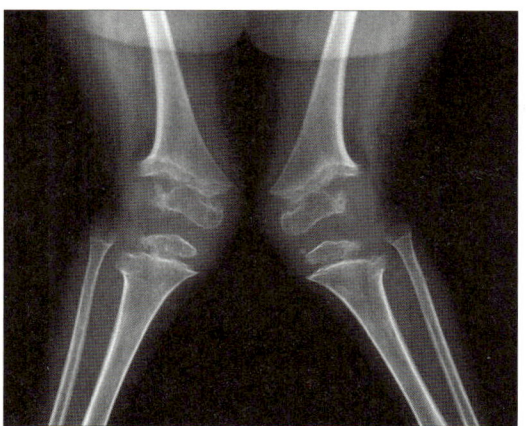

Fig. 40.3: Plain X-ray of genu valgum

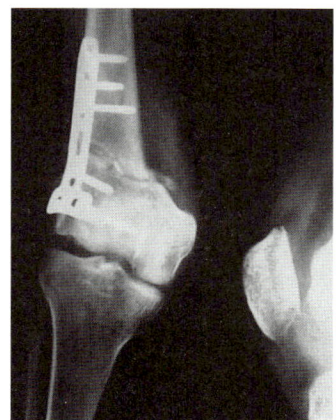

Fig. 40.4: Lateral closed wedge osteotomy

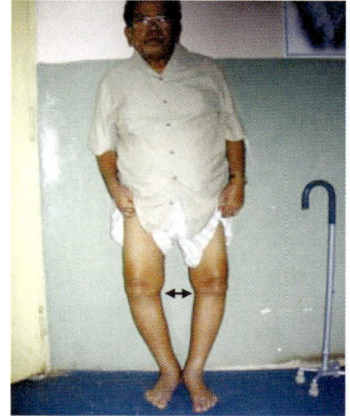

Fig. 40.5: Genu varum with increased intercondylar distance. Genu varum is said to exist if there is approximately 3 cm gap between the medial femoral condyles when the malleoli are together.

no treatment and raising the inner side of the heels by 4 to 5 mm may possibly relieve strain on ankles. The knock-knee braces may be useful.

- *Severe cases:* If by the age of 4 years, intermalleolar distance is 10 cm or more, operation may become necessary.

Surgical Methods

Epiphyseal stapling is done on the medial side before skeletal maturity

Osteotomy: After skeletal maturity a lateral closed wedge osteotomy is done (Fig. 40.4).

GENU VARUM (BOW LEGS)

It is defined as a lateral angulation of the knee. The longitudinal axis of femur and tibia deviates medially. The deformity involves tibia alone or the femur or tibia and fibula both.

Types and Causes

Unilateral
- Due to growth abnormalities of upper tibial epiphysis.
- Infections like osteomyelitis
- Trauma near the growth epiphysis of femur
- Tumors affecting the lower end of femur and upper end of tibia.

Bilateral
a Physiological (is corrected by 4 years).
b. Pathological:
  - Congenital causes
  - Postural abnormalities
  - Developmental disorders
  - Metabolic disorders (rickets rare)
  - Endocrine disorders
  - Degenerative disorders, e.g. osteoarthritis of knee—This is a common cause (Fig. 40.5)
  - Occupational disorders, e.g. in jockeys

- Idiopathic
- Paget's disease
- Blount's disease (tibia vara).

Measurements of the Deformity

Child: The deformity is clinically assessed by noting the inter condylar distance and drawing the plumb line (methods described in clinical examination of the knee)

Adults: The angle of genu varum is calculated on a standing radiograph of the whole limb.

Clinical Features

The primary deformity in genu varum is lateral angulation of the knee. In response to this secondary deformities develop in the tibia and the foot.

Radiology: Plain X-ray helps to evaluate the extent of the deformity (Fig. 40.6).

Treatment

Treatment should be conservative until 4 years of age. Knee-ankle-foot orthoses with the medial bar and the lateral strap is used. Corrective osteotomy like lateral

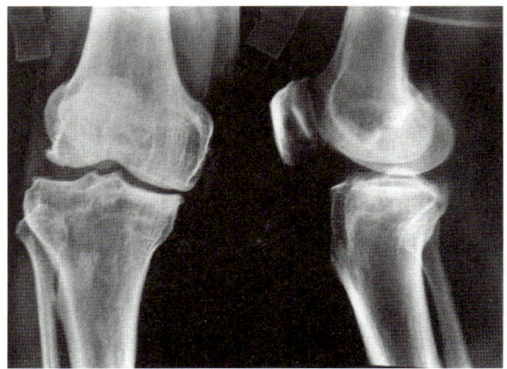

Fig. 40.6: Plain X-ray showing genu varum deformity

closed wedge osteotomy is indicated after skeletal maturity.

GENU RECURVATUM

This is defined as backward bending of the knee (higher extension). The cause could be congenital (Fig. 40.7) or acquired. The common acquired causes are polio and quadriceps contracture due to post-injection contractures in infants.

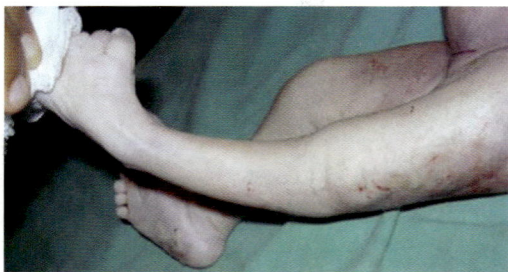

Fig. 40.7: Congenital hyperextension of the knee

Treatment

The treatment is essentially by supportive braces. Severe cases require corrective osteotomy at the supracondylar level.

BURSAE AROUND THE KNEE

Anterior

The following are the bursae around the knees:
- *Suprapatellar bursitis:* Always communicates with the knee joint
- *Prepatellar bursitis* (housemaid's knee) is seen in the lower half of patella and upper half of ligamentum patella (Figs 40.8 and 40.9).
- *Infrapatellar bursitis* seen in the lower half of ligamentum patella (Clergyman's, Parson's, or carpet layer's knee) (Figs 40.10 and 40.11).

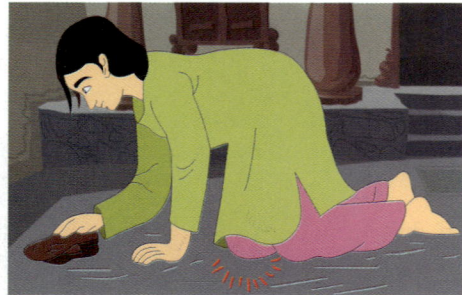

Fig. 40.8: Mechanism of housemaid's knee

Lateral

Cyst of lateral meniscus.

Medial

- Cyst of medial meniscus

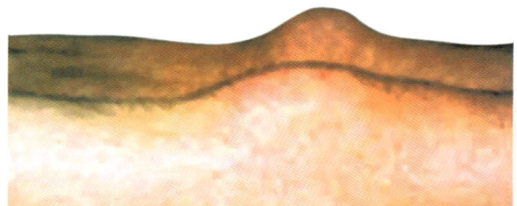

Fig. 40.9: Clinical photograph of housemaid's knee

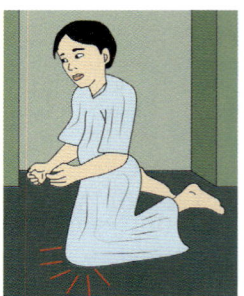

Fig. 40.10: Mechanism of formation of clergyman's knee

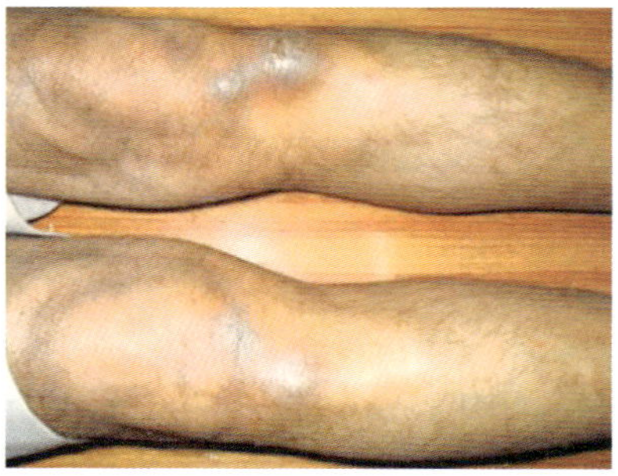

Fig. 40.11: Clergyman's knee

40

- Bursa anserina between the tibial collateral ligament and tendons of the semimembranosus, gracilis, semitendinosus.

Posteriorly

- Semimembranosus bursitis
- Baker's cyst
- Lymphangiectasia
- Aneurysm of popliteal artery
- Neuromyxofibroma.

POPLITEAL CYST (BAKER'S CYST)

This was first described by Adam in the year 1840 and later by Baker in 1877.

Commonly symptoms are seen in the bursa of the medial head of gastrocnemius and semimembranosus bursa.

Causes: Though the exact cause is unknown are children in adults it could be secondary due to rheumatoid arthritis or osteoarthritis.

Clinical Features

These are similar to internal derangement of the knee, like pain, stiffness, swelling, giving way. The swelling is seen in the middle of the popliteal fossa. It disappears on flexion and appears on extension (Fig. 40.12). The fluctuation and transilluminations tests are positive.

Investigations

Plain X-ray of the knee show intraarticular pathology like OA or rheumatoid knee. However, arthrography of the knee gives a better visualization of the herniation of the cyst (Fig. 40.13).

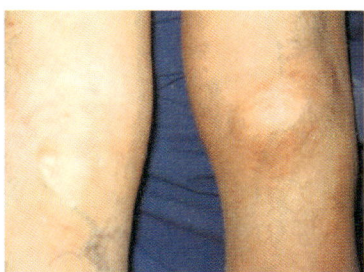
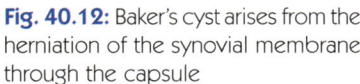

Fig. 40.12: Baker's cyst arises from the herniation of the synovial membrane through the capsule

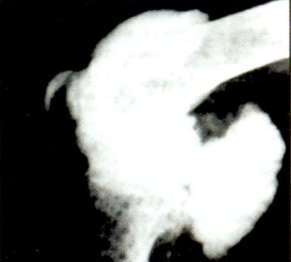

Fig. 40.13: Arthrography showing ruptured popliteal cyst

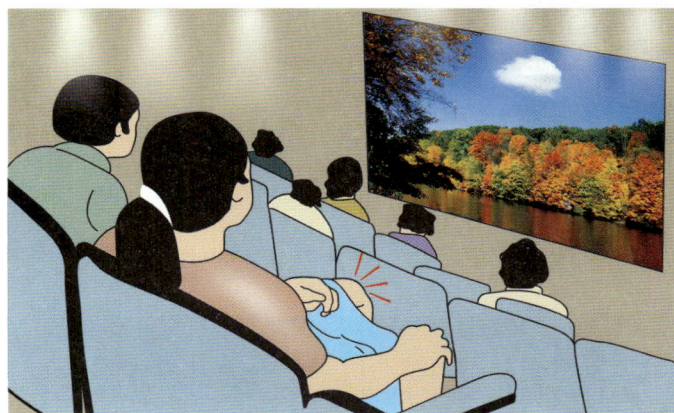

Fig. 40.15: Typical "Movie or theater sign" in chondromalacia patella

Treatment

The treatment of choice is excision of the bursa and closer of the capsular orifice by:

- Scarification of the edges and suture.
- To close the gap by a graft from tendinous part of the gastrocnemius, etc.

> **Remember**
>
> One-third to one-half of patients with Baker's cyst is seen in children. It is rare after seventh year of life. Hence, delay in excision is followed by gradual disappearance of the cyst.

CHONDROMALACIA PATELLA

It is defined as a blistering, cystic change of the patellar cartilage and it usually affects the medial facet of the patella.

Clinical Features

Patient complains of generalized deep pain in the knee. The knee may be swollen with a chronic effusion of synovial fluid and there will be a positive patellofemoral grinding test when the condition is severe (Fig. 40.14).

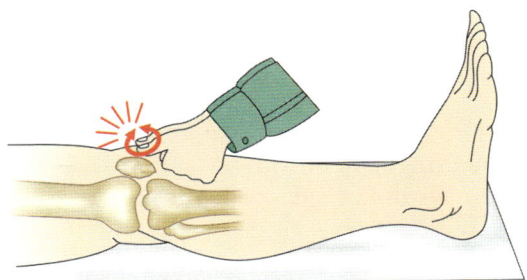

Fig. 40.14: Method of performing a grinding test in chondromalacia patella

The patella will appear out of alignment and there may well be a high 'Q'-angle. The vastus medialis will be weak, radiographs will occasionally show spurring and the patient will be unable to do squats.

Movie sign or theater sign: This is quite characteristic of chondromalacia. Prolonged sitting as in watching a movie heralds the onset of knee pain (Fig. 40.15).

Investigations: Radiograph of the knee shows irregular retro patellar surface (Fig. 40.16). Arthroscopy is an extremely useful diagnostic technique.

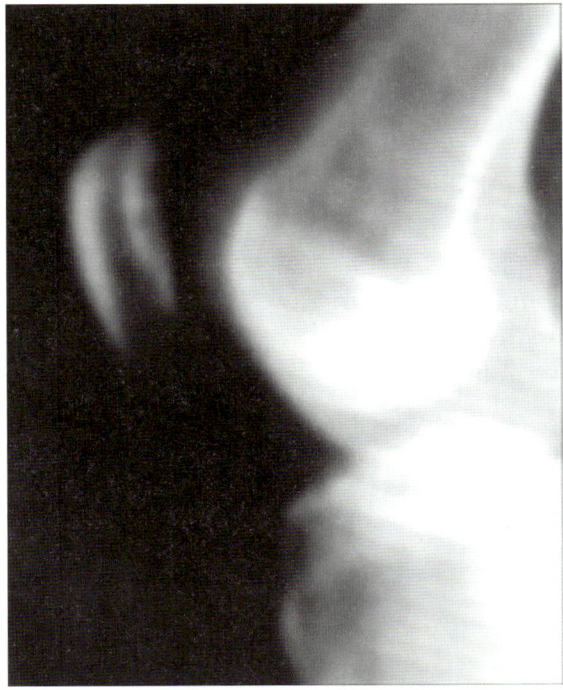

Fig. 40.16: Lateral view showing chondromalacia patellae

Differential diagnosis: Chronic synovitis of the knee, sprain of the retinacula, etc.

Treatment

Treatment consists of ice and ultrasound massage of the painful area, realignment of the maltracking of the patella by orthotic therapy, arthroscopic shaving of the retro patellar surface gives excellent results in cases that are unresponsive to the conventional conservative methods of treatment.

41 Regional Orthopedic Conditions of the Foot

ARCHES OF THE FOOT

The tarsal and metatarsal bones of the foot are bound by ligaments and are arranged in the form of two arches: longitudinal and transverse (Figs 41.1A and B). Integrity of these arches are maintained by shape of the bones, tension of the ligaments and plantar aponeurosis, muscular action of both short muscles and long muscles through bracing action of their tendons. Two conditions of clinical importance discussed in this chapter relates one to exaggerated longitudinal arch called the pes cavus and the other to loss of medial longitudinal arch called the pes planus.

PES CAVUS

Pes cavus is a deformity characterized by an excessively high longitudinal arch that results from an equinus position of the forefoot in relation to the hind foot (Fig. 41.2B).

Note: In this condition finger can be slipped under the navicular bone and it penetrates a distance of greater than 2 cm from the vertical edge of the foot.

Theories of Pathogenesis

Weakness of intrinsic muscles of the foot, over activity of the intrinsics, muscle imbalance, weak anterior tibial muscles and normal peroneus muscle and weakness of the calf muscles can cause it.

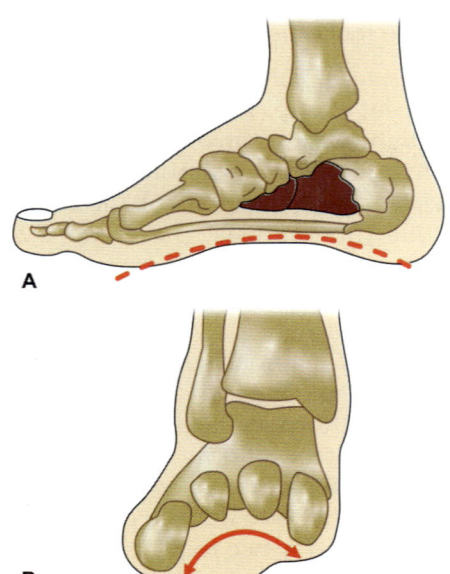

Figs 41.1A and B: Normal foot (A) longitudinal arch (B) transverse arch

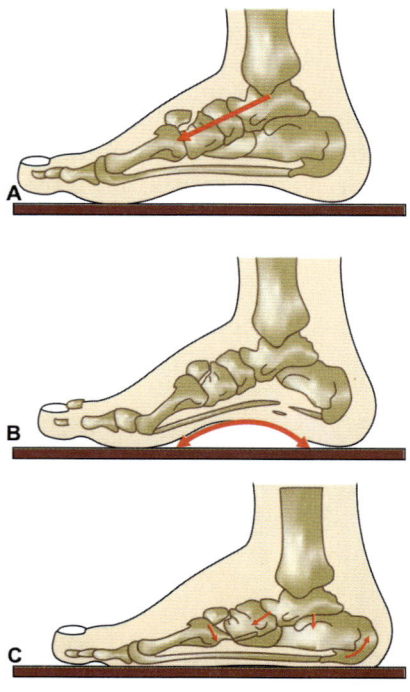

Figs 41.2A to C: (A) Normal foot, (B) pes cavus, (C) pes planus

215

Pathologic Anatomy

This consists of dropping of the foot, contractures of the plantar fascia, varus of the heel, and clawing of the toes.

Causes

In 80 percent of the cases the cause is unknown and is called the idiopathic variety. In the remaining 20 percent of the cases, it could be secondarily due to neurological disorders like cerebral palsy, polio, Friedreich's ataxia or may be due to CTEV or due to trauma to the foot, etc.

Clinical Features

This consists of high medial longitudinal arch, first metatarsal drop and pronation, tight plantar fascia, cock-up deformities of all the toes at the MTP joints, varus heel, and clawing of the toes (late feature) (Fig. 41.3).

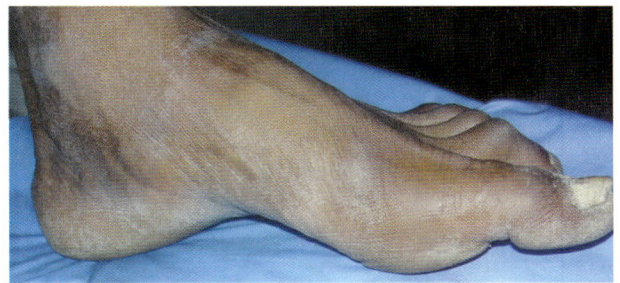

Fig. 41.3: Pes cavus and clawing of toes

Treatment

Correction of the primary deformity, which is equinus and pronation of the foot, is done first. Secondary deformities like, contracted plantar fascia, clawed toes and varus of the heels are corrected next. In the early stages conservative treatment is advocated. In late stages surgery is required and consists of soft tissue release in children, bony surgeries in adults.

PES PLANUS

This refers to loss of medial-longitudinal arch of the foot (Fig. 41.4).

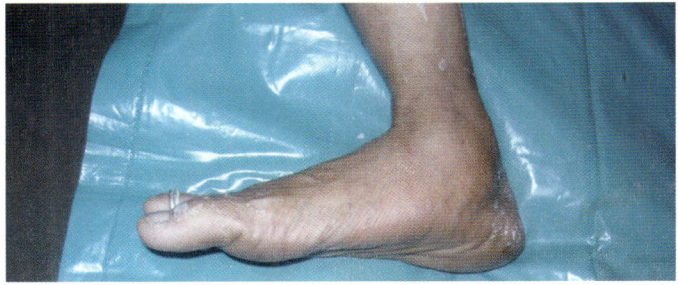

Fig. 41.4: Decreased longitudinal arch of the foot in pes planus

Types of Flatfoot and their Causes

Congenital	Acquired
Causes	*Causes and varieties*
• Calcaneovalgus	• Traumatic flatfoot (fracture calcaneus; Pott's fracture, etc.)
• Vertical talus deformity	• Relaxed or static flat foot (commonest) due to postural abnormalities
• Talocalcaneal bar	• Rigid flatfoot, fibrous or bony ankylosis from any cause
• Congenital ligament laxity	• *Spasmodic flatfoot* due to spasmodic contraction of the peroneal muscles due to rheumatoid arthritis, etc.

Note: However, the most common cause is idiopathic and here the exact cause of the flatfoot is unknown.

Predisposing factors: General muscle hypotonia, excessive fatigue of the foot muscles due to prolonged standing, unsuitable footwear, etc.

Clinical Features

Medial arch is obliterated, navicular bone is prominent, and fingers cannot be inserted under the arch, sole of the foot. Area of weight bearing increases and may show increased callosity. Pes planus could be:

Flexible: On non-weight bearing, normal appearing arch develops.

Rigid: Could be semi-rigid or fixed. During non-weight bearing normal acceptable medial arch does not develop.

Static type: This is the most common type, the reasons could be faulty postural activity of muscles, equinus deformity of the foot, and varus deformity of the foot.

Peroneal or spasmodic flatfoot: This is common in the young adolescent group. Patient complains of acute onset of pain, tightness, spasm of peroneal muscles, and eversion of foot and it is commonly associated with calcaneonavicular bar. It can also be associated with conditions like tuberculosis, rheumatoid arthritis, which causes spasm due to reflex muscle reaction.

Treatment

Conservative methods: It consists of orthopedic shoes with Thomas heels, medial heel wedges and navicular pad. Asymptomatic cases need parent education. Symptomatic cases require orthopedic shoes for mild cases, Custom prosthesis for severe cases. Fifteen to twenty percent adults have flexible pes planus, which are asymptomatic and hence require no treatment.

Surgical correction: This is done to relieve the disabling pain after exhausting every means of conservative management and not for cosmesis alone.

CONGENITAL VERTICAL TALUS (Popularly Known as Rocker Bottom Foot)

Normally talus is placed horizontally in the hind foot. Sometimes due to a congenital abnormality, it may remain vertical. A vertical talus reverses the normal concave arch with the abnormal convex arch (likened to the *Rocker Bottom* of an easy chair) (Fig. 41.5). Additionally the foot may be in severe valgus. X-ray of the foot clinches the diagnosis. The navicle instead of being in front of the talus sits on top of it due to the dislocation of the talonavicular joint.

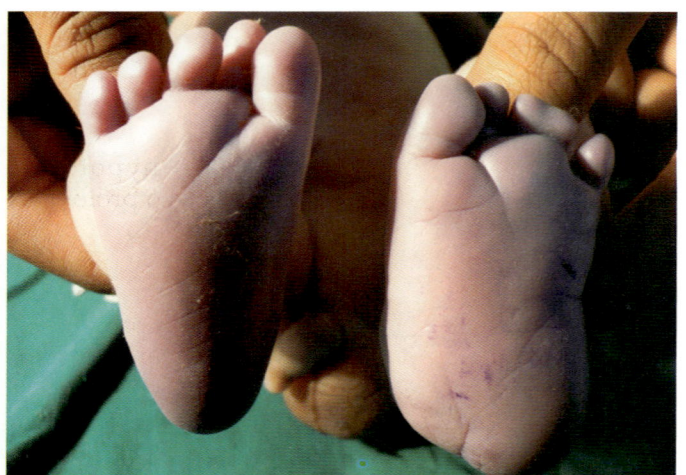

Fig. 41.5: Rocker bottom foot

The views recommended are:
- AP view—Talocalcaneal angle is increased
- Lateral view—Calcaneum and talus vertically placed.
- Plantar flexion view—To assess the talar and metatarsal calcaneal axis.
- Lateral dorsiflexion view—To assess the heel equinus.

Treatment

At birth manipulation of the foot into plantar flexion and inversion is attempted. Footwear correction in mild cases and corrective surgery in severe cases which consists of open reduction and retention done as a single stage or multiple stages after the child attains 1 year age.

CONGENITAL LIGAMENT LAXITY (INFANTILE FLATFOOT)

This is the commonly encountered variety of flatfoot in clinical practice. The anxious parents rush to the orthopedists when they observe that their child on beginning to stand and walk does so on flatfeet. On questioning, they reveal a familial history of flatfoot. The reasons in these cases could be congenital foot ligament laxity.

Treatment

This should be begun early and suitable arches should be provided in the shoes of the child. In the older child, foot exercises may be taught.

FOOT PAIN: METATARSALGIA

It is defined as pain beneath the metatarsal heads or shafts. It may be due to trauma, inflammation, and static causes due to developmental anomalies, obesity, etc.

Clinical Features

Patient complains of pain beneath the metatarsal heads (Fig. 41.6) compression of the foot increases the pain (Fig. 41.7). Splayfoot, atrophy of the interosseous muscles and clawing of the toes are the other features.

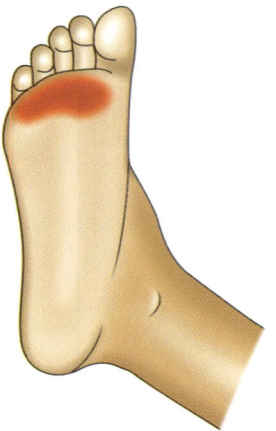

Fig. 41.6: Areas of pain in metatarsalgia

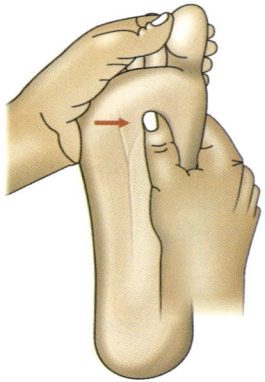

Fig. 41.7: Method of eliciting tenderness in metatarsalgia

Treatment

Treatment consists of intrinsic muscle exercises, well-designed shoes, pad and strapping changed at intervals of one week, support of inner sole with pad and oblique osteotomy of the metatarsal necks for metatarsalgia associated with metatarsal head prolapse.

MORTON'S NEUROMA

In 1876, Morton described a condition of pinching of the lateral plantar nerve in the fourth web space between the mobile fourth to fifth metatarsal heads of the foot (Fig. 41.8).

Clinical Features

Patient complains of pain in the region of the third-and-fourth metatarsal heads, that increases by walking and decreases by rest.

Mulder's click: When neuroma is squeezed between the metatarsal heads a click is felt. This is common in women and is usually unilateral.

41

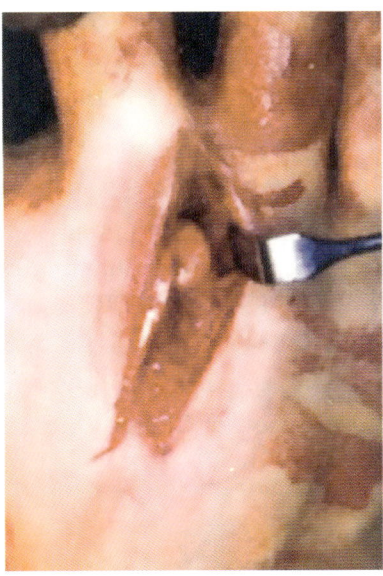

Fig. 41.8: Clinical photograph of Morton's neuroma

Treatment

Nonoperative treatment consists of shoes with metatarsal bars; local infiltration of hydrocortisone, use of wide toe box, etc. (Fig. 41.9).

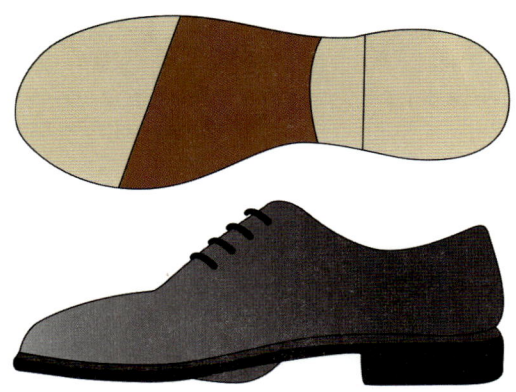

Fig. 41.9: Incorporation of metatarsal bars, under the sole of the footwear

Surgical treatment is mainly excision of the neuroma in the third web space and this has an 83 percent success rate.

COMMON PAINFUL HEEL CONDITIONS

Plantar fasciitis: It is characterized by pain at the insertion of plantar fascia and is due repetitive trauma to the heel (Fig. 41.10). There will be localized tenderness at the insertion of the plantar fascia (Fig. 41.11).

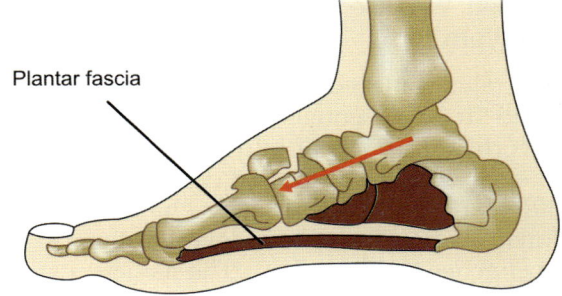

Fig. 41.10: Plantar fascia

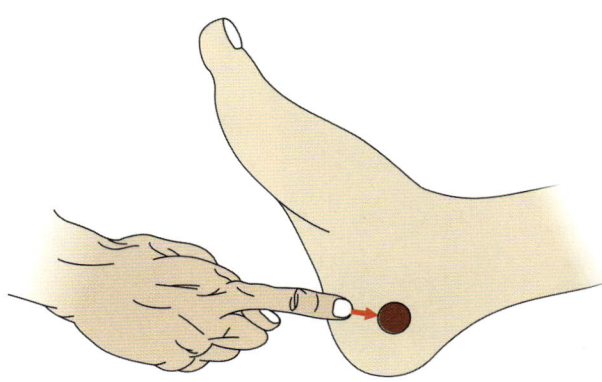

Fig. 41.11: Point of tenderness in plantar fasciitis and calcaneal spur

Treatment

Conservative treatment consists of NSAIDs, local steroids and footwear correction. If it fails, surgical release of the plantar fascia through a proximal medial longitudinal arch incision is contemplated.

CALCANEAL SPURS

It is a spike of extra bone at the anterior edge of the calcaneal tuberosity (usually medial).

Causes: Repeated attacks of plantar fasciitis, repeated micro trauma to the heel, constant pull of the shortened plantar fascia over the heel, ill-fitting footwear, fibromatosis of the plantar fascia are some of the causes.

Clinical Features

Patient complains of pain over ball of the heel, tenderness on plantar aspect of the heel (Fig. 41.11), slight swelling at the attachment of plantar fascia. Typically the patient complains of early morning stiffness of the foot and has difficulty in walking as soon he gets up in the morning. In retrocalcaneal spur patient complains of pain, swelling over (Fig. 41.11) the posterior aspect of the calcaneal.

Radiograph: Lateral view of the heel reveals an extra growth in most cases (Fig. 41.12).

Treatment

Conservative methods include treating the causative factor, rest, NSAIDs, local infiltration of hydrocortisone and microcellular rubber or silicon heel used for the sole of the footwear (Fig. 41.13).

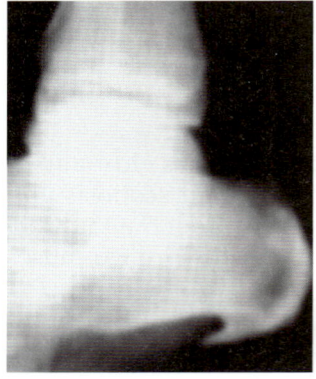
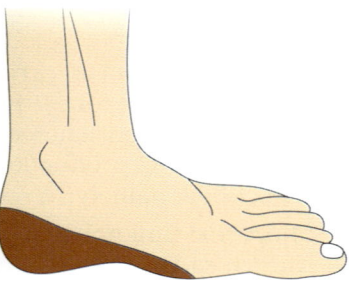

Fig. 41.12: Plain X-ray of the heel lateral view with calcaneal spur

Fig. 41.13: UC-BL shoe inserts to relieve heel stress in plantar fasciitis and calcaneal spur

HALLUX VALGUS

It is a deviation of the great toe at the metatarsophalangeal joint away from the midline (Figs 41.14A and B).

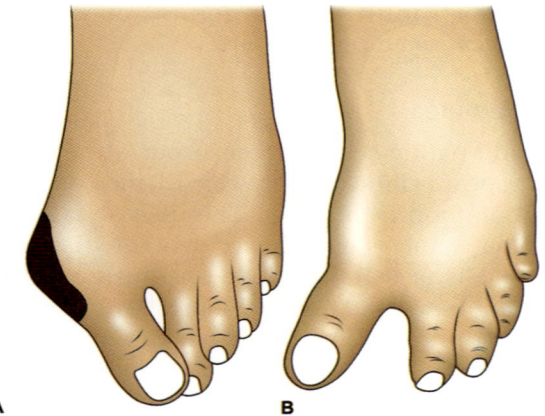

Figs 41.14A and B: Prominent great toe deformities: (A) hallux valgus, (B) hallux varus

Causes

These are some of the important causes of hallux valgus: Wearing of tight socks and footwear, congenital, diseases like gout, rheumatoid arthritis, etc. It is more commonly seen in women (Male: Female = 1:10) (Fig. 41.15).

Treatment

Mild cases: Physiotherapy measures and footwear correction suffices in mild cases:

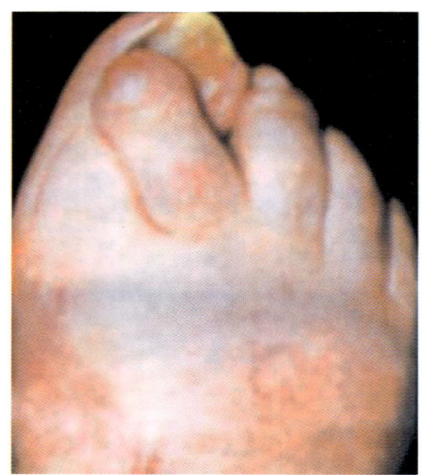

Fig. 41.15: Clinical photograph of hallux valgus

- Relaxed passive stretching of the abductors of great toe.
- Active exercises to the foot intrinsic muscles.
- Proper weight-bearing methods.
- Footwears with straight inner border with a wedge between the I and II toe helps.
- Faradic foot stimulation is recommended.

Severe cases: Surgery is the treatment of choice and includes
- *Keller's operation:* Excision of the head of the first metatarsal and proximal portion of the proximal phalanx.
- *Mayo's operation:* Here only head of the first metatarsal bone is excised.
- *Arthroplasty:* Excision of the first MTP joint with Bunion.
- *Arthrodesis* of the first MTP joint is done in some intractable cases.

HALLUX RIGIDUS

In this condition there is pain and stiffness in the MTP joint of the great toe and is due osteoarthritis.

Causes

Consists of repeated injuries to the great toe, improper footwear, familial and common in females. There may be erosion of the articular cartilage leading to OA and formation of exostosis.

Treatment

Mild cases: Conservative measures like painkillers.

Thermotherapy: Helps to reduce pain and spasm.

Footwear modifications: Like metatarsal bars, soft soles, etc. *POP cast* may be required in some cases.

Severe cases: Arthroplasty or Arthrodesis of the first MTP joint may be required.

41

Scoliosis
Spondylolisthesis
Kyphosis
Lumbar canal stenosis

SCOLIOSIS

By definition, Scoliosis is a lateral curvature of the spine in the upright position. The lateral curvature is usually accompanied by some rotational deformity. The other deformities of spine are shown in Figs 42.1A to E.

Varieties

Nonstructural scoliosis: In nonstructural scoliosis the curves are flexible and readily correctible with side bending. It is frequently seen as a compensatory mechanism to a leg length discrepancy, fixed flexion deformity of the hip (compensatory scoliosis), local inflammation or irritation due to acute lumbar disc disease and prolapsed disc (sciatic scoliosis) or due to poor postural habits (postural scoliosis).

Structural scoliosis: In structural scoliosis the curves are fixed and nonflexible and fail to correct with side bending. Lateral bending of spine is asymmetric or involved vertebrae are fixed in a rotated position or both.

Note
- Postural scoliosis is the most common variety of nonstructural scoliosis.
- Idiopathic scoliosis is the most common variety of structural scoliosis.

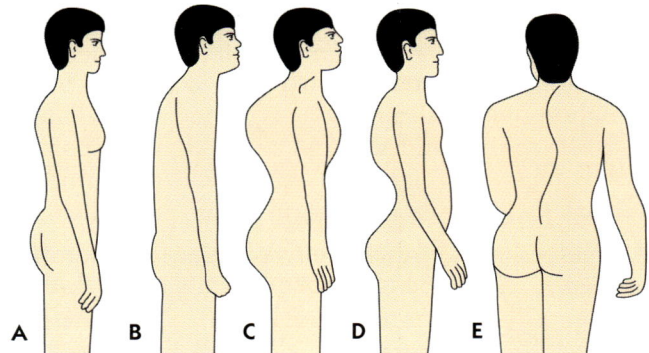

Figs 42.1A to E: Various deformities of the spine: (A) normal, (B) flat back, (C) kyphosis, (D) lordosis, (E) scoliosis

Structural Scoliosis

It may occur from a variety of causes. Idiopathic scoliosis accounts for 90 percent of all scoliosis and appears to represent a hereditary disorder but the exact mechanism of its production is unknown. Two causes are described, namely:

1. Idiopathic (unknown cause)
2. Known cause. The important among these are:
   a. *Congenital scoliosis:* This is due to defect in segmentation, which is usually due to a lateral bar or due to a defect in the formation including hemi vertebrae or double hemi vertebrae.
   b. *Paralytic scoliosis:* This is due to muscle imbalance on either side of the trunk, the most common cause being anterior poliomyelitis. Cerebral palsies, muscular dystrophies, etc. are the other common causes.
   c. *Miscellaneous causes:* This group includes neurofibromas, multiple congenital contractures osteogenesis imperfecta, etc.

Clinical Features

Though idiopathic scoliosis can occur at any age, it usually appears clinically between 10 and 13 years. It is more common in females. The disease is usually asymptomatic and is usually accidentally discovered. The diagnosis is usually made on routine physical examination especially during medical examination at schools. Look for different varieties of curves (Figs 42.3A to D). In long-standing cases, patients may complain of pain, there could be impaired lung function and rarely neurological deficits. But in idiopathic scoliosis deformity is often the only complaint (Figs 42.2A and B).

Scoliotic Facts

Structural curve: This is a laterally curved spine that lacks normal flexibility.

Primary curve: This is the earliest curve to appear.

Compensatory curve or secondary curve: This is the curve, which develops above or below the primary curve in an effort to balance the spine.

Major curve: This is the largest structural curve

Minor curve: This is the smallest curve.

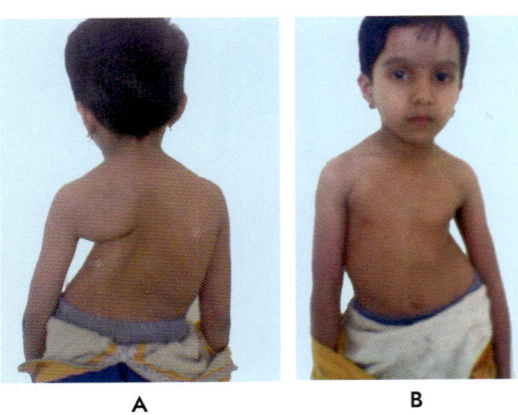

Figs 42.2A and B: Scoliosis is a lateral curvature of the spine (best examined from the back)

Apical vertebra: This is the most deviated vertebra from the vertical axis of the patient.

End vertebrae
a. The uppermost vertebra whose superior surface tilts maximally towards the concavity of the curve.
b. The lowermost vertebra whose inferior surface tilts maximally towards the concavity of the curve.

Radiology

Radiography of the spine is the main investigation tool and the following views are taken (Fig. 42.4).

PA view of the spine, standard lateral radiography of the spine, right and left bending films of spine and the

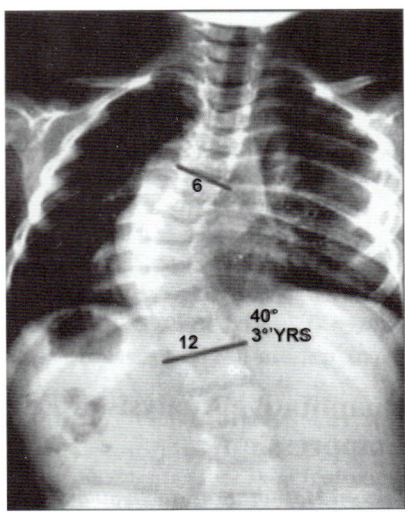

Fig. 42.4: Radiograph showing paralytic scoliosis

stagnara derotation view which is an oblique view of the spine. The radiological parameters of importance are:

Cobb method to measure severity of the curve: The upper and lower vertebrae are identified. Intersecting perpendicular line from the superior surface of the superior end vertebrae and from the inferior surface of the inferior end vertebrae is drawn. The angle of deviation of these perpendiculars from a straight line is the 'angle of the curve' (Fig. 42.5).

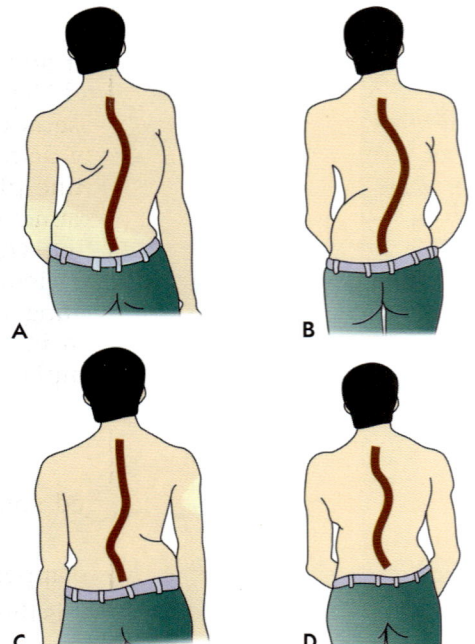

Figs 42.3A to D: Various types of scolistic curves: (A) thoracic curve, (B) thoracolumbar curve, (C) lumbar curve, and (D) double lumbar curve

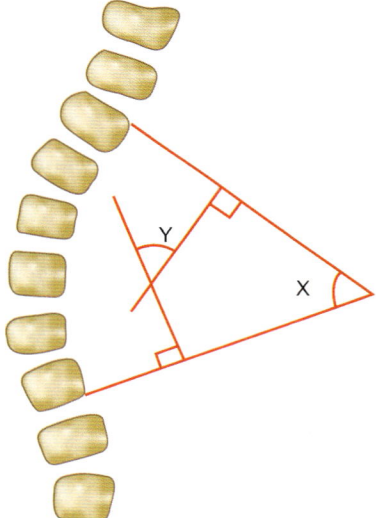

Fig. 42.5: Cobb method of measuring severity of a curve (Y = angle)

Nash and Moe's method to measure vertebral rotation: In the PA view the positions of the spinous process and the pedicles are noted. Normally the spinous process lies in the center but shifted to one side if there is rotation (Fig. 42.6).

42

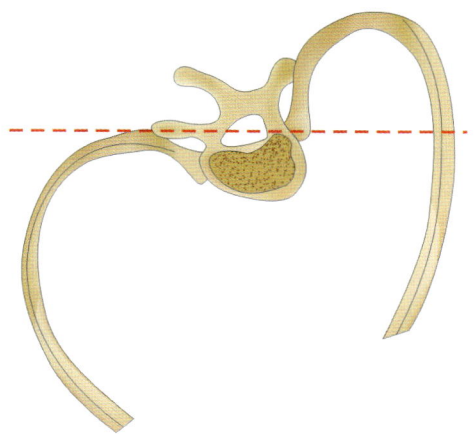

Fig. 42.6: Rib distortion due to vertebral rotation

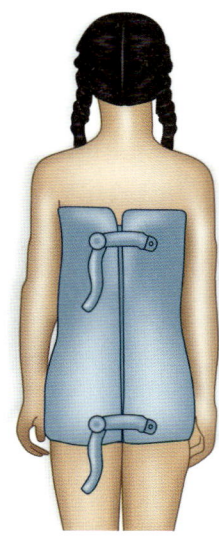

Fig. 42.7: Orthotic treatment of structural scoliosis with Boston brace

Reisser's sign: This is a classification of the ossification of the iliac epiphysis, which usually starts from the anterior superior iliac spine and progresses posteriorly towards the posterior iliac spine. Reisser's stage 4 corresponds with cessation of spine growth and stage 5 correlates with cessation of height increase. The importance of this sign is, the completion of growth can be radiologically assessed which indicates no possibility of the curve progression.

Compensation: If head is to be balanced above the pelvis when the patient is erect, it is done so by any curve or curves that develops in the opposite direction. *The formation of curves in the opposite direction is called compensation.* The angle of secondary curves should be equal to that of the primary curve. If it exceeds it is called over compensation.

Treatment

The most important aspect in the treatment of scoliosis is early detection of the curve. A curve that is obvious in standing position has already approached 30 to 40°. Detecting a curve before it reaches 20° is of utmost importance because curves over 20° tend to progress. Frequent re-examinations are essential. The treatment depends on the age of the patient and the severity of the curve.

Non-surgical Treatment

Observation: This is the primary treatment of all curves especially for curves less than 20 degrees. *At present radiography is the only definite documentation of curve size and progression.*

Orthotic treatment: This is effective in skeletally immature persons. For mild or moderate curves, Milwaukee brace, Boston brace, Reisser's turn buckle cast, localizer cast, etc. are used and the 20° level is considered still for bracing (Fig. 42.7).

Other non-operative measures: Exercises and electrical stimulation have been unsuccessfully tried in adolescent variety.

Surgical treatment: It is indicated for high degree inflexible thoracic curve, curve over 60° and aims at obtaining fusion at the spine (see box). Preoperative traction through the halopelvic traction stretches the contracted structures assures greater success (Fig. 42.8). The correction obtained during surgery is stabilized and maintained internally by Hartshill frame, segmental fusion, etc. (Fig. 42.9).

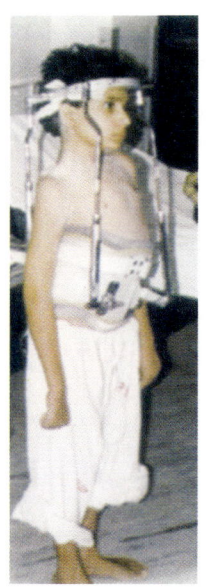

Fig. 42.8: Halo pelvic distraction apparatus used for skeletal traction in correction of structural scoliotic curves

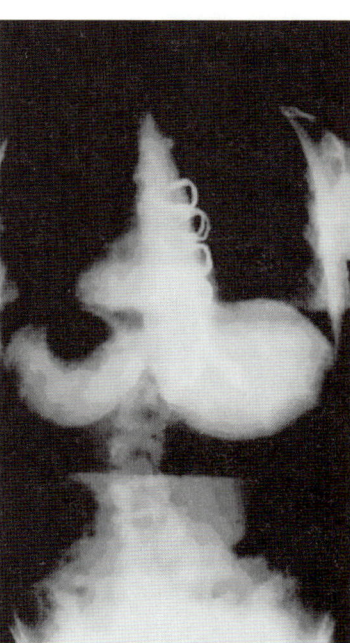

Fig. 42.9: Segmental correction and fusion

- Scoliosis is lateral curvature of the spine.
- Idiopathic variety accounts for 90% of cases.
- Female preponderance.
- X-ray is the only definite documentation of curve size and progression.
- The most important aspect of treatment is early detection.
- Curves < 20° need observation.
- Curves > 20° require treatment.
- Curves between 20 and 40° can be treated by Milwaukee brace, which has to be worn 23 hrs per day for a period of at least two years.
- Curves > 40° need surgical correction and fusion.

Remember: **3 Os in scoliotic treatment.**
Observation (for < 20 degrees curves),
Orthoses (for curves between 20 and 40 degrees),
Operation (for curves > 40 degrees).

SPONDYLOLISTHESIS
(Spondylos—spine; Olisthein—to slip)

It is defined as slow anterior displacement of a vertebra at the lower lumbar spine, generally accepted as, the lowermost vertebra L5 slipping forward on the first sacral segment S1 (Figs 42.10A and B).

Pathogenesis any defect in the chain of structures of the muscles, ligaments, bones allows a vertebra to slip other the other. Defect in the pars seems to be the most common cause (Fig. 42.10A).

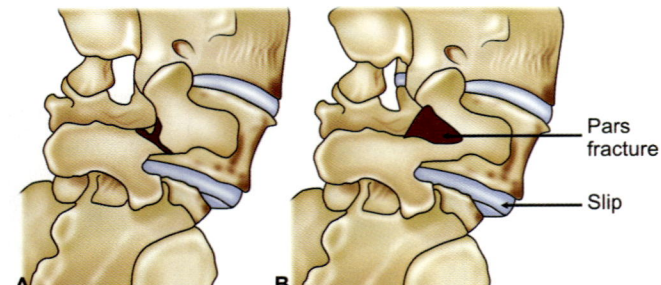

Pars
fracture

Slip

Figs 42.10A and B: (A) Fracture or discontinuity in the pars (spondylolysis), (B) spondylolisthesis

Essential lesion It is the interruption in the concavity of the pars interarticularis.

Spondylolysis: In this the defect in the pars exists but without the forward slipping. This could be due to a fracture, stress fracture or nonunion.
   Note: Retrolisthesis is the opposite of spondylolisthesis. Here the spine has slipped backwards.

Classification (Wiltse, Macnab and Newman)

Five varieties are described (Figs 42.11A to F).

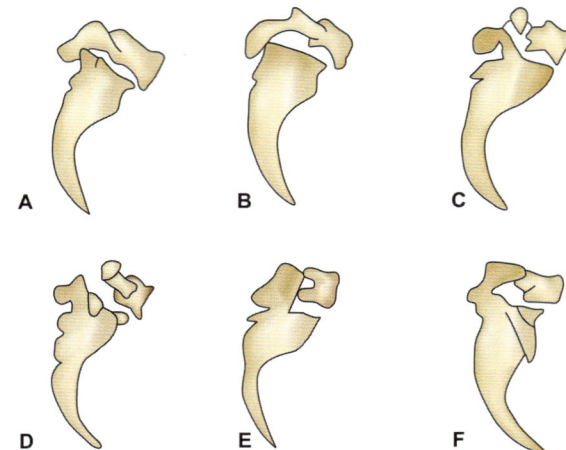

Figs 42.11A to F: Varieties of spondylolisthesis: (A) normal, (B) congenital, (C) isthmic, (D) traumatic, (E) degenerative, and (F) pathological

42

Dysplastic: Congenital abnormalities of the upper sacrum or the arch of L5. These permit the spondylolisthesis to occur.

Isthmic (true) lesion is in pars and is the most common variety in children. Rarely seen before 8 years. At adolescent growth spurt, sudden increase in activity, gymnastics, carrying heavy bags, etc. may lead to a fatigue or stress fracture of the pars, which may give rise to the slip.

Degenerative: Here pars is intact but the facet joints degenerate and allow the forward slip and is seen in the elderly people.

Traumatic: This is due to fracture in other areas of the bony hook rather than the pars.

Pathological: There is a generalized or localized bony disease in this variety.

Note:
Isthmic spondylolisthesis—most common variety.
Dysplastic spondylolisthesis—least common variety.
Other varieties—fall in between.

Clinical Features

Most of the times patient is asymptomatic. Isthmic is the common variety in children and degenerative in adults. Whatever the variety backaches with varying stiffness with or without are the complaints. Movements of the spine are restricted too. All these symptoms increase on standing. Important characteristic clinical signs are increased lumbar lordosis (Fig. 42.12), a prominent transverse furrow, *Step sign*-palpable step usually at L5-S1 level and decreased SLR due to sciatica (Fig. 42.13).

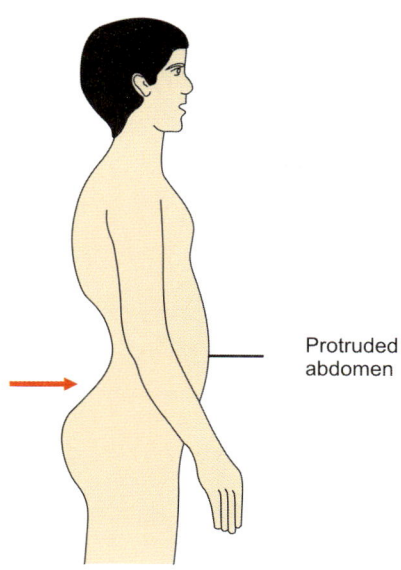

Protruded abdomen

Fig. 42.12: Increased lumbar lordosis in spondylolisthesis

42

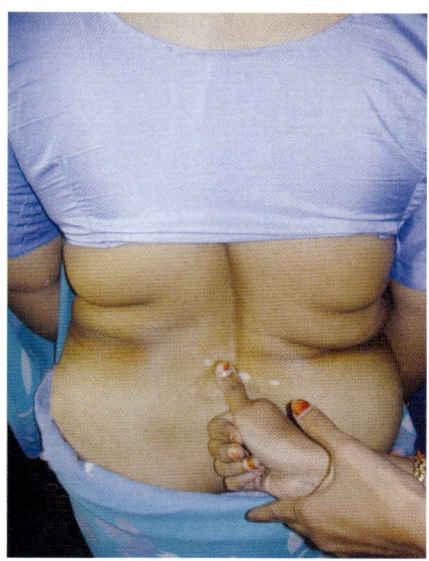

Fig. 42.13: Method of eliciting step sign and the transverse furrow

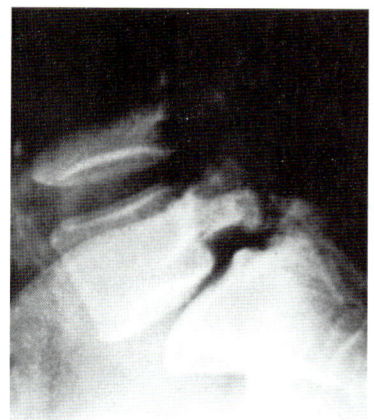

Fig. 42.14: Spondylolisthesis

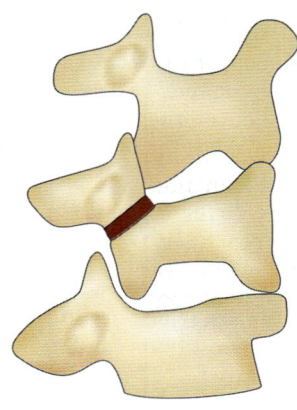

Fig. 42.15: Fracture of the pars. In true spondylosis familiarly known as "Scottish terrier sign".

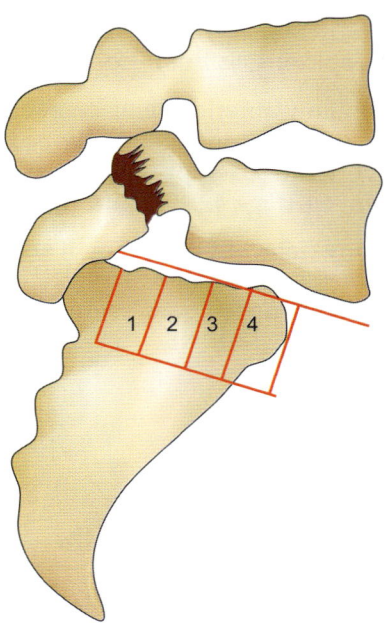

Fig. 42.16: Meyerding's classification of spondylolisthesis. The amount of slippage is graded 1–4.

Radiograph of the spine is the investigation of choice. Anteroposterior and lateral films are helpful (Fig. 42.14). Nevertheless, oblique view of the lumbar spine demonstrates the defect in the pars very accurately as a "Scottie dog" sign. The Scottie dog's neck, which represents the pars defect, is broken in the isthmic variety (Fig. 42.15). The edges of the defect are smooth and rounded and suggest a pseudarthrosis rather than acute fracture.

In the lateral view, forward displacement of the vertebra can be noted with respect to lower vertebra. Depending upon the extent of forward displacement, Meyerding has classified them into four types (See box below and Fig. 42.16).

Meyerding's Grading*
G1   25% forward displacement
G2   25–50%
G3   50–70%
G4   > 75%

Percentage of slip is calculated by the upper vertebral displacement over the lower vertebral body.

Treatment

Clinically spondylolisthesis is divided into three groups, asymptomatic, mild to moderate and severe varieties, based on the severity of symptoms. Table 42.1 shows different methods of conservative treatment to be employed in the above three clinical varieties of

Table 42.1: Different methods of conservative treatment

Asymptomatic	Mild to moderate severe	Severe
• Correction of poor posture • Elimination of stressful occupation • To avoid certain special sports activities	• Alleviation of anxiety • Analgesics and muscle relaxants • Deep heat • Exercises • Brace	• Rest • NSAIDs • Gradual exercises • Brace

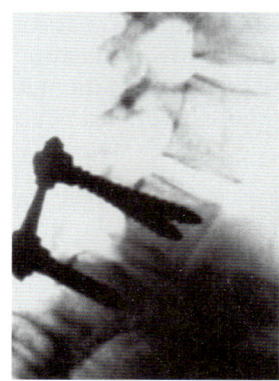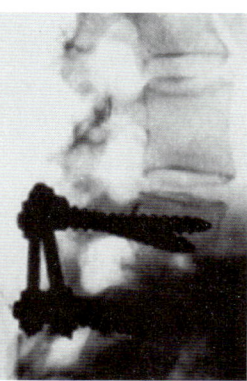

Fig. 42.17: Posterior spinal stabilization by Steffee plate and screws

spondylolisthesis. However, simple measures like exercises NSAIDS, proper postural habits, physiotherapy, braces, etc. are quite effective in mild cases. More severe cases require more aggressive approaches like surgery.

Surgical Management

Indications are failure of conservative therapy, signs of root compression, progressive slipping, slip of more than 30 percent, even when painless, and persistent pain in the back, thigh or persistent sciatica.

Methods of Surgery

1. *Poster lateral fusion* is the best method of fusing the slipped vertebra because it preserves the supporting soft tissues and has a high rate of fusion.
2. *Posterior fusion* here postoperative and additional slip is frequent until the fusion is solid.
3. *Laminectomy* helps relieve neurological deficits and is followed by poster lateral fusion.
4. Laminectomy and intertransverse fusion.
5. *Anterior interbody fusion* is indicated for subtotal spondylolisthesis and is a risky and difficult procedure with doubtful efficacy.

Fusion is achieved in spondylolisthesis by putting autologous cancellous bone graft and stabilization is obtained by Hartshill rectangle frame or Steffee plate and screws (Fig. 42.17).

KYPHOSIS

It is an increase in the normal posterior convexity of the thoracic spine and is referred to as 'hyper kyphosis' (Figs 42.18A and B).

Causes

Localized injury or disease like fracture, Pott's disease, secondaries in the spine, etc.

Generalized bone diseases ankylosing spondylitis, osteomalacia, Paget's disease, acromegaly, etc. are some of the examples.

Defective growth or habit

Children—Stooping posture while reading (postural).

Adolescents—Vertebral epiphysitis (Scheuermann's) seen in boys 14–17 yr.

Adults—Bending occupation, e.g. porter, cobbler.

Elderly—Senile osteoporosis.

Compensatory kyphosis—Due to increased lordosis.

Note: Postural kyphosis is the most common variety.

Types

Knuckle: Prominence of single spinous process indicating collapse of single vertebra, e.g. TB spine/Kummel's disease (Fig. 42.18B).

Angular: 2–3 vertebral body is collapsed, e.g. late stage of TB, secondary carcinoma.

Round: Several vertebrae are involved and hence gives a round appearance, e.g. in children—Scheuermann's disease, in old age—senile kyphosis.

42

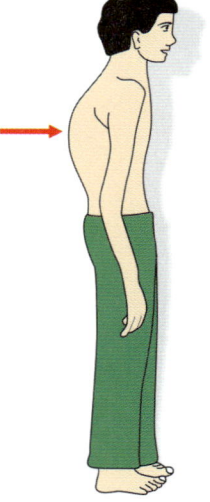

Fig. 42.18A: Thoracic kyphosis arrow showing gibbus

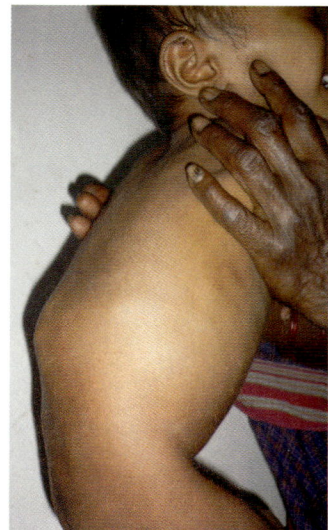

Fig. 42.18B: Angular gibbus

Methods of examination: Look from the side and note if the thoracic curvature is regular, now determine if the kyphosis is mobile or fixed by asking the patient to bend forwards and observe for the disappearance of the deformity.

Investigations: Plain X-ray of the thoracic spine (Fig. 42.19) CT scan, MRI are is some of the important investigation methods to evaluate the severity of kyphosis.

Treatment: In mild deformities, anterior hyperextension bracing is indicated (Fig. 42.20). In severe deformities, surgical decompression and stabilization is advised.

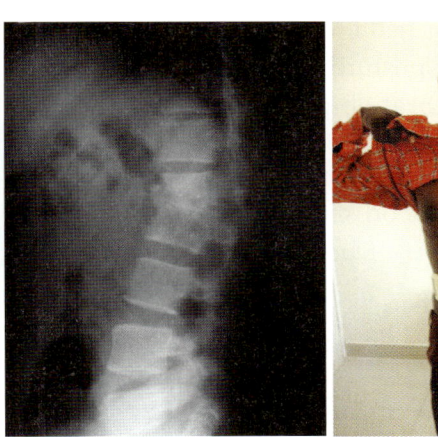 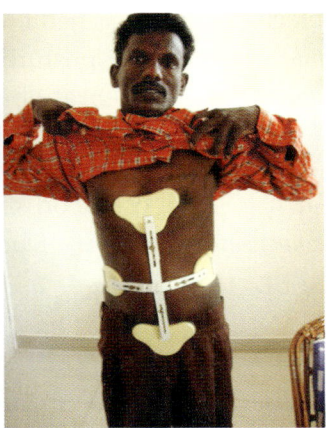

Fig. 42.19: TB spine leading to gibbus   **Fig. 42.20:** Anterior hyperextension brace

LUMBAR CANAL STENOSIS

Lumbar canal stenosis is a cauda equina compression in which the lateral or anteroposterior diameter of the spinal canal is narrow with or without a change in the cross-sectional area (Fig. 42.21).

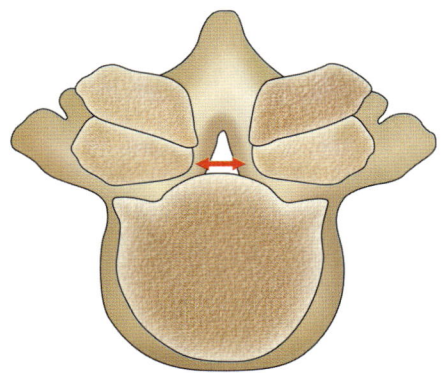

Fig. 42.21: Lumbar canal stenosis

Causes

It could be due to generalized or localized narrowing. The common disorders leading to a reduction in the canal space are disc prolapse, congenital conditions, diseases like Paget's, fluorosis, traumatic conditions.

Clinical Features

It is common in males below 40 years. Usually the symptoms are fewer in number but the patient may complain of low backache. Cauda equina claudication is common and the patient complains of pain in the buttocks and legs after walking, which decreases on sitting, rest and forward bending. Patient may complain of hypoesthesia and paresthesia and has no problem walking uphill or riding a bicycle. Nerve root entrapment in the lateral recess causes claudication and sciatica. Stoop test will be positive.

Investigations

Radiographs of the lumbar spine consisting of AP, lateral and oblique views may show reduced interpedicular distance, reduction in the mid-sagittal diameter, etc. *Myelography may show* waist-like narrowing of the dural sac and indentation of the dural tube due to disc prolapse. *MRI and CT scan* help to diagnose lateral recess stenosis, facet hypertrophy and midsagittal distance (Figs 42.22A to C).

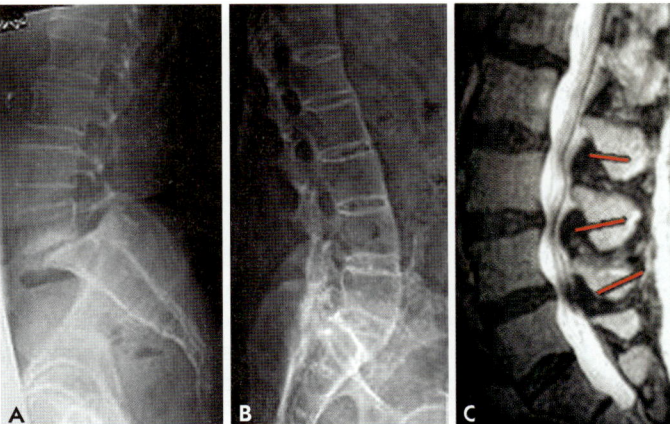

Figs 42.22A to C: Canal stenosis due to: (A) listhesis (B) lumbar spondylosis and (C) disc prolapse

Treatment

Conservative methods: This is the treatment method of choice in the initial stages and consists of rest, NSAIDs physiotherapy and exercises. If these measures fail then surgery is indicated.

Surgical methods: Described for lumbar canal stenosis aim at decompressing the constricted lumbar canal. Laminectomy is useful in central canal stenosis. Discectomy and osteotomy of the inferior articular process to remove the hypertrophic elements.

43 Hand Disorders

Hand is a very important organ of the body. Disorders affecting the hand could lead to loss of hand function in various forms and degrees. Thumb itself accounts for over 40 percent function of the hand. It is imperative that the problems affecting the hand should be diagnosed and managed correctly. The following are the various disorders affecting the hand.

INFECTIONS OF THE HAND

The effects of hand infection can be as devastating as major trauma. Trivial injuries like a scratch, a prick, small punctured wounds, etc. cause hand infections. *Staph. aureus* (80%), *Streptococcus pyogenes* and gram-negative bacilli are the famous trio who inflict the infective unmitigated disaster in the hand. The sequelae of these infections are edema, abscess, necrosis, fibrosis and lastly contractions leading to a grotesque, debilitating hand. The presence of an abscess seems to send a message to the surgeons, *"Drain me or I'll drain myself!"* Hence, an abscess caused should be drained; the surgeon only has to decide the proper time and incisions. Early use of potent antibiotics has considerably downed the threat of serious hand infections.

As elsewhere before we delve into the discussions on individual hand infections, it helps considerably to know the principles of treatment:

- Hands should be kept elevated to facilitate gravity to drain and thereby prevent edema and swelling of the hand.
- Following treatment hand needs to be placed in functional positions for optimum results.

- Early and appropriate use of IV antibiotics prevents pus formation (within 24–48 hrs).
- If pus is formed let it out through proper incisions at the appropriate time.
- Local anesthetic may help the spread of infection and adds more fluid to the already existing swelling. Hence, general anesthesia or regional block is preferred.
- Tourniquet is indicated but exsanguination are not preferred as it helps spread the infection (alternatively, elevation of hand for three minutes is ideal).
- Do not forget the all important hand after care which has a direct bearing on the final outcome of the hand function.

With the principles of treatment as a backdrop let us now consider the important hand infections in order of importance.

PARONYCHIA

Paronychia is an infection of the eponychium and could be acute or chronic (Fig. 43.1). Acute paronychia has the distinction of being the most common infection of the hand. *Staph. aureus* is the culprit and it usually is due to a hangnail, unsterile manicure instruments and reckless nail pairing. The infection normally begins at one corner, tracks down to the opposite end via the eponychium or nail (40%).

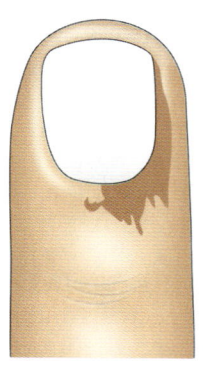

Fig. 43.1: Paronychia

Clinical Features

Agonizing pain, marked tenderness and a conspicuous red looking swelling are the hallmarks of acute paronychia.

Treatment

Conservative measures and early antibiotic therapy is the mainstay of initial treatment. However, if abscess has formed and if the pus is at one end, incise it, if under one nail corner, remove that corner and if it has shifted to the opposite end excise proximal one-third of the nail. If encountered with a floating nail, write its obituary by taking it out totally, as it is dead and gone!

Note: Chronic paronychia which is regarded as a complication of acute paronychia is usually not so! It is usually seen in syringomyelia or in people who do not wear rubber gloves during washing!

APICAL SUBUNGUAL INFECTION

Here the space between the distal phalanx and the nail plate is infected. An injury or pinprick could lead to this. Pain is excruciating and the tenderness is felt most below the nail free edge and the pus is usually left pointing towards this free edge. Initially conservative treatment helps but in the stage of pus formation, drainage is done by a small V-shaped incision. Rarely a chronic sinus develops and the phalanx could develop osteomyelitis.

DISTAL PULP SPACE INFECTION (Syn: Felon)

Next to acute paronychia this is the most common hand infection. It usually follows a pin prick with the index finger and thumb being the common unfortunate victims.

Surgical Anatomy

Multiple fibrous septae travel from skin to bone partitioning the fat filled distal pulp space into tiny compartments (Fig. 43.2). One such septum also cordons of the space at the distal finger flexor crease. The terminal branches of the digital artery after giving a branch to the basal epiphyseal plate runs through this compartment. The evil effects of this arrangement could lead to the following undesirable consequences:

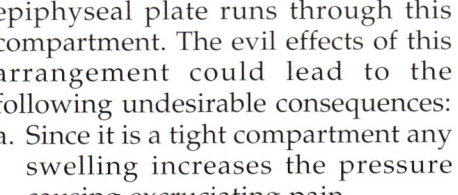

Fig. 43.2: Multiple fibrous septa in distal pulp space

a. Since it is a tight compartment any swelling increases the pressure causing excruciating pain.
b. If superficial, penetrates the skin causing skin necrosis and if deep penetrates the periosteum causing osteomyelitis.
c. Thrombosis of the digital arteries leads to osteomyelitis.
d. It may, in rare events, cause flexor tenosynovitis or infective arthritis of DIP joint.

Clinical Features

Patient initially complains of dull pain more so in the dependent position and swelling. Loss of sleep due to nocturnal pain is a usual feature after about two days. Pressure over the involved part increases pain. Abscess may develop in later stages if left unattended.

Treatment

Treatment consists of antibiotics in the initial stages and if the pain lasts for more than twelve hours, incision helps (Fig. 43.3). If the abscess is pointing volarwards, a longitudinal midline incision is taken and if the abscess is deep, a longitudinal incision at the side cutting through the partitions is preferred. If osteomyelitis develops in the distal phalanx, sequestrectomy is done if the sequestrum is well formed and separated.

MIDDLE AND PROXIMAL VOLAR SPACE INFECTION

Middle volar space is bounded by distal volar crease above and proximal volar crease below. It is a well cordoned of area on both the sides. On the other hand, proximal volar space is well separated at the distal end but at the proximal end, it communicates freely with the corresponding web space. These also follow pin pricks and may be confused with tenosynovitis of the flexor tendons. Spread to the adjacent web space is fairly common. Clinical features and treatment are almost similar (Fig. 43.4).

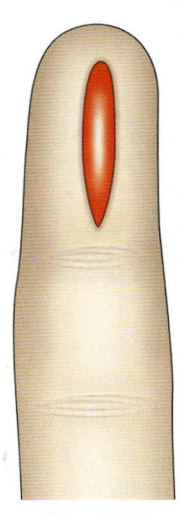

Fig. 43.3: Surgical incision for draining felon

INFECTION OF THE WEB SPACES

What are these web spaces? These are three triangular areas filled with loose fat between the ends of the fingers. Infection reaches these areas either through a skin crack or a blister or through the lumbrical canal courtesy an abscess in the proximal volar space.

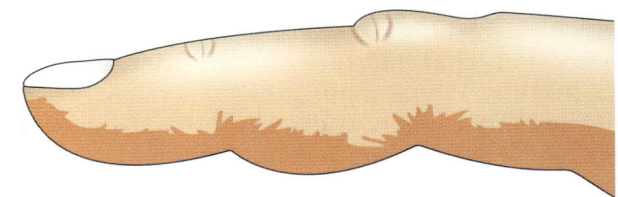

Fig. 43.4: Middle volar space infection

Clinical Features

The patient first presents with severe constitutional symptoms and edema of the back of the hand. Once the infection localizes the following signs become evident:

- The base of the affected finger is swollen.
- In severe cases, the adjacent finger is separated.
- Skin over the affected space shows purplish discoloration.
- A fan-shaped blush extends from the web to the dorsum.
- Maximum tenderness is found in the web and base of the finger.

43

Treatment

Conservative treatment with antibiotics helps in the initial stages. In the later stages incision and drainage becomes very essential. Though the swelling is more towards the dorsum, the dangerous part of the abscess remains nearer the palm. If not incised it may spread into the middle palmar space via the lumbrical canal. Two incisions may be required for drainage, one on the dorsal surface between the metacarpal heads and the other on the palm distal to the distal palmar crease. The web should be left unincised.

DEEP PALMAR ABSCESS

This is rare and accounts for only 1 percent of all hand infections (Fig. 43.5).

Surgical Anatomy

This is a space lined by fascia and in between the flexor tendons above and the metacarpal bones below. The fascia of the hypothenar muscles and its lateral border by the fascia of the adductor and other thenar muscles forms its medial border. A fascia divides this space into middle palmar space and a thenar space.

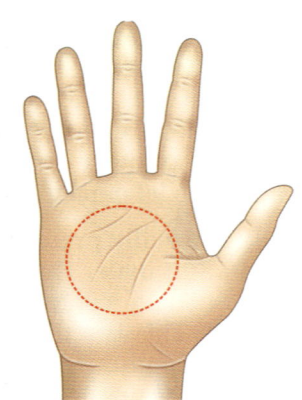

Fig. 43.5: Deep palmar abscess

Clinical Features

The patient usually presents with a severe systemic reaction. There is a local pain, tenderness, loss of active movements of the middle and ring fingers and there is generalized gross swelling of the hand and fingers, which resemble an inflated rubber glove (also called Frog hand). Similar symptoms are seen in a thenar abscess but the thumb web is more swollen, index finger is held flexed and active movements of both the index and thumb is lost. With the increasing swelling, the concavity of the palm becomes flat and later convex before it bursts open.

Diagnostic test: In a deep palmar abscess, passive stretching of the metacarpophalangeal joint is painful while that of interphalangeal joint is painless. In tenosynovitis of the flexor tendons the passive stretching of both the MP and the IP joints are painful.

Treatment

After the initial conservative treatment, the abscess in the middle palmar space is drained by a central transverse incision at the level of the distal palmar crease in line with the middle finger extending ulnarwards towards the hypothenar eminence. Abscess in the thenar space is drained by a curved incision in the thumb web parallel to the border of the first dorsal interosseous muscle.

TENOSYNOVITIS

These are serious infections and are due to infection of the fibrous sheaths and synovial lining of the flexor tendons of the hand.

Surgical Anatomy

The fibrous and synovial sheaths of the flexor tendons of the hand are arranged in two groups: the radial and the ulnar bursae (Figs 43.6A and B). The radial bursa is the smaller of the two and it lines the flexor tendon of the thumb and extends 1–2 cm above the wrist up to the distal end of the tendon. The ulnar bursa encloses the synovial sheaths of the index, middle, ring, and little fingers. Distally those for the index, middle and ring fingers it extends up to the level of transverse palmar crease and for the little finger it extends throughout the length of the tendons. The ulnar bursa encloses tendons of flexor digitorum superficialis and profundus of the above fingers. These two bursae may communicate with each other.

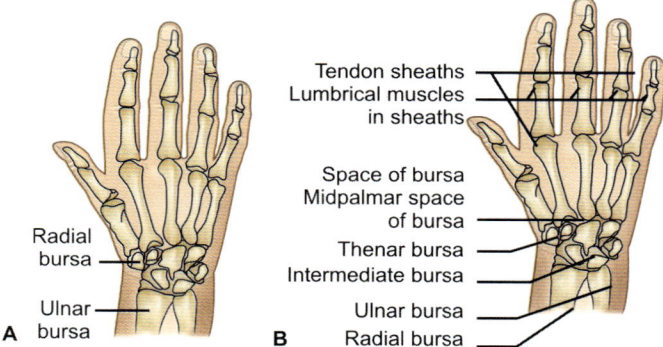

Tendon sheaths
Lumbrical muscles in sheaths

Space of bursa
Midpalmar space of bursa
Thenar bursa
Intermediate bursa
Ulnar bursa
Radial bursa

Radial bursa
Ulnar bursa

A   B

Figs 43.6A and B: (A) Radial, (B) ulnar bursae of the hand

Etiology: The causative organisms are usually due to *Staph. aureus* or *Streptococcus pyogenes*. Penetrating injuries of the tendon sheaths, extension of the infection from its terminal pulp space, etc. are some of the common modes of infection. The consequences of tenosynovitis are disastrous, as it may lead to adhesions, rupture if infection is severe and loss of gliding movements.

Clinical Features

Patient complains of pain, swelling, and the affected finger is motionless. Active or passive extensions of the fingers are very painful. The classical local signs include the swelling of the finger through its entire length, flexion of the finger with marked pain on extension, and tenderness over the sheath.

43

In tenosynovitis of the little finger (Fig. 43.7), tenderness can be elicited at a point in between the two palmar creases. This is called the 'Kanavel's sign' (Fig. 43.8).

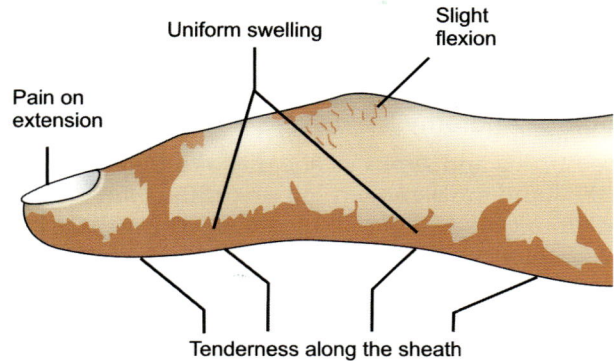

Fig.43.7: Tenosynovitis of a finger showing its four typical features

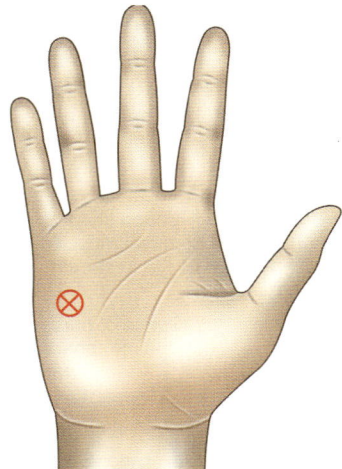

Fig. 43.8: Kanavel's sign

Treatment

Early treatment with antibiotics is started. In the early stages of pus formation abscess is drained by a transverse incision at the distal palmar crease and the proximal edge of the sheath is opened. Then the sheath is opened distally through a midcarpal incision over the middle phalanx. If the infection has progressed far, then a full midlateral incision may be required. Sloughed tendons require excision.

INJURIES OF THE HAND

These are discussed in a separate chapter.

ARTHRITIC HAND

The following arthritic conditions affect the hand
Rheumatoid arthritis: The rheumatoid hand is discussed on page no. 306.

Osteoarthritis: The distal interphalangeal joints are more commonly affected than the proximal interphalangeal joints. Heberden's nodes are seen in DIP joints. Carpometacarpal joint of the thumb may also be affected. Cartilage destruction, spur formation and limited motion are the common sequel.

Lupus erythematosus: This involves the skin over the nose as well as tendons and joints. Periarticular soft tissue and tendons are affected very severely, joints are grossly deformed at the metacarpophalangeal joints.

Psoriasis: Psoriatic arthritis has an incidence of about 7 percent and the deformities are similar to rheumatoid arthritis.

Reiter's syndrome: This is described as a triad of conjunctivitis, urethritis and synovitis. Synovitis is asymmetrical and heel pain, back pain and nail deformities are seen. More common in young males it attacks the lower limbs more than the upper limbs. More than 90 percent resolve on its own.

Gout: It usually presents as a single, painful, red joint in an adult male. The joint is swollen, hot and tender and is usually confused to a cellulitis or abscess and drained. This is a disease due to massive deposits of monosodium urate crystals around the joints.

PARALYTIC HAND

This is mainly due to peripheral nerve involvement of the upper limbs. Discussed at great length in the chapter on peripheral nerve injuries.

IMPORTANT CONGENITAL ANOMALIES OF THE HAND

- *Polydactyly:* Duplication of one or more fingers
- *Syndactyly:* Fusion of fingers especially the middle and ring fingers
- *Macrodactly:* Enlargement of the finger
- *Congenital trigger finger:* Contracture of the distal joint especially of the thumb
- *Streeter's dysplasia:* Construction and the hand
- *Camptodactyly:* Flexion contracture of the PIP joint especially the little finger
- *Cleft hand:* Division of hand into two parts
- *Mirror hand:* Here ulna and corpus or reduplicated
- *Congenital radioulnar synostosis:* Discussed on page no. 257
- *Madelung's deformity:* Discussed on page no. 257
- *Congenital absence of radius and ulna:* Absence of radius is more common than ulna
- *Kirner's deformity:* Spontaneous injury to the hip of the fifth digit.

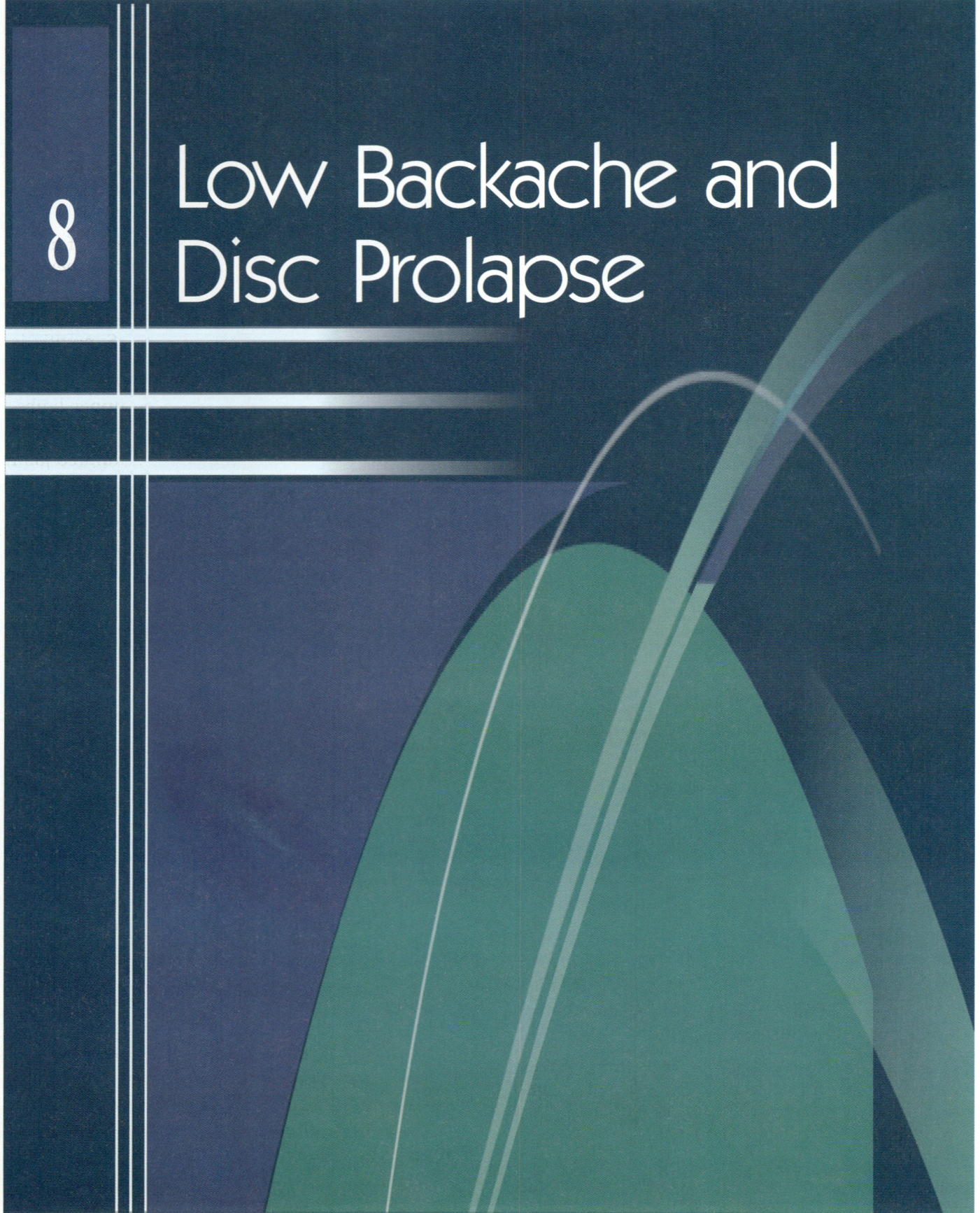

Low Backache and Disc Prolapse

8

Low Backache

Approach to a Patient with Low Backache

Backache, which was known as an ancient curse, is now known as a modern international epidemic. It is an extremely common malady afflicting the human race across the globe cutting the geographical boundaries, race, culture, etc. Eighty to ninety percent of the human population will suffer from some form of backache, mild or severe in their lifetime. Among the galaxy of causative factors, both spinal and extra spinal, the most common cause of low backache seems to be mechanical or common low backache due to postural problems.

Posture: Posture is defined as the positional relationship of the different regions of the body to each other. Proper posture is about maintaining an erect and balanced spine. Thus, it can be concluded that postural defects, overloading and abrupt unbalanced movements are frequently responsible for backache.

Remember

- Posture is an entity seen only in human beings, thanks to the two-legged posture.
- Backache is a very common malady next only to head-ache and affects nearly 80 percent of the population.
- Most common cause of backache is bad posture, which increases the strain on the discs and ligaments causing faster disc degeneration.
- Any abrupt, unbalanced and unwarranted movements upset the stabilizing function of the back muscles increasing load on the discs.
- Hence bad posture, overloading and abrupt unbalanced movements are the causes of disc rupture or prolapse.

Causes of Backache

A variety of conditions related and unrelated to spine cause backache (See box). The common causes of backache are:

Unaccustomed activities: A sedentary person suddenly adopting an active form of life, etc.

Poor posture: Improper posture during sitting, walking, standing, working places enormous load on the back and results in backache. *This is by far the most common cause of low backache* (Figs 44.1A to F).

Occupational backache: Certain occupation places enormous stress on the back, e.g. garbage collectors, porters.

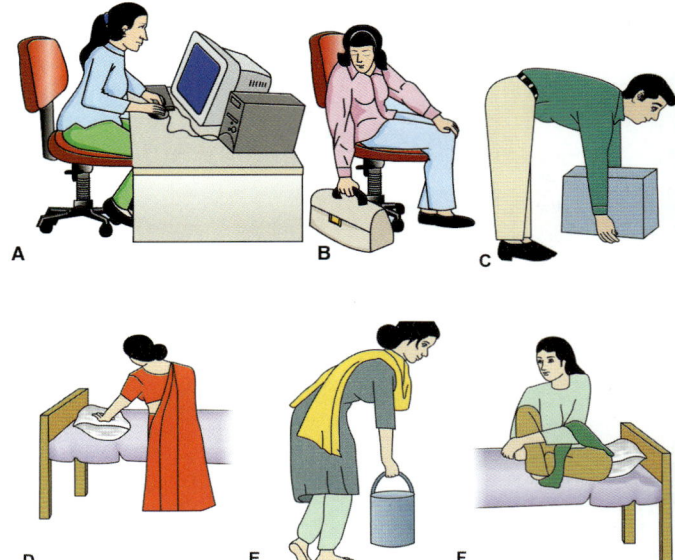

Figs 44.1A to F: Improper postural habits causes common low back pain

Obesity: Protruding abdomen places enormous strain on the back. *The facet joint osteoarthritis* due to old age, repeated bending and twisting activities lead to arthritis of facet joints.

Other Important Causes for Low Backache

Uncommon causes: These are due to diseases of the spine like congenital anomalies, inflammatory conditions, infections, tumors (See box).

Spinal stenosis: Due to degenerative process is another common cause.

Structures Involved in Backache (Figs 44.2A to C)

Vertebral bodies: Micro crush fractures, and spondylosis.

Intervertebral discs: Disc degeneration and prolapse.

Posterior intervertebral joints: Degenerative lesions, synovitis, sprain, etc.

Ligaments and small intervertebral muscles: Elongation, excessive use, reflex contractures.

Posterior longitudinal ligament: Elongation and irritation by discal protrusion.

Nerves: Irritation or compression of the spinal nerve roots by disc herniation or irritation of the sensory nerves of the various para vertebral structures.

Common low backache (Accounts for 80%): This includes back muscle strain, ligament sprain and prolapsed disc:

- *Muscle strain:* Acute backache is due to strain of the back muscles during, sudden unaccustomed activity, sports, trauma, etc.
- *Ligament sprain:* The back ligaments are strained during sudden lifting or twisting activities.
- *Prolapsed lumbar intervertebral disc:* This is the second most common cause for low back pain after muscle strain. Discussed at great length earlier.

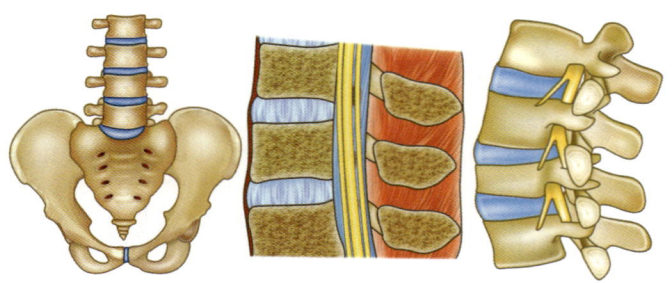

Figs 44.2A to C: Structures involved in common low backache: (A) Osteophytes seen in lumbar spondylosis, (B) Compression on PLL and nerves due to disc protrusion, and (C) Disc disease and facet joint arthritis

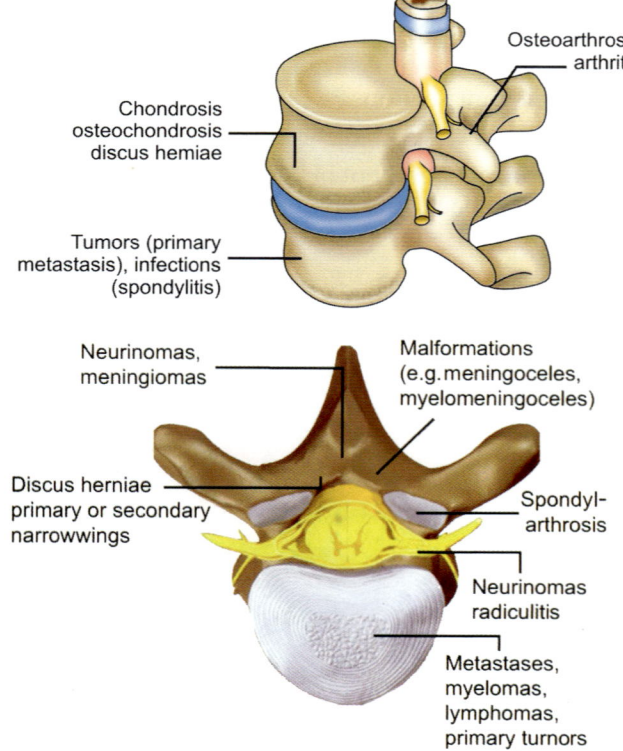

Fig. 44.2D: Structures involved in uncommon low backache: Tumors and other conditions

Common causes
- Back muscle sprain and ligament sprain
- Prolapsed lumbar intervertebral disc. This with the above two causes of back muscle strain and ligament sprain account for 80% of the causes of low backache.
- Obesity
- Poor posture
- Facet joint arthritis
- Unaccustomed activities
- Occupational causes

Uncommon causes
Congenital causes (4 'S')
- **S**coliosis
- **S**pondylolisthesis
- **S**pina bifida
- **S**pondylolysis

Infective conditions
- Osteomyelitis
- Tuberculosis
- Brucellosis

Traumatic causes
- Vertebral body injuries, posterior arch fractures
- Muscle sprain/strain
- Prolapsed disc

Inflammatory causes
- Rheumatoid arthritis
- Ankylosing spondylitis and other SSA's

Neoplasms
- Benign—osteoid osteoma
- Malignant—secondaries, multiple myeloma, etc.

Metabolic causes
- Osteoporosis
- Osteomalacia

Degenerative conditions
- Osteoarthritis
- Lumbar spondylosis

Referred pain from
- Gynecological diseases
- Genitourinary diseases
- Gastrointestinal conditions, etc.

Clinical Features

Age: Backache is more common in middle-aged and elderly people (usually degenerative). In young adults, it is due to trauma and in children; it is usually due to organic lesions like TB.

Sex: Osteoporosis, rheumatoid arthritis, etc. are more common in females. Ankylosing spondylitis, trauma, secondaries, etc. are more common in males.

Occupation: People with sedentary jobs and heavy manual laborers are frequently prone for backache.

Presenting Complaints

Pain: Over 90 percent of the patients complain of pain in the back. The following points should be enquired.

44

Nature of pain: Is it sudden (trauma) or gradual (spondylosis)? Did weight lifting, sudden bending, etc. precede it? Is there remissions and exacerbations (disc disease) or is it continuous (tumors)? Is there history of night cries (e.g. TB spine)? Does rest relieve it? Does it radiate to the lower limbs? etc.

> *Note:* In Ankylosing spondylitis and other SSA, pain becomes worse after rest! In common low backache rest relieves pain and muscle spasm.

Site: Is the pain in the middle of the spine or Para vertebral muscles. Is it in the dorsolumbar spine (trauma or tumor) or in the lumbar spine (disc disease)?

Sciatica: Sciatica is defined as a radiating pain along the course of the sciatic nerve and is felt in the back, buttocks, posterior of the thigh, legs and the foot. It is commonly due to disc prolapse.

Neurological symptoms: These consist of paresthesia, muscle weakness, disturbance of sphincters, cauda equina syndrome, etc.

Facet syndromes: Here patient complains of chronic backache, early morning stiffness, difficulty in getting out of bed, standing, sitting or climbing.

Other complaints: There may be history of stiffness, pain in other joints (e.g. rheumatoid arthritis), constitutional symptoms (e.g. tuberculosis, malignancy), genitourinary complaints, etc.

Physical Signs

Stance and gait: Does the patient stand with a normal stance or has deformities like scoliosis, kyphosis, lordosis or pelvic tilt. Is the gait normal or altered?

Spasm: This is seen in acute painful conditions of the spine. The patient complains of pain in the Para vertebral muscles and painful restriction of all the spine movements.

Movements: There may be restriction of the spine movements due to the organic lesions affecting the back or due to muscle spasm, disc lesions, etc.

Swelling: It may be due to cold abscesses following TB spine.

Tenderness: It may be present over the spinous process, in between the spinous processes, over muscles, ligaments, facet joints, etc.

Neurological examination: This consists of examinations of the various dermatomes for sensations, myotomes for muscle power and reflexes.

SLRT: This is to know the effects of disc prolapse on the sciatic nerve and is already discussed.

Other examinations: Like examination of the adjacent joints, peripheral pulses, abdominal, rectal or paravaginal examinations.

Investigations

Blood tests: These are useful in detecting metabolic, hormonal, infective and malignant conditions.

Radiology: Routine plain radiographs of the lumbar spine are advised. Both anterioposterior and lateral views are usually required. Oblique views are helpful in detecting the fracture of pars. Though X-rays are not very helpful in detecting the disc prolapse, it is of value in diagnosing metabolic, degenerative, inflammatory, malignant conditions affecting the spine.

Myelography: This procedure is not routinely used any more because of its complications. However, it has a role in demonstrating blocks due to disc prolapse.

CT scan: It is a noninvasive procedure and helps to identify the bone and soft tissue problems with greater accuracy.

MRI scan: This is the gold standard in the investigations of the spine. It is noninvasive and is better than CT scan in diagnosing the bone and soft tissue problems around the spine. However, its high cost is prohibitive and is available only in major cities and centers.

Treatment: The underlying cause has to be detected and managed accordingly. The general treatment for backache consists of drugs like NSAIDS, muscle relaxants, physiotherapy, traction (Fig. 44.3A), use of belts and corsets (Fig. 44.3B). Proper postural habits, back exercises and back education go a long way in preventing the backache. Surgery is done for specific indications and specific surgical techniques have been dealt in relevant sections.

Ways to prevent recurrence: This is the most important aspect of the management of backache. Like in all other diseases, so in backache prevention is better than cure.

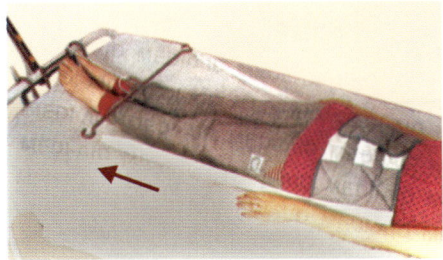

Fig. 44.3A: Lumbar traction

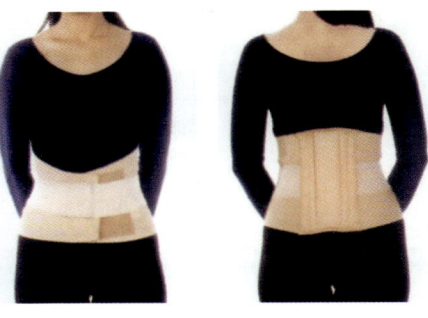

Fig. 44.3B: Belts and corsets are useful in acute low backache

Backache can be prevented largely by observing the following measures (Table 44.1):

- Adopting proper posture and creating awareness that it is in the erect position that the back can withstand strain the best.

- *Back education:* Stress on the back is less when it is properly used during sitting, walking, etc. These proper habits have to be cultivated with practice (Figs 44.4 to 44.10).

Table 44.1: Proper postural habits

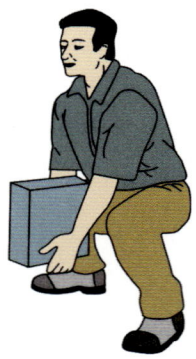

Fig. 44.4: *Lifting objects—* Bend at your knees and not at your waist. Hold the object you are lifting close to your body, not higher than your chest. It is easier to push rather than pull heavy objects, e.g. furniture, and keep the knees bent while pushing

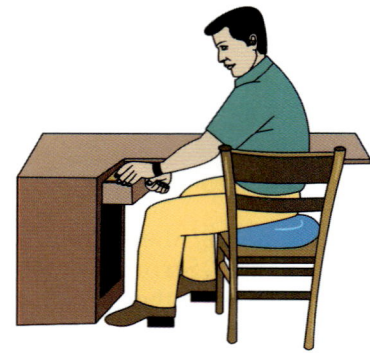

Fig. 44.7: *Turning and reaching out—* do not twist your waist. Rather, turn by moving your feet. Keep the phone and such like objects within easy reach; do not strain to reach them. Stand on a stool to reach high objects.

44

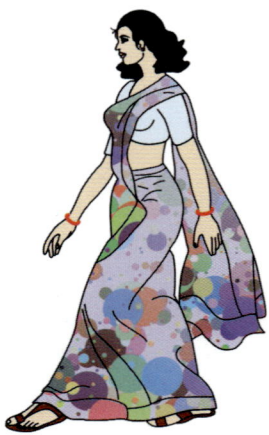

Fig. 44.5: *Walking—*walk well with your head high, chin tucked in, toes pointing straight in front. Wear comfortable footwear. Take steps of a natural, comfortable length. Swing the arms naturally.

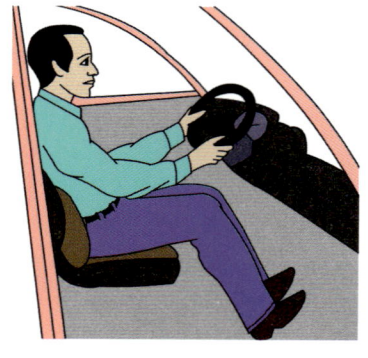

Fig. 44.8: *Sitting and driving habits—*right and wrong.

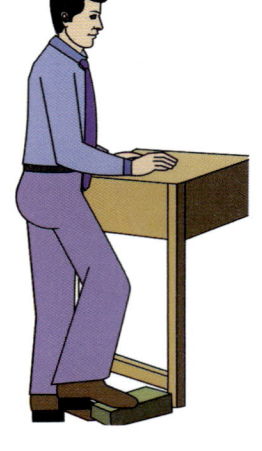

Fig. 44.9: *Standing—*keep one foot in front and knees slightly bent while standing upright. If you have to stand for a long time, try keeping one foot higher than the other does, on a low stool. Change your position often.

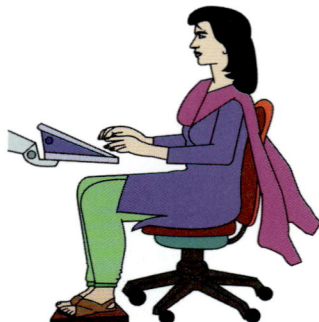

Fig. 44.6: *Sitting—*Ensure your back is firmly touching the back of the chair. Keep the knees slightly higher than the hips, e.g. by using something to prop up your feet. Sit close to your desk or table to avoid bending forward. Do not sit for too long. And when driving, move the front seat close to the steering wheel and both hands should be kept on the wheel.

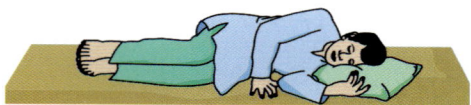

Fig. 44.10: *Sleeping—*if you sleep on your side, keep knees and lower body bent a little. On your back, put a pillow under your knees. Try not to sleep on your stomach—but if you must, put a pillow under your waist not under your head. Use a firm mattress—neither soft/squashy nor very hard.

Remember

Do's
- Forward bent attitude
- Body eight borne on the heels
- Proper eight lifting as shown early
- Sit with buttocks tucked under
- While driving push the seat forwards to raise the knees and decrease the lordosis.
- Flex the knees and hip hen lying on the side.
- Turn to the side and then up

Don'ts
- Sleep in the prone position
- Rise from a sitting position suddenly
- Bend over a washbasin

- Wear high heels as pelvis is thrust forward and the spine bends backwards
- Use too high a chair
- Use soft mattress which increases the lumbosacral extension. A firm mattress encourages lumbar spine to be straight.

Bs in backache
- **B**ad posture
- **B**ed rest
- **B**elts
- **B**ack education
- **B**eck exercises
- **B**ed choice

- *Back exercises:* These aim to strengthen the abdominal, pelvic, back and thigh muscles. Strong healthy muscles reduces load on the discs and other structures
- To avoid all sports including the aerobic ones. Swimming and walking are encouraged.

Other Important Causes of Backache

- Spinal stenosis
- Spondylolisthesis
- Tuberculosis of spine
- Spine injuries
- Lumbar spondylosis
- Osteomalacia
- Osteoporosis
- Ankylosing spondylitis
- SI joint arthritis
- Scoliosis
  These are discussed in appropriate sections.

44

Lumbar Disc Prolapse

Disc prolapse
Approach to a patient with low backache

DISC PROLAPSE

Lumbar disc disease is an important cause of low backache so much so that people have perceptions that all low backache is due to disc prolapse. Now let us study about the disc and its role in backache.

BRIEF ANATOMY

Disc Anatomy and Physiology

Development of spine starts from the third week of intrauterine life and continues until third decade of life. There are 23 discs throughout the spine, absent only in atlantoaxial articulation. It is thinnest in the thoracic region and thickest in the lumbar (Figs 45.1A and B).

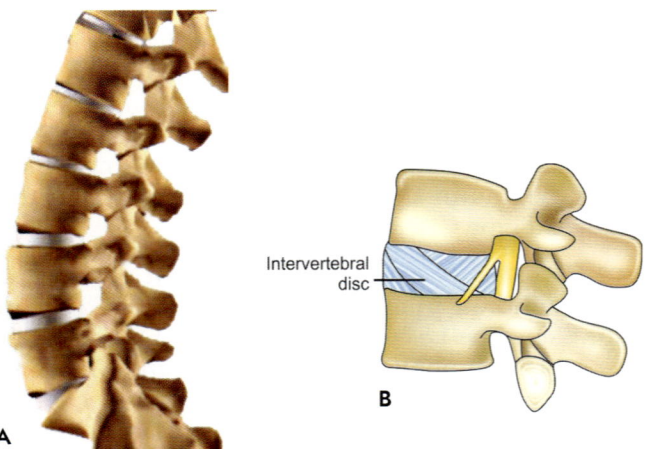

Figs 45.1A and B: (A) Lumbar spine with their intervertebral discs, (B) intervertebral disc

The disc consists of two parts centrally it is nucleus pulposus, which is made up of collagen fibrils, fibrocytes, chondrocytes, gelatinous matrix, water and salt. Peripherally it has annulus fibrosus, which is a fibrocartilaginous tissue. It is thick anteriorly and thin posteriorly more so in the posterolateral aspect. Hence posterolateral disc prolapse is more common. The fibers of annulus are joined by diagonal fibers also known as Sharpe's fibers.

Neural fibers in the outer rings of the annulus contain branches of the Sino vertebral nerve dorsally and ventrally branches from the sympathetic chain.

With age, water content of the disc decreases, fibrous tissue and cartilage cells increase, and the nucleus becomes granular and friable. Disc apart from giving the spine its mobility functions as a shock absorber. The related structures around a disc are shown in Fig. 45.3.

Classification of disc Prolapse

Intervertebral disc prolapse usually refers to the escape of the central nucleus pulposus through a rent in the peripheral annulus fibrosus (Fig. 45.2). It passes through the following various stages before it finally breaks down (Fig. 45.4).

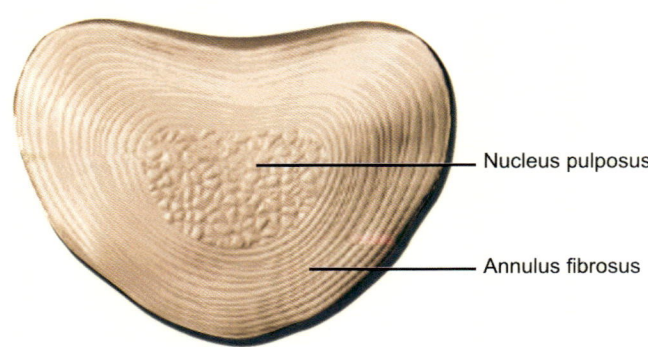

Nucleus pulposus

Annulus fibrosus

Fig. 45.2: Cross sectional structure of a disc

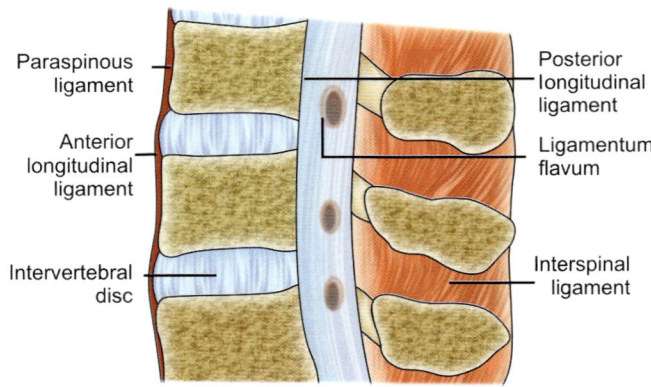

Paraspinous ligament

Anterior longitudinal ligament

Intervertebral disc

Posterior longitudinal ligament

Ligamentum flavum

Interspinal ligament

Fig. 45.3: Various ligaments of the spine

Disc bulging or protrusion is eccentric accumulation of nucleus pulposus with slight deformity of the annulus due to weakness in its fibers. This is usually preceded by degeneration of the nucleus.

Prolapsed disc: The posterior and lateral aspects of the annulus are weak and it is through this 'weak' spot that the nucleus usually herniates.

Extruded disc: Here the disc comes out into the canal lies behind the posterior longitudinal ligament and impinges on the cord or adjacent nerve root (Fig. 45.5).

Sequestrated disc: Here the nuclear material has separated from the disc itself and potentially migrates, down into the canal.

Etiology of disc herniation: The etiology consists of risk factors and the definitive causes resulting in disc herniation.

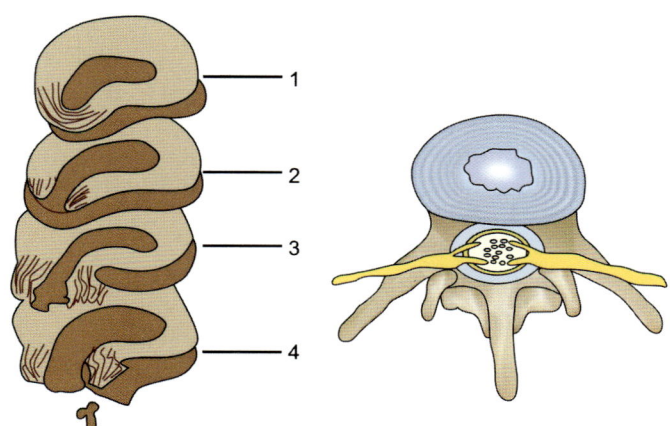

Fig. 45.4: Types of prolapse disc: (1) bulge disc, (2) prolapse disc, (3) extruded disc, and (4) sequestrated disc

Fig. 45.5: Exiting nerve roots

Risk Factors

- Jobs requiring heavy and repetitive weight-lifting.
- Use of machine tools.
- Operation of motor vehicles.
- Cigarette smokers and tobacco consumers.
- Anxiety and depression.
- Stressful occupation as in doctors, police, etc.
- Women with greater number of pregnancies.
- Obesity and other cardiovascular risk factors.
- Monotonous work, working overtime, etc.
- Improper postural habits.

Definitive Causes

- Degenerative changes make the disc susceptible to trauma. Any trauma, which suddenly increases the pressure, will result in rupture of the posterior fibers of the annulus, e.g. weight-lifting, fall on the buttocks, direct trauma to the back, twisting movements and occupation involving flexion and lifting motions (Fig. 45.6).

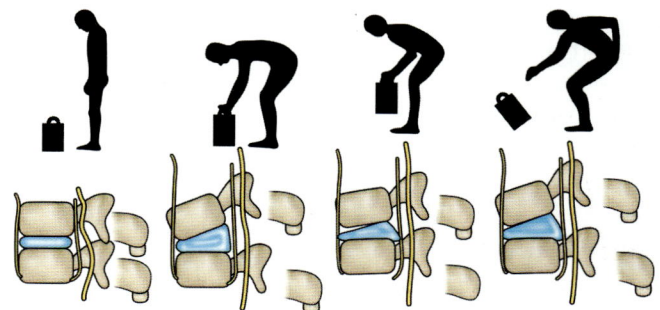

Fig. 45.6: Common mode of disc prolapse due to sudden and improper weight-lifting.

- Disc may also rupture during pregnancy, labor and after prolonged bed rest due to disc softening.
- Disc rupture without any cause is due to degenerative process.

Clinical Features

Clinical features can be discussed under three headings (Figs 45.10A to D):

Low backache: Back pain is common in the second decade, disc disease and disc herniation in the third or fourth decade. *The usual history of lumbar disc herniation is of repetitive low back pain, radiating to the buttocks and decreased by rest.* Pain is increased by flexion episode, sitting, straining, sneezing, coughing, etc. Pain is decreased by rest and in semifowler position.

Radiculopathy: This refers to pain in the distribution of the sciatic nerve and is invariably due to disc herniation. This is called as *sciatica* and leg pain equal to or more than the back pain is due to the radicular pain from the nerve root compression due to herniated disc. The radicular pain usually extends below the knee. Pain usually begins in the lower back radiating to the sacroiliac regions, buttocks and thigh.

Nerve root compression: About 95 percent of the disc prolapse takes place through the L4–5 region compressing the L5 nerve root (Fig. 45.5). The other nerve roots commonly involved are L4 and S1 due to disc prolapse between L3–4 and L5–S1 respectively. Table 45.1 shows the various clinical manifestations following nerve root compression.

Remember one question test: Radicular pain
Between the knee and the ankle, where is the pain?
- Front → L4
- Side → L5
- Back → S1

Examination of the back: (*Also see section on clinical methods*) (Table 45.2)
- *Note any postural defects* like scoliosis, lordosis or kyphosis.
- *Tenderness:* It is usually diffuse and in rare instances could be localized (Fig. 45.17).

- *Movements*: All the movements of the spine are painfully restricted (Figs 45.12 to 45.16).
- *Evaluation of neurological system:* The dermatomal and the myotomal distribution are carefully analyzed to detect the level of lesion (Table 45.1) (Figs 45.7 to 45.9).
- *Straight leg raising test (SLRT):* It helps to evaluate sciatica and its causes. Patient is in supine position; the examiner raises the leg straight one after the other (Fig. 45.17). Up to 30° nerve is not put under stretch. Between 30 and 70° nerve encounters the prolapsed disc and the patient complains of pain. Beyond 70° if patient complains of pain it is usually not due to disc prolapse but could be due to sacroiliac joint involvement (Fig. 45.20).
- *Femoral nerve stretch test (reverse SLRT):* Here the patient is in prone position and is asked to lift the leg straight. This puts a stretch on the femoral nerve. If the patient complains of pain, it indicates a high-level disc prolapse (L1–2–3) (Fig. 45.19 and Table 45.2).

Note: Remember the hallmark of disc disease is repetitive low backache and buttock pain, which is relieved by rest.

Investigations

Radiography of the back is not very reliable as normal findings are observed in 7 to 46 percent of the cases. Disc space is reduced in old cases but in acute cases, it is maintained. Oblique view is recommended to rule out spondylolysis (Fig. 45.21).

Myelography: This is helpful in detecting the intraspinal lesions, spinal stenosis and cases of previously operated backs. It is now replaced by noninvasive procedures like CT scan and MRI (Fig. 45.22).

CT scan: It is a very useful noninvasive, painless outpatient procedure. It gives a cross-sectional study of the pathology. It however fails to detect intraspinal lesion, arachnoiditis and scar from disc herniation (Fig. 45.23). It helps to detect the foraminal stenosis and the lateral disc prolapse.

MRI: This is also an extremely useful, painless, non-invasive outpatient procedure. It helps to detect the intraspinal lesion, helps to examine the entire spine and identifies degenerative disc (Fig. 45.24). However, it is expensive and hence prohibitive.

Discography: A radiopaque dye is injected into the space. This reproduces the pain experienced by the patient

45

Table 45.1: Nerve root compression in disc prolapse						
Disc prolapse between	*Pain*	*Radiation*	*Sensory loss*	*Motor loss*	*Reflexes loss*	**SLRT*
L3 and L4 L4 nerve root is involved	Lumbar region	Along the antero-medial aspect of the thigh	Medial shin	Quadriceps	Knee jerk	Normal
L4 L5 L5 root involved 95% disc prolapse occur here	Lumbar region, groin, sacroiliac region	Lateral thigh, leg, dorsum of the foot and hallux	Hallux area	Extensor hallucis muscle	Medial hamstrings	Reduced
L4 and S1 S1 root is involved	Same as above	Buttocks, posterior thigh, leg and lateral foot	Lateral foot	Gastrocnemius	Ankle jerk	Reduced

Easy way to remember
L_4 root involvement—remember '4' heads of quadriceps. Hence knee jerk lost (Fig. 45.6)
L_5 root involvement—remember '5' toes—Great toe and lateral 4 toes lose extension (Fig. 45.7)
S_1 root involvement—remember of 'S' of tendo Achilles. Hence, ankle jerk lost (Fig. 45.8)
* SLRT—straight leg raising test

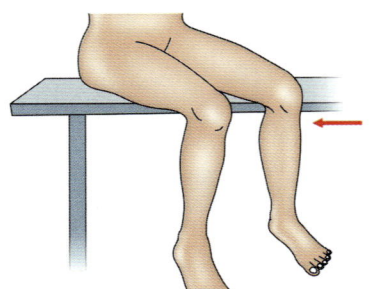

Fig. 45.7: Involvement of L4 myotome

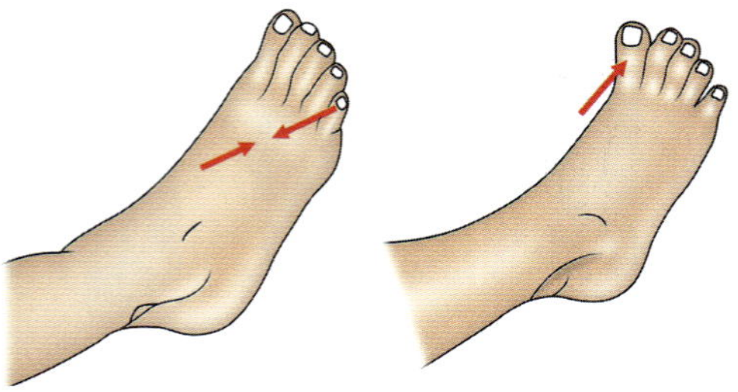

Fig. 45.8: Involvement of L5 myotome, Patient is unable to extend the toes

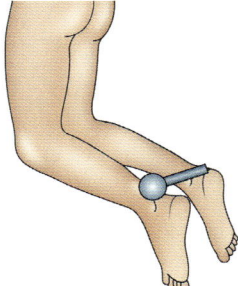

Fig. 45.9: S_1 myotomal involvement loss of ankle jerk

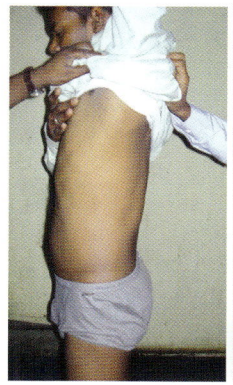

Fig. 45.10A: Loss of lumbar lordosis

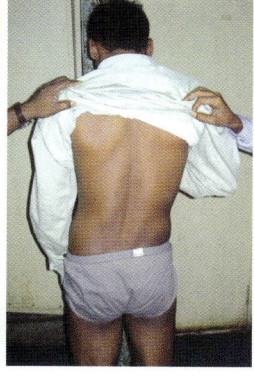

Fig. 45.10B: Paraspinal muscle spasm

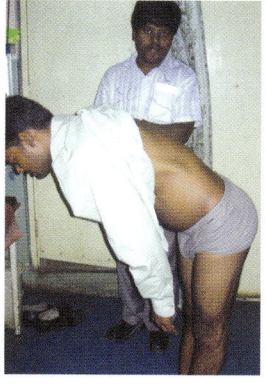

Fig. 45.10C: Severe restriction of forward flexion

Fig. 45.10D: Back completely touches the bed

Table 45.2: Clinical examination of the back

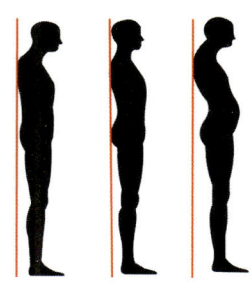

Fig. 45.11: Inspection with the patient in standing position look for ostural abnormalities. The figure from left to right depict thoracic hyperkyphosis, normal spine and exaggerated lumbar lordosis (Fig. 45.9).

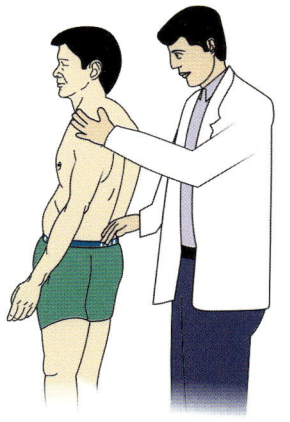

Fig. 45.16: At the waist as far backward as possible. Normal range Presence of pain in the anterior 30°.

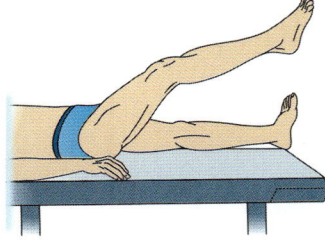

Fig. 45.17: SLRT with the patient in the supine position raise his or her leg to the point of pain or 90° whichever comes first. Inference: localized pain indicates a disc lesion, while radiating pain indicates sciatic radiculopathy. Dull posterior thigh pain indicates tight hamstrings. If the test is positive for sciatic radiculopathy do Lasegue test, buckle sign, etc.

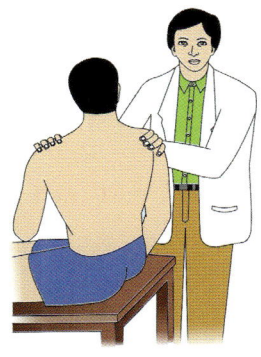

Fig. 45.12: Rotation Instruct the patient to rotate from the waist to the left and to the right as far as possible. Normal range is 45° per side. Note: In all the movements of the spine the neutral position is 0°.

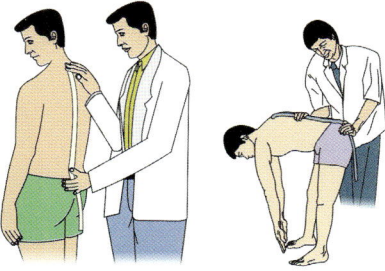

Figs 45.13 and 45.14: Movements of the spine 1. To test flexion Instruct the patient to bend forwards as much as possible at the waist. Normal flexion is 80° or fingertips 3 to 4 inches from the floor

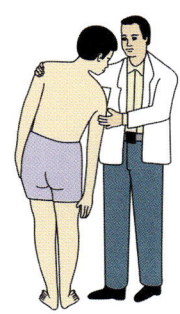

Fig. 45.15: Lateral flexion Instruct the patient to bend to the left and to the right as far

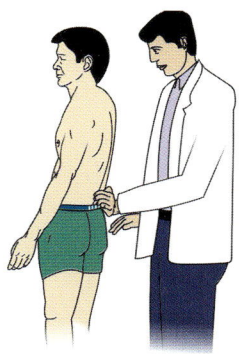

Fig. 45.18: Site of pain and sciatic radiculopathy in disc prolapse

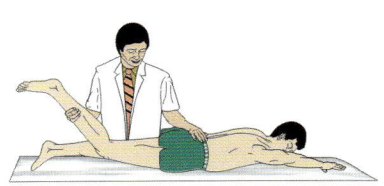

Fig. 45.19: Test Patient is instructed to lift the leg straight in prone position. Presence of pain in the anterior aspect of thigh indicates high level disc lesion

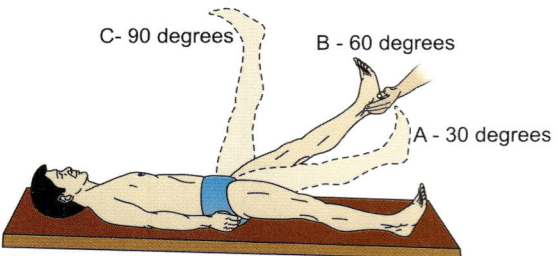

C- 90 degrees B - 60 degrees A - 30 degrees

Fig. 45.20: Method of performing SLRT

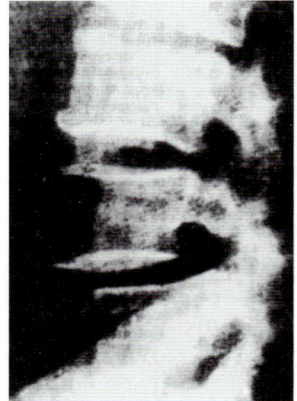
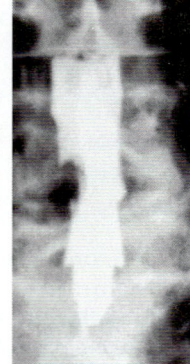

Fig. 45.21: Radiograph of LS spine showing lumbar disc disease

Fig. 45.22: Myelographic study of the lumbar spine

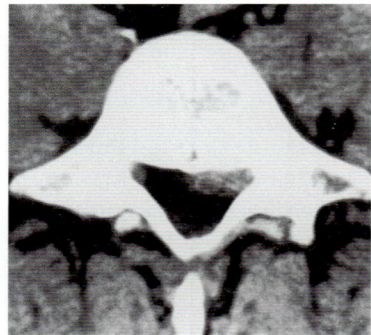
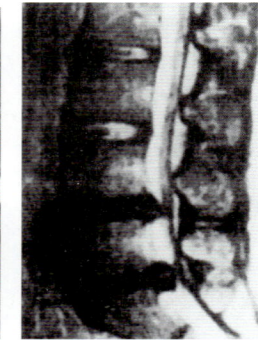

Fig. 45.23: CT scan showing posterolateral disc herniation

Fig. 45.24: MRI of lumbar spine with L4 disc prolapse compressing the spinal cord.

previously and is relieved by injecting xylocaine. It is a painful procedure and can introduce infection into the disc. Hence, it is less practiced.

Other tests of diagnostic importance are *bone scans, EMG,* routine laboratory studies, injection studies etc.

Treatment

Conservative therapy: Absolute bed rest is the best treatment for acute low backache due to IVDP, ice packs, non-

Table 45.3: Treatment plan of disc prolapse	
1. Conservative	• Absolute bed rest • Traction • NSAIDs • Belts
2. Epidural steroids	• For sub acute and chronic cases • Long-acting steroids + Local anesthetics • Reduces dependence on narcotics • Effect lasts for 3 weeks
3. Surgery	• Done in proper indications • Open or microscopic lumbar discectomy
4. Chemonucleolysis	• Same indications as for surgery • Limited only to lumbar spine • Drug used is chymopapain
5. Physiotherapy	• Active and passive physiotherapy • Flexion or extension exercises
6. Recurrence	• Back education prevention • Proper postural habits • Back exercises • Avoid all sports

steroidal anti-inflammatory drugs (NSAIDs), muscle relaxants, anti-depressants are recommended. Bucks extension skin traction and pelvic traction help to relieve pain. As the pain decreases, walking within limits of comfort is also encouraged. Sitting and riding in a car is discouraged. Back braces or belts are recommended in acute stages. They are discarded as soon as symptoms decrease otherwise muscles become weak and hasten the degeneration.

Role of exercises: Isometric abdominal and lower extremity exercises are begun. Lower extremity exercises increase the strength and relieves the stress on the back.

Back education and importance of proper posture is taught. See the pictorial display of proper postural habits and back exercises recommended for prevention of low backache (Table 45.3).

Epidural steroids: Epidural steroids are a symptomatic method of treatment, and consist of injecting a long-acting steroid and a local anesthetic. Its effect lasts for three weeks and is useful for sub acute and chronic cases. It also reduces dependence on narcotics in chronic cases.

Surgery: Indications
• Failed conservative management.
• Marked progressive weakness of muscles.
• Progressive neurological deficit.
• Cauda equina paralysis.

Principles of surgery: The principle of surgery is to see that the pressure on the nerve root is relieved by

45

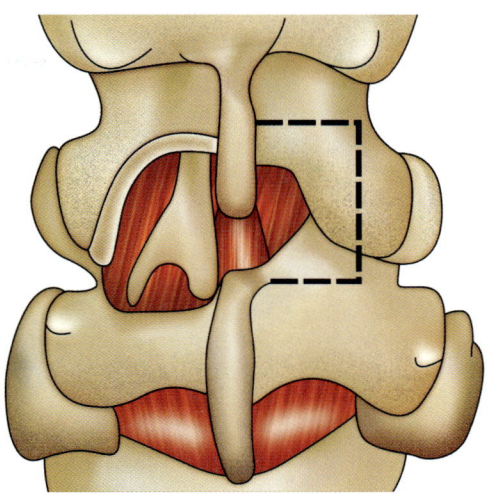

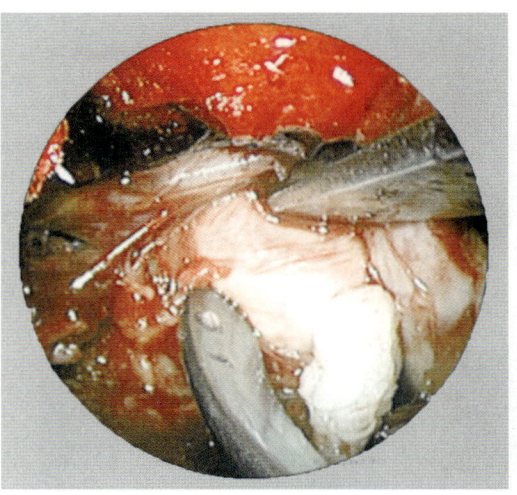

Fig. 45.25: Hemilaminectomy technique for decompressing the spinal cord

Fig. 45.26: Microscopic lumbar discectomy

45

removing the prolapsed disc. Dissection of muscles and bone removal should be kept at a minimum to prevent weakening of the spine.

Surgical methods
- *Laminectomy and disc excision:* Earlier this was the surgery of choice but now it is no longer resorted to as it makes the spine unstable.
- *Hemilaminectomy:* Here part of the lamina is removed. (Fig. 45.25).
- *The fenestration surgery:* Here the spine is approached unilaterally and the spine on the opposite side is not exposed. Here only the contiguous margin of upper and lower laminae is removed and medial facetectomy is done. The disc is now excised.
- *Microscopic or endoscopic lumbar discectomy:* Using an operating microscope or an endoscope the disc can be excised through a very small incision (< 3.5 cm) with minimum damage to the structures and minimal blood loss (Fig. 45.26).

Chemonucleolysis: Indications are the same as for surgery. It is limited to lumbar spine. Drug used is chymopapain.

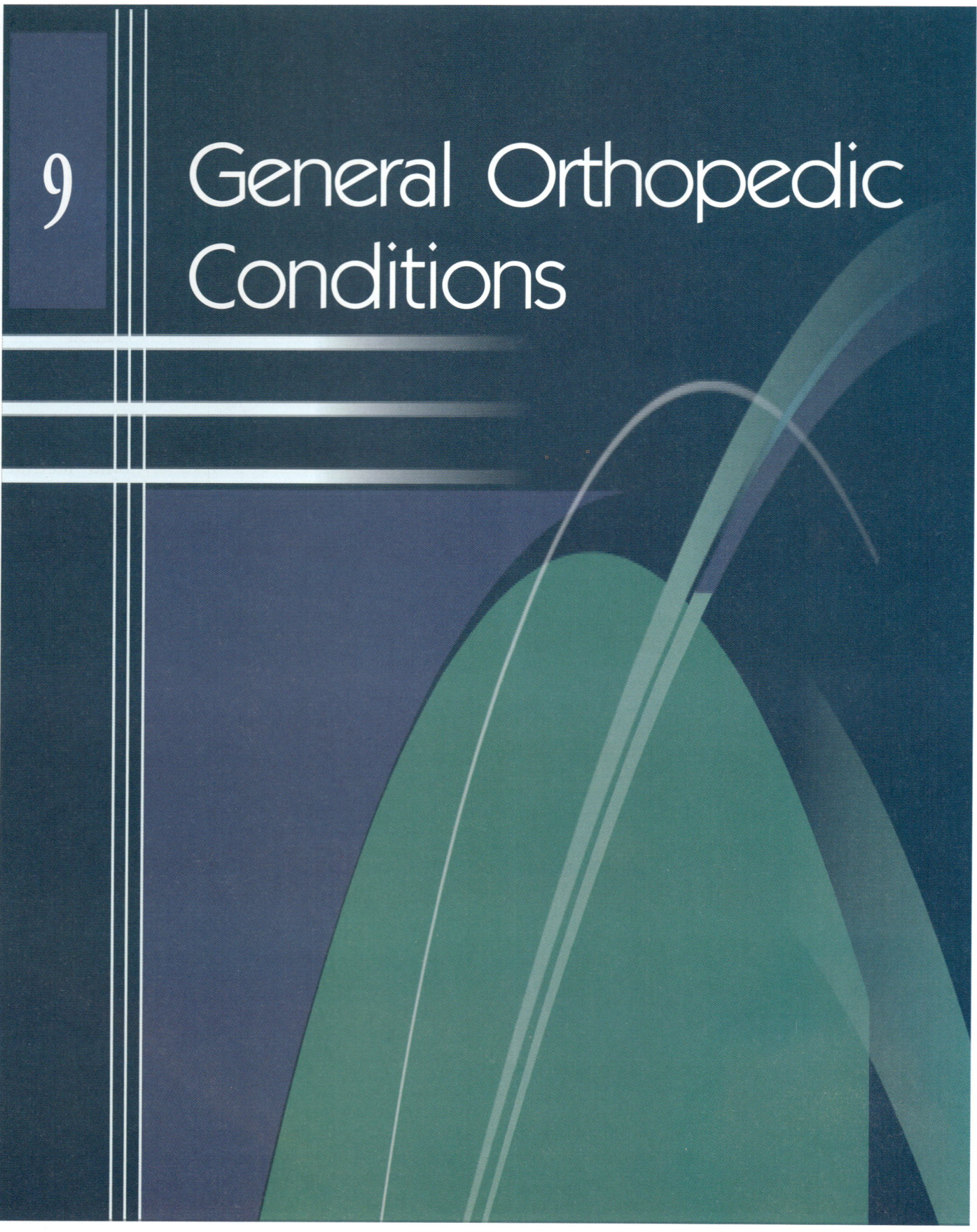

9 General Orthopedic Conditions

Congenital Disorders Developmental Dysplasia of Hip

46

Earlier known as Congenital Dislocation of Hip (CDH). Developmental dysplasia of hip is defined as partial or complete displacement of the femoral head from the acetabular cavity since birth.

Risk Factors (4 F's)

- **F**emales
- **F**irst borns
- **F**amilial
- **F**aulty intrauterine position (e.g. breech).

Theories of Etiology

- *Genetic theory:* Dysplastic trait is found in families.
- *Hormonal theory:* Hormone induced joint laxity. The hormone which is the culprit is the maternal hormone "Relaxin". This is supposed to help in the relaxation of the pelvic joints to facilitate normal labor. Nevertheless, if this hormone stumbles across the placental barrier and enters the fetal blood, it produces the same effect, i.e. excessive joint relaxation. This hormonal misadventure is however undesirable as the excessive joint laxity results in dislocation of the joint, especially the hip.
- *Mechanical theory:* Faulty intrauterine positions particularly in the first born like breech (confinement theory).
- Primary acetabular dysplasia.

Note: DDH is two times more common in breech prescription than vertex

Remember

The incidences in DDH
- 1 per 1000 live birth
- Left hip affected in 67% of cases
- Family history present in 20%
- Incidence of breech 30 to 50%
- 1:3 cases are bilateral
- Female preponderance (3 to 5 times more common)
- Faulty intrauterine position (Breech).

Pathology: The following pathological changes are observed in DDH (Fig. 46.1) and the severity varies according to the stages of the disease.

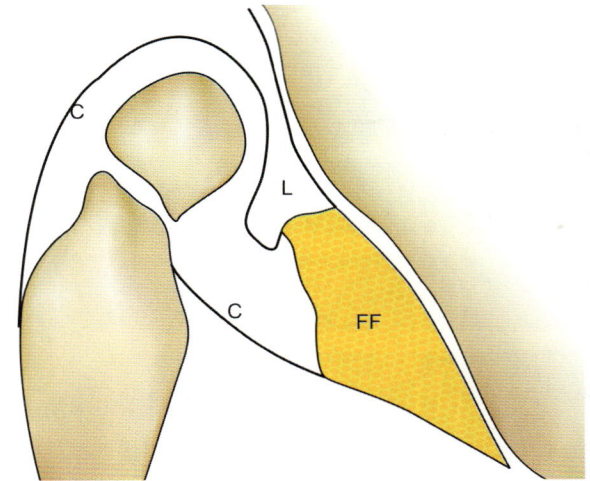

Fig. 46.1: FF shows the fibro fatty tissue within the acetabulum, L shows the limbus is inverted and C show the capsule is stretched

Bone

Acetabulum: There could be a primary acetabular dysplasia and the acetabulum is shallow. There could be a gap or groove at posterosuperior aspect. The triangular outer surface of ilium and acetabulum are in the same line. Above the acetabulum there is a depression containing the head of the femur. The acetabular cavity is shallow and has a steep slope.

Head of femur: The dislocated head of femur at first appears normal, ossification is delayed, later head is flat on its posterior and medial aspect. Femoral head when present in the ilium is buffer or conical shaped.

Neck of femur: There could be shortening and anteversion.

Pelvis: The pelvis is usually tilted forwards, it is small and atrophied. There is lordosis and it may be more vertical than normal.

Capsule: The capsule could show *hourglass constriction*, one containing head and the other containing the acetabulum. Constriction is produced by iliopsoas and the ligamentum teres passes through this constriction and it is hypertrophied.

Muscles

Pelvifemoral group: Adductors, sartorius, gracilis, rectus femoris, hamstrings, tensor fascia lata muscles. These muscles are shortened and they prevent reduction of the head.

Pelvitrochanteric group (obturators, quadratus femoris, iliopsoas): These are elongated and the psoas forms an obstacle to reduction.

Glutei muscles: show little organic change but power is diminished.

Remember

Conditions due to packaging problems (i.e. decreased intrauterine space)
- DDH
- Torticollis
- Metatarsus adductus
- Increased type III collagen

Stages of DDH (3Ds)

There are three stages in DDH as shown in Fig. 46.2.

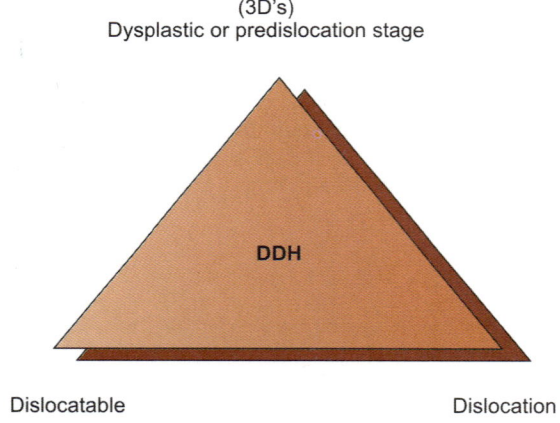

Fig. 46.2: Stages of developmental dysplasia of hip

Clinical Features

The clinical features vary in infants, children and adults.

In infants First a thorough clinical examination is carried out to detect the presence of any other congenital anomalies. If the hip is dislocated, all features of dislocation are present. The glutei and thigh folds are not symmetrical. The perineum is widened and abduction of the hip is decreased by 50 percent while the internal rotation movement is increased. Radiographic examination in infants is of little value, but von Rosen's line is helpful in making an early radiological diagnosis in this age group (Figs 46.3A and B).

Due to the paucity of the clinical findings during this period, more reliance is placed on certain clinical tests like the Barlow's Test, Ortolani's Test, and Galeazzi's

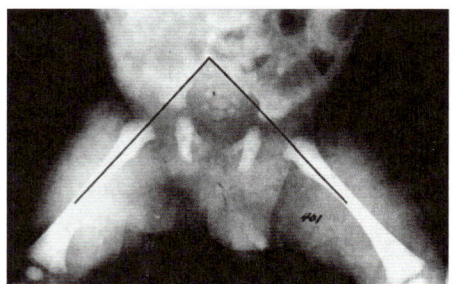

Fig. 46.3A: Plain X-ray showing von Rosen's line

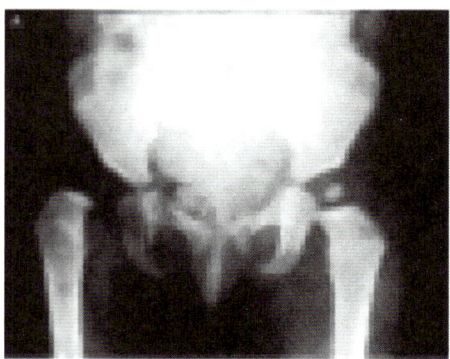

Fig. 46.3B: Radiograph showing congenital dislocation of hip

Test. These tests help us to identify the hidden DDH (Table 46.1 and Figs 46.6 to 46.8).

Children and Adolescents

Here the patient shows a waddling or sailor's gait. There is an increased lumbar lordosis (Fig. 46.4). The deformity frequently encountered in unilateral cases is shortening. In bilateral cases, the lower limbs are short, perineum is wide, and buttocks are broad and flat. Femoral artery is prominently felt. Abduction and lateral rotation movements of the hip are decreased (Fig. 46.5). *Telescopy and Trendelenburg tests* are positive. Clinical tests of importance in infants are not of relevance in this age group (Table 46.1).

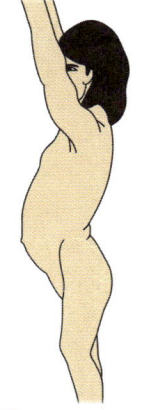

Fig. 46.4: Exaggerated lumbar lordosis indicating the presence of flexion deformity in a neglected bilateral DDH

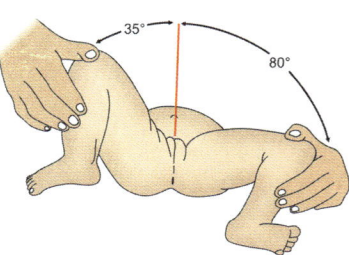

Fig. 46.5: Limitation of abduction of the involved right hip

46

Clinical tests	How to perform?	Inference
Barlow's test (Fig. 46.6) 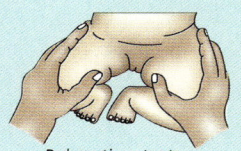 Relocation test	This test is done within 2 to 3 days of birth. The infant is supine with the knees fully flexed and the hip at 90° of flexion. The hip is slowly adducted and the head is slowly pushed backwards and outwards from the acetabulum by the fingers.	This test is positive when the joint is dislocated and the femoral head pops out of the acetabulum with a click or jerk. Reliable and useful upto 6 months after which the greater trochanter cannot be held with tip of the middle finger.
Ortolani's test (Fig. 46.7) 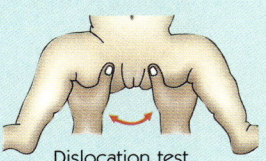 Dislocation test	This test is done between 3 and 9 months and is not satisfactory in a newborn. Here the infant is supine, with the hip and knee flexed. The hip is slowly adducted and abducted to detect any reduction of the femoral head into the acetabulum.	This test indicates the reduction of the dislocated hip. These two tests are generally reliable and should be performed as a screening tests in all cases of suspected CDH. They are misleading if abduction is restricted due to adduction contractures.
Galeazzi or Allen's sign (Fig. 46.8) 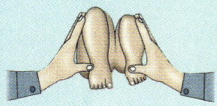	The child is in supine position with both the hip and the knee in flexion. The level of both the knee joints are noted with reference to a horizontal line.	Normally both the knee should be at the same level. In DDH the affected knee is seen beneath the horizontal line indicating femoral shortening. The shortening is in the supratrochanteric region and can be assessed by the Bryant's triangle.
Skin fold test of thigh (Fig. 46.9) 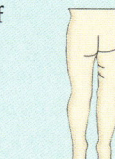	The child is completely stripped and in the vertical position the levels of the thigh folds studied.	Normally, the thigh folds are symmetrical in nature. In DDH they are no longer symmetrical due to the shortening of the affected limb.
Skin fold test of glutei region (Fig. 46.10) 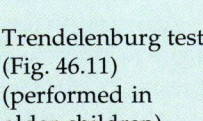	The procedure is similar to the one performed above, but here the levels of the gluteal folds are noted.	Normally, the thigh folds are symmetrical in nature. In DDH they are no longer symmetrical due to the shortening of the affected limb.
Trendelenburg test (Fig. 46.11) (performed in older children) 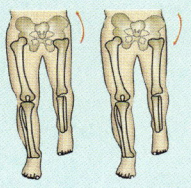 (A) Normal (B) Positive test	The patient is made to stand first on the normal limb and then on the affected limb. The contralateral leg is then raised from the ground.	When standing on the normal limb, the opposite hip is in a higher position, but when the patient or the child stands on the affected limb, the opposite pelvis drops indicating impairment of abductor mechanism due to DDH. This test cannot be performed in infants.
Fig. 46.12 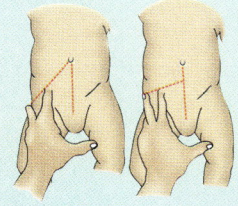	Klisic test	Normally an imaginary line between the greater trochanter and ASIS cuts through the umbilicus. In DDH, it cuts midway between the umbilicus and pubis.

Radiographic Study

Unlike in infants radiographs of pelvis show important features in this age group. The following radiological parameters should be noted: the primary ossific center of the head of the femur appears late and is poorly developed (Fig. 46.3B)

Perkins's line: This is a vertical line drawn at the outer border of the acetabulum.

Shenton's line: This is a smooth curve formed by the inferior border of the neck of the femur with the superior margin of the obturator foramen.

Hilgenreiner's line: This is a horizontal line drawn at the level of triradiate cartilage.

Acetabular index: Normal value is less than or equal to 30°.

CE angle of Wiberg: The normal value is 15–30°.

The Hilgenreiner's line and the Perkins's line helps to assess the position of the femoral head (Figs 46.14A and B). Normally the head lies in the lower and inner quadrant formed by these two lines. In DDH the head lies in the upper and outer quadrant, the continuity of Shenton's line is broken in DDH (Fig. 46.13). The acetabular index and the CE angle of Wiberg help to assess the acetabulum.

In adults all the features seen in adolescents are seen. In addition, patient will have features of secondary osteoarthritis of the hip namely pain, stiffness, limp, crepitus, restricted movements, etc.

Treatment

The aim of treatment in DDH is to achieve and maintain an early concentric reduction to prevent future degenerative joint disease. The methods to obtain

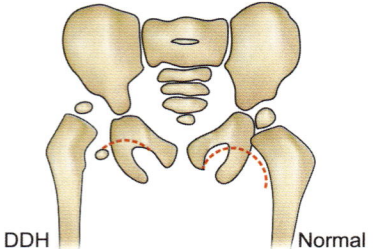

Fig. 46.13: Shenton's line broken in CDH

reduction of the head into the acetabulum vary according to the age groups.

In infants Reduction can be obtained and maintained by Pavlik harness which was first described by Arnold Pavlik of Czechoslovakia in the year 1958, von Rosen splints and other splints. Pavlik harness (Fig. 46.15) is the most important appliance useful in this age group. *This is the only harness that promotes spontaneous reduction of a dislocated hip and maintains the reduction, whereas other appliances only maintain the reduction. Hence Pavlik harness is called as "dynamic flexion abduction orthoses".* This is useful in children less than 6 months of age. Apart from the reduction and the immobilization, it allows active movements in all directions except extension and adduction. Nappies can be changed easily. The success rate of this harness is 85 to 95 percent. However as the age advances, soft tissue contractures develop along with secondary changes in the acetabulum, which bring down the success rate of Pavlik harness. Complications include osteonecrosis and failure of reduction.

Between 6 and 18 months as mentioned earlier Pavlik harness has no role in the treatment of DDH in this age

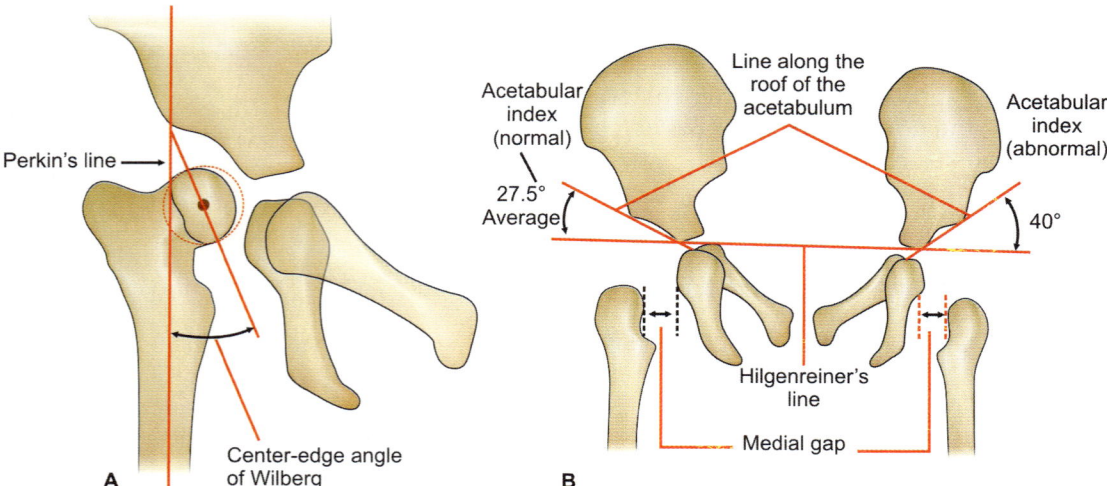

Figs 46.14A and B: (A) Center-edge of Wilberg: It is an angle formed between the Perkin's line and the line drawn from the lateral lip of the acetabulum passing through the center of the femoral head. In older children (10–13 year) the angle should always be more than 10°, (B) acetabular index. This is an angle formed between a line drawn along the margin of the roof of the acetabulum and Hilgenreiner's line average angle in newborn is about 27.5°. It decrease with age. *Medial gap:* This is the distance between the inner margin of the tear drop and the inner margin of the neck of the femur. The gap increases in dislocation. Always compared with the opposite hip. Not useful in bilateral cases.

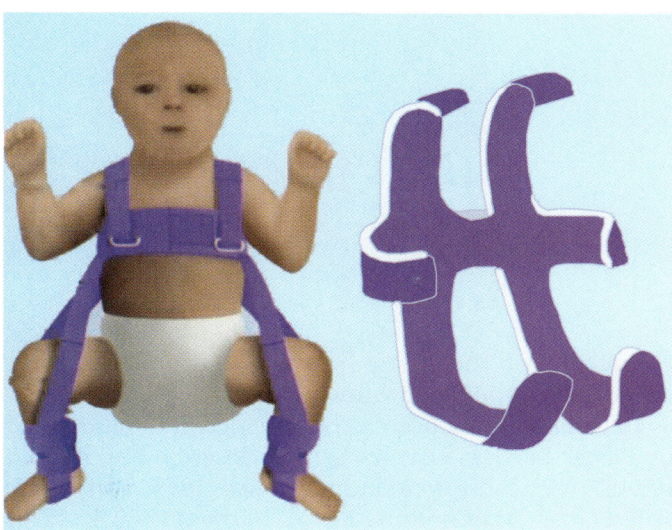

Fig. 46.15: Pavlik harness in DDH

46

group. Here the treatment of choice is gentle closed reduction and hip spica application (A frog leg or Lorenz cast and a Batchelor cast, Fig. 46.16). Open reduction is done if this method proves unsuccessful.

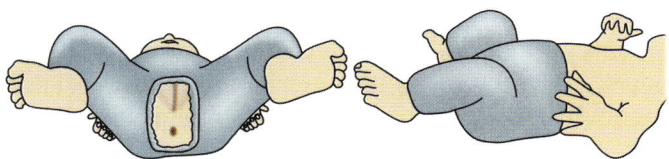

Fig. 46.16: DDH treated with plaster cast in frog leg position

Between 18 and 36 months: In this age group open reduction is the treatment of choice as closed reduction is often not successful. Open reduction is to be followed with either pelvic or femoral osteotomy to provide concentric reduction of the femoral head within the acetabulum. Preoperative traction Byrant or follows helps to stretch the contracted structured.

Remember

Why close reduction fails?
- Due to persistent dislocation soft tissue contractures develop preventing closed reduction attempts.
- Threat of AVN if head is forcibly reduced into the acetabulum.

Role of Osteotomies

Osteotomies are done for instability, failure of acetabular development or progressive head subluxation after reduction. They are done only if congruent reduction is possible, if there is satisfactory range of movements and if the femoral head has a reasonable sphericity. The osteotomies could be femoral or pelvic

and the choice is usually left to the surgeons, but there are some guiding principles.

Pelvic osteotomies: These are chosen if there is severe dysplasia and radiographic changes on the acetabular side.

Femoral osteotomies: This is the procedure of choice if there are changes in the femoral head and if there is increase in ante/version of the neck.

Between 3 and 8 years: Here open reduction is followed either by femoral shortening or pelvic osteotomies.

Between 8 and 18 years: In this age group open reduction is followed by femoral shortening or pelvic osteotomies. If osteoarthritis of the hip develops, total hip replacement is the surgery of choice. Arthrodesis of hip is rarely done. Both these surgeries are planned once the child reaches the adult stage.

Remember
- **Important radiological parameters in DDH**
- < 6 m: von Rosen's line
- > 6 m: Perkin's line, Shenton's line, acetabular index and delayed ossification.

Innominate Osteotomy in DDH (Acetabular Reconstruction)

Salter's osteotomy: This is indicated in patients with instability after reduction or in persistent DDH between 18 months and 6 years. The procedure consists of using the symphysis pubis as a hinge, osteotomising the acetabulum and turning it to cover the head (Fig. 46.17).

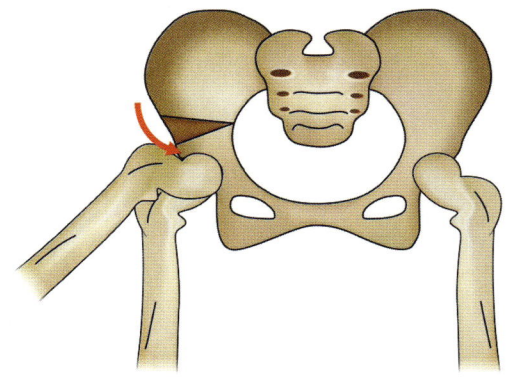

Fig. 46.17: Salter's osteotomy

Pemberton's pericapsular osteotomy: It is indicated in paralytic dislocation and in postacetabular deficiency between 1 and 10 years. Here the osteotomy is done through the acetabular roof using triradiate cartilage as the hinge.

Steel's osteotomy: This is useful in older children when symphysis pubis and the triradiate cartilage are fused. This is a triple innominate osteotomy.

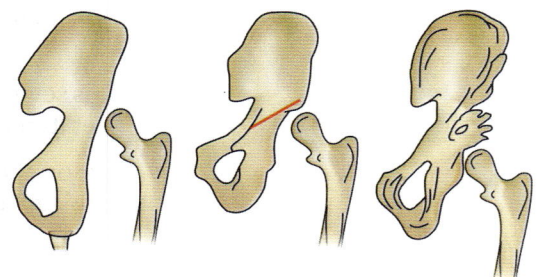

Fig. 46.18: Acetabular shelf operation

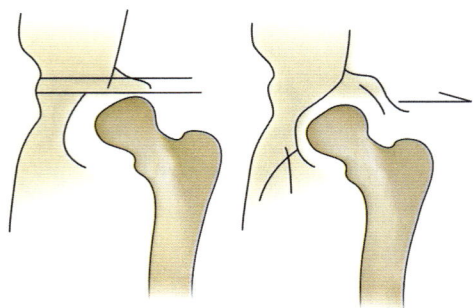

Fig. 46.19 Chiari's osteotomy

Shelf operation: It is indicated in CDH with recurrence. Here the acetabulum is extended laterally and anteriorly by bone graft (Fig. 46.18).

Chiari's pelvic displacement osteotomy: This is a salvage procedure and is indicated in children older than 4 years. Here the osteotomy is done through the ilium above the acetabulum and the distal fragment is pushed medially (Fig.46.19). The upper fragment deepens the acetabulum.

46

47 Congenital Talipes Equinovarus (CTEV) Foot

One may pride in having flat foot, agile foot, nimble foot, but look at the tale of woes a clubfoot presents to the unfortunate victim affected with this malady!

Clubfoot: It is so called because severe untreated talipes equinovarus has a club-like appearance. This is the most common among various foot deformities (Figs 47.1A to I)

This is the most common congenital foot disorder. *Incidence* is 1.2/1000 live births.

Sex: Males are more commonly affected than females.

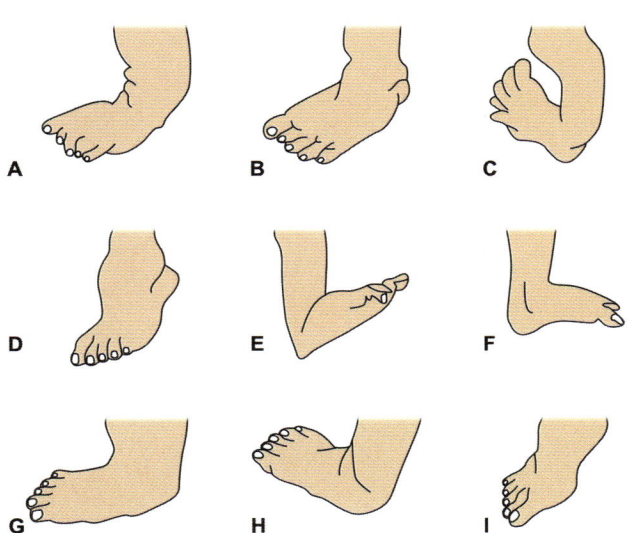

Figs 47.1A to I: Different varieties of foot deformities: (A) varus, (B) equinovarus, (C) calcaneovarus, (D) equinus, (E) calcaneus, (F) cavus, (G) valgus, (H) calcaneovalgus, and (I) equinovalgus

Etiology of CTEV

This could be primary or secondary. In the primary variety exact cause is unknown, while in the secondary variety the causes could be polio, spina bifida, etc.

Interesting Features of CTEV

Talipes: It is a Latin word derived from Talus = ankle, pes = foot
Original meaning: A deformity that causes the patient to walk on the ankle.
Present day meaning is any variety of clubfoot.

Types of CTEV (Etiology)

- Osseous type — Clubfoot is associated with absence of tibia and fibula
- Muscular type — Arthrogryposis multiplex congenital or multiple congenital contractures
- Neuropathic type — Due to spina bifida, etc.
- Idiopathic type — No apparent cause, commonest variety

IDIOPATHIC CTEV

This is the most common type of CTEV one encounters in clinical practice. There is no apparent cause and hence various theories are proposed.

Pathology: The pathology in CTEV affects all the bones and joints of the foot with corresponding soft tissue contractures especially of the posteromedial structures. The primary problem usually lies in the bones with secondary soft tissue contractures (Fig. 47.2). However, sometimes the primary pathology may be in the surrounding soft tissues, which brings about secondary changes in the bones, however, the later event is rare. Table 47.1 shows the bony changes and the structures involved in the posteromedial aspect of the ankle and foot in a case of CTEV. All these contracted soft tissue should be released during surgery to bring back the bones to normal alignment.

Clinical Features

Congenital talipes equinovarus is a grotesque looking deformity of the foot. In idiopathic variety deformity is the only complaint. The diagnosis is fairly simple and

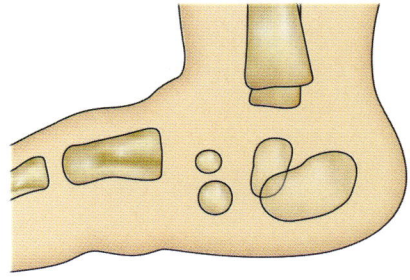

Fig. 47.2: Bony arrangements in CTEV

Table 47.1: Bony and soft tissue changes in CTEV

Bones and joints (bony)	Muscles, capsules, ligaments (soft tissues) (Figs 47.1A to C)
• Calcaneus is in varus position • Talus displaced medial and plantar wards • Navicular medially displaced and rotated • Cuboid displaced medially and articulates with the non-articular surface of the calcaneus (Known as cuboid sign or locked cuboid) • Metatarsals deviates medially at Tarsometatarsal joints • Talocalcaneal articulation is a ball and socket joint. The anterior and middle articulation of the calcaneum forms the socket and the head of the talus forms the ball which is dislocated in CTEV. • Tibia usually shows medial torsion, rarely lateral torsion. In short all the above bones are displaced down and medial in a case of CTEV.	Structures contracted on the medial side (3) Rule of 3 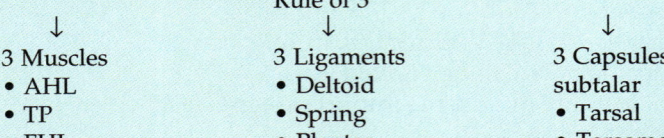 3 Muscles 3 Ligaments 3 Capsules • AHL • Deltoid subtalar • TP • Spring • Tarsal • FHL • Plantar • Tarsometatarsal joints • FDL Structures contracted on the posterior side (2) Rule of 2 2 Muscles 2 Ligaments 2 Capsules • Tibialis posterior • Talofibular • Ankle joint • Tendo Achilles • Calcaneofibular • Subtalar joint Structures involved on the Anterior side (1). Rule of 1 1 Muscle 1 Ligament 1 Capsule • Tibialis anterior • Superior peroneal • Calcaneocuboid, joint • Inserted abnormally Retinacula

47

straightforward. *Five classical primary deformities are seen and in response to this, secondary deformities develop. These primary and secondary deformities together form the clubfoot complex* (Table 47.2). A detailed examination of the foot is necessary to detect the full spectrum of deformities in CTEV (Figs 47.3A to C).

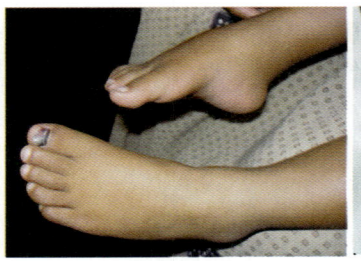
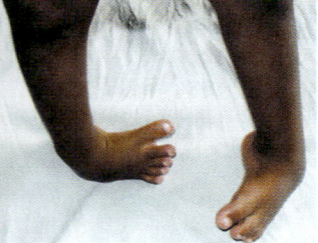

A   B

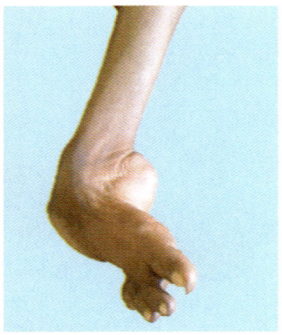

C

Figs 47.3A to C: Clinical photograph showing clubfoot (A) Unilateral (B) Bilateral (C) Neglected clubfoot

Table 47.2: Clubfoot complex

Deformities in clubfoot

Primary deformities	Secondary deformities
• Equinus	• Foot size is decreased to 50%
• Varus	• Medial border is concave, lateral border is convex
• Cavus • Forefoot adduction	• Forefoot is plantar flexed upon hind foot
• Internal tibial torsion • Skin is stretched over the dorsum of the foot	
Late changes	
• Degeneration of joints	• Callosities are the dorsum of the foot
• Fusion of joints	• Stumbling gait • Hypotrophic anterior tibial artery • Atrophy of muscles in anterior or posterior compapartments of the leg • Tight plantar fascia and tendo Achilles on attempting correction. • Transverse skin crease. • Heel is small and is impalpable.

With advancing age, the cosmetically unsightly club-foot starts posing functional problems like altered gait (stumbling gait), callosities, degeneration and arthritic changes in the ankle and foot joints. Correction is a must to restore normalcy.

In other varieties of CTEV, clinical features peculiar to the etiological factors can be elicited.

Two clinical tests are of extreme importance in CTEV and are described below:

Dorsiflexion test: In a newborn child it is possible to dorsiflex the foot till its dorsal surface comes in contact with the anterior surface of the tibia. This is not possible in CTEV and this can be used as a screening test (Fig.47.4) in a newborn child.

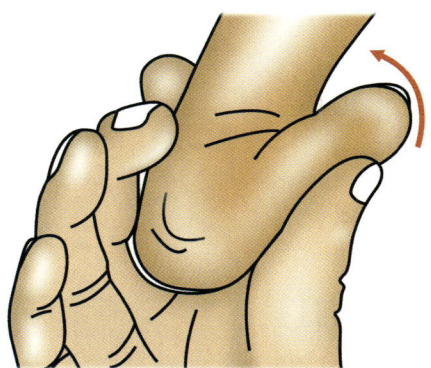

Fig. 47.4: Dorsiflexion test in a newborn

Plumb line test: This test helps to detect the tibial torsion in an older child (Fig. 47.5). The child is made to sit on a table with both the lower limbs hanging from the edge. A line drawn from the center of the patella to the the tibial tubercle when extended down, should cut the foot at the first or second intermetatarsal space normally. This is called the plumb line. In CTEV with medial rotation of the tibia it cuts the fourth or fifth intermetatarsal space and vice versa in lateral rotation of the tibia.

> **VITAL FACTS**
> Undetected muscle imbalance and tibial torsion are the important causes of recurrence of the treated and corrected clubfoot. Hence the importance of these tests.

Investigation

Since CTEV is a mechanical problem, laboratory investigations are less useful. Radiography is by far the most important investigation. It helps to know the exact angles of each deformity seen clinically in CTEV. In anterioposterior view the angles formed between the long axis of the talus and the calcaneum (talometatarsal angle), the talus and the metatarsals are evaluated Talometatarsal angle. This helps to know the angle of

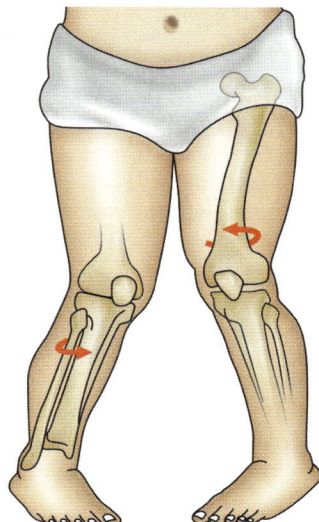

Fig. 47.5: Internal tibial torsion

varus and the forefoot adduction (Figs 47.6A and B). In the lateral view, the angle formed between the talus and the tibia, and talus and calcaneum helps to know the extent of equinus and varus respectively. It is a simple fact that all angles should be restored back to normal following treatment. Any residual uncorrected angle is a future pointer to relapse. In neglected clubfoot all these angles are grossly distorted (Fig 47.7).

Management

Broadly speaking CTEV can be managed by three methods.
- Conservative management
- Surgical management
- Management by external fixators.

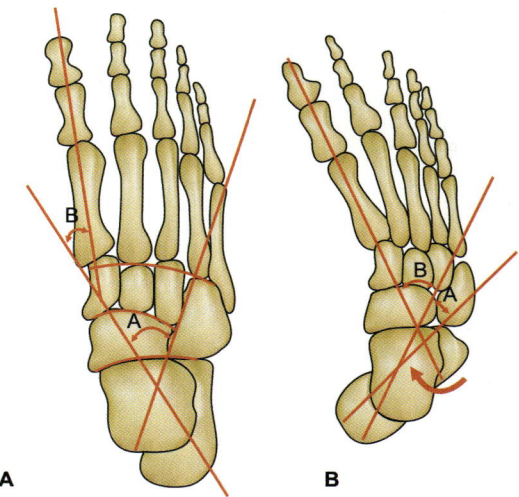

Figs 47.6A and B: Important radiological lines: (A) talocalcaneal angles, (B) talometatarsal angle

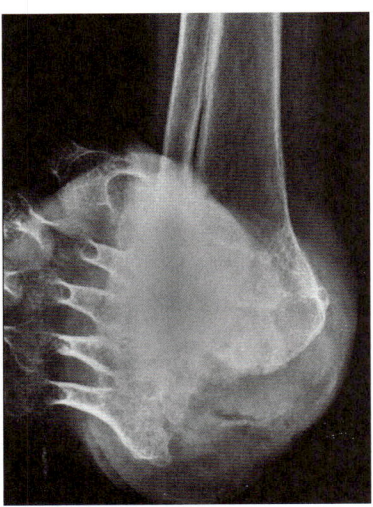

Fig. 47.7: Neglected clubfoot

Conservative management: It is the treatment of choice in infants less than 6 months of age. The recommended regime is as follows (after Kite and Lovell).

First 6 weeks of life (Kite's method): Weekly serial manipulation of the deformities and above knee casting for the first 6 weeks of life. Later, it is done every fortnightly till correction is achieved. Manipulation by mother is usually not sufficient (Fig. 47.8). Success rate of serial manipulation and casting ranges from 15 to 80 percent. If correction is achieved in first 6 months of age, Phelps Brace is used during day time and Denis Browne splint during the night time from 6 to 18 months to prevent recurrence. After 18 months, below knee walking calipers are given up to 4 years of age. From 4 years to skeletal maturity regular followup is advised.

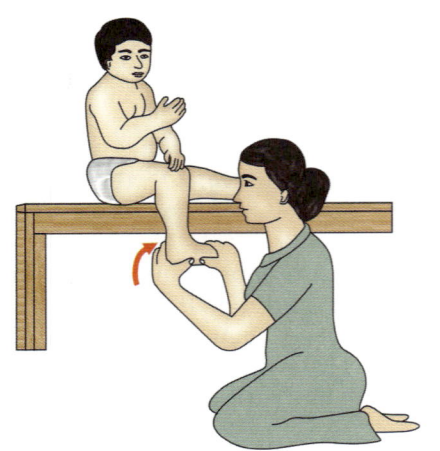

Fig. 47.8: A mother manipulating her child's clubfoot

PONSETI TECHNIQUE

Ponseti in the year 1950 described a very effective conservative method of treating a clubfoot with very few recurrence rates. There is an extremely high success rate for correcting clubfoot using the Ponseti method for non-surgical cast correction of clubfoot. Of late lot of interest is being revived with this technique of clubfoot management. Here the success of the reduction is 90–98 percent and is better than the Kite's regime. It is mooted as a better alternative to the more cumbersome surgical correction. It can be used in older children of 2 years age and also after failed previoius nonoperative techniques and thus has a wider application.

Treatment Phase

Ideally, it is begun, as soon as possible after birth. The treatment involves weekly stretching of the foot deformity in the clinic, followed by the application of long leg plaster casts. The cast is changed every 1 or 2 weeks, and a newborn with a congenital clubfoot should expect the deformity corrected in about five to six weeks. Before the application of the final cast, the physician usually performs a tenotomy, an Achilles tendon lengthening using non-invasive surgery. The incision is so small that no stitching is required. The child wears a final cast for three weeks to allow the tendon to heal.

Maintenance Phase

The child then wears a corrective foot orthosis full time (23 hours a day) for three months, followed by night and naptime wear for up to four years to prevent the deformity from recurring.

Benefits of the Ponseti Method

The Ponseti method delivers excellent correction of clubfoot without the associated risks and complications of major foot surgery. Parents, as much as the child, appreciate the fact that clubfoot can be corrected successfully without surgery. Moreover, studies show that patients treated with the Ponseti method enjoy a more flexible foot and ankle than those treated surgically. Long-term studies of the Ponseti method have demonstrated that cast correction of clubfoot not only helps dramatically during childhood, but also in adulthood.

47

Remember
Order of correction of deformity
The mnemonic **ADVERB** helps to remember the order of correction.
AD   Forefoot adduction is corrected first
V   Correction of heel varus next
E   Lastly correction of hindfoot equinus
RB   This order is followed to prevent "**Rocker Bottom Foot**" which develops if foot is dorsiflexed through hindfoot rather than midfoot.

Surgical methods: Soft tissue procedures are advocated for children less than 4 years. Bony procedures are added later on. For mild CTEV with no severe internal rotation deformity of calcaneus, a one-stage posteromedial release of TURCO is preferred.

Structures Released in Turco's Procedure (Posteromedial release)

1. *On the posterior side*
   a. Z-plasty of tendo Achilles to lengthen it (Fig. 47.9).
   b. Posterior capsulotomy of the ankle and subtalar joints.
   c. Release of posterior talofibular and calcaneo-fibular ligaments.

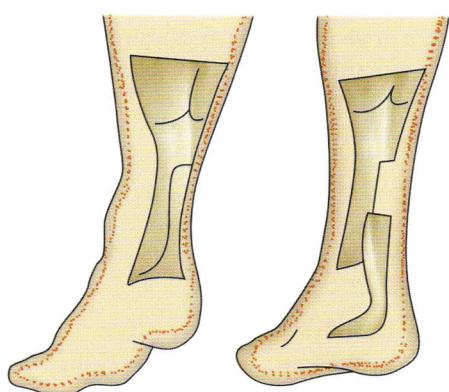

Fig. 47.9: Tendo Achilles lengthening by Z-plasty for clubfoot

2. *One the medial side*
   a. Lengthening of the tibialis posterior, flexor hallucis longus and flexor digitorum longus muscle.
   b. Release of talonavicular ligament, spring ligament and the superficial part of deltoid ligament.
   c. Release of interosseous talocalcaneal ligament, capsules of naviculocuneiform and first metatarso-cuneiform joints.
3. *On the plantar side*
   a. Plantar fascia.
   b. Release of abductor hallucis and flexor digitorum brevis.

For severe deformities with severe internal rotation of calcaneum—a one-stage modified Mc-Kay procedure of both posteromedial and posterolateral release is preferred.

Bony Procedures

These are added to the soft tissue procedures after 4 years of age. Dwyer's lateral closed wedge osteotomy (Fig. 47.10) helps correct the varus deformity, Evan's and Davis' operations also help to correct varus in slightly older child. Triple arthodesis is recommended after skeletal maturity.

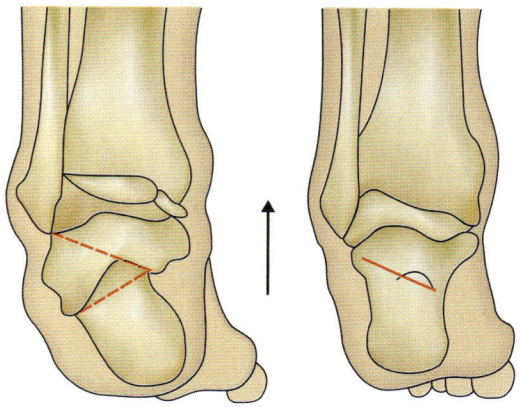

Fig. 47.10: Dwyer's lateral closed wedge osteotomy

Surgeries for Uncorrected Clubfoot

In older children and adolescents

Triple arthrodesis: Indicated for children more than 10 years. It is functionally and cosmetically superior. Lateral closed wedge osteotomy through subtalar and midtarsal joints is done to fuse all the three joints of the foot namely the subtalar, talonavicular and calcanecuboid joints (Figs 47.11A and B).

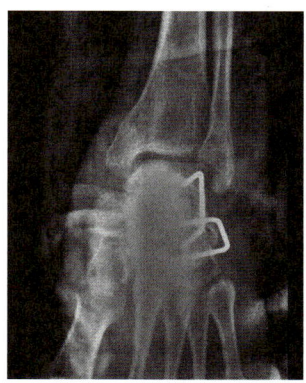 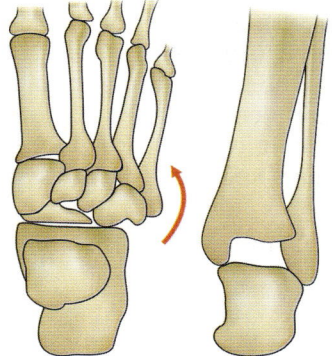

Fig. 47.11A: Triple arthrodesis   **Fig. 47.11B:** Triple arthrodesis in CTEV indicated in neglected clubfoot

Talectomy: It is a salvage procedure and is indicated for severe uncorrected clubfoot. It is also indicated in those cases previously corrected and unsuccessful. For uncorrectable CTEV by any other procedure, talectomy is useful as a salvage procedure.

Tendon transfers: It is indicated for recurrent clubfoot (recurrence is due to muscle imbalance, here peroneals are weak and invertors are strong).

Garceaus method: Transfer of tibialis anterior to middle cuneiform bone.

Modified garceaus method: Transfer of tibialis anterior to base of fifth metatarsal bone.

SURGICAL MANAGEMENT INDICATIONS (5 Rs)

- **R**esponse not obtained to conservative treatment after 6 months.
- **R**igid clubfoot (means forefoot deformities are corrected but hindfoot deformities remain uncorrected after conservative treatment).
- **R**elapsed clubfoot (means deformities are corrected initially, but relapse later, either partial or total).
- **R**ecurrent clubfoot (it is type of relapse, the cause being muscle imbalance which was overlooked initially).
- **R**esistant clubfoot (very resistant to correction).

Surgery for correction of tibial torsion in clubfoot (Sell's criteria) more than 15° torsion should be corrected by derotation osteotomy. Otherwise all deformities will recur due to the pressure of the caliper on the lateral border of the foot.

Caliper is used after the correction to maintain the correction of deformities obtained either by conservative or surgical measures.

Treatment by external fixators: This is a recent concept in the management of CTEV and is reserved for difficult cases. There are two types of external fixator frames; Ilizarov, a Russian orthopedic surgeon design and Indian orthopedic surgeon Dr BB Joshi has designed the second. This frame is known as Joshi's external stabilization system popularly called as JESS (Fig. 47.12).

When done in properly indicated cases, external fixator produces excellent results. It is a semi-invasive, bloodless surgery and can be done without a tourniquet. Though technically very demanding it avoids all the complications of surgery and a postoperative scar. It is known to correct all the components of the deformities both bony and soft tissues. The rate of relapse or recurrence is comparatively less and even if it does occur, the options of surgery are always open.

> **Remember**
>
> **Three Is for relapse**
> - **I**mproper and inadequate conservative treatment and also surgical release of contracted structures
> - **I**mbalance of foot muscles if left uncorrected
> - **I**nternal torsion of tibia if overlooked

Retention of CTEV Correction

Whatever may be the methods of correction of CTEV whether conservative, surgical or external fixators, retentions of the corrected deformities should be done by one of the following methods to prevent relapse.

a. Denis Browne splint is used usually during the night (Fig. 47.13).
b. Phelps's brace is used mainly in the daytime.
c. Below knee walking calipers.
d. CTEV shoes are mainly used when the child starts walking and up to 5 years of age (Fig. 47.14).

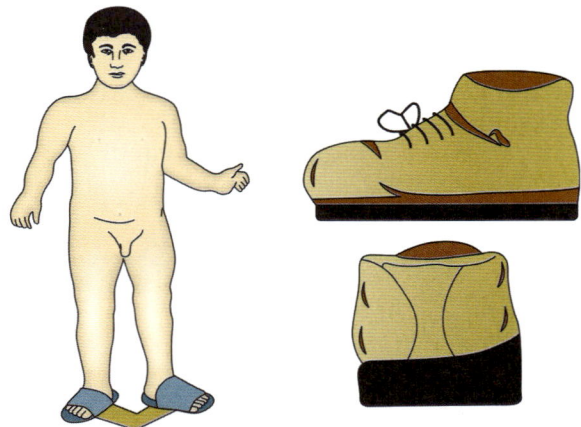

Fig. **47.13:** Denis Browne splint   Fig. **47.14:** CTEV shoes

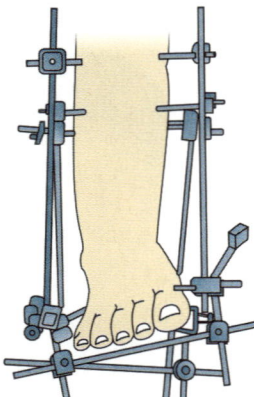

Fig. **47.12:** Correction of CTEV using Joshi's external fixator frame

QUICK FACTS

Do you know how does a CTEV shoe differ from an ordinary shoe?
- It has a straight inner border which helps prevent forefoot adduction
- It has an outer shoe raise and this helps prevent foot-inversion
- There is no heel and this helps prevent equinus.

47

48 | Other Congenital Disorders

CONGENITAL TORTICOLLIS (WRYNECK)

- Contracture of the sternocleidomastoid muscle on one side since birth (Fig. 48.1).
- *Exact* cause is *not* known.
- Tumor is palpable at birth.
- It may be due to *birth* trauma also.
- Deformity is the *only* complain initially.
- Later facial asymmetry and macular problems in the retina develop.
- During infancy, consevative tyreatment, like stretching of the muscle is done.
- If it persists for more than 1 year it should be surgically released.

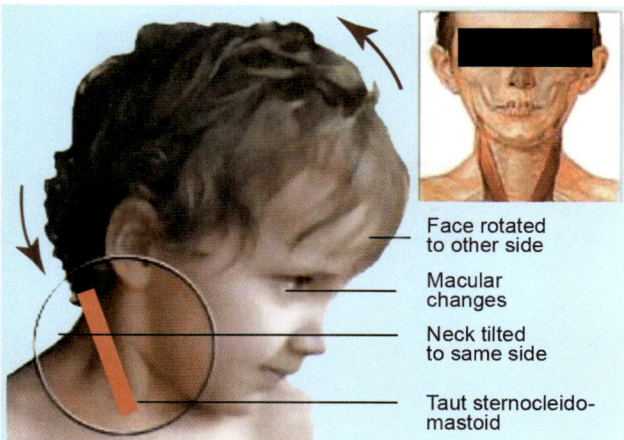

Face rotated to other side

Macular changes

Neck tilted to same side

Taut sternocleido-mastoid

Fig. 48.1: Wryneck

CONGENITAL ELEVATION OF THE SCAPULA (SPRENGEL SHOULDER)

- It is due to the imperfect descent of the shoulder girdle by the third month (Figs. 48.2A and B).

- The scapula is high by 2 to 10 cm.
- Deformity is the only complaint.
- There is no functional impairment.
- No treatment is required in mild cases.
- In severe cases, surgical release of the muscles from the scapula is indicated after 3 years.

CLEIDOCRANIAL DYSOSTOSIS

- Here clavicle is absent either partially or wholly.
- Exact cause is not known.

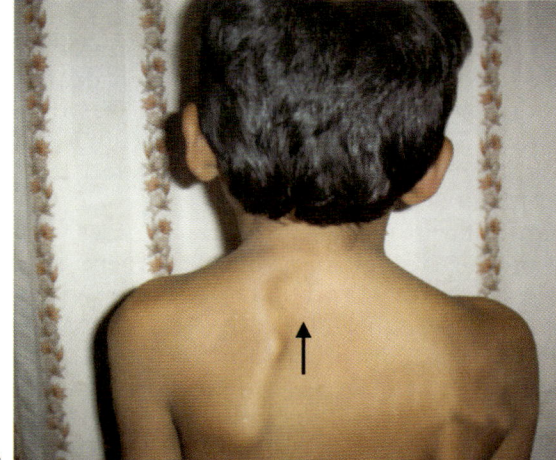

A

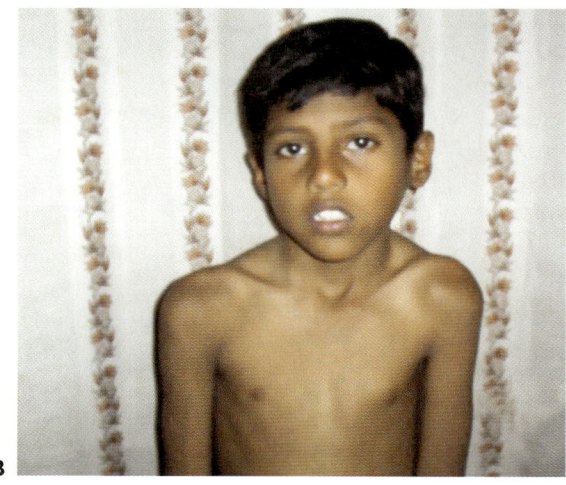

B

Figs 48.2A and B: Congenital elevation of scapula: (A) view from the back, (B) view from the front

- Accidentally discovered.
- No functional impairment
- Tips of the shoulder can be approximated to each other (Fig. 48.3)
- Plain X-ray shows absence of clavicle (Fig. 48.4)
- No treatment is required in most of the cases
- Surgically removed if there is pain due to pressure of one or both the ends.

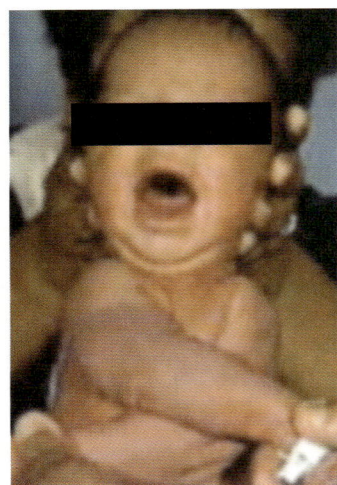

Fig. 48.3: Cleidocranial dysostosis

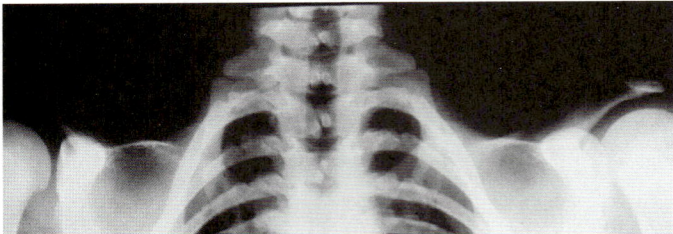

Fig. 48.4: Absence of clavicle

CONGENITAL RADIOULNAR SYNOSTOSIS

- This involves the proximal ends of radius and ulna.
- The forearm is fixed in pronation.
- It is usually bilateral.
- There is a familial tendency.
- Plain X-ray helps to determine the level and extent of fusion of radius and ulna (Fig. 48.5)
- Treatment is limited to osteotomy, to place the forearm in mid-prone position for better function.

MADELUNG'S DEFORMITY

- This *is an abnormality* of the *palmar;* ulnar *aspect* of the distal
- There is *progressive ulnar and volar tilt resulting* in dorsal subluxation of the distal ulna.
- It consists of *volar* subluxation of the hand, prominence of the distal ulna, and volar and ulnar angulation of the distal radius.

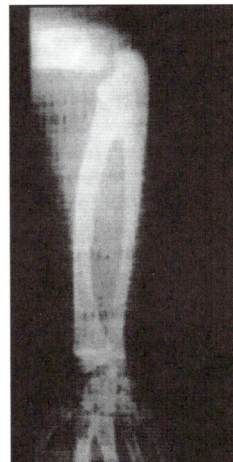

Fig. 48.5: Congenital radioulnar synostosis

- Commonly bilateral.
- Girls are more affected.
- There is a positive family history.
- There is minimal *pain* and excellent function. Hence conservative treatment is considered initially.
- Plain X-ray helps to assess the deformity (Fig. 48.6)
- Surgery is considered for severe deformity or persistent pain.
- In children, Milch Resection (radial osteotomy with ulnar shortening) is the commonly performed surgery.
- In adults Osteotomy and Darrach's procedure are done.

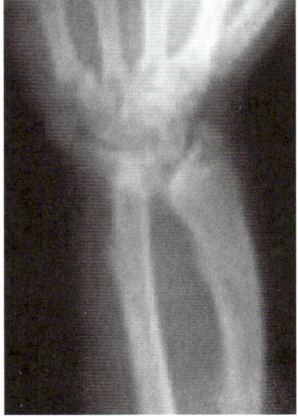

Fig. 48.6: Madelung's deformity

CONGENITAL ABSENCE OF RADIUS (Radial clubhand)

- Failure of the formation of the parts along the preaxial or radial borders of the upper *extremity.*
- Deficient or absent thenar muscles, short or absent thumbs, short or absent radius (Fig. 48.7A).
- Complete radial absence is more common than partial.

48

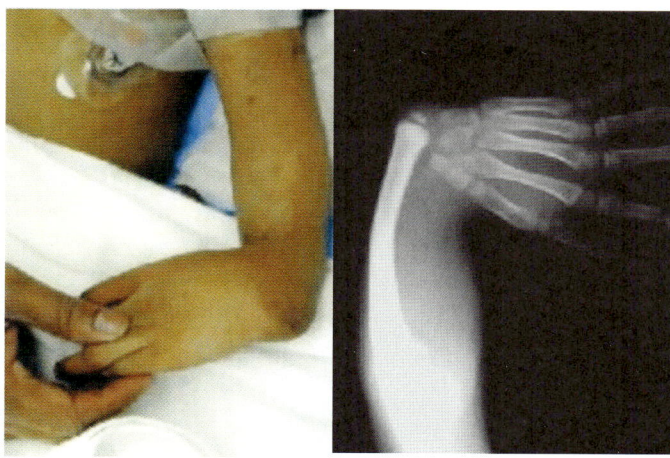

Figs 48.7A and B: Radial clubhand (A) clinical photo (B) plain X-ray

- Right side is more common.
- Plain X-ray shows the absence of radius (Fig. 48.7B)
- Important surgical correction methods include centralization of the hands, pollicization, etc.

CONGENITAL PSEUDARTHROSIS OF TIBIA

- It is a rare condition with an incidence of 1 in 2.5 lac births radius.
- In 50–60% of cases neurofibromatosis is present.
- There is anterior bowing of the tibia with varying sclerosis, cyst, etc.

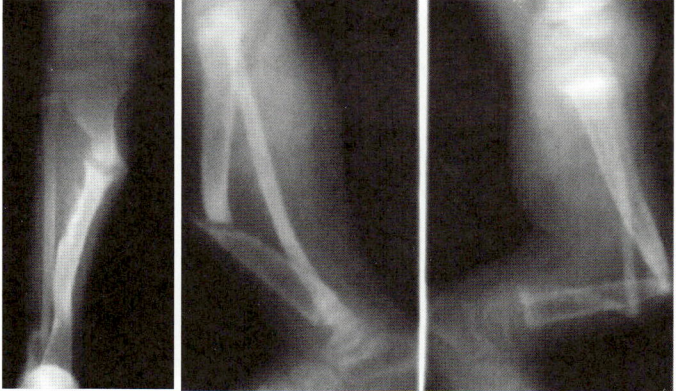

Fig. 48.8: Plain X-ray showing congenital pseudarthrosis of tibia

- Plain X-ray helps to detect the extent of bowing, cyst, fracture, etc. (Fig. 48.8).
- Treatment is essentially surgical and consists of bone grafting operations, Sofield's multiple osteotomies with internal fixation by intra-medullary nails, etc.

CONGENITAL DISLOCATION OF THE KNEE

- It is mostly due to malposition *in utero*.
- Quadriceps contracture and absence or hypo plastic anterior cruciate ligament is another important cause.
- Plain X-ray helps to detect the dislocation (Fig. 48.9).
- Serial casting for mild cases.
- Severe cases managed surgically by Z-plasty of the quadriceps (Neibeuer and King's technique.)

CONGENITAL ABSENCE OF FIBULA

- This is partially or completely absent more often than any other long bones in the body.
- In mild variety, leg is marginally short, in severe varieties, there is equinovalgus deformity of the ankle
- Wiltse's osteotomy to correct the valgus deformity in skeletally mature patients is done.

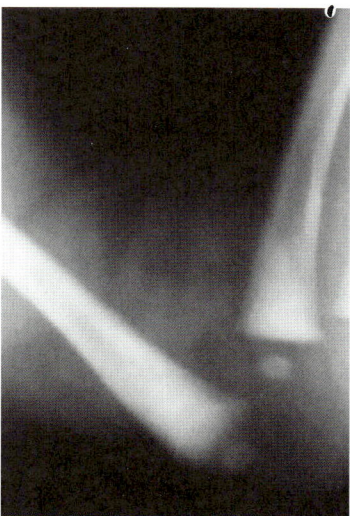

Fig. 48.9: Plain X-ray showing congenital dislocation of the knee joint

Developmental Disorders

ACHONDROPLASIA

It is a defect in the endochondral ossification of the bone, with the membranous ossification being normal. This is the most common type of dwarfism one encounters in clinical practice. The limbs are short and the head is big, because, along with the growth of the limbs, growth of the base of the skull is affected but the membranous bones of the vault escape.

Incidence: It is around 1.5–2/10,000 live births.

Clinical Features

The patient is a short-limbed dwarf. The fingers are short and stumpy (star fish hand) and do not reach below the upper one-third of the thigh as he stands (Fig. 49.1). Patient can kiss his toes with the knees straight. Head is large, nose is flattened but the length of the trunk may be normal and occasionally may show kyphoscoliosis or lordosis. Cervical lordosis and increased lumbar lordosis develop in the later stages of the disease (Fig. 49.2). The intelligence and sexual developments are normal.

X-ray findings: Ilium is quadrilateral in shape, coxa vara. Scalloping of the vertebral body, narrow spinal canal and foramen magnum, widened metaphysis at the ends of long bones, etc. (Fig. 49.3) are seen.

QUICK FACTS

Do you know the common causes of dwarfism?
- Achondroplasia
- Cretinism
- Diaphyseal aclasia
- Hunter, Hurler and Morquio's disease
- Malnutrition, etc.

Treatment

No treatment is required as the patient is able to lead a normal life. However, limb-lengthening procedures to increase the height (Ilizarov's technique) could be an option of the patient desires so. Canal stenosis at the cervical and lumbar level may need decompression at later stages of life.

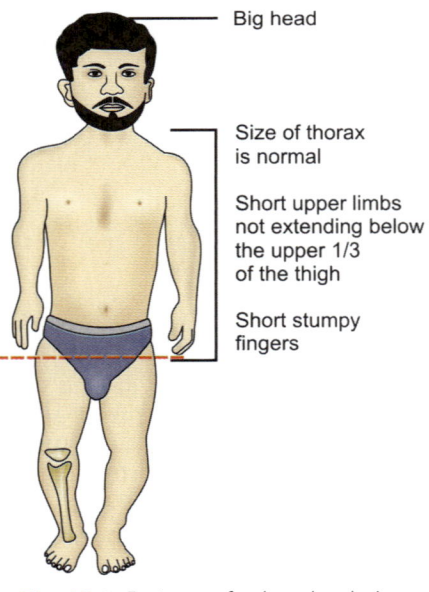

— Big head

— Size of thorax is normal

— Short upper limbs not extending below the upper 1/3 of the thigh

— Short stumpy fingers

Fig. 49.1: Features of achondroplasia

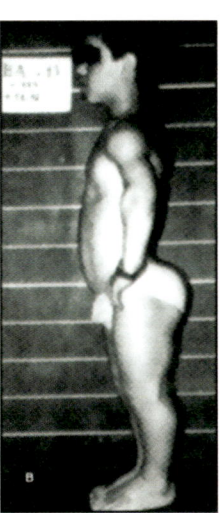

Fig. 49.2: Clinical photo-graph showing features of achondroplasia

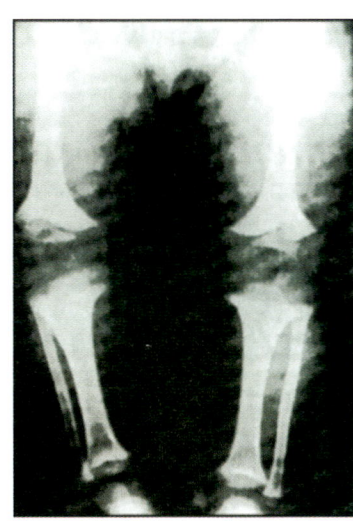

Fig. 49.3: Radiograph features in achondroplasia

Remember

About achondroplasia
- Failure of endochondral ossification
- Commonest type of dwarf
- Normal intelligence
- Usually employed as a clown
- Limb lengthening procedures help

OSTEOGENESIS IMPERFECTA

It is a hereditary condition characterized by fragility of bones, deafness, blue sclera, laxity of joints and a tendency to improve with age. It is a disease of the mesodermal tissues with deposition of normal collagen in bone, skin, sclera and dentine.

Etiology

The etiological factors could be heredity, Mendelian recessive—in prenatal cases, and Mendelian dominant—in postnatal cases.

49

Pathogenesis and Pathology and Intramembranes

Primary defect is failure of osteoblast formation during endochondral ossification; osteoid formation does not take place and the trabeculare are thin and break easily.

Classification: Shapiro's types:
1. *Osteogenesis imperfecta congenita:* Here fractures occur at utero or at birth
2. *Osteogenesis imperfecta tarda:* Here fractures can occur after birth either before or after the patient starts walking.

Clinical Features

Patient presents with blue sclera, dentinogenesis imperfecta and generalized osteoporosis (Figs 49.4A and B). Blue sclera is seen only in 92 percent of cases, while the other two features are seen in almost all cases. Osteoporosis gives rise to bowing and multiple fractures. Fractures are usually due to trivial trauma but surprisingly heals well. Other features include deafness due to otosclerosis, laxity of joints, dwarfism, broad skull, poorly calcified decidual teeth but permanent teeth are normal and the blood chemistry is normal, pencil thin cortex, plastic bowing, etc.

Remember

The mnemonic **BLOOD** in osteogenesis imperfecta
- **BL**—Blue sclera
- **O**—Otosclerosis
- **O**—Osteoporosis
- **D**—Dentinogenesis imperfecta.

QUICK FACTS

Do you know the **4 Os** responsible for easy fracture?
- Osteoporosis
- Osteopetrosis

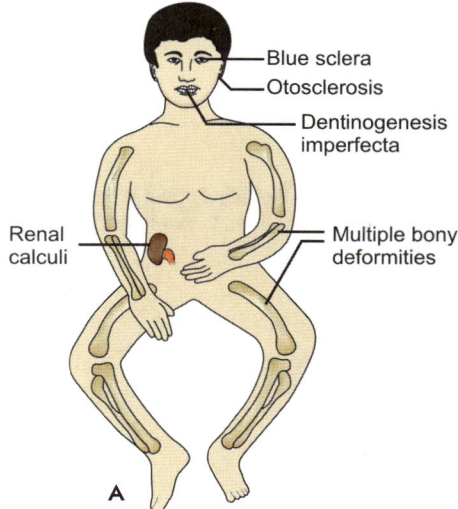

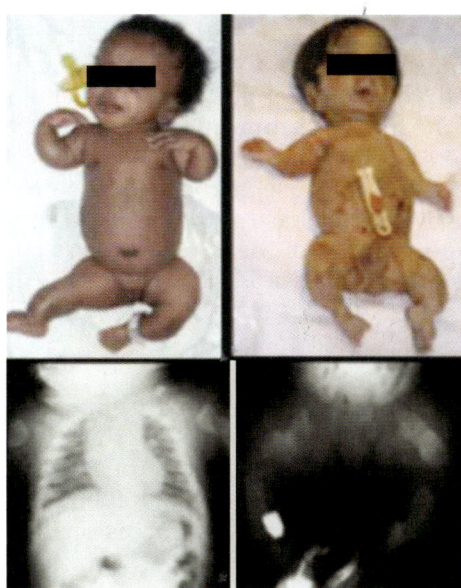

Figs 49.4A and B: (A) Features of osteogenesis imperfecta, (B) clinical photograph and X-ray findings

- Osteomalacia
- Osteogenesis imperfecta

3 Fs in osteogenesis imperfecta
- Fragile bones
- Fractures—multiple and frequent
- Fetal variety is fatal

Laboratory Investigations

There is no specific laboratory test for this disease but alkaline phosphatase. Prenatal determination of the probability of osteogenesis imperfecta on the fetus can be achieved by amniocentesis and estimation of *inorganic pyrophosphate*. This compound is elevated 3 to 4 times the normal value. Plain X-ray shows multiple malunited fractures at different sites (Fig. 49.5).

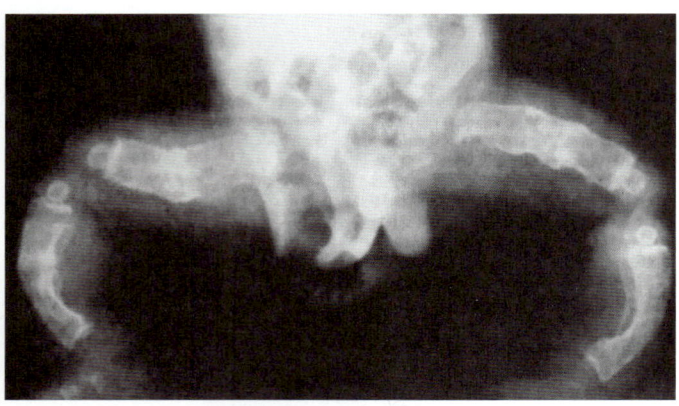

Fig. 49.5: Radiograph features in osteogenesis imperfecta

Treatment

Principles

Protect the child until the tendency of the fracture lessens as age advances.

Administer vitamins, biphosphonates estrogens and androgens.

Operate in infantile type as the tendency to fracture is much higher and hence the treatment of choice is multiple osteotomies with intramedullary nailing.

Hereditary multiple exostosis (Diaphyseal aclasia) is autosomal dominant and there is a failure of bone remodeling, excess of metaphysis is not resorbed, but forms irregular cartilage capped exostosis.

Clinical Features

Skull and spine are normal but the patient is slightly short stature and may present with multiple bony lumps in the following areas: upper humerus, lower end of radius and ulna, around knee, around ankle and flat bones.

FIBROUS DYSPLASIA

Fibrous dysplasia is a rare disease with fibrous replacement of bones. It may be *monostotic or polyostotic.*

Etiology

It is unknown, begins in childhood, progresses beyond puberty and has equal incidence in both sexes.

Pathology

Gross: Bone is irregular and bent, long bones are shortened, pathological fractures heal readily, **shepherd crook deformity** (shaft of femur bowed, varus neck) is seen in upper femur and is the hallmark of this disease and base of skull becomes hyperostotic.

Microscopy: This shows dense collagen tissue, giant cells are sparse, and islands of cartilage is seen in only 10 percent cases.

Clinical Features

Clinical features in early childhood are mild and asymptomatic. Onset is seen in less than 10 years of age. Patient may present with limp, pain, and fractures. Females have abnormal vaginal bleeding. Bending deformity and shortening of the bones are common features and lengthening is rare. *Shepherd crook deformity is quite characteristic*. There is asymmetry of the head and face and local irregular brown patches if seen are associated with polyostotic types. Sexual precocity is typical in females.

Albright's Syndrome

It is a unilateral polyostotic fibrous dysplasia with sexual precocity in females.

Mazabrand Syndrome

This is polyostotic fibrous dysplasia with myxoma of the skeletal muscles.

Laboratory Investigation

Serum calcium, phosphorus, alkaline phosphatase are normal. In severe cases alkaline phosphatase may increase.

Radiology

Localized lesions are cystic, multilocular, and show ground glass appearance, pathological fracture may occur. Shepherd crook deformity (Fig. 49.6) and Harrison's grooves following rib fractures, intrapelvic protrusion of acetabulum, and hyperostosis at the base of the skull, are the other important features.

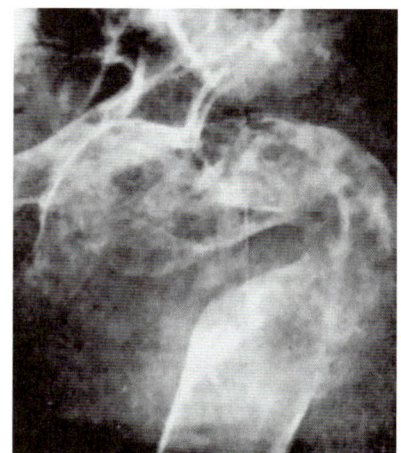

Fig. 49.6: Shepherd crook deformity in fibrous dysplasia

4 Ss in fibrous dysplasia
- **S**hepherd crook deformity
- **S**exual precocity in females
- **S**erum investigations are normal
- **S**urgery is the treatment of choice

49

Treatment

Surgery is the treatment of choice in fibrous dysplasia and consists of open reduction and internal fixation with bone grafting.

PAGET'S DISEASE

Paget's disease is seen after 40 years of age and is more common in males. There is impairment in the bone resorption and bone formation due to defective osteoclastic functions. As a result of this bone gets thickened and bent more so the tibia. Bone is soft in the initial stages and dense later.

Clinical Features

The affected bones are thickened and bent. Patient complains of dull bone pain and deformities (Fig. 49.7) of the long bones. Headache, dizziness, neuritic and arthritic pains, etc. are the other complaints.

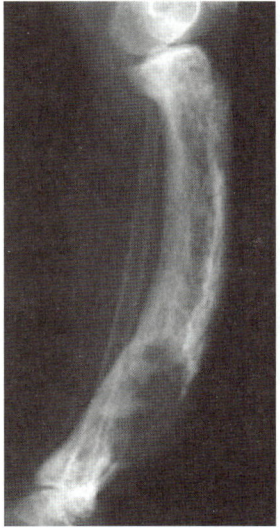

Fig. 49.8A: Plain X-ray of Paget's disease

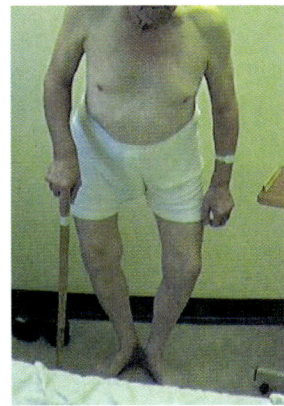

Fig. 49.7: Clinical photograph of Paget's disease

Investigations

Serum alkaline phosphatase serum and urinary hydroproline are increased, calcium and phosphorous are normal.

Radiology

Shows multiple lytic areas with intervening newbone formation (Figs 49.8A to C).

Treatment

This is essentially conservative and the drugs of choice are calcitonin or diphosphonate.

OSTEOCHONDRITIS

These are disorders of the growing epiphysis in children and adolescents. The affected epiphyses are softened and are vulnerable to be deformed due to pressure. Among various sites, femoral head affection (Perthes' disease) is the commonest and has been dealt in detail earlier. Table 49.1 shows other types of ostoechondritis:

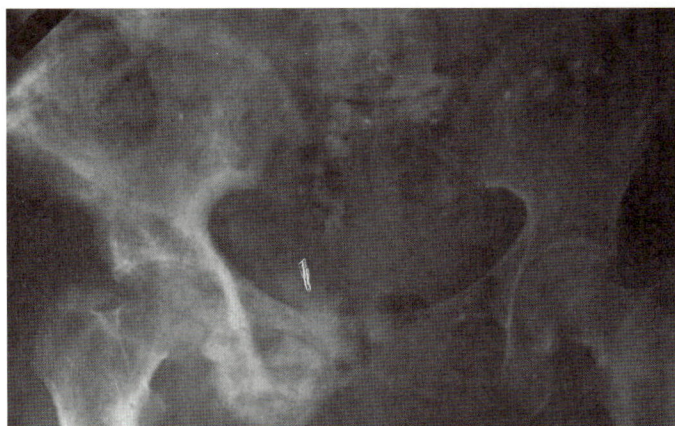

Fig. 49.8B: Plain X-ray of Paget's disease

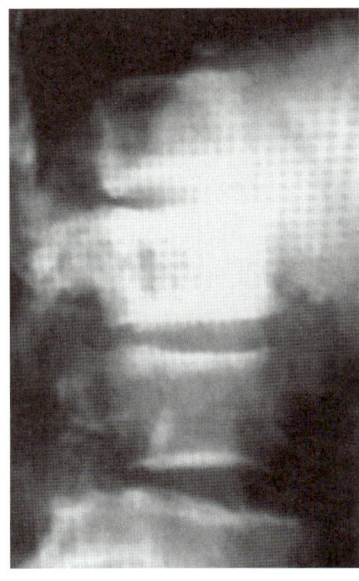

Fig. 49.8C: Radiograph features in Paget's disease

49

Table 49.1: Types of osteochondritis

Diseases	Bone attacks
• Prieser's disease	Scaphoid
• Panner's disease	Capitulum
• Keinbok's disease	Lunate
• Frieberg disease	2nd metatarsal head
• Kohler's disease	Navicular bone
• Calve's disease	Centred vertebral epiphysis
• Perthes' disease	Upper femoral epiphysis
• Scheuermann's disease	Vertebral ring epiphysis
• Osgood-Schlatter	Tibial tuberosity
• Sever's disesae	Calcaneal epiphysitis

QUICK FACTS: OTHER IMPORTANT DEVELOPMENT DISORDERS IN A NUTSHELL

I. Mucopolysaccharide Disorders

1. *Morquio-Brailsford disease*
   • Normal development till 5 years.
   • Dwarfism present
   • Manubriosternal angle greater than 90 degrees (Pathognomonic)
   • Flat vertebra with narrow tongue of bone projecting forwards (Platyspondyly)
   • Keratin sulphate in urine.
2. *Hurler's disease* (Gaegoylism)
   • Rarely survive into adulthood.
   • Mental retardation
   • Dermatin and Heparin sulphate in urine.
   • Coarse skin, wide set eyes and corneal opacity.
3. *Hunter's disease*
   • Less severe than Hurler's
   • All patients are males.

II. Epiphyseal Dysplasias

1. *Epiphyseal Dysplasia Multiplexa*
   • Very rare
   • Epiphysis appears early and closes early leading to deformities
   • Familial
2. *Epiphyseal Dysplasia Punctata*
   • Variation of the above.
   • More severe
3. *Conradi's Disease*
   • Mental retardation

   • Dwarfism, cataract
   • Congenital heart disease
4. *Epiphyseal Hemimelia*
   • Only ankle, knee of one limb involved.
   • One half of the epiphysis either medial or lateral is involved.

III. Metaphyseal Dysplasia

1. *Pyle's Disease*
   • Autosomal recessive
   • Failure of remodeling of the metaphysis
   • Erlenmeyer flask deformity of the distal femur and proximal tibia.
   • Genu valgum
2. *Cranio-Metaphyseal Dysplasia*
   • Autosomal dominant
   • Confused with Pyle's disease
   • Metaphyseal widening
3. *Metaphyseal Chondrodysplasia*
   • Autosomal dominant
   • Metaphysis is irregular and lytic

IV. Diaphyseal Dysplasia

1. *Engelmann's Disease (Progressive Diaphyseal Dysplasia)*
   Fusiform widening and sclerosis of the shafts of the long bones.
   • Long bones are symmetrically affected.
2. *Craniodiaphyseal Dysplasia*
   • Expansion of the long bone shafts
   • Gross thickening of the skull and face.

V. Miscellaneous

1. *Nail Patella Syndrome*
   • Autosomal dominant
   • Nails are hypoplastic
   • Patella is small and absent
2. *Marfan's Syndrome*
   • Autosomal dominant
   • Defect in the elastin collagen
   • Ocular lens dislocation
   • Tall with disproportionate legs
   • Aortic aneurysm
3. *Apert's Syndrome (Acrocephalosyndactyly)*
   • Autosomal dominant
   • Head is tower-shaped
   • Syndactyly of fingers and toes are seen.
4. *Carpenter's Syndrome:* This is Apert's syndrome with polydactyly.

49

50 Metabolic Bone Disorders

Rickets
Osteomalacia
Hyperparathyroidism
Osteoporosis
Scurvy
Fluorosis
Lathyrism

RICKETS

It is a metabolic bone disease of childhood in which, the osteoid, the organic matrix of bone, fails to mineralize due to interference with calcification mechanism. It is usually common between six months and two years.

Causes

Four main causes
1. *Vitamin D deficiency*
   - Reduced dietary intake*
   - Reduced amount of sunlight*
   - Pigmented skin
2. *Malabsorption due to*
   - Celiac disease
   - Hepatic osteodystrophy
3. *Renal disease:*
   - Glomerular failure
   - Renal osteodystrophy
4. *Antiepileptic drugs* favors formation of hepatic enzyme, which prevents conversion of calciferol.

> **Remember: About Vitamin D**
> - Two principal vitamin D's nutritionally useful are calciferol D2 and cholecalciferol D3.
> - 1, 25-dihydroxy vitamin D is formed in the kidney and is in the active form.
> - It aids in the absorption of calcium from the gut.
> - It is necessary for calcium deposition in bone.
> - Its lack upsets the calcification of cartilage and mineralization of osteoid.

Metabolic Abnormality in Rickets

Vitamin D 1, 25 (DH) 2-D3 Calcium
Absorption → Hypocalcemia PTH
Ca level → Bone resorption increased
Compensatory attempts to bone formation

Alkaline phosphatase negative Ca and P level
Ca level is increased by mobilization of bone stock, increased intestinal absorption, decreased renal excretion and decreased phosphate absorption.

> **QUICK FACTS**
> Do you know the daily requirements of calcium?
>
> | | |
> |---|---|
> | Adult | 50 mg |
> | Child | 00 mg |
> | Adolescent | 1000–1300 mg |
> | Pregnant women | 1500 mg |
> | Lactating women | 2000 mg |
> | Postmenopausal women | 1500 mg |
> | Major fracture | 1500 mg |

Pathology

Bones of the skeletal system: Bones are soft and porotic and bend easily. Epiphyseal line of 2 mm is normal but in rickets it forms a wide irregular band. Metaphysis is broad and irregular. Bony trabeculae are weak and continued stimulation makes the connective tissue hyperplasic, so that the extremity of bone appears misshaped and unmodelled.

These changes are most marked at the actively growing part of the bone and only affect the bone being deposited during the active phase of the disease. Bone formed before and after the active phase is normal.

Types of Rickets

Fetal rickets is commonly seen in osteomalacic mothers.

Infantile rickets (nutritional rickets) this is rare before 6 months and is the most common form of rickets seen in 6 months to 3 years of life.

Late rickets or rachitis tarda this is late onset rickets, familial and it is vitamin D resistant rickets.

> **QUICK FACTS**
> **Varieties of rickets**
> Type I This is due to dietary deficiency or defects in metabolism of vitamin D.
> Type II This is due to low serum phosphorus due to dietary phosphate deficiency or defective tubular resorption. This is vitamin D resistant rickets and is also called hypophosphatemic rickets.
> *Type I Dietary deficiency of vitamin D is the most common variety of rickets.*

Clinical Features

Symptoms: Patient complains of bone pain during rest, and excessive perspiration in upper half of the body. He or she loathes using the limb and the weakness of proximal muscles of the lower limbs produces waddling gait. There is evidence of catarrh of mucus membranes (recurrent diarrhea, constipation, bronchitis). Irritability of CNS produces convulsions, laryngismus, spasmophilia, Chvostek's sign, opisthotonos, etc. (Fig. 50.1).

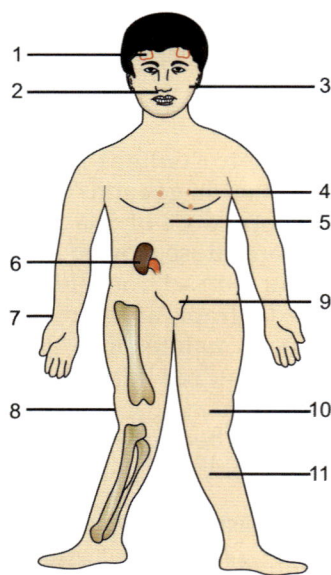

Fig. 50.1: Nutritional rickets: (1) frontal bossing, (2) dentition changes, (3) Chvostek's sign, (4) chest changes, (5) malabsorption, (6) aminoaciduria, (7) expanded wrist, (8) genu valgum, (9) pelvic obliquity, (10) myopathy, (11) skin changes

Deformities of Rickets (from head to toe)

Skull

- Broadened forehead
- Skull squared (caput quadratum)
- Frontal and parietal bossing—seen after the age of 6 months.
- Craniotabes is a ping-pong sensation on compressing the membranous bones of the skull.
- Spine kyphoscolosis

Chest (Fig. 50.2)

- Pigeon chest due to prominent sternum.
- Narrow chest.
- Rickety rosary (enlargement of costochondral junction).
- Harrison's sulci due to diaphragmatic pull on the soft ribs.

Bones

- *Enlargement of the metaphysal segments* of long bones like radius, tibia, costochondral junction, etc. are seen in children between 6 and 9 months of age.
- *Vertebral columns* show exaggerated curvature.
- *Pelvis* is trefoil shaped.
- *Coxa vara*
- *Femur* is bent anteriorly and laterally.
- *Bowed tibia* (Fig. 50.3).
- *Knock knee (genu valgum) more so in renal rickets* (Fig. 50.4).

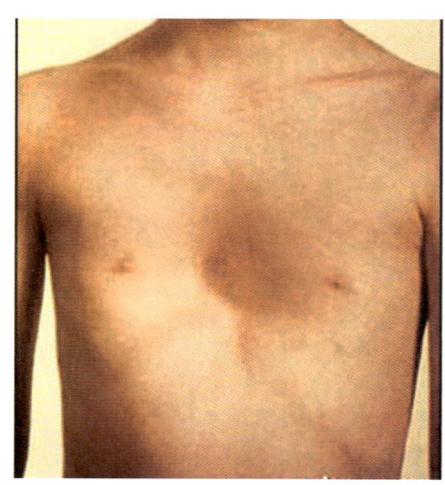

Fig. 50.2: Chest changes

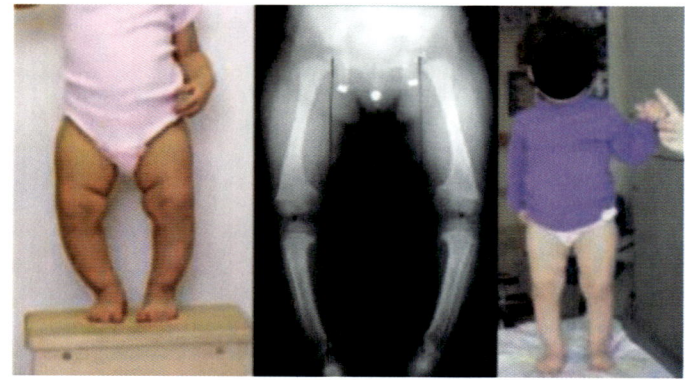

Fig. 50.3: Clinical photograph and X-ray showing knee changes in rickets

Other Features

Other features encountered in rickets are wizened look, delayed dentition, prominent abdomen, separation of recti, pale and flabby skin and incomplete fractures, etc.

Investigations

X-rays of the distal end of the forearm, and around the knees show characteristic changes typical of rickets (Figs 50.5 and 50.6). These changes help in the early detection of ricket (See box).

50

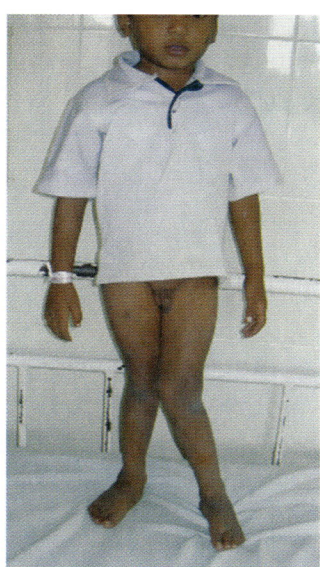

Fig. 50.4: Genu valgum in renal rickets

50

Remember

Characteristic X-ray findings
- Delayed appearance of epiphysis and widening of the epiphyseal plates.
- Champagne glass appearance (widening and cupping of the distal ends of long bones) also called 'trumpeting'.
- Space between diaphysis and epiphysis is increased.
- Deformity and bowing of the ends of long bones.
- Thickened epiphysis.
- Decreased density of cortex (rarefaction).
- Trabecular pattern is course.

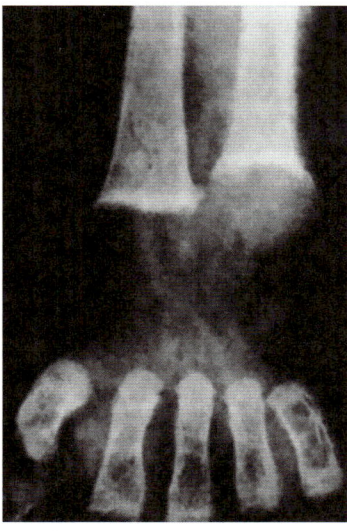

Fig. 50.5: Typical X-ray of the wrist metaphyseal cupping and irregularity of epiphyseal plates seen in rickets

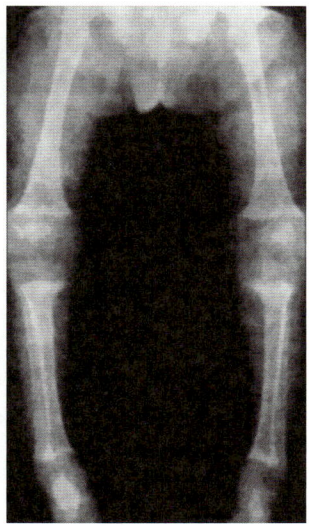

Fig. 50.6: Radiographic features of the knee in rickets

Biochemistry

- Calcium is normal or decreased (due to compensatory hyperparathyroidism).
- Serum phosphorus is low.
- Alkaline phosphatase is normal.
- Urinary calcium is low (excretion less than 5 mg/kg/24 hr).
- Levels of 2, 5-hydroxyl D if low will indicate effectiveness of treatment.

Note: Importance of biochemical values in this condition is their return to normal upon correct therapy.

Treatment

Adequate exposure to sunlight is desirable. Medical treatment in the initial stages aims to bring about quick healing. A single oral dose of 6 lac IU of vitamin D is given. A second same dose may be required after 3 to 4 weeks of treatment if no sclerotic (healing sign) change is seen on the radiograph at the metaphyseal side of the growth plate. A maintenance dose of 4000 IU of vitamin D may be required if the child responds to the above treatment regimen.

Absolute and strict bed rest, ricket splints, etc. helps in prevention of deformities.

Treatment of Established Deformity

Correction by splints (Mermaid splint) this is mainly useful when the disease is active and if the deformity is slight. It is very effective in children and in preventing deformities concerning the lower limbs. However, it is slow and requires continual supervision.

Correction by osteotomy is indicated when deformity is near the joint and when the growth stops. It is done during III stage (Lovett's) (nonunion follows if done before). The procedure of choice is medial closed wedge osteotomy of the lower end of femur (MacEvans osteotomy).

Note: At least 6 months of medical treatment should have elapsed before contemplating surgical correction.

Differential Diagnosis

Acute poliomyelitis, congenital syphilis, septic arthritis, infantile scurvy, etc.

OSTEOMALACIA

It is the adult counterpart of rickets and is characterized by failure of mineralization and an excess of osteoid due to an interference with calcification mechanism. *The osteoid is increased at the cost of mineralized bone. It is primarily a vitamin D deficiency disease* (Figs 50.7A and B).

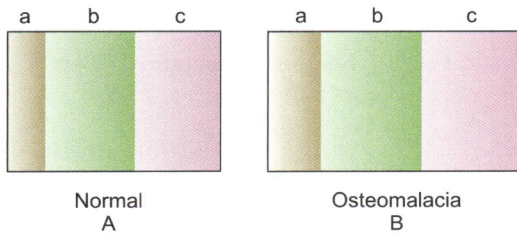

Figs 50.7A and B: (a) Osteoid, (b) bone, and (c) marrow

Etiology

- Decreased vitamin D intake or defective absorption from the intestine.
- Derangement of vitamin D and phosphorus metabolism (hereditary or acquired).
- Lack of exposure to sunlight: This is common in Muslim women who practice purdha system and this remain unexposed to sun for greater part of their lives.

Clinical Features

Patient complains of generalized skeletal pain and muscle weakness. There may be acute pain due to fracture. Other symptoms related to causative factors like dietary, renal and GIT may be seen. The following deformities are encountered, scoliosis, kyphosis, coxa vara, protrusio acetabuli, thighs and legs are bent, pelvis is trefoil, etc.

Radiographic features: Reveal generalized demineralization, loss of transverse trabeculae, no subperiosteal resorption of bone, etc. Presence of Looser's zones is quite characteristic of osteomalacia (Fig. 50.8).

They heal when osteomalacia is treated:

Spine: The bodies of spine are biconcave and are called "codfish spine".

Hip show protrusio acetabuli and triradiate pelvis.

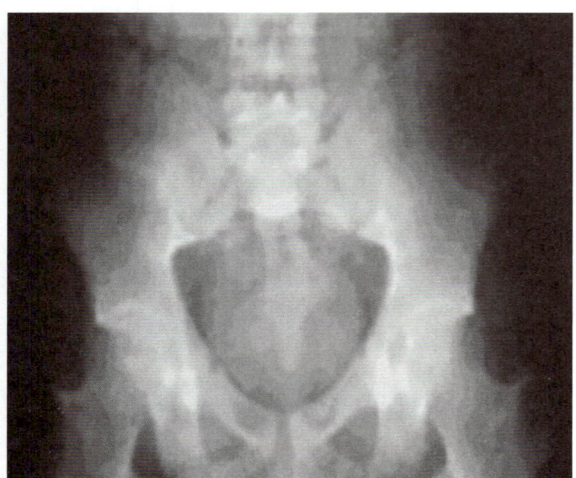

Fig. 50.8: Radiographic changes in osteomalacia

Remember

About looser's line

- Looser's line (Syn: Pseudo fracture, Milkman's line). It is transverse, bilaterally symmetrical and incomplete.
- Fractures healed with defective callus.
- Sometimes only evidence of osteomalacia in treated cases.

Sites: They commonly occur at sites of stress like:

- Axillary borders of scapula
- Ramus of pubis or ischium
- Neck of femur
- Ribs

Laboratory Investigations

Serum calcium is normal or decreased, serum phosphatase is normal or decreased, alkaline phosphatase is slightly increased (rarely exceeds 200 IU) and serum PTH is increased.

Conservative Treatment

Calcium is given at 0.5 to 3 gm/day, vitamin D 10,000 IU/day, and high protein diet. In vitamin D deficiency, 10,000 IU of vitamin D followed by a daily maintenance dose of 400 IU is recommended. In renal diseases, alfa-calcidol is the drug of choice. Calcium needs to be supplemented in daily divided doses of 0.5 to 3 gm. The gastrointestinal tract errors are also corrected simultaneously.

HYPERPARATHYROIDISM

Parathyroid secretes parathyroid hormone, excessive secretion of which results in hyperparathyroidism. It may be *primary or secondary.*

PRIMARY HYPERPARATHYROIDISM (Osteitis Fibrosa Cystica, von Recklinghausen's Disease)

Parathormone *increases serum calcium and decreases serum phosphorus through its action on kidney, bone and intestines (See Box).*

Remember

About parathormone

- Secreted by principal or chief cells of parathyroid
- Maintains serum calcium level
- Lowers serum phosphorus level
- Increases diuresis of phosphorus
- Promotes renal and intestinal reabsorption of calcium
- Stimulates action of osteoclasts
- It will directly affect dissolution of bone
- Inhibits calcifying effect of vitamin D
- Increases solubility of calcium and phosphorus

Pathogenesis

Rise in the level of parathormone causes increased osteoclastic activity, which resorbs the bone.

50

Consequently, there is increased osteoblastic activity resulting in fibrous replacement of bone and consequent weakening.

Pathology

An adenoma in the parathyroid glands is usually seen.

Causes

Adenoma accounts for more than 90 percent of the cases, carcinoma is rare and hyperplasia of the chief cells is seen in 6 percent of the cases.

Clinical Features

This disease equally affects both sexes. It is common in middle-aged women. Patient complains of severe pain and tenderness over the back and lower limbs, generalized muscle weakness and hypotonia. Pathological fractures and delayed union may be seen. Deformities of limbs and spine are common features. Hyperphosphaturia, polyuria, polydipsia, renal calculi are some of the urinary complications.

Skeletal changes seen are diffuse bone resorption due to increased osteoclastic activity, multiple deformities (because bone is soft due to replacement with fibrous tissue), pathological fractures, marrow fibrosis, brown tumor due to cavities filled with blood, multiple bone cysts, etc. Fracture healing is normal.

Radiology

Radiographic features show generalized rarefaction, trabeculae and cortex are thin, cysts and bending deformities, diffuse osteoporosis of skull, pin head stippling of skull (also called salt and pepper appearance), vertebrae are porotic and indented by discs, demineralization of mandible, disappearance of lamina dura in the tooth. Subperiosteal resorption of the phalanges is quite characteristic (Fig. 50.9).

> **Remember**
>
> **Radiological highlights in hyperparathyroidism**
> - *Skull:* Salt and Pepper appearance or also called pinhead stippling.
> - *Tooth:* Loss of lamina dura (a thin cortical sheet surrounding the tooth).
> - *Spine:* Central vertebral body collapse and biconcave discs.
> - *Phalanges:* Subperiosteal resorption.
> - *All bones:* Diffuse ground glass appearance.

Laboratory Investigations

Increased calcium and decreased phosphorus levels in the serum, hypercalciuria, hyperphosphaturia and increased alkaline phosphatase are some of the important laboratory findings.

Treatment

Medical treatment consists of providing large doses of calcium, phosphorus and vitamin D. Treatment of choice is parathyroidectomy. For hyperplasia, three glands and a portion of the fourth are removed. Preoperative calcium is avoided.

Orthopedic management consists of support by splints and corrective osteotomies for bony deformities.

Secondary Hyperparathyroidism

Normal kidneys eliminate phosphorus easily. When kidney is diseased, phosphorus is not excreted. Increased levels of phosphorus in serum results in increased calcium and phosphorus levels in the serum and the excess is deposited in the tissues. This is the pathogenesis in secondary hyperparathyroidism and is seen in certain diseases of the kidney.

Eventual result is renal rickets in a child and renal osteomalacia in an adult. This is high phosphorus rickets compared to normal or low phosphorus rickets in vitamin D deficiency (Fig. 50.10).

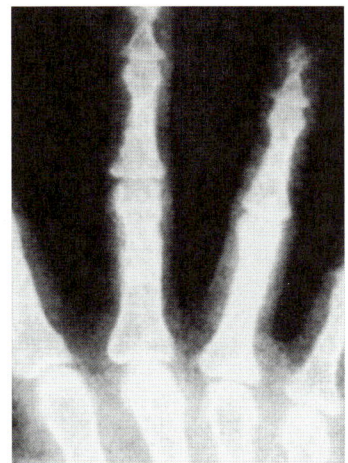

Fig. 50.9: Extensive subperiosteal resorption of bone in hyperparathyroidism

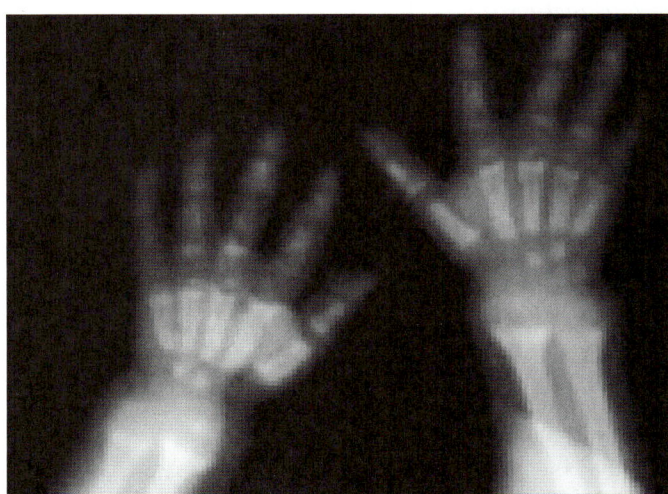

Fig. 50.10: Radiological features in secondary hypoparathyroidism

OSTEOPOROSIS

It is a generic term referring to a state of decreased mass per unit volume of a normally mineralized bone due to loss of bone proteins (Fig. 50.11).

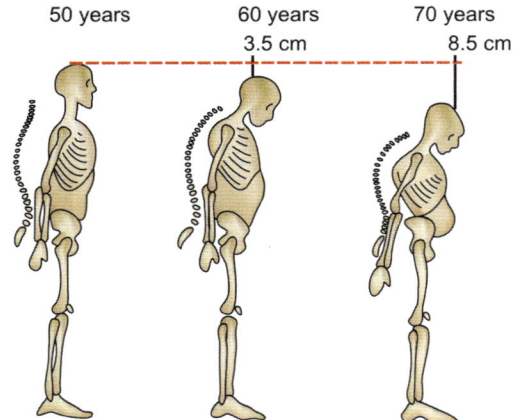

Fig. 50.11: Progressive loss of height in osteoporosis

Causes

1. Senility
2. Postmenopausal women
3. *Disuse*
   - Prolonged bed rest or inactivity
   - Prolonged casting or splinting
   - Paralysis, space travel, etc.
4. *Diet*
   - Calcium, protein, vitamin C low in the diet
   - Chronic alcoholism
   - Anorexia nervosa.
5. *Drugs* whose prolonged use causes osteoporosis are heparin, methotrexate, ethanol, glucocorticoids, etc.
6. *Idiopathic* variety is seen in adolescent and middle-aged male population.
7. *Genetic* role is seen in osteogenesis imperfecta.
8. *Chronic illness* like rheumatoid arthritis, cirrhosis, sarcoidosis, renal tubular acidosis.
9. *Neoplasm* like bone marrow tumors (myeloma, lymphoma, leukemia).
10. *Endocrine abnormalities* Hyperparathyroidism, increased levels of glucocorticoids, estrogens, etc.

Remember

In osteoporosis
- Decreased density is due to deficiency of protein matrix in which calcium is laid down
- Here rate of bone resorption is greater than bone formation
- Most commonly it is due to aging process
- But the most common cause is involutional bone loss in perimenopausal women

---

About osteopteorosis
It is the most common skeletal disorder in the world, next only to arthritis. In osteoporosis, there is a long latent period before clinical symptoms develop. Most prevalent complications are fractures of vertebral bodies, ribs, proximal femur, humerus, distal radius with minimal trauma. Most common cause is involutional bone loss in perimenopausal age group.

Clinical Features

Osteoporosis most of the times does not produce any symptoms and hence is called a "silent disease". However in the event of complications, patient presents with the following complaints.

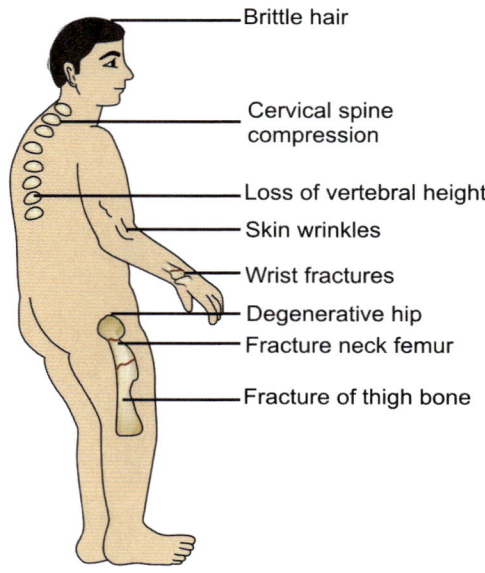

Fig. 50.12: Clinical findings of osteoporosis

Early symptoms: Patient complains of acute pain in middle or low thoracic or high lumbar region. Sudden movement, sitting, sneezing, cough, etc. increases pain. Rest relieves it. However, in some cases, fractures of axial skeleton may be seen with trivial trauma. Round type of gibbus due to compression of thoracic vertebrae is commonly seen. Patients with osteoporosis exhibit progressive loss of height. Other features of osteoporosis are as shown in Fig. 50.12. *Most common symptom of osteoporosis is back pain secondary to vertebral compression* (Fig. 50.13).

Investigations

This consists of plain X-rays, bone densitometry studies and laboratory tests
Radiology: Changes seen in the spine are:
- Loss of vertebral height due to symmetric transverse compression.
- Biconcave central compression (codfish spine) due to the pressure of the bulging disc into the bodies.
- Anterior wedge compression (Fig. 50.14).

50

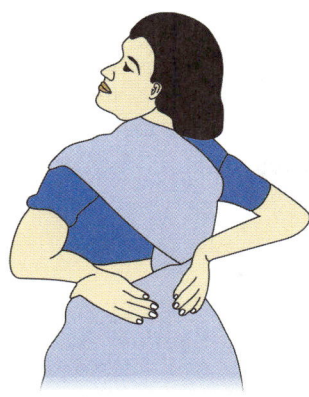

Fig. 50.13: Backache is the most common presentation in osteoporosis

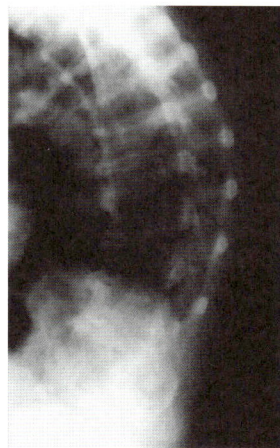

Fig. 50.14: Anterior wedge compression

Other bones
- Ground glass appearance due to generalized rarefaction.
- *Singh's index* this is the grading of trabecular pattern of the neck of femur from 1 to 6.
- Metacarpal index, etc.
- Pathological fractures.

Densitometry: This is the investigation of choice in osteoporosis
a. Single photon absorptiometry is used to assess the amount of cortical bone mineral in appendicular skeleton.
b. Dual photon absorptiometry and quantitative CT scan helps to assess the mineral status of axial skeleton.

> *Note:* Dual photo absorptiometry is the Gold Standard.

c. Total body neutron activation analysis to determine calcium content of the entire body.
d. *Transiliac bone biopsy:* It is an important diagnostic tool in patients of more than 50 years in postmenopausal diseases (Fig. 50.15).

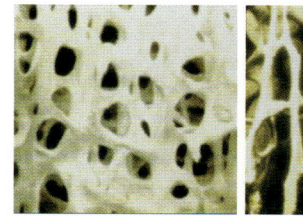
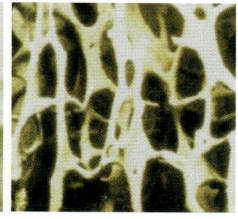

Normal bone   **Osteoporosis**

Fig. 50.15: Skeletal changes in osteoporosis

e. *Blood chemistry:* Serum calcium, phosphorus and alkaline phosphatase levels are normal.

Management of Osteoporosis

The following treatment regimen is recommended:
- *High protein diet* will help increase the organic matrix of the bone.
- *Diet:* Calcium rich foods like ragi, dairy products like milk, curds, butter, cheese.
- *Calcium supplementation* in those who do not take calcium rich foods. Calcium carbonate is the most commonly used calcium supplement.
- *Rest and drugs* like analgesics and anti-inflammatory drugs. Muscle relaxants and supports like belt, collar.
- *Spinal orthosis* when patient is erect and mobile to prevent and correct spine deformities.
- *Postural exercises* and back care (Figs 50.16A to C).

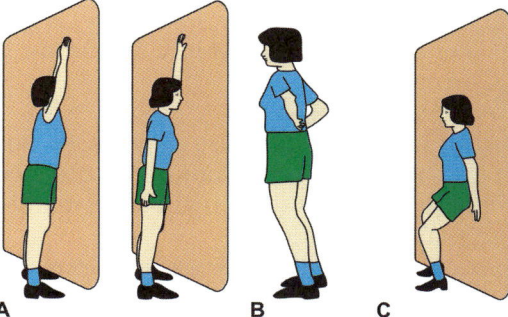

A   B   C

Figs 50.16A to C: Various posture correction exercises in osteoporosis patient (A) wall arching, (B) back bending (C) wall sliding exercises

Drug Therapy

- *Hormone replacement therapy (HRT):* Estrogen supplementation is the single most effective measure to prevent postmenopausal osteoporosis. It preserves positive calcium balance by bone remodeling.
- *Alendronate:* It is a biphosphonate drug and is useful in male patients and in those women who refuse HRT or in whom HRT is contraindicated.
- *Calcitonin:* It has been recently used for prevention of postmenopausal osteoporosis. It inhibits bone loss by preventing bone resorption.

- *Vitamin D and calcium* intake in sufficient quantities.
- *Regular exercises* like walking, swimming helps (Fig. 50.17) to improve the bone strength.
- *Fluorides* are beneficial in the treatment, but not in prevention as it stabilizes the bone mineral and stimulate osteoblasts to form new matrix.

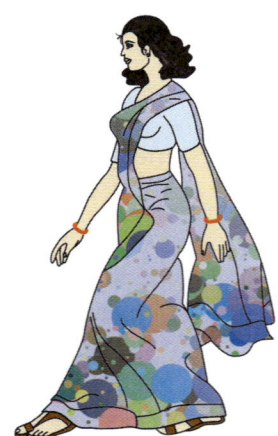

Fig. 50.17: Regular exercises like walking is of great help in elderly patients suffering from osteoporosis

SCURVY

It is a nutritional disorder caused by deficiency of vitamin C and is characterized clinically by a generalized hemorrhagic tendency. The severe form of disease is rare and mild varieties are more common. Deficiency targets the cells of skeletal system more often.

Etiology

- It is most frequent between 5 and 10 months in artificially fed infants.
- Children who take vitamin C-deficient diet.
- When seen with rickets it is called *Barton's disease*.

Pathology

Cohesive property of the matrix of connective tissue and endothelium is impaired resulting in capillary hemorrhage leading to gum bleeding, subperiosteal hemorrhage, etc.

Clinical Features

The affected child is restless, pale and febrile. The affected limb is swollen, tender, and painful, muscles are in spasm and the child loathes using the limb. This voluntary immobilization of the extremities is called *pseudoparalysis*. The gums display a bluish, spongy swelling especially around the upper central incisor teeth. Brittle and loose teeth, ecchymosis beneath the skin, hematemesis, hematuria, anemia, weight loss, anorexia, etc. are the other features (Fig. 50.18). Sometimes even death supervenes.

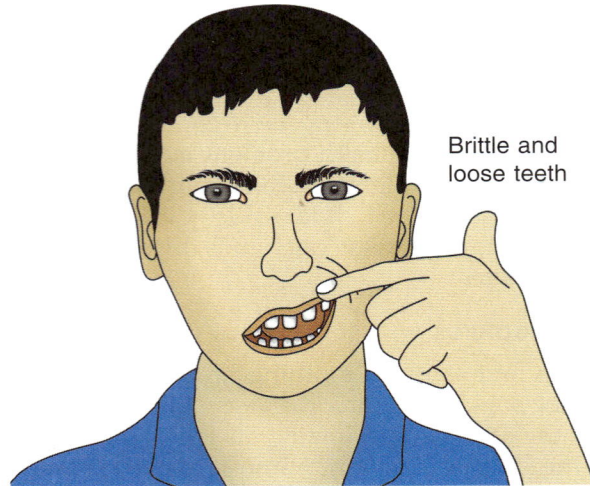

Brittle and loose teeth

Fig. 50.18: Clinical features of scurvy

The lower femur, the upper tibia and the upper humerus are favored sites for epiphyseal fracture separation. Costochondral separation is typical. Mild forms of scurvy are more common. In adults pain and tenderness over the bone and fracture with mild trauma is suggestive.

Investigations

Blood ascorbic acid level is normal and is around 0.5 mg/dl (N = 1 gm/dl)). Anemia is common.

Radiology

- Characteristic lines are seen (Fig. 50.19).
- Ground glass appearance of the bone.
- Subperiosteal fractures are seen.
- Epiphyseal fracture separation, etc. results.

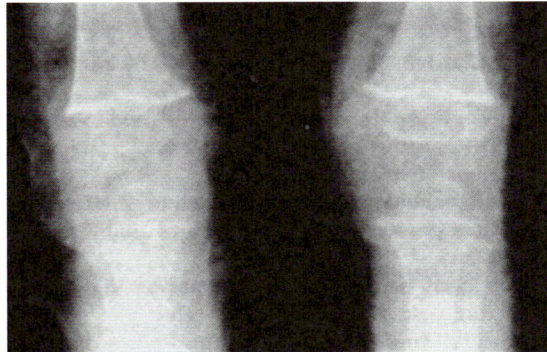

Fig. 50.19: Radiological lines in scurvy—white line of Frankel and Winberger's line

Treatment

Treatment is essentially conservative and consists of supplementing vitamin C in the diet and encouraging the child to take foods rich in other vitamins. The painful

50

joints and the fractures need to be immobilized with plaster splints.

FLUOROSIS

Fluorosis is a pubic health problem in our country in states like Andhra Pradesh, Tamil Nadu. It results when the fluoride content of drinking water exceeds 1 PPM. As a result, excess calcium is deposited in bone and soft tissues.

Clinical Features

Fluorosis first starts as mottling of the enamel of the upper incisors. Dental fluorosis results in the destruction of the tooth and ultimately its loss (Fig. 50.20).

In the skeletal system, spine is more commonly affected. The posterior longitudinal ligament is thickened and may compress the cord. This may lead to spastic paraparesis. Genu valgum is commonly seen (Fig. 50.21).

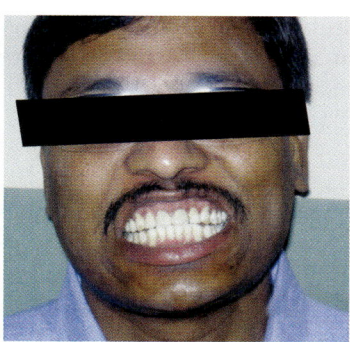

Fig. 50.20: Dental fluorosis

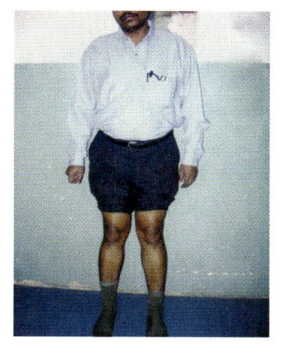

Fig. 50.21: Skeletal changes in fluorosis

Investigations

Tests reveal high fluoride levels in blood and urine. Radiographs show calcification at posterior longitudinal ligament in spine and intraosseous membrane in the leg and forearm. Pelvis, spine and other bones show increased density. Bone biopsy clinches the diagnosis.

Treatment

The patient is encouraged to drink defluorinated water. Preventing the disease by defluorination of drinking water is by far the best measure to tackle this menacing problem.

QUICK FACTS

Fluorosis is one of the leading causes of osteosclerosis. Do you know other conditions?
Remember the mnemonic **PRISM** to recall these:
P—Paget's disease
R—Renal rickets
I—Ingleman's disease
S—Secondaries are the bones from prostate, breast, etc.
M—Marble bone disease (Osteopetrosis)

LATHYRISM

In this condition the bones lose their customary hardness and become abnormally soft. Their blood vessels, especially the arteries, likewise develop aneurysm. All this is due to consumption of toxic foods containing lathyrisms which are known to alter the collagen of bones at other connective tissues.

50

51 Osteomyelitis

INTRODUCTION

Osteomyelitis is defined as a suppurative process of the bone caused by pyogenic organisms or simply a pyogenic infection of the cancellous portion of the bone.

Classification

Three types are described based on duration of symptoms, route of spread of infection and host response (Table 51.1).

Table 51.1: Classification of osteomyelitis		
Duration	*Route of spread Waldogel's*	*Host response*
1. Acute (<2 weeks)	1. Hematogenous (most common)	1. Pyogenic
2. Subacute (2–3 weeks)		2. Non-pyogenic
3. Chronic (>3 weeks)	2. Direct	
4. Residual	3. Contiguity	

Hematogenous spread with primary infection being elsewhere like tonsillitis, ASOM, pyoderma, etc. is the common mode of spread. Spread from neighboring infective sites like septic arthritis and direct inoculation of infecting organisms by way of penetrating wounds, punctured wounds, trauma, etc. come second.

ACUTE OSTEOMYELITIS

Etiology, the etiological factors causing osteomyelitis can be best understood if discussed under the following heads (Fig. 51.1).

Agent factors the following myriad of incriminating organisms is responsible for its causation:
- *"S" series organisms* ('S' denotes severe osteomyelitis and those organisms causing it start with the letter "S").
- *Staphylococcus aureus (60–85%).*

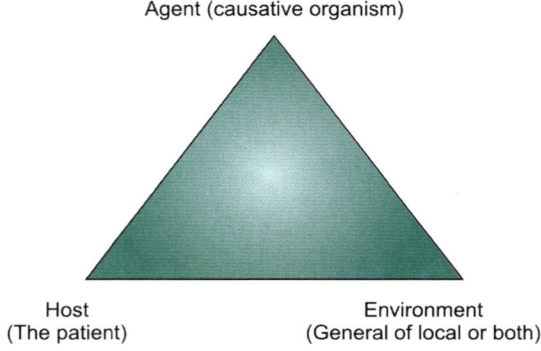

Fig. 51.1: Etiological factors causing osteomyelitis

This is the most common organism causing acute osteomyelitis.
- *Staphylococcus haemolyticus (8–10%).*
- *Salmonella* osteomyelitis is relatively rare and presents an interesting picture as most of its features start with "S".
  - Several bones involved
  - Symmetrical involvement of bones
  - Severe osteomyelitis
  - Spine may be involved
  - Sickle cell anemia present
  - Stool culture may be positive.
- *P-series organisms* (their mode of entry is through punctured wounds)
  - *Pseudomonas*
  - *Pneumococcus*
  C-series ('C' denotes compound fractures)
  - *Clostridium welchii*
  - Coliforms *(E.coli).*
  B-series
  - *Brucella bacillus.*
  H-series
  - *Haemophilus influenzae* (7 months to 4 years)
  This is known to cause osteomyelitis in the age group of 7 months to 4 years.
  T-series
  - *Treponema pallidum* (syphilitic osteomyelitis)
  - Tubercle bacillus (*Mycobacterium*).
  Fungal osteomyelitis (ABC)
  - Actinomycosis
  - Blastomycosis

– Cryptococcosis and coccidiodomycosis
These usually cause chronic osteomyelitis.

Host Factors

Age: In children the incidence is 88 percent (because more prone for injury and fall). *In adults,* it is 12 percent. Hence, it is predominantly a disease of childhood.

Sex: Male preponderance (? more playful).

Economic status: Low socioeconomic groups are more susceptible.

Environmental Factors

General factors: All the above mentioned general factors bring down the resistance of the patient thereby making them susceptible for infection (See box).

Local factors: All are extremely important in localizing the infection to the metaphysis (See box).

Hairpin bend of the metaphyseal vessels: This slows down the circulation for a moment, which is sufficient for the organisms to escape out (Fig. 51.2).

51

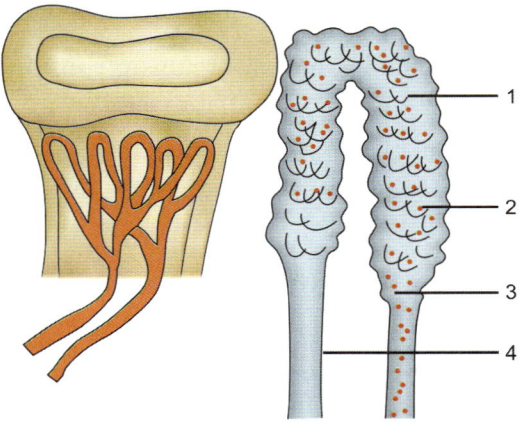

Fig. 51.2: Microanatomy of the hairpin bend vessels: (1) thrombosed vessel, (2) bacterial colonies, (3) artery, and (4) vein

Metaphyseal hemorrhage: Results from the bleeding due to microscopic trauma. The blood clot so accumulated acts as an excellent culture media for the escaped organisms to grow.

Defective phagocytosis: WBCs here are busy removing the debris of the decalcification due to growth process. Therefore, their function of eliminating the offending organism is slightly impaired.

Rapid growth at the metaphysis: Makes the cells more susceptible to the action of bacterial toxins as the cells are immature.

Vasospasm: Though protective as it arrests further bleeding from the traumatized vessels it also causes anoxia and failure of antibiotics and other defense cells from reaching the area.

Anoxia: It is due to vasospasm and it helps the bacteria grow.

Thus, acute osteomyelitis develops because of the combination of agent, host and environment factors.

QUICK FACTS

General factors	Local factors
• Anemia	• Responsible for localization of infection at metaphysis
	• Debility especially in children
• Infection	• Hairpin bend vessels
	• Poor nutrition
• Metaphyseal hemorrhage	• Poor immune status
• Defective phagocytosis	
• Rapid growth at metaphysis	
• Necrotic tissue acts as a culture media	
	• Anoxia
	• Vasospasm

Pathophysiology: The infection results in the formation of abscess at the region of metaphysis. The pus so formed finds its way out through the *area of least resistance*. In children less than 2 years, periosteum is loosely attached to the cortex and hence forms a potentially weak point. The subperiosteal abscess so developed will either spread through the soft tissues or drain to the outside by forming a sinus breaking the skin or it will percolate down towards the diaphysis between the periosteum and the cortex and enter the shaft through the widened haversian pores due to anoxia. The growth plate limits spread to the joint. Between 2 and 16 years, periosteum is firmly attached to the cortex and with the growth plate still present, the pus has to spread towards the diaphysis at a slow pace. Above 16 years the growth plate has disappeared, the periosteum is firmly adherent, and the pus spreads towards the diaphysis very slowly (Figs 51.3A to C, and 51.4).

QUICK FACTS: SPREAD IN ACUTE OSTEOMYELITIS

< 2 years	2–16 years	> 16 years
• Subperiosteal	• Subperiosteal	• Diaphysis (common (common) (rare) but very slow)
• Diaphysis (rare)	• Diaphysis	• Joint space involved
• Joint space (rare)	(common but slow) (rare)	• Extraperiosteal

Clinical Features

Acute osteomyelitis is a clinical catastrophe. It presents in the following manner.

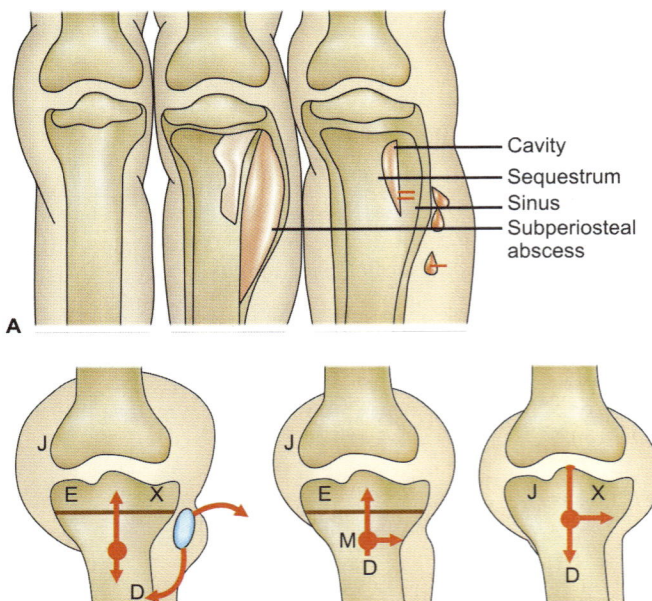

A

B **C** **D**

Figs 51.3A to D: (A) Pathological sequence in osteomyelitis (B) spread of pus from the metaphysis in children of less than 2 yr. Subperiosteal common, joint involvement rare but still joint can be involved in two ways: (1) If the capsule encloses the metaphyseal region, (2) Through the common blood supply from the nutrient vessel which gives rise to metaphyseal and epiphyseal vessels; (B) spread in children between 2–16 yr. In this age group, diaphyseal spread is common; and (C) spread in patients > 16 yr. In this age joint involvement may be direct because the growth plate has disappeared J joint, E epiphysis, M metaphysis, D diaphysis, and X no spread

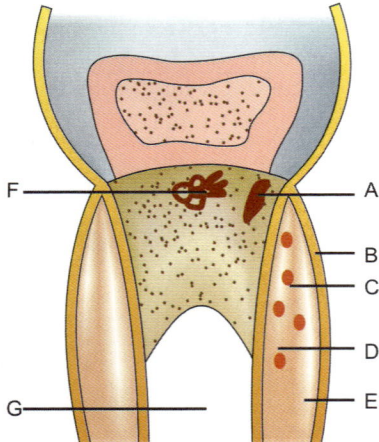

Fig. 51.4: Entire spectrum of pathological changes in osteomyelitis: (A) sequestrum, (B) periosteum, (C) pus, (D) cortex, (E) involucrum, (F) bone abscess, and (G) medullary cavity

Fever: This is the most common presenting symptom. The child usually has very high fever and is associated with profuse sweating, chills and rigors. Sometimes the presentation is so acute that the child may be in shock and unconscious.

Swelling: This usually follows the fever and may affect the ends of long bones. The swelling may be acutely painful and the skin may appear red.

Limitation of movement: The child may not move the joint near the affected bone due to pain and swelling. In fact, the child may lie still without moving the joint and this is sometimes called a state of pseudoparalysis.

Clinical Signs

General features of anemia, dehydration, pyrexia, pulse rate, shock and toxicity may be present.

Local features: The local swelling may show increased temperature may be tender to touch, and the skin is stretched. Movements of the neighboring joints are decreased and there may be effusion in them too.

Investigations: The investigations of acute and chronic osteomyelitis is compared for easy remembrance and understanding (Table 51.2). In general, in acute osteomyelitis laboratory investigations and bone scan are more useful while radiology is of much help in chronic osteomyelitis. Plain X-rays show subperiosteal reaction (Fig. 51.5).

51

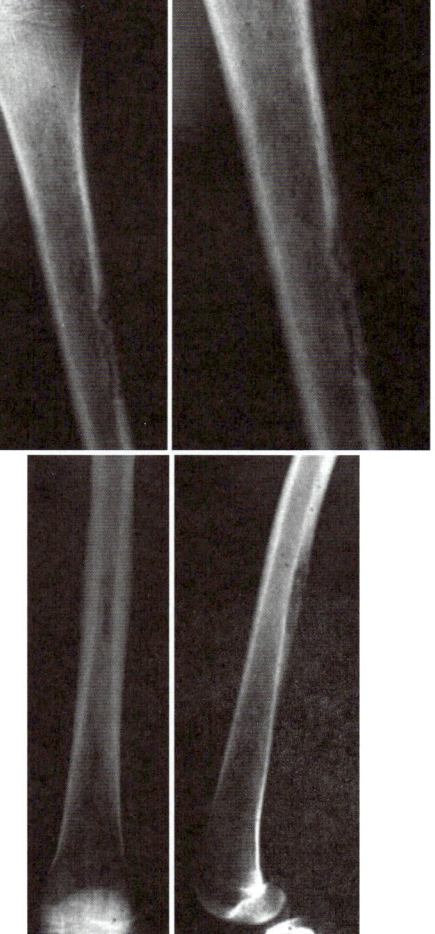

Fig. 51.5: Acute osteomyelitis

51

Table 51.2: Investigations in osteomyelitis

General	Acute osteomyelitis	Chronic osteomyelitis
Haemoglobin (%)	Normal or decreased	Decreased
ESR	Normal or increased	Increased
WBCs	Neutrophils Increased	Lymphocytes are increased
X-rays	< 48 hr	• Sequestrum identified by the denser X-ray shadow. The density is because of the impermeability for the X-rays.
	Few changes	
	• Rarefaction is the earliest sign	
	• Loss of demarcation of line between subcutaneous shadows and muscles	• Involucrum (new bone surrounding the sequestra)
	• Appearance of transverse lines of increased densities outward from the muscles > 2 weeks Periosteal new bone formation is seen	• Cloacae (holes through which sequestra is released)
		• Irregular bone thickening
	• Rarefaction	• ? Pathological fracture
Bone scan (Technetium 99m, GA-67, Indium-111- Labeled Leucocytes)	• Confirms diagnosis as early as 24–48 hr after the onset in 90–95% of cases in early stages	• Useful in detecting sequestrum
	• Focal area of early uptake	
	• But it cannot distinguish a tumor from infection (Non-specific)	
Blood culture (taken at three different times at least two hours apart)	Positive in 60%	—
Gram's staining (aspirate from infected bones) Sinograms	Helps choose the appropriate antibiotics	—
		• Methylene blue
		• Radiopaque dyes to identify sinus tract before doing sequestrectomy
Cement beads	—	• To identify avascular bone from vascular bone

Note: In acute osteomyelitis bone scan helps in early diagnosis with almost 100% accuracy. X-ray has its limitation. Chronic osteomyelitis can reasonably be diagnosed well on X-rays.

Management: Acute osteomyelitis is an orthopedic emergency, which needs in-patient admission. The management can be discussed as general and local.

General management (Fig. 51.6) Conservative management is the mainstay of treatment.

The mnemonic **RESTS** sums up the conservative line of treatment:

Rest in bed: Protect affected part with splints to alleviate pain and spasm.

Elevation of the part, warm and moist packs to reduce the swelling.

Systemic treatment consists of blood transfusion, intravenous fluids to correct shock and hypovolemia.

Treatment: With antibiotics discussed below helps to reduce toxicity.

Surgery: Properly indicated and timed to prevent complications.

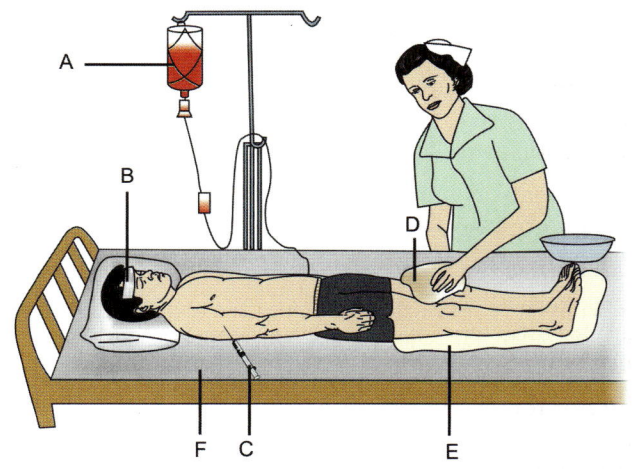

Fig. 51.6: Principles of treatment in acute osteomyelitis: (A) IV fluids and blood transfusion, (B) tepid sponging, (C) intravenous antibiotics, (D) cryotherapy, (E) splints and elevation of the affected part, (F) rest in bed and hospitalization

Drug Therapy

The drugs of choice are a combination of Cefotaxime (100–150 mg/kg body weight) and Amikacin (15 mg/kg body weight) for the first two weeks, are found to be very effective though penicillin G is still the drug of first choice in our country. Fusidic acid is preferred in the western countries.

Current trends in antibiotic therapy: This consists of a short course of intravenous antibiotics for a period of 2 weeks. Followed by oral antibiotics for further 4 weeks. Proper monitoring of the serum antibiotic level is very much essential to obtain good results.

Local management: The focus here is on well-timed surgery if any one of the following indications is present.

Nade's indications for surgery
- Abscess formation.
- Severely ill and moribund child.
- Failure to respond to intravenous antibiotics for more than 48 hr.

Surgical Methods

Depending upon the situation any one of the following surgical methods could be employed:
- *Aspiration* it helps in decompression and the material so obtained may be used to identify the organism and check for antibiotic sensitivity.
- *Incision and drainage* helps to drain the subcutaneous abscess.
- *Multiple drill holes* if the abscess is subperiosteal. This technique helps to drain the pus by making multiple holes in the cortex.
- *Small bone window* if the multiple drill holes do not drain the pus, a small window of bone is removed from the cortex and the pus is evacuated.

Differential Diagnosis

Acute septic arthritis: Here the infection is in the joint, in osteomyelitis it is in the bone near the joint. Hence, joint movements are severely restricted and more painful in acute septic arthritis.

Scurvy: Features of pseudoparalysis, bleeding gums, tender limbs, etc. are the features.

Acute anterior poliomyelitis: Here pain and tenderness are spread throughout the muscle mass whereas in osteomyelitis tenderness is greatest on direct pressure over the bone.

Cellulitis: It is difficult to differentiate from acute osteomyelitis; however, cellulitis has no edge, no fluctuation, no pus and no limits.

Other differential diagnosis: Erysipelas, erythema nodosum, Ewing's sarcoma, sickle cell anemia, etc. are some of the possible differential diagnosis.

Complications (seen in 5% of cases)

- Septicemia, pyemia are the common general complications.
- Septic arthritis due to extension of the neighboring foci of infection into the joint.
- Chronic osteomyelitis develops due to improper and inadequate treatment. The incidence rate is 5 to 10 percent.
- Pathological fractures and growth disturbances are relatively rare.
- Mortality rate is less than 2 percent due to early antibiotic therapy.

Characteristic points in acute osteomyelitis
- Disease is common in children.
- *Staphylococcus aureus* is the common organism.
- Metaphysis is involved.
- Fever is the common presenting symptom.
- Bone scan helps in early diagnosis.
- Conservative management is the mainstay of treatment and ninety percent resolve.

SUBACUTE OSTEOMYELITIS

Subacute osteomyelitis is caused by *Staphylococcus aureus*. Patient complains of pain without constitutional symptoms. Temperature may be increased or normal. It is not detected until at least two weeks has elapsed. Blood culture is positive in only 60 percent of cases, and WBC and ESR are raised in only 50 percent of the cases.

SUBACUTE OSTEOMYELITIS IS DUE TO
- Increased host resistance.
- Lowered bacterial resistance.
- If antibiotics are administered before symptoms appear.

CHRONIC OSTEOMYELITIS

Any osteomyelitis lasting for more than three weeks is termed as chronic. Chronic osteomyelitis can arise from any one of the following ways:
- Improper, inadequate and delayed treatment of the initial acute infections.
- Sequel of acute osteomyelitis (5–10%)
- Following compound fractures
- Following surgery on bones and joints
- Chronic from the beginning (e.g. tuberculosis, syphilis, Brodie's abscess)
- Anaerobic organisms (sclerosing osteomyelitis of Garre)
- Fungal osteomyelitis.

QUICK FACTS
Salient features in chronic osteomyelitis
- Systemic symptoms would have disappeared.
- One or more foci in the bone containing pus, sequestra or draining sinuses, etc.

51

- Acute exacerbation is due to trauma, lowered resistance, etc.
- Sites: Lower end of femur is the commonest site.

Clinical symptoms are very few. Fever, pain, swelling are seen in acute exacerbation of chronic osteomyelitis.

Signs

Irregular thickening of bone develops due to unequal pace of destruction of bone and new bone formation. This is a characteristic feature of chronic osteomyelitis.

Sinuses are usually multiple and are fixed to the underlying bone. The presence of sinuses indicates unabsorbed sequestra, unobliterated cavities and presence of anaerobic organisms. They are immobile and adherent to the bone. They heal and unheal periodically. The discharge through the sinus varies from serous to purulent (Figs 51.7A and B).

51

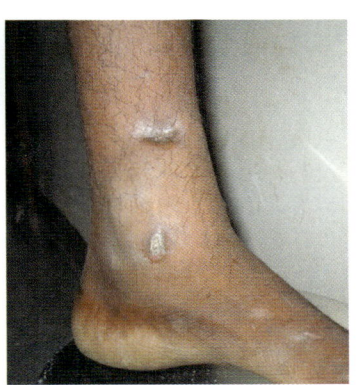

Fig. 51.7A: Chronic osteomyelitis

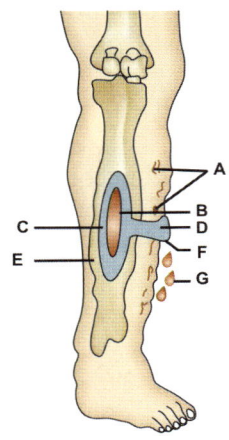

Fig. 51.7B: Features of chronic osteomyelitis: (A) multiple scars and sinuses, (B) sequestrum, (C) cavity, (D) cloacae, (E) irregular thickening of bone, (F) sprouting granulation tissue, (G) discharge of pus and bony spicules

Note: History of discharge of tiny bony spicules through the sinus, clinches the diagnosis of chronic osteomyelitis with certainty.

Scars and muscle contractures develop due to the spread of infection from the bones to the muscles and the consequent fibrosis.

Tenderness is present on deep palpation.
- *Joints in* the adjoining areas may be stiff due to soft tissue contractures.
- *Shortening or lengthening* of the bones may occur due to the affection or stimulation of the growing epiphysis respectively.
- *Deformities and decreased movements* develop due to scars and contractures.

- *Pathological fractures* may occur either due to chronic osteomyelitis, which weakens the bone, or due to extensive *debridement during surgery, which leaves a thin layer of bone* (Fig. 51.8B).

Note: Sequestra it is a dead bone within a living bone and is defined as an infected granulation tissue. The inflammatory foci are surrounded by sclerotic bone supplied with blood and covered by periosteum, scarred muscle and subcutaneous tissues.

QUICK FACTS: SEQUESTRA TYPES

Disease		Type of sequestra
TB osteomyelitis	→	Sandy or rice grains
Actinomycosis	→	Black
Pin tract infection	→	Ring
Chronic osteomyelitis in children	→	Diaphyseal
Syphilitic osteomyelitis	→	Ivory
Amputation stumps	→	Crown
TB Ribs	→	Feathery

Investigations

X-ray, tomography, sinogram, CT scan, gallium-67 and Indium-111-labelled leukocyte scan, etc. can identify sequestra. X-ray changes (Fig. 51.8A) have been enumerated in Table 51.2.

Management of Chronic Osteomyelitis

Goal is eradication of the infection by achieving a viable and vascular environment. This can be done by radical debridement by way of sequestrectomy and resection of scarred and infected bone and soft tissue. Appropriate antibiotic is also required. Finally, reconstruction of both the bone and soft tissue defects may be needed.

Principles of treatment: As is evident from the goal, surgery is the treatment of choice.

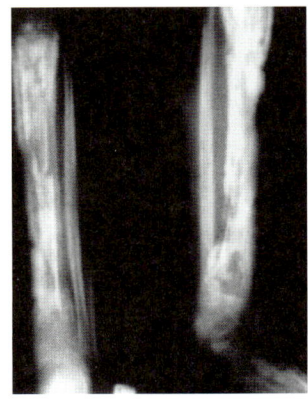

Fig. 51.8A: Chronic osteomyelitis with diaphyseal sequestrum of tibia

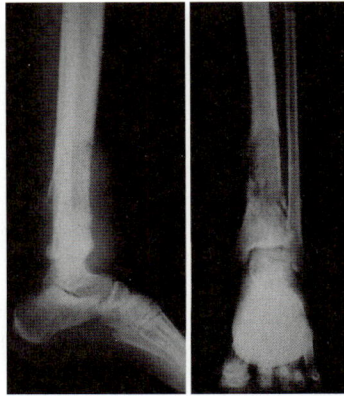

Fig. 51.8B: Chronic osteomyelitis pathological fracture

- *Surgery* is to be undertaken only when fever and infection has subsided, living bone can be distinguished from the dead bone and when involucrum appears sufficient to maintain length and contour of the bone after excision of any large sequestra.
- Secondary infection is usually present. When surgery is indicated culture is done and antibiotics started at least 4 days before surgery and is continued for 2 weeks.
- When acute exacerbation fails to respond to conservative treatment, incision and drainage have to be done.

Surgery Methods

Sequestrectomy and saucerization (Fig. 51.9) Sequestrum is identified on the X-ray, as it is denser and lies free in the cavity. It takes 2 to 3 months before it is isolated, separated and easily seen on the X-ray and only then, sequestrectomy is planned. All the sinus tracts are injected with methylene blue 24 hours before surgery. By making multiple drill holes, the cortex is removed in a rectangular fashion. Sequestrectmy is done next. The cavity is curetted until fresh bleeding occurs and the deep shape of the cavity is converted into a shallow cavity (called saucerization).

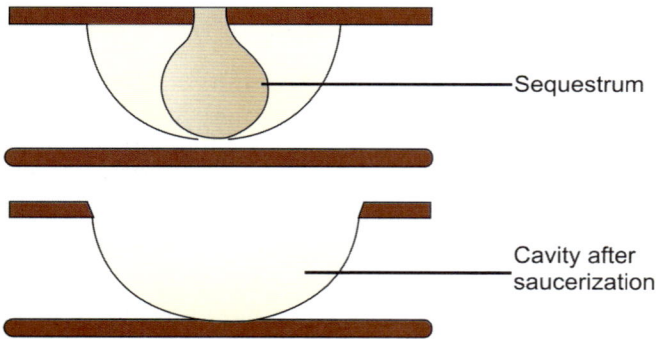

Fig. 51.9: Sequestrectomy and saucerization

Note: Sequestrectomy usually leaves a deep cavity beneath which are potentially a dead space favoring collection of pus and other debris. To prevent this from happening the deep cavity is made shallow for effective drainage of the collected materials.

After sequestrectomy, there is a huge gap in the bone due to its non-collapsing walls and there are four basic methods of immediate biological management of dead space so left:

1. Local closure if the space left is very small.
2. Myoplasty for slightly larger space, surrounding muscles can be packed into the cavity.
3. Cancellous bone grafts for a space less than 2.5 cm.
4. Free vascularized bone graft for larger areas.

Note: About saucerization. Imagine a 'cup and saucer' you normally use to drink tea. The process of changing a 'deep' cup into a 'shallow' saucer is called saucerization.

Other Methods of Treatment

- Papineau et al described an open grafting technique for chronic osteomyelitis.
- Hyperbaric oxygen therapy.
- Closed suction drainage (Fig. 51.10). After sequestrectomy, the wound is closed over a suction drain. Through an inlet tube, an irrigation fluid consisting of saline, antibiotics and detergent is pushed into the medullary cavity and drained out through an outlet tube to which a slow suction is applied. This enables the wound to be continuously bathed in this antibiotic solution and is usually done for 4–8 days.

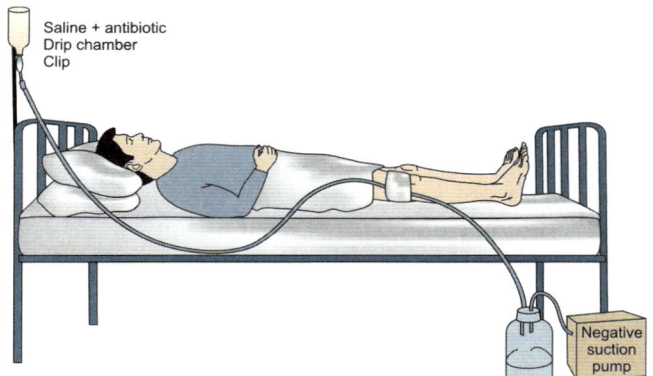

Fig. 51.10: Closed suction drainage

- Amputation is done rarely in the following circumstances: If patient's life is endangered by infection or in extensive infection. Lot of circumspection should be used while deciding upon amputation for chronic osteomyelitis. It should be the last choice and not the first.
- *Ilizarov's method* it has been found to be a very effective method of managing chronic osteomyelitis of late. Though technically very demanding, if planned and executed properly, it gives very good results in bad cases of chronic osteomyelitis.
- Excision of bones can be done, if smaller bones are involved like phalanges, carpal bones.

Complications

1. *Most common complications:* Pathological fracture is by far the most common complication. The incidence is 5 to 10 percent. It requires Papineau treatment comprising thorough debridement, grafting and stabilization of fracture fragments by external fixators.
2. *Common complications*
   a. *Acute exacerbation* of existing chronic disease initiated by a change in bacterial flora or by

51

decrease in the general resistance of the patient, which flares up the dormant infection.

b. *Growth disturbances* Usually the growth is not affected (64%), more commonly shortening may be seen (64%) due to the arrest of the growth plate by the neighboring infection and very rarely there may be stimulation of the growth plate resulting in lengthening (5%) of bones.

c. *Deformities* develop due to soft tissue, muscle and joint contractures and due to growth plate disturbances.

d. Joint stiffness due to extraarticular soft tissue contractures.

3. *Rare complications: Amyloidosis* due to long-standing infection. *Epithelioma* of the sinus tract due to chronic discharging sinus which induces metaplasia and formation of squamous cell carcinoma (incidence < 1%).

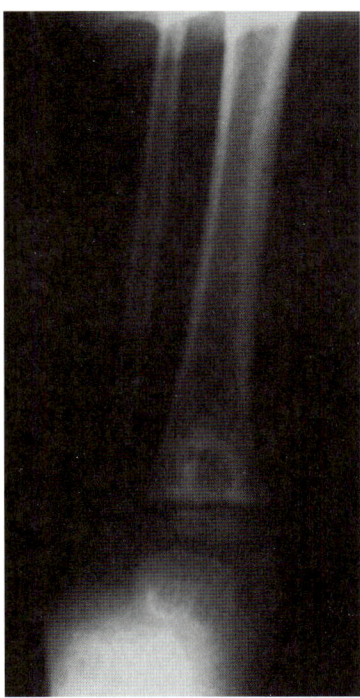

Fig. 51.11: Brodie's abscess

51   OSTEOMYELITIS OF SPECIAL IMPORTANCE

BRODIE'S ABSCESS

Brodie's abscess is a localized form of chronic osteomyelitis, involves metaphyseal and diaphyseal area, and is common in young adults. Patient complains of intermittent pain of long duration and local tenderness. Causative organism is low virulence *Staph aureus* in 50 percent of the cases.

Investigation

Radiograph shows varied appearance: Usually a cavity a surrounded by a slerotic bone is seen at the metaphysioepiphyseal junction (Fig. 51.11). It frequently requires biopsy for diagnosis.

Treatment: Consists of a long-term appropriate antibiotics, curettage and bone grafting, and the wound is loosely closed over a drain.

SCLEROTIC OSTEOMYELITIS OF GARRE

It is a chronic or subacute form of osteomyelitis and affects the subperiosteal region of the bone. Bone is

thickened. It affects children and young adults. The cause is unknown but it could be due to low-grade anaerobic infection. A secondary infection may occur at a distant site.

Clinical features: The patient may complain of intermittent pain, swelling, tenderness and low-grade fever, etc.

Investigations: Radiographs show expanded bone with generalized sclerosis. ESR is usually raised. Biopsy is definitive and confirmatory. Bone scan and pet scan also helps.

Treatment: It consists of fenestration of sclerotic bone and appropriate antibiotics should be given.

TUBERCULAR OSTEOMYELITIS

Discussed in chapter on tuberculosis of bones and joints.

52 | Skeletal Tuberculosis: General Principles

INTRODUCTION

Though ubiquitous in distribution, tuberculosis has firmly entrenched itself with the Third World, thanks to the illiteracy, poverty, poor hygienic conditions and a host of other favorable factors. India is infamous for hosting nearly one-fifth of the thirty million people suffering from tuberculosis throughout the world. Though largely preventable, tuberculosis can be successfully combated by an effective chemotherapy. The bugbears of treatment being its long duration, poor patient compliance, emergence of drug resistance and others. Skeletal tuberculosis mercifully is not as common as pulmonary tuberculosis and accounts for only 1 to 3 percent of the cases.

Tuberculosis, being mainly the disease of Third World, it is no wonder that India has produced pioneers like Dr Tuli, Dr Kumar, Dr Shanmugasundaram, and others whose work on skeletal tuberculosis has been acknowledged worldwide.

HISTORY

- Hippocrates [460–370 BC] was the first to suggest the relationship between pulmonary disease and spinal deformity.
- Percivall Pott [1714–1788] described the "gibbus" deformity and its sequelae. He did not describe the disease or its tuberculous nature.
- Laennec [1781–1826] described the basic microscopic lesion, **the tubercle**.
- Drugs Streptomycin was first used in 1947, PAS in 1949, and INH in 1952.

Skeletal tuberculosis is always *secondary,* the primary foci being either in the lungs, lymph nodes or gastrointestinal tract. The incidence of bone and joint tuberculosis is 2 to 3 percent. Fifty percent of these cases are found in the vertebral column. The other major areas affected in order of predilection are hip, knee, foot, elbow, hand, shoulder, etc.

Skeletal tuberculosis occurs mostly in the first three decades of life but no age is immune.

Etiology

1. *TB bacillus*
   a. Human variety, *Mycobacterium tuberculosis* (more common)
   b. Bovine (rare)
2. *Route:* Always secondary, may spread to the bone through:
   a. Blood, e.g. through Batson's plexus in tuberculosis of spine
   b. Lymphatic spread
   c. Direct
3. *Precipitating factors*
   a. General factors like anemia, debility, etc. help precipitate the infection.
   b. Local factors like trauma etc. localize the problem to the bone.
4. *Local trauma:* Causes vascular stasis and intraosseus hemorrhage.

How does osteoarticular tubercular lesion develop?
Primary focus
Maybe active or quiescent (lungs, tonsils, mediastinum, mesentery, etc.)
↓
Bacillemia
↓
Through the arteries and veins
(e.g. Batson's plexus in the spine)
↓
Reach the skeletal system
↓
Tubercle develops

Pathology

Pathology following a minor skeletal injury, the vessels ruptures and there is hemorrhage. The tubercle bacilli present in the circulation settle and proliferate in the blood clot so formed. A tubercle follicle is formed and it consists of lymphocytes, giant cells, and endothelial

52

cells. Small such tubercle follicles coalesce to form a larger follicle which undergoes caseation at the center and fibrosis at the periphery. The caseation at the center of the affected bone breaks down forming pus. It spreads towards the subperiosteal region, breaks the periosteum and tracks along the lines of least resistance. It reaches the skin and forms a cold abscess (not warm). Later on it breaches the skin forming a sinus.

Changes in the marrow: In the early stages there is increase in the polymorphs. In the later stages, it is replaced by lymphocytes. The marrow is slowly surrounded by fat cells and is replaced by fibrous tissue.

Lamellae: There may be osteoporosis due to the action of osteoclasts or due to metaplasia. Osteosclerosis may also be seen.

Periosteum: Increased vascularity in the periosteum leads to new bone formation and the consequent subperiosteal thickening.

Joint involvement: Joints may be affected due to direct spread from the vicinity of a tubercular bone infection or more commonly from a synovitis. Unlike septic arthritis, synovitis is low grade here. The pannus causes a slow destruction of the cartilage and other structures of the joints. This slow destruction mostly leads to fibrous ankylosis and very rarely to bony ankylosis. Eventually various deformities may develop and the pus so formed may burst open through the skin forming a cold abscess.

Note: In skeletal tuberculosis, healing is usually by fibrous ankylosis except in spine where bony ankylosis is more common.

Clinical Features

The diagnostic triad (Fig. 52.1) best sums up the clinical features.

Insidious onset: Skeletal tuberculosis does not happen suddenly. It takes months and sometime years to develop wreaking havoc with the affected bones. Slow

to affect and even slower to regress is the hallmark of the disease.

Monoarticular: The patient usually complains of pain in one joint, which is dull aching and chronic in nature. He or she may give history of night cries which is due to the rubbing of inflamed articular surfaces against each other due to the release of muscular spasm at rest. The joint movements are decreased in all directions, initially due to muscle spasm and later due to arthritis. The wasting of the limb muscles is gross and is out of proportion. Regional lymph nodes may be enlarged.

Constitutional symptoms: This is present in approximately 20 percent of the cases. It consists of low-grade fever, lassitude in the afternoon, loss of appetite and weight, night sweats, anemia, tachycardia and evening rise of temperature.

Laboratory investigations: These consist of hemoglobin estimation, total and differential count, raised ESR, urine routine tests, etc.
Other investigations

Positive evidence of the disease
a. Identification of organism on culture from the joint, histology, etc.
b. Reproduction of disease by inoculating guinea pigs.

ZN stains for acid-fast bacilli in aspirate or excised tissue.

Guinea pig Test

Mantoux test is significant only in the first 3 to 4 years of life, adults are usually positive. Negative test does not rule out tuberculosis.

X-ray
• No typical finding for tuberculosis.
• Earliest sign is decalcification of bones (rarefaction).
• Late signs are joint destruction.

Biopsy of regional lymph nodes may show "tubercles".

Exploratory arthrotomy is the certain way of ascertaining diagnosis. The tissue may be cultured or may be injected into a guinea pig.

Serum ELISA test: This helps to detect the antibodies against *Mycobacterium* bacteria.

Note: Do not forget to take a chest X-ray in skeletal tuberculosis.

Treatment

Principles of Treatment

General treatment: This includes rich protein diet, hematinics, adequate exposure to sunshine. The general treatment aims at building up the general resistance and immunity of the patient.

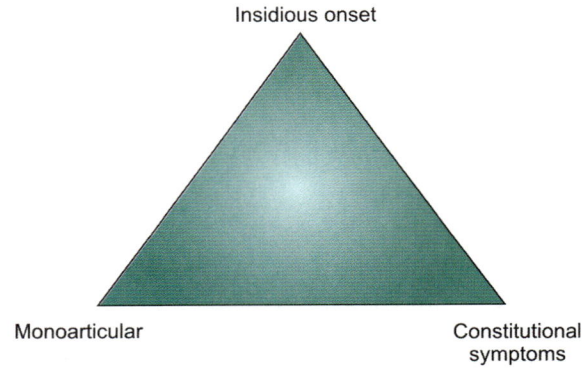

Insidious onset

Monoarticular   Constitutional symptoms

Fig. 52.1: Diagnostic triad of skeletal tuberculosis

Chemotherapy: This is the mainstay of treatment and is discussed in detail below.

Local treatment: Aims to prevent, correct, or decrease the deformities, by positioning the joints in appropriate functional position by proper splints. If the disease is osseous, aim at ankylosis in functional position by immobilization. If the disease is synovial aim at mobility by traction.

Operative treatment: It consists of biopsy partial capsulectomy, synovectomy, osteotomy, curettage, joint debridement arthrodesis, etc. depending on the stage of tuberculosis.

Treatment of tubercular abscess: Conservative treatment is recommended in most of the cases. Aspiration is done if the abscess is tense.

Chemotherapy: Drugs used for the treatment of tuberculosis are grouped as follows.

First line of drugs: These have the greatest level of efficiency and have an acceptable degree of toxicity.

The following are the first line of drugs used in tuberculosis (mnemonic **PRISE**).

P Pyrazinamide
R Rifampicin
I INH
S Streptomycin
E Ethambutol.

Second line of drugs: These are useful if the patient develops resistance to the first line of drugs (mnemonic **CAKECA**).

C Capriomycin
A Amikacin
K Kanamycin
E Ethionamide
C Cycloserine
A Aminosalicylic acid (PAS).

Second line of drugs is used only for treatment of diseases caused by resistant microorganisms or by non-TB mycobacterium. All drugs are given parenterally and are potentially ototoxic and nephrotoxic. Hence, no two drugs from this group should be used simultaneously. These are not used with streptomycin for the same reasons.

Table 52.1 outlines the chemotherapeutic drugs in skeletal tuberculosis.

Chemotherapy Regimes

- *Nine-month regime:* Nine months of rifampicin and INH are effective for all forms of disease.
- *Six-month regime*
  First two months, INH + Rifampicin + Pyrazinamide
  Next four months, INH + Rifampicin
  When the primary resistance to INH is high, therapy is usually initiated with first four line drugs.
- *Third regime:* Here three to four drugs are used in the first four months, two to three drugs in the second four months, one or two drugs in the third four months and one drug (i.e. INH) in the last three to four months of treatment.

QUICK FACTS: SKELETAL TUBERCULOSIS (GENERAL)

- Incidence is 2 to 3 percent
- Usually monoarticular
- Always secondary
- Spine is affected commonly
- Only 20 percent show constitutional symptoms
- Cold abscess is a feature
- Chemotherapy is the mainstay of treatment.

52

Table 52.1: Chemotherapeutic drugs in skeletal tuberculosis						
Drugs	Antibacterial activity	Mechanism	Absorption	Chemistry	Dose	Untoward effects
1. INH (primary drug for chemotherapy of tuberculosis)	Bacteriostatic for resting bacilli	Inhibits bio synthesis of mycolic acid, a constituent of the cell walls	Gets rapidly absorbed, diffuses into all body fluids and cells, penetrates the caseous material	Hydoxide of Isonicotinic acids	• Adults 5 mg/ kg body wt • Children 10–20 mg/kg body wt	• Rash 2% • Fever 1.2% • Jaundice 0.6% • Peripheral neuritis 0.2%
2. R-cin (Rifampicin)	Inhibits most of gram +ve, gram -ve, and myco TB, bactericidal	Inhibits RNA synthesis	Peak action in 2–4 hr	Semi synthetic derivative of Rifampicin	10 mg/kg	• Hepatitis • Orange color to urine, etc. Well tolerated
3. Ethambutol	Bacteriostatic, suppresses growth of most INH and SM resistant TB	Inhibits incorporation of mycolic acids	Absorbed well from GIT		15 mg/kg (not used in children < 5 yr)	• Optic neuritis • Urate conc. increase in blood in blood

Contd.

Contd.

Drugs	Antibacterial activity	Mechanism	Absorption	Chemistry	Dose	Untoward effects
4. Streptomycin		It usually suppresses growth of most INH resistant TB bacilli		Acts only on extracellular microbes	20–35 mg/kg	• 8.2% incidence, Involves auditory and vestibular actions of 8th cranial nerve
5. Pyrazinamide			Well absorbed	Synthetic analogue of nicotinamide	20–35 mg/kg	Injury to liver hepatitis
6. Ethionamide	Suppressor	Inhibits acetylation of INH	Rapid and well absorbed		250 mg/BD 15–20 mg/kg	Metallic taste hepatitis
7. PAS	Suppressor	Inhibits PABA	Readily absorbed	Structural analogue of PABA	Daily dose of 14–16 gm	Epigastric pain, Nausea, anorexia
8. Cycloserine			Rapidly absorbed		15–20 mg/kg	CNS toxicity
9. Kanamycin					1 gm/day	Ototoxic/ nephrotoxic
10. Capreomycin					15–30 mg/kg	
11. Amikacin						

52

53

Tuberculosis Spine

Tuberculosis spine
TB spine with paraplegia

TUBERCULOSIS SPINE (Known after Sir Percivall Pott)

This is the most common form of skeletal tuberculosis constituting about 50 percent of all cases.

Regional distribution
- Cervical—12%
- Cervicodorsal—5%
- Dorsal—42%
- Dorsolumbar—12%
- Lumbar—26%
- Lumbosacral—3%

As is evident from the above table spinal tuberculosis commonly affects the thoracic, thoracolumbar and lumbar vertebra accounting for nearly 80 percent of the cases. The reasons cited for this area of predilection are:
- Large amount of spongy tissue within the vertebral body.
- Degree of weight bearing which is comparatively more.
- More vertebral mobility is seen here.

Sites of Involvement within the vertebra: It is observed that spinal tuberculosis could start in any of the part (Fig. 53.1) of the vertebra (95% anterior; 5% posterior elements).

1. *Central:* This is less common and is known to produce central or *concertina* collapse of the vertebra
2. *Metaphyseal or intervertebral space (98%):* This is the most common area of involvement and is not without reason. Embryological development explains the reasons for this.
   Lower half of one vertebra and upper half of the adjacent vertebra with the intervening disc all develop from one sclerotome, which has a common source of blood supply (Fig. 53.2)? Hence bacillemia involves this embryological section more often.
3. *Anterior or periosteal:* Here anterior surface of vertebral body is involved and it may give rise to anterior wedge compression of the vertebra.
4. *Appendiceal:* Here occasionally transverse process and rarely vertebral arch are affected.

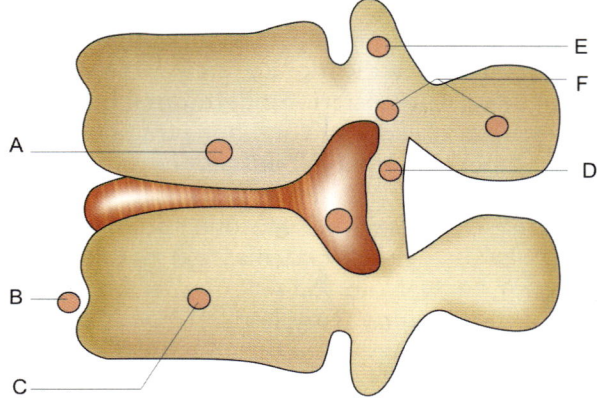

Fig. 53.1: Sites of involvement of TB spine: (A) metaphyseal, (B) anterior, (C) central, (D) true arthritis, (E) appendiceal, and (F) posterior spinal elements

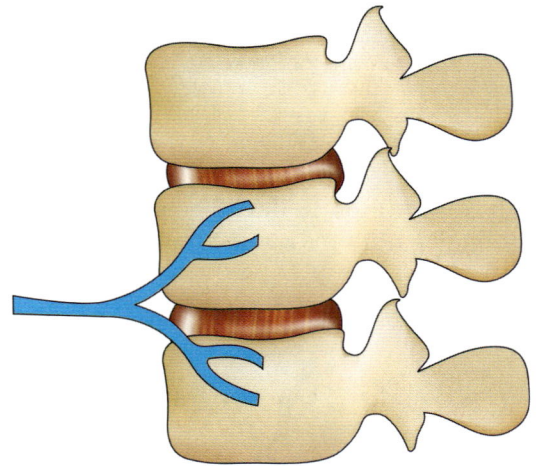

Fig. 53.2: Blood supply of vertebrae

5. *True tubercular arthritis* is seen in the atlantoaxial and at atlanto-occipital joints.

Sequences of pathological events: As mentioned earlier due to primary foci in the lungs, lymph nodes or abdomen, bacillemia develops and the organisms reach the spine through the Batson plexus.

Tuberculous endarteritis which develops following the infection results in marrow devitalization. Later on the tubercular follicle develops. Lamellae are destroyed due to hyperemia causing osteoporosis. As a result of

this the vertebral body gets easily compressed. In the thoracic vertebrae because of the normal kyphotic curve, anterior wedge compression is more common. In the lordotic cervical and lumbar vertebra, wedging is minimal.

This non-pyogenic infection results in formation of cold abscess which penetrates the epiphyseal cortex and involves the adjacent disc and the vertebra. It may also spread beneath the anterior longitudinal ligament and reach the neighboring vertebra. When it spreads posteriorly it may cause pressure on the spinal cord which is more common in the thoracic area as the spinal canal is small here. The posterior longitudinal ligament limits the spread of sequestra and bone fragments into the joints. Sometimes the cold abscess may penetrate the anterior longitudinal ligament and migrate along the *lines of least resistance*—(i.e. along the fascial planes, blood vessels, nerves) and may get manifested elsewhere far away from the original lesion (Fig. 53.3). Healing in the spine is by bony fusion. Cold abscess can spread to the abdomen through the diaphragmatic orifices (Fig. 53.4). Flow chart 53.1 shows the spread of cold abscess in the cervical, thoracic and lumbar tuberculosis.

Note: Cold abscess consists of serum, WBCs, caseous material, granulation tissue and tubercle bacilli. It is so called because there are no signs of inflammation.

Clinical Features

Tuberculosis of spine is usually insidious in onset although sometimes it may present acutely. The constitutional symptoms almost always antedate local

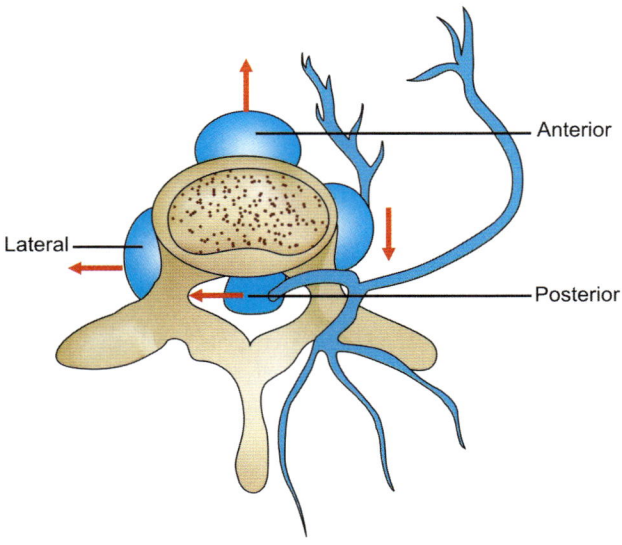

Fig. 53.3: Spread of the cold abscess

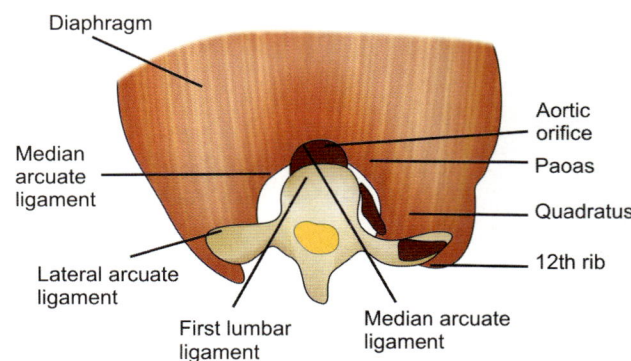

Fig. 53.4: Spread of the cold abscess through the diaphragmatic orifices

spinal involvement. Weakness, anorexia, night sweats and cries, evening or afternoon rise of temperature, loss of appetite and weight are some of those.

Patient may complain of back pain, which is localized over the site of vertebral involvement or is referred depending on the specific nerve root irritation. Thus if cervical roots are involved pain radiates to the arm, if dorsal roots are involved patient complains of girdle pain, if lumbar nerve roots are involved patient complains of radiating pain to the groin and if sacral roots are involved patient complains of sciatica.

Back stiffness is another common earliest complaint given by the patient. Patient is unable to bend and pick up the objects on the ground. Patient may give history of night cries. If the patient complains of stiffness, weakness, awkwardness of lower extremities, it heralds the onset of paraplegia. In more severe cases patient may present with cold abscess or paraplegia.

Physical Findings

The patient has a very protective attitude and has a very cautious and careful gait. The muscle spasm straightens out the spine. The spinous process of the involved vertebra is tender to percuss and when an attempt is made to rotate the vertebra. Back movements are decreased in all directions especially forward, flexion. There is pronounced wasting of the back muscles. The clinical attitude of the patient varies according to the region involved (See box). Cold abscess may be seen as Para vertebral swelling or in areas already described. Patient may develop or present with neurological complications like spastic or flaccid paraplegia. Of the various deformities of spine due to tuberculosis, *kyphotic* deformity is the most common and is seen in over 95 percent of the cases (Fig. 53.5).

General examination reveals signs of anemia, debility, involvement of lungs, lymph nodes, etc.

Flow chart 53.1

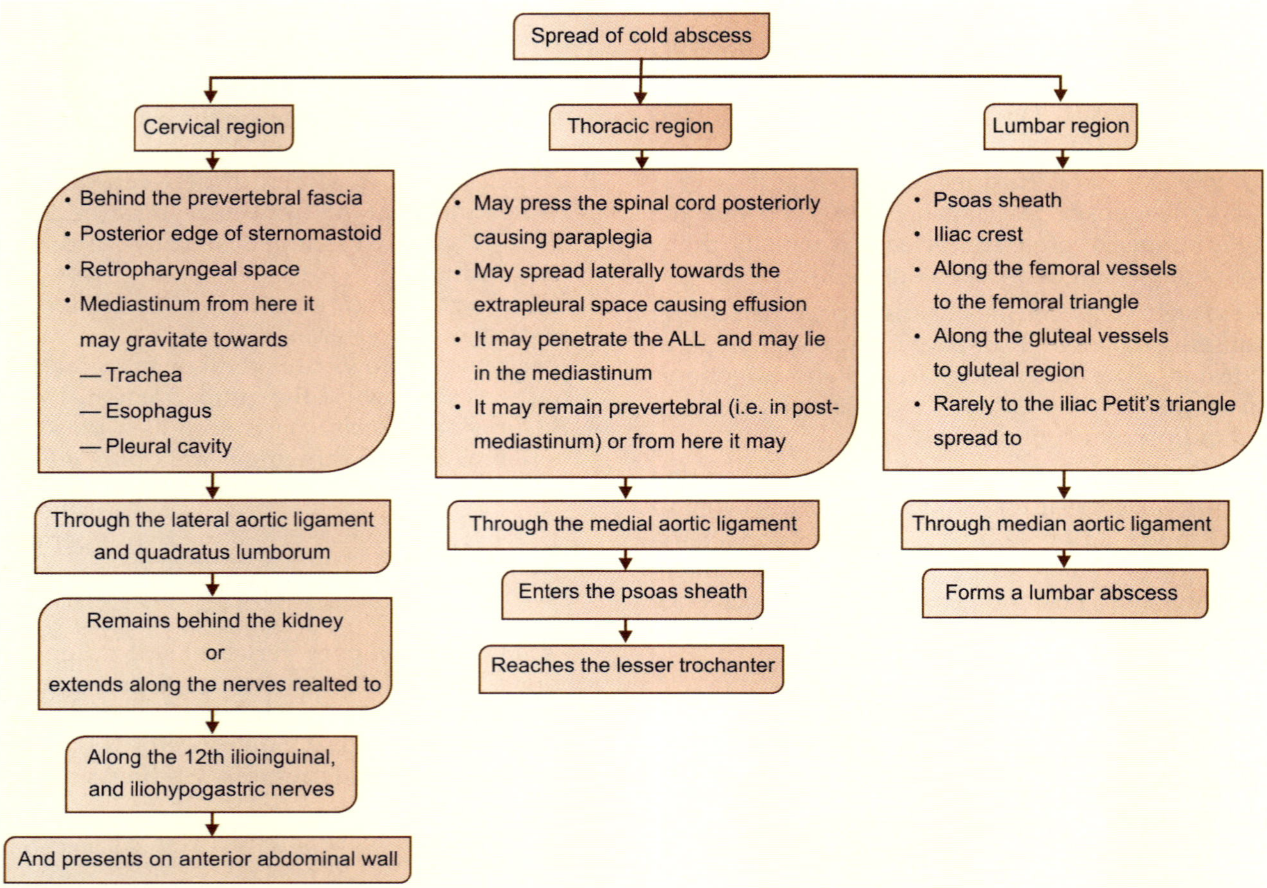

```
                        Spread of cold abscess

        ┌──────────────────────┼──────────────────────┐
   Cervical region         Thoracic region         Lumbar region
```

Cervical region	Thoracic region	Lumbar region

• Behind the prevertebral fascia
• Posterior edge of sternomastoid
• Retropharyngeal space
• Mediastinum from here it may gravitate towards
  — Trachea
  — Esophagus
  — Pleural cavity
	• May press the spinal cord posteriorly causing paraplegia
	• May spread laterally towards the extrapleural space causing effusion
	• It may penetrate the ALL and may lie in the mediastinum
	• It may remain prevertebral (i.e. in post-mediastinum) or from here it may
		• Psoas sheath
		• Iliac crest
		• Along the femoral vessels to the femoral triangle
		• Along the gluteal vessels to gluteal region
		• Rarely to the iliac Petit's triangle spread to

Through the lateral aortic ligament and quadratus lumborum	Through the medial aortic ligament	Through median aortic ligament
Remains behind the kidney or extends along the nerves realted to	Enters the psoas sheath	Forms a lumbar abscess
Along the 12th ilioinguinal, and iliohypogastric nerves	Reaches the lesser trochanter	
And presents on anterior abdominal wall		

Note: Cold abscess is called "cold" because it is not associated with features like redness, heat, etc. as in pyogenic abscess

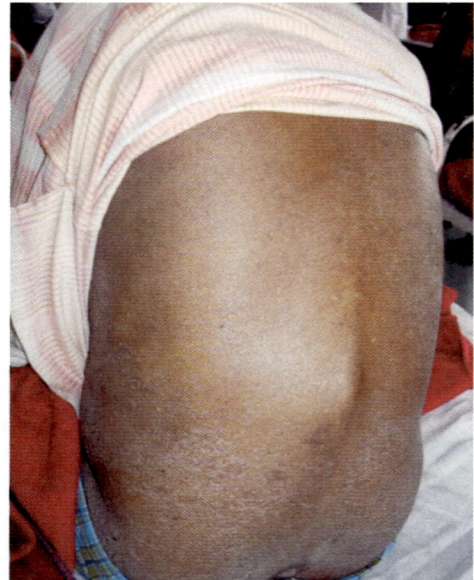

Fig. 53.5: Kyphotic deformity in tuberculosis of spine

QUICK FACTS: TYPICAL ATTITUDES IN SKELETAL TB
- Upper cervical → Wryneck
- Lower cervical → Military position
- Lower thoracic → Alderman's gait
- Upper lumbar → Prominent abdomen
- Lower lumbar → Increased lordosis

QUICK FACTS: SPINE IRREGULARITIES IN SKELETAL TB
- Kyphosis (95%)
- Scoliosis (5%)
- Lordosis
- Boarding
- Paravertebral thickening

Other Features
- Muscle spasm
- Wasting of all spinal muscles
- Spastic or flaccid paraplegia (20%)
- Cold abscess (20%)
- Sinuses (13%)
- Complications of skeletal TB.

53

Investigations

Laboratory tests: These tests show anemia, lymphocytes, hypoproteinemia, mild increase in ESR, etc. Mantoux test is helpful especially in children below 2–3 years but is not diagnostic. The importance of general tests lies in indicating chronic disease.

Radiographs: X-ray of the affected vertebrae is a very important diagnostic test and it is observed that the average number of affected vertebra is usually three. The following changes are seen on the X-ray.

Earliest change: This consists of disc space narrowing and subsequent loss of disc space in the common paradiscal lesions. The bones look rarefied and osteopenic (about 40 percent of calcium loss must take place to show a radiolucent sign on the X-ray).

Late changes: This includes anterior wedge compression in anterior vertebral involvement (Fig. 53.7A) central vertebral body collapse also called as "concertina collapse" (Figs 53.6A and B) in central involvement, destruction of the posterior elements in the posterior affection, etc.

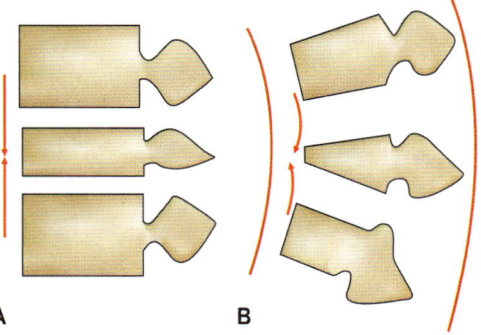

A   **B**

Figs 53.6A and B: (A) Concertina collapse, and (B) anterior wedge compression

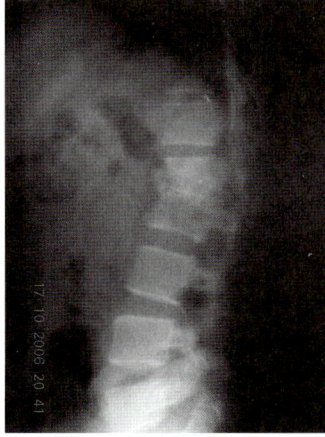 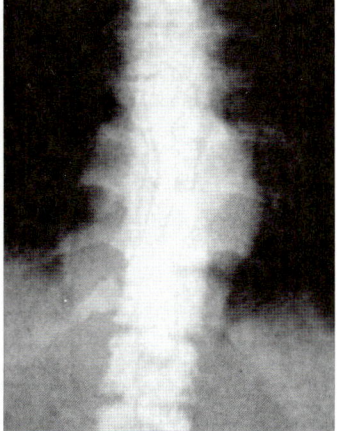

Fig. 53.7A: TB spine   **Fig. 53.7B:** Tense Para vertebral abscess of tuberculosis of the dorsal spine

Soft tissue swelling and its calcification are highly predictable of tuberculosis. In the healing stages, the vertebral body and the posterior elements may appear denser due to sclerosis.

Para vertebral shadow: If seen on the X-ray indicates cold abscess (Fig. 53.7B)
1. *Cervical region* it is seen in between the vertebral bodies and pharynx (retropharyngeal).
2. *Upper thoracic* V-shaped shadow and widened mediastinum.
3. *Below fourth thoracic vertebra* shows a fusiform or bird nest shadow appearance.
4. *Psoas abscess* shows unilateral or bilateral widening of psoas shadows in the lumbar region.
5. *Aneurysmal phenomenon* is seen as a tense thoracic vertebral abscess showing a scalloping effect.
6. Sclerosis and bony ankylosis indicate healing.

> *Note:* The most common is paradiscal, rarest is appendiceal involvement in spinal tuberculosis.

CT scan identifies para vertebral soft tissue swelling more readily than X-rays. It helps to assess the degree of neural compromise and helps in better evaluation of the pathologic process. Some prefer CT to X-ray to determine the clinical progress. Findings are similar to X-rays.

> *Note:* The only detectable abnormality on plain X-ray and CT scan specifically related to tuberculosis is fine calcification in the Paravertebral soft tissue shadow.

CT are also helpful in detecting tubercular affection of posterior spinal elements, craniovertebral and craniodorsal region, sacrum and sacroiliac region.

MRI helps in further delineation of the disease and helps to detect the cord compression. It does not eliminate the need for biopsy. It is 94 percent accurate (Fig. 53.9). Small calcifications seen on X-rays are not seen on MRI.

Ultrasound is useful to detect size of cold abscess in lumbar vertebral disease.

Gallium scanning is useful in disseminated TB.

Biopsy no one diagnostic test is 100 percent accurate for definitive diagnosis. Hence diagnosis is dependent on culture of the organism and requires biopsy by percutaneous technique with CT control.

Treatment

General Measures

This form of treatment has already seen discussed.

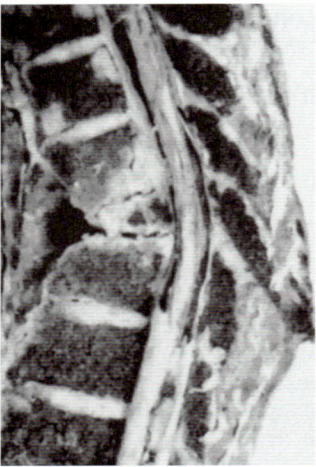

Fig. 53.8: Specimen of tuberculosis spine showing destruction and collapse of a vertebra

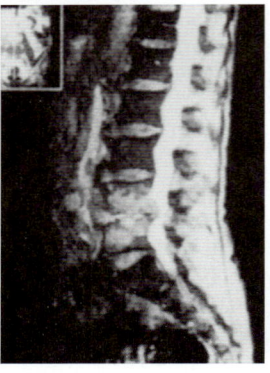
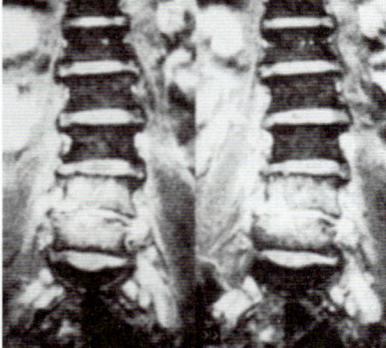

Fig. 53.9: Magnetic resonance imaging (MRI) of lumbar spine showing tubercular lesion of L$_4$ and L$_5$ vertebra

Local Measures

- *Rest and immobilization*: Bed rest helps considerably in the initial stages. A plaster of Paris body cast helps to immobilize the spine. Collar and Minerva Jacket helps to immobilize the cervical spine.
- *Mobilization*: As the disease subsides, patient may be mobilized with a brace. Collar for cervical spine, ASH brace for the thoracolumbar vertebra are the preferred braces and they need to be worn at least for 2 years.
- *Chemotherapy:* Definitive diagnosis by biopsy and culture is necessary before starting the treatment, because of the toxicity of the chemotherapeutic regime and length of the treatment required.

Surgery

Indications for Surgery

- Neurological symptoms.
- Kyphosis with several vertebral involvement, severe kyphosis, progressive kyphosis, etc.
- Resistance to chemotherapy.
- Recurrence of disease.
- Cord compression.

- Progressive impairment of pulmonary function.
- Spinal instability.

Surgical procedures: The following surgical procedures are described.

Aspiration: This technique is useful to aspirate the contents of a cold abscess through a thick bored needle. The needle should be inserted below the abscess to enable the gravity to help drain the contents.

Minimal debridement: This consists of evaluating the cold abscess through costotransversectomy or decompression. Here the contents are evacuated, the walls thoroughly curetted and bone grafting is done if necessary. Recently evacuation and debridement of a thoracic cold abscess through a thoracoscope has been successfully tried.

Radical debridement: This is done through the anterior approach and is invariably followed by spinal fusion with a strut graft involving rib or fibula after a thorough debridement.

Objectives of surgery: Surgery helps to excise the infected tissue, decompress the intraspinal neural elements, reduce the spinal instability and provide stability by spine fusion techniques.

> *Middle path regime:* Tuli and Kumar advocated triple drug therapy without surgery. In their series, operative treatment was reserved for patients:
> - Not responding favorably to drug therapy after 6 months of treatment.
> - Recrudescence of the disease.
> - Patient with neural complications.
> - Operative treatment is combined with six to twelve months of bed rest, followed by eighteen to twenty-four months of spinal bracing.

Complications of Tuberculosis Spine

- Paraplegia
- Cold abscess
- Sinuses
- Secondary infection
- Amyloid disease
- Fatality

TB SPINE WITH PARAPLEGIA

The incidence of this complication is 10 to 30 percent and it is most often associated with tuberculosis of the dorsal spine.

The following are the reasons cited for this
- TB is more common in dorsal spine.
- Spinal cord terminates below L1.
- Spinal cord is smallest in this region.

53

- Normal curve of the thoracic spine encourages marked kyphosis.
- Anterior longitudinal ligament in the dorsal region loosely confines the abscess.

Pathology

Paraplegia could result due to inflammatory causes, mechanical causes, and intrinsic causes and due to spinal tumor disease.

Classification

Seddon's Classification

- Early onset paraplegia is associated with the active disease. It is seen within two years of onset of the disease.
- Late onset paraplegia is associated with healed disease. It is seen after two years after the onset of disease.

Clinical Features

Rarely paraplegia may be the presenting symptom. Late onset paraplegia may be associated with clumsiness, twitching, increased reflexes, clonus, positive Babinski's sign, etc. Motor functions are usually affected first. The paralysis usually follows the following stages in order of severity—muscle weakness, spasticity, in coordination, paraplegia in extension, flexor spasms, paraplegia in flexion (severe form), and flaccid paraplegia lastly.

Kumar's Grading of Paraplegia

Grade I   Negligible, patient is unaware, physician detects ankle clonus, and up-going plantar.

Grade II   Mild, patient aware but walks with or without support.

Grade III   Moderate, non-ambulatory, paralysis in extension. Sensory deficit < 50 percent.

Grade IV   Severe grade III + severe paraplegia + sensory deficit more than 50 percent.

Note: Clonus is the first most prominent early sign of Pott's disease. Sense of position, vibration are last to disappear.

Investigation

These are the same as described for TB spine. MRI is the gold standard among the investigations for paraplegia due to TB spine.

Principles of Treatment

Three schools of thought are described for management of paraplegia due to tuberculosis.

Bosworth: Immobilization and early posterior arthrodesis.

Hodgson radical: Anterior decompression and arthrodesis.

Tuli and Kumar's: Middle path regime.

WHAT IS MIDDLE PATH REGIME?

- Admission, rest in bed or plaster of Paris cast.
- Chemotherapy.
- X-ray and ESR once in three months. Gradual mobilization in the absence of neurological complications.
- Spinal braces—18 months to 2 years.
- Abscesses are aspirated or drained.
- Sinuses heal within 6 to 12 weeks.
- If no neural complications develop, if response is obtained within 3 to 4 weeks of triple drug therapy, surgery is unnecessary.
- Excision surgery for posterior spinal disease.
- Operative debridement for patients who do not show arrest of disease after 3 to 6 months of chemotherapy.

Treatment of Pott's Paraplegia

The following measures are adopted in the treatment of Pott's paraplegia.

Conservative treatment: Chemotherapy is the mainstay of this method and has already been described. Immobilization of the spine to provide rest and thereby promote healing is done by traction (in cervical region) plaster cast or brace (in dorsal region), etc. Management of bedsores, bladder and bowel management is done as already discussed in the management of spinal injury. Physiotherapy and occupational therapy helps in the treatment of the paralyzed lower limbs.

Surgical treatment: The incidence of surgery has considerably decreased as chemotherapy is found to be successful in treating Pott's paraplegia. Only 5 percent of the cases require surgery in uncomplicated cases and 60 percent of the cases with neurological deficits require surgery.

Main Indications for Surgery

- Failed conservative treatment: If the patient does not respond to conservative treatment even after 3 to 6 months.
- In doubtful diagnosis.
- Fusion for mechanical instability by some grafts, implants, etc. either by the anterior or posterior approach.
- Recurrence of the disease after treatment.
- In rapid onset paraplegia.
- In disease secondary to cervical disease and cauda equina paralysis.

Other Indications

- Recurrent paraplegia.

- Painful paraplegia due to root compression, etc.
- Posterior spinal disease involving the posterior elements of the vertebra.
- Spinal tumor syndrome resulting in cord compression.
- Rapid onset paraplegia due to thrombosis, trauma, etc.
- Severe paraplegia.
- Secondary to cervical disease and cauda equina paralysis.

Surgical Techniques

Costotransversectomy: This is indicated for a tense para vertebral abscess. As the name suggests excision of the transverse process of the affected vertebra and about an inch of the adjacent rib to facilitate the drainage of abscess is done (Fig. 53.10). If pus is yielded under pressure, one has to wait up to six weeks for improvement. If no improvement occurs anterolateral decompression is done.

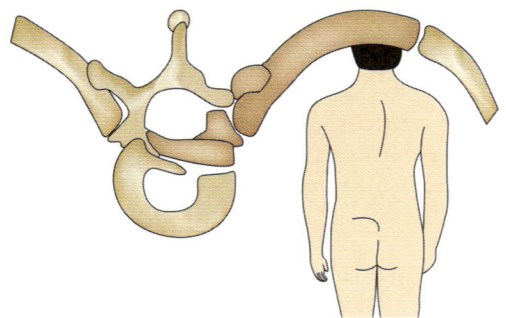

Fig. 53.10: Structures removed in costotransversectomy

Anterolateral decompression (ALD): The structures removed in this procedure is posterior part of the rib, transverse process, pedicle and part of the vertebral body anterior to the cord (Fig. 53.11). This is the surgery of choice for Pott's paraplegia. It helps to effectively remove the solid and liquid debris. ALD is done through an extra pleural mediastinal approach. Bone graft may be inserted if needed.

Anterior decompression: This is technically more demanding. Here the affected vertebra is approached through a transpleural or transperitoneal route, diseased tissue is curetted and a bone graft is inserted (Fig. 53.12).

Laminectomy: In Pott's paraplegia, anterior part of the cord is predominantly affected and laminectomy does not decompress this part of the cord. Moreover, it makes the spine unstable as it removes the healthy areas of the vertebrae. Hence, this procedure is not commonly recommended.

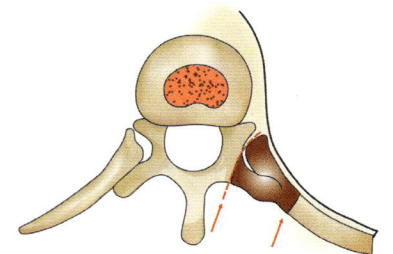

Fig. 53.11: Structures removed in ALD

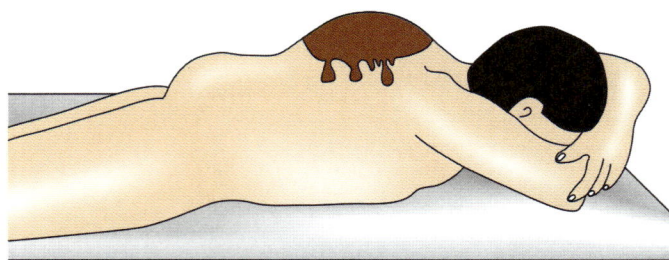

Fig. 53.12: Approach for ALD and costotransversectomy

53

If arthrodesis of the spine is required after the above procedures, anterior arthrodesis is normally preferred. Posterior spinal arthrodesis has limited value and is usually done to stabilize the craniovertebral region. Paralysis secondary to cervical disease is treated by either laminectomy and posterior arthrodesis or radical debridement and anterior arthrodesis. Severe cauda equina paralysis requires lumbar transversectomy.

Prognosis in paraplegia is better in
- Central cord involvement.
- Early onset paraplegia.
- If general condition is good.
- In children response to the treatment is better.
- Sudden onset paraplegia is prognostically poor.
- Motor paralysis alone suggests favorable prognosis.
- Sensory, bladder and bowel involvement indicate poor prognosis.

Cold abscess is another complication. It can present as one of the **3 P**s
- **P**alpable tumor in neck, back, thigh, etc.
- **P**ressure symptoms on the cord.
- **P**resent on radiographs of spine (no symptoms).

Treatment methods: Early aseptic evacuation is indicated.
- Aspiration if the contents are very fluid.
- Majority require open surgery for evacuation, e.g. costotransversectomy for tense paravertebral abscess, ALD for less than tense paravertebral abscess.

Tuberculosis of Joints and Bones

TUBERCULOSIS HIP JOINT

Tuberculosis of hip joint is ranked next to spinal tuberculosis (10:7) and it constitutes 15 percent of all osteoarticular tuberculosis. It is always secondary. The initial focus of infection could be either in the (i) acetabular roof, (ii) epiphysis, (iii) metaphyseal region, (iv) greater trochanter, (v) synovial membrane (rare), and (vi) trochanteric bursae (Fig. 54.1).

Pathogenesis

Tuberculosis elsewhere like lungs, tonsils, GIT, etc. spreads through the hematogenous route, the tubercular infection develops in any one of the six sites already mentioned. Synovial membrane is the one most commonly affected. Here the tubercle formation causes synovial hypertrophy resulting in pannus formation. This pannus destroys the articular cartilage resulting in the development of fibrous ankylosis of the hip. Bony ankylosis rarely develops.

Microscopy

It shows tubercle formation, giant cells and lymphocytes. Upper end of the femur is intracapsular and the joint gets rapidly involved. On the contrary, the joint involvement in acetabular lesions is rare.

The smaller tubercles coalesce, undergo caseation and forms a cold abscess. This cold abscess tracks down along the areas of least resistance and may point in any one of following sites (Fig. 54.2): (i) femoral triangle, (ii) inguinal region, (iii) medial side of the thigh, (iv) greater trochanter, (v) glutei region, (vi) ischiorectal fossa, (vii) lateral and posterior aspect of thigh, and (vii) pelvis.

Healing as already suggested takes place by developing a fibrous ankylosis.

Clinical Features

Tuberculosis of hip is common in the first three decades of life. Patient usually presents with *painful limp* and is the most common earliest symptom. He or she has an antalgic gait with a short stance phase. Pain is

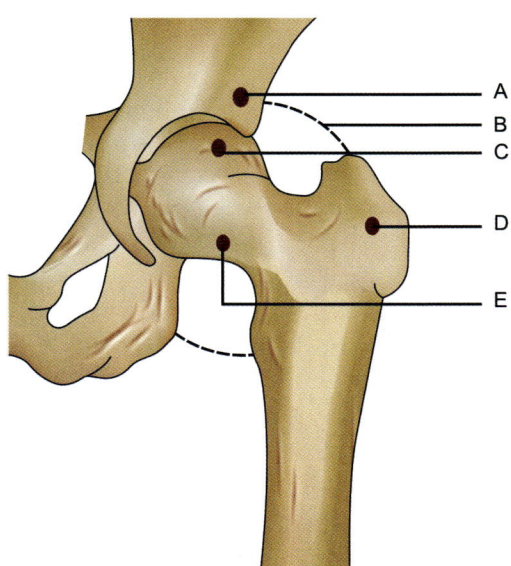

Fig. 54.1: Sites of common tubercular infection of the hip (A) acetabular roof, (B) synovium, (C) epiphysis, (D) metaphysis, and (E) greater trochanter

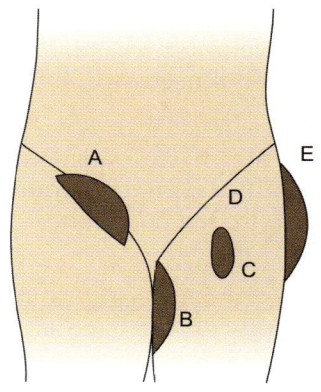

Fig. 54.2: Sites of cold abscess: (A) inguinal region, (B) medial side of thigh, (C) femoral triangle, (D) gluteal region, and (E) lateral aspect of thigh

maximum towards the end of the day and there is a history of *night cries*. There is *marked wasting* of the thigh and glutei muscles. There may be presence of *scars and sinuses.*

About 8 percent of the patients may develop *cold abscess* in the regions shown in the figure above and 10 percent may show pathological subluxation. Tenderness can be elicited by direct pressure in the femoral triangle or by bitrochanteric compression. The *attitude* differs depending upon the stage of the disease, which is discussed later. The following *deformities* may develop in tuberculosis hip.

- *Flexion deformity:* In the initial stages of the disease patient keeps the hip in flexion, as this is the position of ease and of maximum joint capacity. Soft tissue contractures convert this into a fixed flexion deformity (FFD) making locomotion impossible. FFD is concealed by increased lumbar lordosis. Thomas Test helps reveal the conceal FFD of the hip.
- *Adduction deformity:* Soft tissue contractures convert the adduction position adapted by the patient due to the spasm of the adductor muscles following damage to the articular cartilage, to one of fixed adduction deformity (Fig. 54.3A).
- *Abduction deformity:* In the initial phases of the disease because of the increase in the joint space due to effusion, the limb assumes a position of flexion, abduction and external rotation. If fixed in this position by soft tissue contractures patient develops a fixed abduction deformity (Fig. 54.3B).

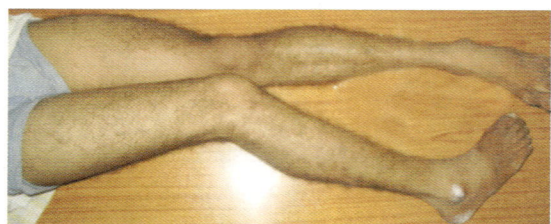

Fig. 54.3A: TB hip (Flexion adduction and internal rotation)

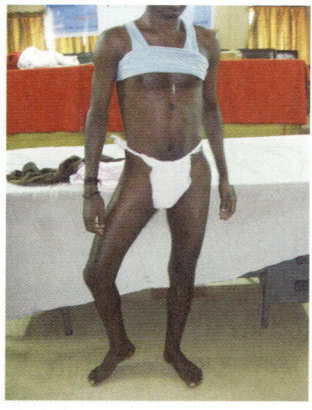 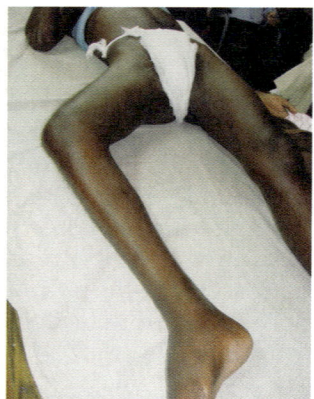

Fig. 54.3B: Deformities in TB hip   **Fig. 54.3C:** TB hip

(Flexion, abduction and external rotation)

The methods of unveiling and recording of fixed flexion, adduction and abduction deformities are discussed in patients in clinical examination of the hip joint.

Limb length discrepancy: In the initial stages there may be apparent lengthening but in the advanced stages patient develops true shortening.

Movements of the hip joint: Both active and passive movements of the hip joint are restricted in all directions, initially due to muscle spasm and later due to ankylosis.

Stages of Tuberculosis Hip

The following stages are described in tuberculosis hip (Figs 54.4A to C).

Stage I (Stage of synovitis): Here the disease is synovial with the patient assuming flexed, abducted and external rotated position of the limb due to increased synovial fluid effusion into the joint. There is *apparent* lengthening. There is no real shortening and the extremes of movements are decreased and painful (here apparent length is more than true length).

Stage II (Stage of early arthritis): Here the cartilage gets involved. The local signs are exaggerated. The spasms of the adductors and flexors result in flexion, adduction and internal rotation of the affected limb. There is apparent shortening; significant muscle wasting and hip movements are decreased in all directions. True shortening may be less than 1 cm (here apparent length, less than true length).

Stage III (Advanced arthritis): The flexion, adduction, internal rotation deformity found in Stage II are exaggerated. There is a true shortening with considerable restriction of hip movements and muscle wasting. There is gross destruction of the articular cartilage of the head of the femur and acetabulum (apparent length is less than true length).

Stage IV (Advanced arthritis with subluxation of dislocation): Migrating acetabulum, frank pathological posterior dislocation, mortar and pestle hip, protrusio acetabuli are the features in this stage.

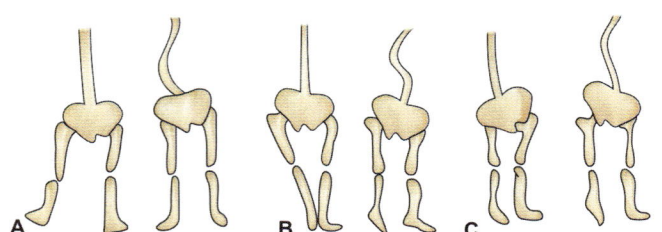

Figs 54.4A to C: Stages of tuberculosis hip: (A) stage of synovitis, (B) stage of early arthritis, and (C) stage of advanced arthritis

54

The Trendelenburg test is positive in all the above stages.

Investigations

Laboratory tests: These tests show anemia, lymphocytosis, increased ESR, etc.

Radiograph of the hip: In the early stages, the radiographs show rarefaction of the bones and in advanced stages, there may be reduction in the joint space. Depending upon the radiological features. Shanmugasundaram has described seven types of tuberculosis hip in advanced stages of arthritis (Figs 54.5A to E).

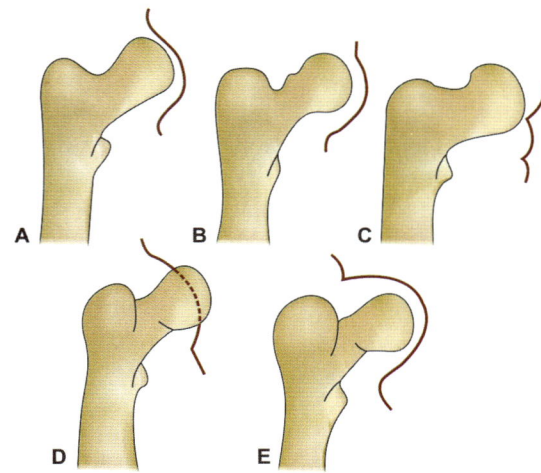

Figs 54.5A to E: Shanmugasundaram's radiological types of TB hip: (A) normal type, (B) traveling acetabulum, (C) dislocated type, (D) protrusio acetabuli, and (E) mortar and pestle

- *Normal appearance:* Here the hip almost looks normal but for some rarefaction.
- *Traveling or wandering acetabulum:* Here because of the destruction of the joint due to arthritis and due to the muscle spasm, the head of the femur comes to lie in the region of the ilium (Fig. 54.6).
- *Dislocated hip:* In this condition, there is pathological dislocation of the hip joint.

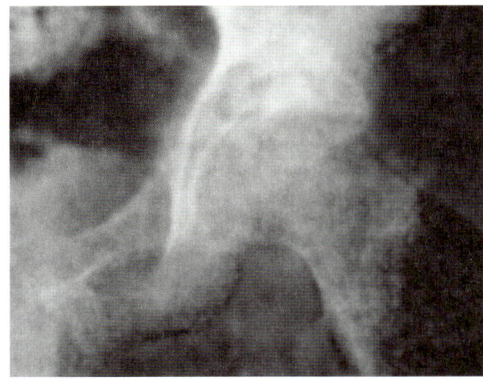

Fig. 54.6: Advanced stage of TB hip, sequestra seen in the acetabulum

- *Perthes type:* Here the head of the femur is dense and there could be collapse.
- *Atrophic type:* Here the head of the femur is small and atrophic.
- *Protrusio acetabuli type:* Here there is gross reduction of the joint space and head of the femur threatens to protrude through the acetabulum into the pelvic cavity (Fig. 54.7).
- *Mortar and pestle type:* In this condition the head of the femur is small (pestle) and the acetabular cavity (mortar) is wide.

This classification helps to assess the severity of the affection of the hip due to the disease.

Other investigations synovial: Fluid analysis (estimation of protein, lymphocytes, sugar, etc.), synovial biopsy, Mantoux test, arthrography, etc. may help in the diagnosis.

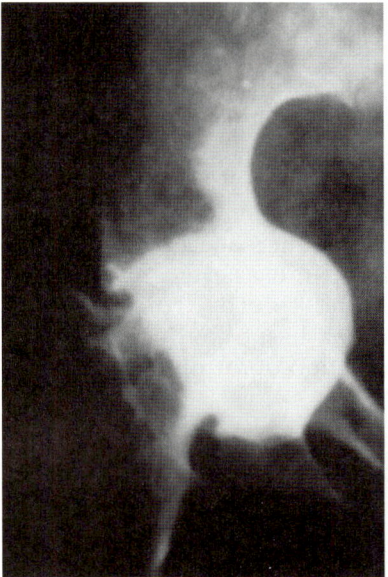

Fig. 54.7: Protrusio acetabuli

Treatment

General measures: These proceed on the same lines as suggested earlier.

Definitive measures: In the early stages (synovitis and early arthritis) the patient is put on chemotherapy and traction. Traction reduces the muscle spasm, prevents or corrects the deformity and maintains the joint space. If favorable clinical response is obtained the hip is gradually mobilized. If the disease is not responding favorably then synovectomy and arthrotomy are carried out in the synovitis stage. Synovectomy and thorough joint debridement is done in cases of early arthritis (Flow chart 54.1).

Late stages (stage of advanced arthritis): The end result of this stage is fibrous ankylosis and the patient is put on chemotherapy and traction. Once gross ankylosis is

Flow chart 54.1: Early stages (TB hip) synovitis and early arthritis

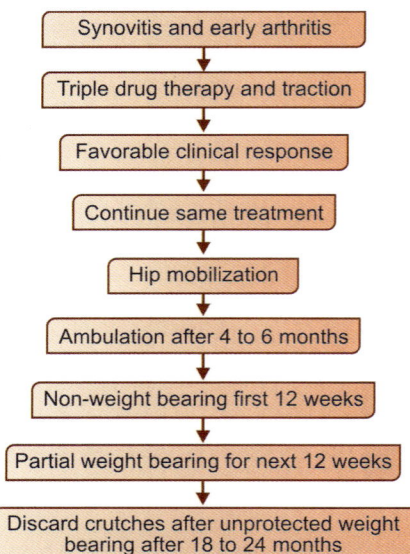

accepted and if the limb is in proper position (10° to 30° of flexion, 5 to 10° of external rotation and neutral between adduction and adduction) patient is immobilized in plaster of Paris spica and later the patient is made to bear weight. If the limb is not in functional position, then corrective osteotomy and arthrodesis in proper position are carried out (Flow chart 54.2).

Flow chart 54.2

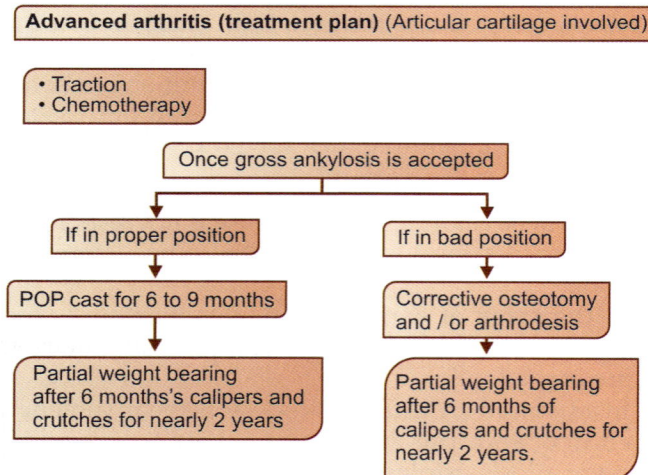

Surgical Treatment in Tuberculosis Hip

Synovectomy and arthrotomy: This is done in synovitis stage when the disease is not responding favourably to conservative treatment. Partial synovectomy, joint drainage and lavage are done.

Synovectomy and joint debridement: This is preferred in early arthritis. The joint is exposed through the posterior approach, thorough debridement of the joint is done by evacuation and the walls are curetted and washed.

Osteotomy: This is an upper femoral corrective osteotomy and is indicated in sound ankylosis in bad position in flexion adduction contractures. This helps to correct the deformity and change the line of weight bearing.

Displacement osteotomy: This is done in fibrous ankylosis with gross deformity.

Arthrodesis: This is indicated in adults with painful fibrous ankylosis with active or healed disease. This procedure converts a painful hip to painless stable hip. The procedure could either be intraarticular or extraarticular or both.

Arthroplasty: Stiff hip is a gross disability and is particularly not acceptable by Indian patients because they cannot squat on the ground and use the Indian toilet. Here girdle stone excision arthroplasty is preferred and it can be done in active or healed disease after the growth stops. This gives a mobile painless hip joint apart from controlling the infection and correcting the deformity. However, it leaves the hip unstable.

Total hip replacement: It is rarely done in tuberculosis hip. It is suggested after 10 years after the last evidence of active infection.

Amniotic arthroplasty: It has been tried in tuberculosis hip. Nevertheless, the results are far from satisfactory.

54

QUICK FACTS: TUBERCULOSIS HIP
- Second in frequency in skeletal tuberculosis
- Limp is the earliest symptom
- Three classical deformities
- Passes through four pathological stages
- Fibrous ankylosis is the result.

Differential Diagnosis

In adults: Chronic septic arthritis, osteoarthritis hip, rheumatoid arthritis, psoas abscess and inguinal lymphadenitis

In children: Perthes, DDH, Congenital coxa vara, etc.

All these conditions are discussed in detail in relevant sections. Students are instructed to please go through them.

TUBERCULOSIS KNEE

This is the third common site for skeletal tuberculosis. Incidence is 10 percent. It is also always secondary and may start in any one of the following sites in the knee joint.

Sites

- Synovium (common).
- Subchondral bone (of distal femur, proximal tibia or patella).
- Juxta-articular osseous foci.

The infection so developed results in tubercle formation and the synovium undergoes hypertrophy forming a pannus, which destroys the articular cartilage of the joint and results in fibrous ankylosis. In some cases pus may develop within the joint and may lead to the formation of a cold abscess. If this bursts a chronic discharging sinus may develop. Figures 54.8A to C show the clinical stages of TB knee.

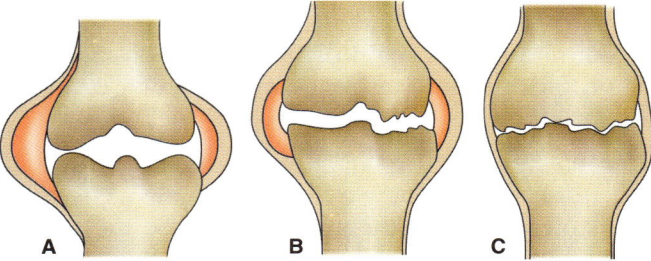

Figs 54.8A to C: Stages of TB knee: (A) synovitis, (B) early arthritis, and (C) advanced arthritis fibrous ankylosis

54

Clinical Features

The disease is insidious in onset, showing systemic and local features of tuberculosis. The joint shows effusion and evidence of synovial hypertrophy. The swelling is white in color. There is tenderness along the joint line and synovial reflections. During the synovial stage, the movements are reduced and painful. In the arthritis stage the joint movements are grossly restricted with painful spasm. There is gross quadriceps atrophy and lymphadenopathy. In the growing child, transient limb lengthening may be seen due to juxta-epiphyseal hyperemia. Triple displacement may develop in advanced cases (See box) (Fig. 54.9).

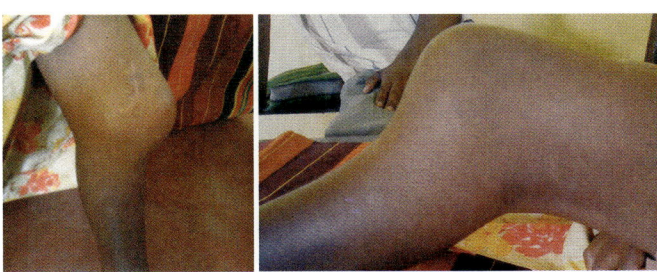

Fig. 54.9: TB knee showing triple displacement

FIVE CLASSICAL DEFORMITIES IN TB KNEE
- Flexion
- Posterior subluxation
- Lateral subluxation
- Lateral rotation
- Abduction of tibia
  The above deformities are due to initial spasm and later contractures of the hamstring muscles.

Investigations

- *General investigations:* It reveal the chronicity of the infection.

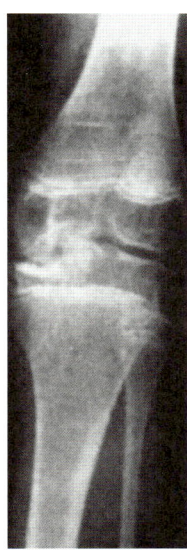

Fig. 54.10: Radiological features in tuberculosis of the knee

- *Radiographs:* Show osteoporosis in the bones adjacent to the joint. In advanced stages, there is reduction of the joint spaces and later triple subluxation (Fig. 54.10).
- *Biopsy:* Gives definitive diagnosis and the material is obtained either by incisional biopsy, aspiration cytology or by needle biopsy.

Treatment

Non-operative treatment: This is indicated in children and in the stage of synovitis. It consists of chemotherapy, traction, and joint aspiration. Skin traction helps to prevent triple deformity, corrects the deformities and to keep the joint surfaces distracted. Immobilization of the knee in Thomas splint is an age-old, time tested, successful treatment regimen for TB knee.

Surgical treatment:
- In the synovial stage if the disease is not responding favorably, arthrotomy and partial synovectomy are done.
- In the stage of early arthritis synovectomy, joint debridement and curettage of the juxta-articular foci are carried out.
- In advanced arthritis, arthrodesis is the treatment of choice and the indications being, advanced tuberculosis, triple deformity, gross instability and painful ankylosis after earlier synovectomy.

Role of supracondylar osteotomy: This is indicated in the situations where the disease has healed with painless range of movements in an unacceptable position and in valgus or varus deformity. Arthroplasty is also being tried without much success.

TUBERCULOSIS SHOULDER

This is quite uncommon and accounts for only 2 percent of the cases. It is more common in adults. Incidence of

concomitant pulmonary tuberculosis is high. The tuberculosis of the shoulder could start in any one of the following sites:

- Synovium
- Glenoid
- Head of humerus.

Pathology

Same as in other forms of skeletal tuberculosis.

Clinical Features

Tuberculosis of the shoulder rarely presents at the stage of synovitis. Abduction and external rotation movements of the shoulder are grossly decreased. There is wasting of the deltoid and supraspinatus muscles. *Common variety is dry type and is called as caries sicca since there is no effusion into the joint.*

Cold abscess if formed could present at:

- Supraspinous fossa
- Deltoid
- Biceps.

Late stages: In the late stages destruction of the upper end of humerus and glenoid cavity are seen. Fibrous ankylosis is the result.

Radiology

Radiographs show generalized rarefaction, articular cartilage erosion, cavities in the head of the humerus and little periosteal reaction. In advanced cases, there is inferior subluxation of the humeral head (Fig. 54.11).

Treatment

It is essentially as in other forms of tuberculosis. Chemotherapy is the mainstay of treatment. The shoulder is immobilized in shoulder spica in a saluting position (70 to 90° in abduction and 30° in flexion) to encourage ankylosis in functional position. The shoulder is put in abduction frame after 3 months. As a rule, sufficient compensatory movements develop at the scapulothoracic joint. Generally, a sound fibrous ankylosis develops and since this is a non-weight bearing joint, a sound fibrous joint is acceptable.

Indications for arthrodesis are painful ankylosis, uncontrolled disease, recurrence, etc.

TUBERCULOSIS ANKLE

This is very uncommon, and the incidence is only 5 percent. Sites of involvement could be:

- Synovium
- Distal end of tibia
- Malleoli
- Talus
- Rarely calcaneum.

Clinical Features

Pain in the region of the ankle, limp, swelling over and front of the joint, malleoli and tendo Achilles. Ankle joint is held in plantar flexion. In the late cases, there is pathological anterior subluxation of the ankle joint. Ankle movements are decreased. There is gross wasting of calf muscles, and evidence of sinus formation

Radiology

Radiographs in the early stages show marked osteoporosis of the ankle bones and in the late stages there is destruction of ankle joint (Fig. 54.12).

Treatment

Conservative Therapy

Aim: Here the aim is to achieve painless ankylosis in neutral position of the ankle. This is achieved by observing the following principles. Chemotherapy as is already discussed, immobilization in below knee plaster

54

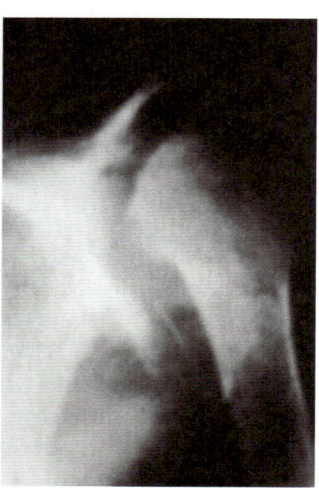

Fig. 54.11: Radiographical features of tuberculosis of the shoulder

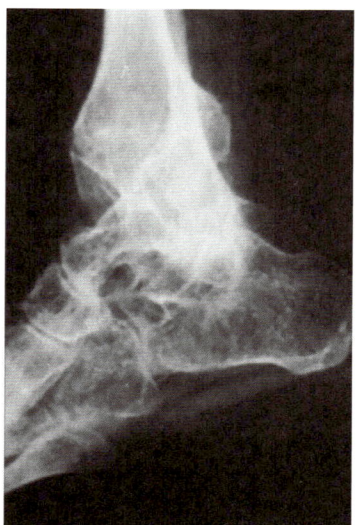

Fig. 54.12: Radiographical features of tuberculosis of the ankle

cast in neutral position crutch walking for first 8 to 12 weeks with plaster on and after 6 months below knee caliper is worn for 2 years.

Surgery

Indications: When the conservative treatment fails or when the diagnosis is in doubt.

Methods

- Synovectomy and joint debridement during the stages of synovitis and early arthritis.
- Arthrodesis for advanced and persistent diseases.

TUBERCULAR OSTEOMYELITIS OF LONG BONES

Here the onset of tuberculosis foci is within the bone, because of deficient anastomosis of the osseous arteries in the childhood, thrombosis caused by tubercular pathology may lead to sequestration of a major part of the diaphysis. This can occur in any of the long tubular bones and the incidence is 2 to 3 percent and 7 percent occurring at multiple sites.

Clinical Features

The patient complains of pain in the affected bone. Swelling is warm and tender. There may be cold abscess or sinus formation or ulcer may be present. Enlargement of regional lymph nodes are seen.

Radiology

Radiographs of anterioposterior and lateral views of the affected part show irregular cavities, little sclerosis (honeycomb appearance) and soft tissue swelling.

DISSEMINATED SKELETAL TB

This is very rare with 7 percent incidence only. It may be due to hematogenous spread or may be due to repeated impregnations at different sites. Rarely it may present as multiple cystic lesions called as osteitis tuberculosa multiplex cystioides.

Treatment

Chemotherapy is the mainstay of treatment and radiographs are taken once in 6 months. Surgical treatment consists of curettage and excision of the lesion.

TUBERCULOSIS OF SHORT TUBULAR BONES

This involves metacarpals and metatarsals. Calcaneum is another common site. In phalanges it is uncommon after the age of 5. This is called tubercular dactylitis. Hand is more frequently involved than foot. Multiple discharing sinus and slabs seen (Fig. 54.13).

Pathogenesis: Due to lavish blood flow through a large nutrient artery entering almost in the middle of the bone:

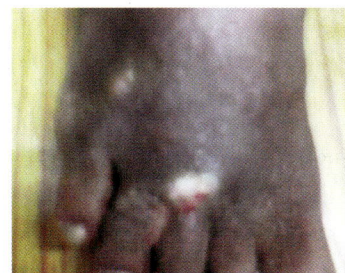

Fig. 54.13: Tubercular dactylitis

- The first inoculum of infection are lodged in the center of marrow cavity, which leads to a spindle-shaped expansion of bone called *spina ventosa.*
- There is subperiosteal new bone formation, abscesses and sinus formation is seen.
- Secondary infection causes further thickening of the bones.

Pathogenesis

Tuberculosis of the phalanges is of two varieties:
- *Tubercular dactylitis:* Here phalanges are affected and is uncommon after the age of 5.
- *Spina ventosa type:* Here phalanges develop small cavities, which are containing soft feathery sequestra. Subperiosteal new bone formation is present. If it is complicated by sinus or secondary infection, intense reactive sclerosis, sequestra and pathological fractures are seen.

Radiographs

Lytic lesions in the middle of the bone, subperiosteal new bone formation is present, soft cork-like sequestra and spina ventosa honeycomb type are some of the important radiological features (Fig. 54.14).

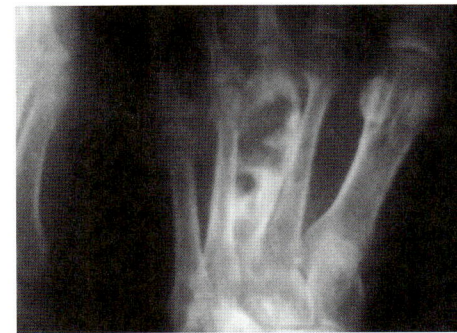

Fig. 54.14: Radiological features in tubercular dactylitis

Treatment

Chemotherapy is the mainstay of treatment and has been already discussed. Surgical treatment consists of the curettage of the lesions followed by histopathological examination of the debris.

55 Disorders of Joints

INTRODUCTION

Arthritis

It is a non-specific term denoting acute or chronic inflammation of the joint. Clinically arthritis falls into the following groups.

Osteoarthritis
- Primary
- Secondary

Rheumatoid arthritis
- Adult
- Juvenile

Infective arthritis
- Acute
- Chronic

Metabolic arthritis
- Gout
- Pseudo gout

Non-specific monoarthritis
- Neuropathic joint disorders (e.g. Charcot's) Special forms:
- Hemophiliac arthritis
- Psoriatic arthritis
- Psychogenic arthritis
- Nearly 10 percent of the population suffers from one form of the arthritis or the other.

INFECTIVE ARTHRITIS

Pyogenic Infection of Joint or Septic Arthritis

Septic arthritis is defined as a bacterial infection of the joint, which causes an intense inflammatory reaction with migration of polymorph nuclear leucocytes and subsequent release of proteolytic enzymes. This could lead to destruction of the articular cartilage and later the joint.

Causative Organisms

The most common offending organisms are *Staphylococcus aureus* (50%), *Streptococcus* (20%), pneu-mococcus (10%), gonococcus, *E. coli*, etc. *H. influenzae* is very common in children less than 2 years. Blood culture is positive only in 60 percent of cases.

ROUTES OF ENTRY FOR ORGANISMS: 6 Ps
- **Primary** focus is in RS, GIT, etc.
- **Pyogenic** osteomyelitis
- **Punctured** wounds
- **Pneumonia,** typhoid, etc.
- **Primary** focus within the joint, absent in few
- **Physician**-iatrogenic, following intraarticular injections, etc.

Predisposing Factors

The predisposing factors are trauma, diabetes, steroid therapy, malignancy, etc. It is more common in children and males.

SITES OF INVOLVEMENT OF THE JOINT
In adults
- Knee (53%)
- Hip (20%)
- Elbow (17%)
- Shoulder (10%)

In children
- Knee (39%)
- Hip (32%)

Remember

Ninety percent of cases of septic arthritis are monoarticular and 10 percent are polyarticular.

Pathology

The organism, which gains entry through one of the above routes, reaches the synovium. Synovitis this develops and leads to the following pathological changes:
- *Exudation into joint* this could be serous, sero-fibrinous or purulent depending upon the severity of infection.
- *Destruction of articular cartilage* by plasmin, cathepsin, prostaglandins, etc.
- Capsules, ligaments are destroyed by pus.

Stages: The stages of infective although are stage of synovitis, stage of arthritis, and stage of recovery or stage of bony ankylosis.

Clinical Features

Septic arthritis usually presents as monoarticular affection in 90 percent and polyarticular in 10 percent of cases and fever is seen in only 50 percent of the cases. Pain, swelling, redness, loss of movements (Figs 55.2A and B) and limp are common complaints. The severity of clinical manifestation depends upon the severity of disease (Table 55.1).

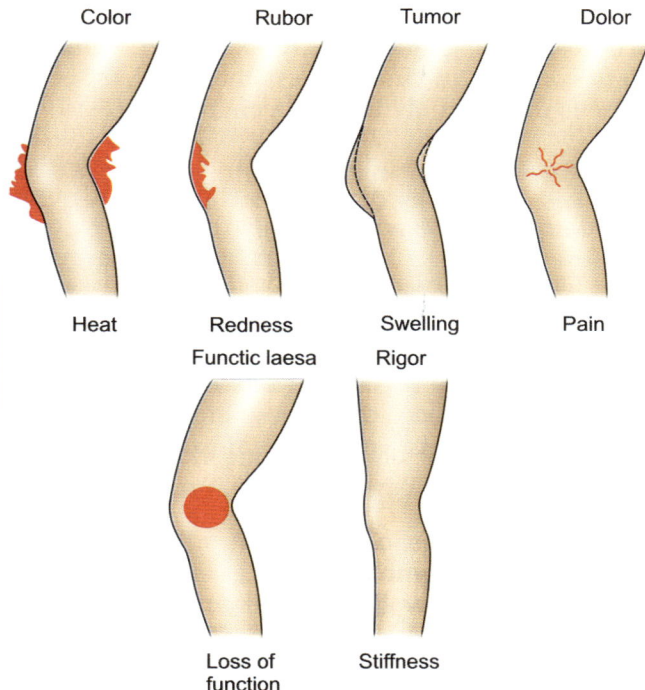

Fig. 55.1: Cardinal signs of inflammation

Table 55.1: Stages of infective arthritis		
Serous	*Serofibrinous*	*Purulent*
• Pain is less	• Tenderness +ve	• Patient is very ill
• Movements of the joint ↓	• Fever +ve	• Pain +ve (severe)
• Local temperature↑	• Night pains +ve	• Wasting +ve
• Flexion deformity	• Movements of joints reduced	• Temperature ↑
	• Pain is less	• Movements of joints severely reduced

Note: Nearly one-third of patients affected with bacterial arthritis suffer loss of joint function.

Investigations

Joint aspirate and synovial fluid analysis: This is the most accurate diagnostic tool for septic arthritis. The synovial fluid is tested for cells, sugar and proteins. Gram staining is positive in 60 percent of the cases for gram-positive cocci.

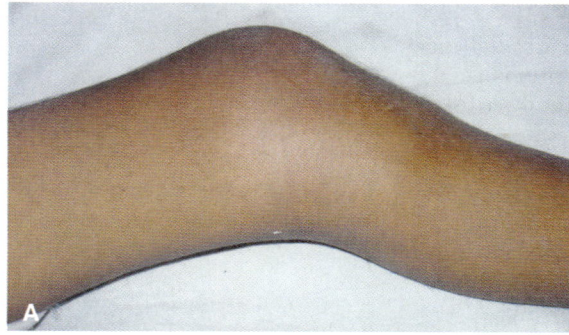

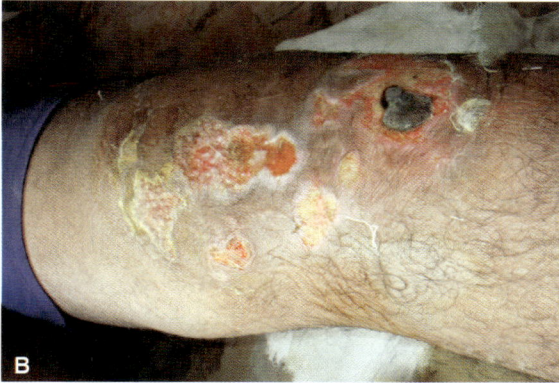

Figs 55.2A and B: Septic arthritis of the knee (A) deformity of the knee (B) skin ulceration of the knee

Laboratory investigations: WBCs (polymorphs) are raised to 50,000 to 1,00,000 (80% of cases), ESR increased more than 20 mm/hr (in 50% of cases), Hb percentage decreases. Blood culture is positive in 35 to 50 percent of the cases.

Radiology
- *Early stages:* It may be normal in some cases. In others earliest findings in the radiographs are soft tissue swelling and periarticular osteoporosis (Fig. 55.3).
- *Late stages:* In the later stages cartilage destruction, loss of joint space, necrosis of bone, epiphyseal disturbances, fibrous ankylosis, and bony ankylosis may be seen.

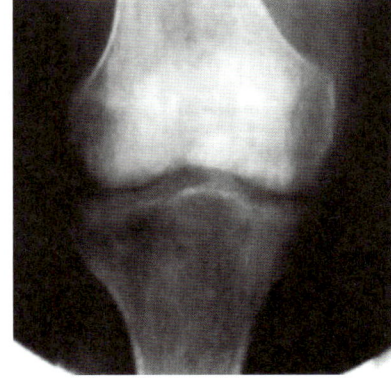

Fig. 55.3: Plain X-ray showing infective arthritis of the knee

Treatment

- *Arthrotomy or joint drainage:* The joint is aspirated first, if pus is present, open arthrotomy is indicated. The pus is cultured and is subjected to Gram staining. Appropriate antibiotics are then chosen and are given intravenously before surgical drainage. Antibiotics are used for a minimum period of 2 to 4 weeks. IV Amikacin (15 mg/kg) and Cefotaxime (100–150 mg/kg) are the drugs of choice in the initial stages.
- *Immobilization* of the joints by using plaster of Paris splints in functional position reduces pain and prevents deformities.
- *Radical treatment* is reserved for all except, very early cases, which do not respond rapidly within 24 hours to antibiotics and immobilization.
- If cartilage is destroyed, aim for ankylosis in functional position by plaster casts.

Complications

- Joint destruction.
- Pathological dislocation.
- Osteoarthritis in later years.
- Ankylosis—fibrous or bony.
- Acute osteomyelitis.
- Amyloidosis very rarely develops.
- Septicemia, pyemia, etc.

> **Remember**
>
> Tom Smith arthritis is a septic arthritis of the hip joint seen in infants. It is often confused with CDH. Arthroscopic joint drainage is the treatment of choice.

Differential Diagnosis

- TB arthritis
- Hemophilia
- Rheumatic arthritis
- Acute osteomyelitis
  Please refer appropriate sentence for details.

Sequelae of Infective Arthritis

What happens when one develops an infective arthritis? Well three things may happen, there may be complete resolution, fibrous or bony ankylosis (Figs 55.4A to C).

QUICK FACTS
- Sites of septic arthritis in parenteral drug abusers:
  - Sacroiliac joint
  - Sternal articulations
  - Pubis symphysis
- Organisms responsible are:
  - *Staphylococcus aureus*
  - *Pseudomonas aeruginosa*
  - *Serratia marcescens*
- In sickle cell anemia, *Salmonella* is the organism causing septic arthritis
- In nail pricks *Pseudomonas aeruginosa* is the organism. The most common site is the second metatarsophalangeal joint

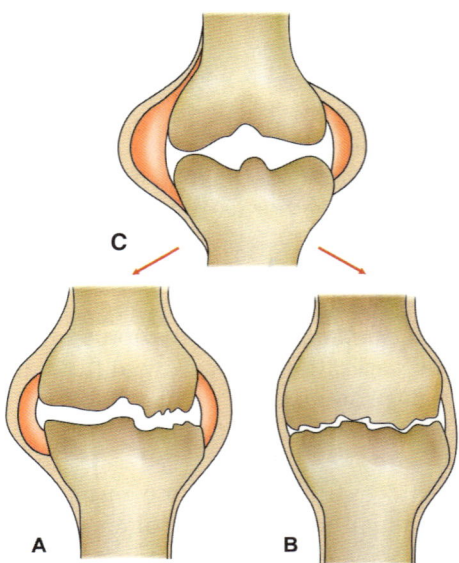

Figs 55.4A to C: Sequelae in infective arthritis: (A) No residual effect leaving back a normal joint, (B) Features suggestive of fibrous ankylosis, (C) Bony ankylosis

55

GONOCOCCAL ARTHRITIS

The incidence of gonococcal arthritis is less than 1 percent and it is familiarly known as a three-week infection. The male to female ratio is 5:1 and the age of predilection is between 20 and 30 years. It usually results due to lack of treatment for gonorrhea. Forty percent of the cases are mono-articular, knee being the most common site.

Pathology

Gonococcal arthritis can present as acute, subacute and chronic. The important pathological features are synovitis, effusion, cartilage erosion, and destruction of cartilage.

Clinical Features

Gonococcal arthritis is usually sudden in onset. Patient presents with chills, fever, pain and swelling of the joint. On examination there is raised temperature and tenderness. There may be history of urethral discharge. The disease may become chronic due to inadequate and improper treatment.

Treatment

The treatment methods consist of local measures like splints, chemotherapy by intravenous penicillin G, rest to the part, aspiration with a thick bored needle and arthrotomy to clear the joint debris.

SYPHILIS OF JOINTS

The incidence of syphilis of the joints is definitely on the decline due to the early use of antibiotics. Syphilitic

arthritis is caused by *Treponema pallidum* and is classified as congenital or acquired (Table 55.2):

Clinical Features

A painless swelling is the hallmark except during the early stages swelling, deformity, loss of movements, etc. are some of the other feature.

Investigations

- Wassermann's test is positive.
- *Treponema pallidum* immobilization test is positive.
- Joint fluid aspiration and synovial fluid analysis for cell, sugar, protein, etc.

Treatment

Antisyphilitic treatment is done but it is often not successful. Penicillin is the drug of choice.

NEUROPATHIC JOINTS (CHARCOT'S)

55

This causes extensive destruction of the joint as it is painless. The following are some of the important causes of neuropathic joints.
- Syringomyelia (25%)
- Tabes dorsalis (4–10%)
- Syphilis
- Rheumatoid arthritis
- Intraarticular steroids
- Traumatic division of sciatic nerve
- Chronic liver disease
- Prolonged administration of drugs like indomethacin, etc.

Sites: Knee, ankle, hip, elbow, shoulder, wrist and intervertebral joints in that order. It is rare before 40 years.

Table 55.2: Types and clinical features in syphilis of joints

Congenital	Acquired

• **Parrot's**
  – Syphilitic joint
  Features
  – Epiphysitis
  – Effusion
  – Separation of
    serous synovitis
2. **Clutton's joints**
  Features
  – Symmetrical
  – Hydrarthrosis
  – Painless
  – 8 to 16 years
    of age
	Early
	• Arthralgia
	  – Secondary stage of syphilis
	  – Nocturnal pain is present
	  – Spasm of muscles
	• Hydrarthrosis epiphysis
	  – Late symmetrical involvement
	• Gummatous arthritis
	  – Synovial form
	  – Osseous form usually affects the knee, resembles osteoarthritis, painless polyarthritis, etc.
	• Charcot's joint is a neuropathic joint

Pathology: The pathological changes seen in the joint are gross destruction of the joint, the capsules are thickened, osteophyte formation is seen, joint cavity is distorted and the loose bodies are present.

Clinical features: In this condition premonitory signs are rare; onset is usually sudden and unexpected. Gross swelling and lax joint are commonly seen (Fig. 55.5).

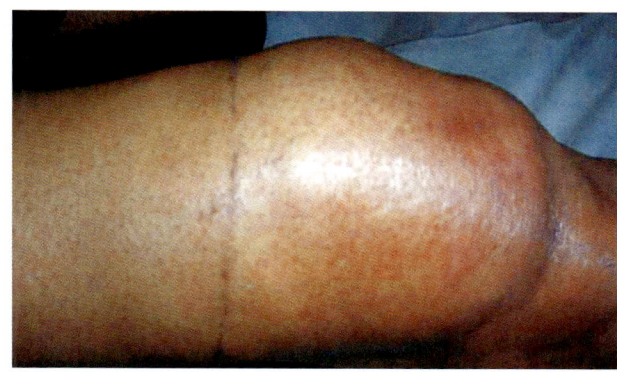

Fig. 55.5: Clinical photograph of a neuropathic knee joint

In the later stages of the disease the following features are seen, lax joints, *striking absence of pain*, joint becomes flail and there is a diffuse erythema around the joints.

Plain X-ray of the affected joint shows gross destruction of the joint (Fig. 55.6).

Treatment

The treatment of choice is Charnley's compression arthrodesis but efficient bracing still has a major role to play (Figs 55.7A and B).

HEMOPHILIC ARTHRITIS (BLEEDER'S JOINTS)

It is a hereditary coagulative disorder characterized by hemorrhages, which is spontaneous and is due to trivial trauma. It is X-linked, carried by female, manifest in

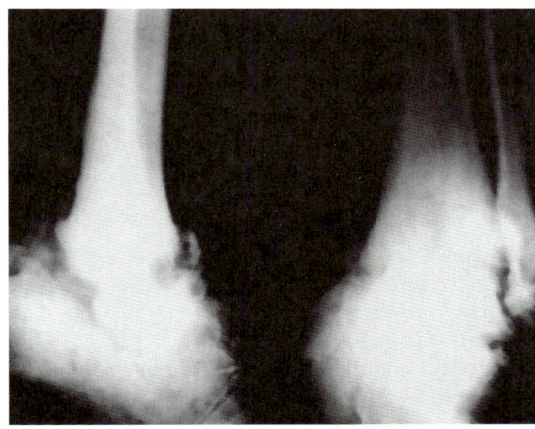

Fig. 55.6: Radiological features of a neuropathic ankle joint

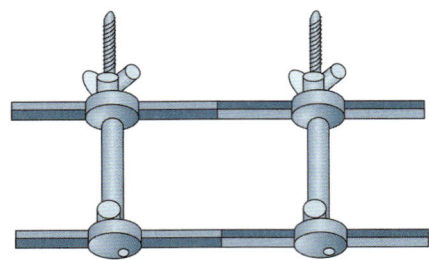

Fig. 55.7A: Charnley's compression clamp with 2 pins

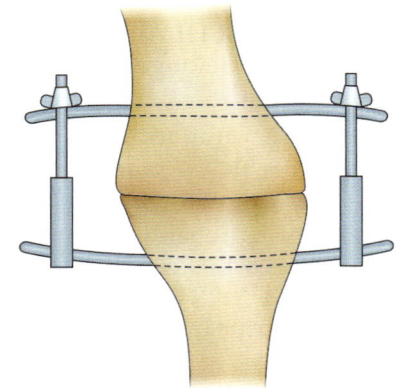

Fig. 55.7B: Charnley's compression arthrodesis

male, cause being prolonged clotting time. Incidence is 3 to 4 per one lakh population.

Pathology

The defective blood interacts with the synovial fluid and causes irritation to the synovial membrane. Due to the proliferation of the macrophages, there is synovial hyperplasia and pannus formation which ultimately causes destruction of the articular cartilage of the joint.

Clinical Features

Bleeding is spontaneous and is usually due to trivial trauma. Acute hemarthrosis occurs within hours. The joint is warm, tender and flexion attitude develops. Acute phase lasts for few weeks. With each attack joint movement decreases, fixed flexion deformity occurs, degenerative arthritis sets in and results in fibrous ankylosis. There is gross muscle atrophy (Fig. 55.8).

Laboratory investigations: The classical feature of this disease is, bleeding time is normal but the clotting time is prolonged.

Radiology: This shows soft tissue swelling, juxtaepiphyseal osteoporosis, squaring of the patella, widening of the intercondylar notch of the femur, subchondral cysts and features of ankylosis (Fig. 55.9).

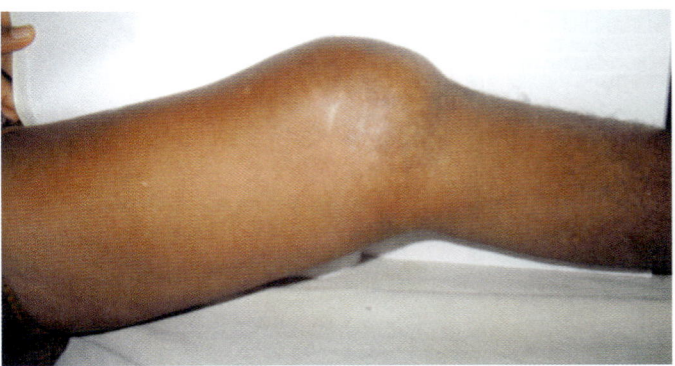

Fig. 55.8: Hemophilic arthritis

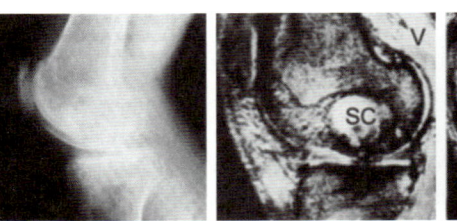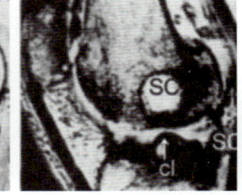

Fig. 55.9: Plain X-ray of MRI changes in hemophilic arthritis

55

Treatment

This varies according to the stages of the disease.

Acute stage: For injuries of less than four hours, the patient is treated on OPD basis. Factor VIII is replaced and is discharged home on the same day.

Late cases: Treated as in-patient, trial aspiration prolonged immobilization, factor VIII replacement and later mobilization with calipers and splints are recommended.

Chronic Hemarthropathy

In chronic hemophilic arthritis the treatment could be conservative or surgical.
Conservative methods:
• *For recent contractures:* Plaster immobilization, dynamic traction and physiotherapy.
• *For post subluxation of tibia:* Dynamic traction
• *For painful unstable joints:* Orthotic splintage

Surgery

Surgery is indicated for painful, stiff joints, stiff contractures and recurrent bleeding into the joint.

Surgical methods: These include synovectomy, internal fixation for fracture nonunion. Supracondylar osteotomy for severe flexion contractures of knee, arthrodesis for severely disorganized joints, total hip replacement for pain in the hip in advanced stages and tendo Achilles lengthening for tendo Achilles contractures, etc.

56 | Rheumatoid Arthritis

INTRODUCTION

The rheumatic diseases embrace an amazing array of hereditary and acquired disorders with a wide variety of clinical features. As per the present understanding rheumatic disorders can be classified under three broad headings.

Diffuse systemic
- Rheumatoid arthritis
- Seronegative spondyloarthritis
- Systemic lupus erythematosus (SLE)
- Polymyositis
- Scleroderma

Localized articular
- Osteoarthritis
- Crystal induced arthritis
- Traumatic arthritis

Non-articular
- Fibromyalgia
- Low back pain
- Tenosynovitis.

RHEUMATOID ARTHRITIS

Rheumatoid arthritis is the most common inflammatory disease of the joints. It is a systemic disease of young and middle-aged adults characterized by proliferative and destructive changes in synovial membrane, periarticular structures, skeletal muscles and perineural sheaths. Eventually joints are destroyed, fibrosed or ankylosed. It is a widespread vasculitis of the small arterioles.

EPIDEMIOLOGY

Incidence is 3 percent.
Sex: Eighty percent affected are women;
Male: Female ratio is 1:3
Age: No age is exempted, mean age is 40 years.

Etiology: The exact cause is unknown but genetics and malfunction of the cellular and humoral arms of the immune system are cited as the probable cause.

Genetics: The presence of HLA-drw-4 and HLA-DR 1, strongly suggests the role of genetics in the causation of rheumatoid arthritis.

Current hypothesis: An initiating antigen triggers an aberrant response, which becomes self-perpetuating long after the offending antigen has been cleared.

Antigenic agents: Which probably act as predisposing factors are viruses: (rubella, Epstein-Barr, etc.) genetic (common in people with HLA DR4 60%), psychological stress, allergic factors, endocrine factors and metabolic factors.

Pathogenesis

Against unknown exciting antigenic agents rheumatoid factors (mainly the Fc fragment of IgG) are elaborated. Rheumatoid factors (autoantibodies) are synthesized in rheumatoid synovial tissue and are mainly IgM in 70 to 90 percent of cases. In the remainder 10 to 30 percent it could be IgG, IgA or IgE. This rheumatoid factor along with IgG triggers off a complement cascade. The WBCs engulf this immune complex and elaborate lysosomes. Neutrophils release procollagenase, which is converted into an active collagenase by the synovial fluid. This splits the collagen of the articular cartilage. The neutral proteases complete the degradation of the collagen fibrils (Fig. 56.2).

Pathology

As explained earlier due to the synthesis of autoantibodies, against unknown antigenic agents in the synovium, primary synovitis sets in. This primary synovitis gives rise to pannus, which in turn forms the villus. This villus migrates towards the joint causing its destruction and ankylosis, fibrous in the early stages followed by bony ankylosis in the late stages.

Pathogenic Spectrum (Fig. 56.1)

Microscopy

It reveals rheumatoid units, which are an area of fibrinoid necrosis surrounded by fibroblasts, arranged radially and it is surrounded by a fibrous capsule (Fig. 56.3). This rheumatoid unit is found in the muscle, vessels, nerves, synovium, etc.

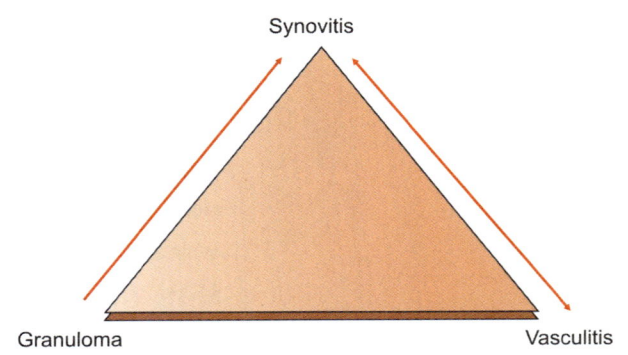

Fig. 56.1: Rheumatoid arthritis = Synovitis + Vasculitis + Granuloma

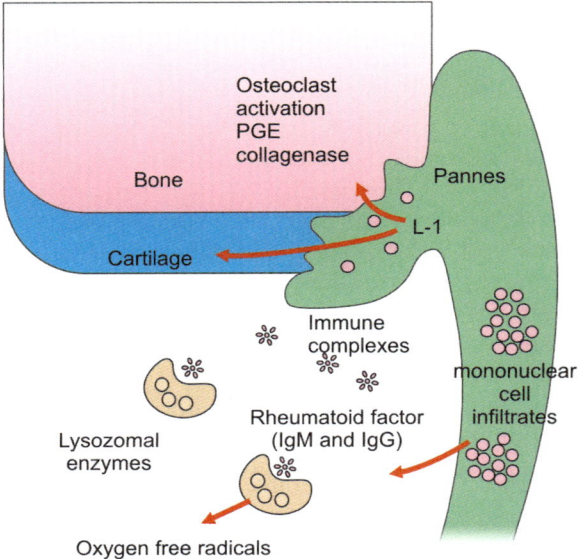

Fig. 56.2: Pathogenesis in rheumatoid arthritis

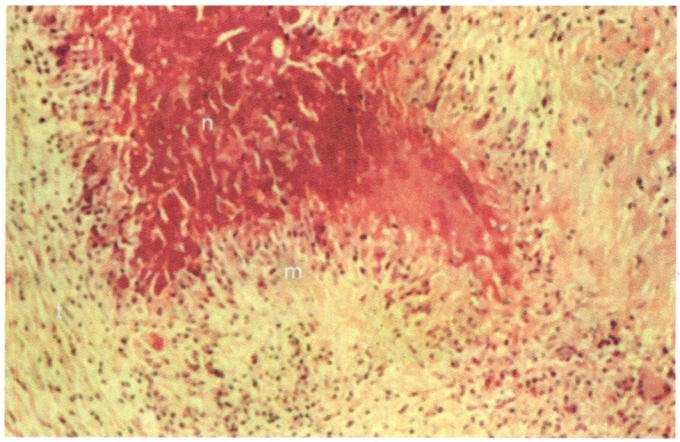

Fig. 56.3: Microscopic feature of a rheumatoid unit

According to American college of rheumatology in 1987 revised criteria at least 4 out of 7 criteria should be fulfilled to make a diagnosis of rheumatoid arthritis.
- Morning stiffness.
- Arthritis or swelling of 3 or more joints for > 6 weeks.
- Arthritis or swelling of hand joints (wrist metacarpal) for more than 6 weeks.
- Symmetrical swelling (arthritis of same joint areas) more than 6 weeks.
- Serum rheumatoid factor present.
- Radiographic features of RA.
- Rheumatoid nodules.

Note: How accurate are these criterias? Sensitivity is 93% and Specificity is 90%.

Clinical Features

Rheumatoid arthritis usually presents in three forms:

Classical presentation: In this group patient is usually a woman in her mid-thirties. Pain, swelling, stiffness of the small joints of hands and feet are the common presenting complaints. Other joints are also affected with varying frequency. Patient also gives history of weight loss, lethargy and depression. Joint swelling could be symmetrical and the patient presents with deformities of bones and joints in the late stages. The patient gives history of remission and exacerbation of symptoms with seasonal variations. This is a very classical complaint in the absence of which diagnosis of rheumatoid arthritis should be carefully made. Symptoms fluctuate from day to day.

Other presentations: This consists of palindromic presentation involving one or two joints, systemic presentation and is usually seen in middle-aged men presenting with pleurisy, pericarditis, etc. It mimics malignancy. It may present as polymyalgia particularly in elderly patients. It may present as monoarthritic swelling. Sometimes the presentation may be very explosive unlike the usual chronic presentation. In some cases it may present as PUO (Pyrexia of Unknown Origin).

Extraarticular features: Two or more features are present in 75 percent of the cases. Rheumatoid factor is invariably present and it indicates a bad prognosis.
- Subcutaneous nodules are present in 25 percent of the cases. It is seen over the elbow (Fig. 56.5E), sacrum and occiput. Nodules may also be present in lungs, eyes, hearts, etc. When present over flexor tendon it may cause trigger finger.
- Widespread vasculitis leading to Raynaud's phenomenon, digital arteritis, necrotizing arteritis, peripheral neuritis, etc.

56

- Blood abnormalities commonly encountered in rheumatoid arthritis are chronic anemia, iron deficiency anemia, vitamin B12 and folate deficiency, leucocytopenia, thrombocytosis and marrow hypoplasia.
- Osteoporosis could be generalized or localized in bones around the joints.
- Eye changes seen are kerato-conjunctivitis sicca or Sjögren's syndrome, episcleritis (common), scleritis (serious problem), secondary glaucoma and scleromalacia perforans.
- Lung affections are pleurisy, pleural effusion, Caplan's syndrome (RA + pneumoconiosis involving the upper lobes) and fibrosing alveolitis in 2 percent.
- Heart affections in rheumatoid arthritis are pericardial friction (10%), pericardial effusion (30%), arrhythmias and heart block.
- Neuromuscular system involvement includes carpal tunnel syndrome, mononeuritis multiplex, muscle wasting, subluxation of C1 and C2, etc.
- Reticuloendothelial system affections include splenomegaly (5%), Felty's syndrome in 1% (RA+ splenomegaly + Neutropenia), generalized lymphadenopathy and painless pitting edema of the feet and ankles.

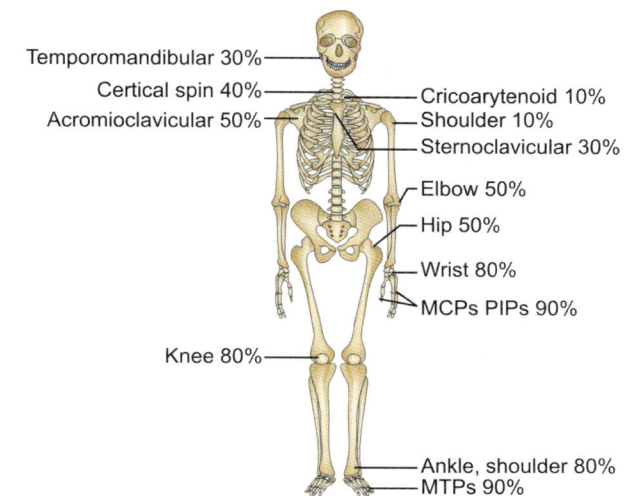

Fig. 56.4: Frequency of involvement of different joint sites in established RA

QUICK FACTS: STAGES IN RHEUMATOID ARTHRITIS

Reversible: Here disease is only synovial. Cartilage is spared.

Not totally reversible: Here disease spreads to the cartilage apart from the synovium. However the affection is mild.

Totally irreversible: Here there is destruction of the cartilage and other structures leading to fibrous or bony ankylosis.

Orthopedic deformities in rheumatoid arthritis: Rheumatoid arthritis can affect any joint in the body. *It involves the peripheral joints more often and very rarely affects the larger joints.* Of particular importance are the affection of the temporomandibular joint and atlantoaxial joint, which can prove lethal due to the cord compression (Fig. 56.4).

QUICK FACTS
- Joints involved in rheumatoid arthritis
- Metacarpophalangeal and interphalangeal joints of the hand.
- Shoulder elbow and wrists.
- Hip, knee and ankle.
Others: Temporomandibular joint, atlantoaxial joints and facet joints of the cervical spine.

Rheumatoid hand: The following are some of the very common deformities seen in the hand (Figs 56.5A to F).

- *Symmetrical peripheral joint swelling* of metacarpophalangeal and interphalangeal joints (Fig. 56.5A).
- *Ulnar deviation* of the hand is due to rupture of the collateral ligaments at the metacarpophalangeal joints, which enables the extensor tendons to slip from their grooves towards the ulnar side (Fig. 56.5C).

- *Boutonnière deformity* is due to the rupture of central extensor expansion of the fingers resulting in flexion at the PIP joint (Fig. 56.5D).
- *Swan neck deformity* is due to the rupture of the volar plate of the PIP joints which enables the tendons to slip towards the dorsal side (Fig. 56.5B). This is also known as *intrinsic plus deformity*. Here there is hyperextension of the PIP joint and flexion of the DIP joints.
- *Trigger fingers and trigger thumb* are due to nodules over the tendons.

Rheumatoid foot: It affects the forefoot, midfoot, and hind foot. In the forefoot patient may develop hallux valgus deformity of the great toe, claw toes, callosity over the dorsum and the sole, widening of the forefoot, etc. The heel may show valgus deformity.

Other joints: In the knee initially there is a gross soft tissue swelling due to synovitis and in the later stages, the patient may develop fibrous ankylosis or bony

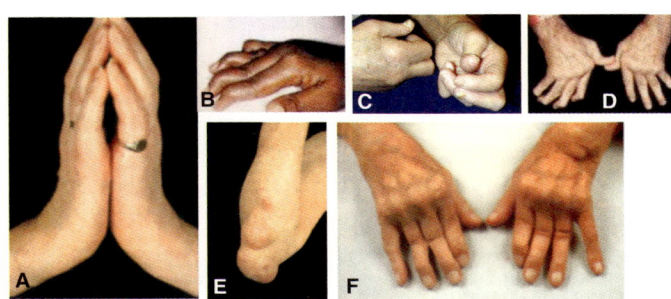

Figs 56.5A to F: Various orthopedic deformities in rheumatoid arthritis: (A) symmetrical swelling of peripheral joints (B) swan neck deformity, (C) ulnar deviation of the fingers, (D) swan neck deformity thumb and boutonnière deformity of the fingers, (E) subcutaneous nodules over the elbow, (F) bilateral symmetrical involvement

ankylosis due to widespread destruction of the articular cartilage by the pannus. Similarly, other major joints of the body like the hip, ankle, shoulder, and elbow could be involved.

Laboratory Investigations: Hb percentage is low and shows normochromic, hypochromic anemia. WBCs are decreased or normal, there are increased lymphocytes and the ESR is raised.

Serological Tests

RA test: It usually detects only IgM type of rheumatoid factor.

Basis: Rheumatoid patient's serum contains RA factor, which in the presence of γ-globulin agglutinates certain strains of streptococci sensitized by sheep cells and latex particles.

a. *Latex fixation test:* Unknown serum + 7-globulin latex suspension

b. *Inhibition test:* This test uses the characteristics of euglobulin from unknown serum. Euglobulin from normal serum neutralizes the rheumatoid factor thereby inhibiting agglutination. Euglobulin from rheumatoid serum has no effect on the rheumatoid factor and agglutination occurs. *This is the most sensitive test.*

Remember

RA factor is found in:
- 75% of rheumatoid arthritis cases
- 10% in healthy elderly people
- 10% in malaria, etc.

Thus, not all cases of Rheumatoid arthritis have positive. Rheumatoid factor and vice versa.

Radiological features: X-rays of the hand (Fig. 56.6) and feet and other joints show the following changes:

- Soft tissue swelling.
- Juxta-articular osteoporosis.
- Erosion of joint margins.
- Joint spaces are decreased.
- Deformities.
- Atlantoaxial subluxation.
- Subchondral erosions and cyst formation.
- Fibrous and bony ankylosis develops in the late stages.

Other common abnormalities: These include increased C reactive protein (CRP), increased alkaline phosphatase, increased platelets, and decreased serum albumin, citrulline antibody is present in most early cases.

Synovial fluid analysis: This is not performed routinely for diagnostic purposes but performed to exclude other causes of inflammation such as infection. Synovial fluid in RA is typically yellow, watery and turbid due to high WBC and has low sugar content.

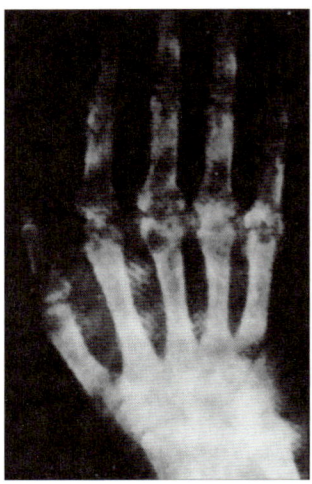

Fig. 56.6: Radiological features of rheumatoid arthritis

QUICK FACTS OF RHEUMATOID ARTHRITIS
- Most common chronic inflammatory disorder.
- 80% in women.
- Exact cause is not known.
- Rheumatoid unit is present.
- History of remissions and exacerbations present.
- Symmetrical peripheral joint involvement.
- Rheumatoid arthritis factor is +ve in 70%.
- Inhibition test is most sensitive.
- Extraarticular features are seen in 75%.

Management

Aims of treatment
- To keep inflammatory process at a minimum, thereby, preserving joint motion, maintaining healthy muscles and preventing secondary joint stiffness and deformity.
- To keep constitutional symptoms at a minimum.
- The possible deformities are anticipated and prevented by appropriate splinting.
- Finally surgical measures to correct the deformities, eliminate pain and provide stability are undertaken.

General measures: It aims at improving the general condition of the patient and to keep the joints properly splinted in functional position to guard against the ensuing ankylosis.

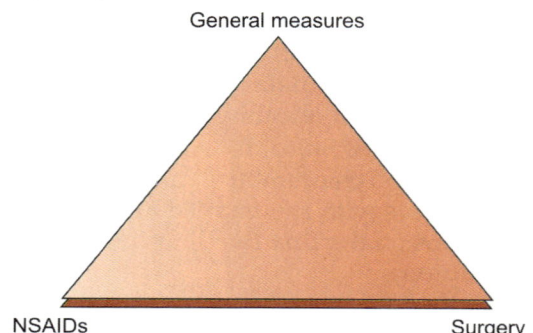

Fig. 56.7: Treatment triad for rheumatoid arthritis

56

56

- Rest in bed.
- Good diet, rich in proteins and minerals.
- Transfusion and hematinics to correct the anemia.
- Hormones combination of estrogen and androgen to improve the bone stock.
- Removal of infective foci.

Splints: These are known to serve three main functions:
- Rest and relief of pain *(rest splints).*
- Prevention and correction of deformity *(corrective splints).*
- Fixation of damaged joint in a good functional position *(fixation splints).*

Splinting in the functional position helps in the event that ankylosis ensues. The splint is removed daily. Hot packs are given or patient is placed in Hubbard tank at (92.6–102°F) and the joints are put into full range of motion. While the joints are immobilized, muscle-setting exercises are advocated. After removal of the splints, resistance exercises are begun.

Drug therapy is the mainstay of treatment in rheumatoid arthritis. Three classes of drugs are used regularly.
- Analgesics
- Anti-inflammatory drugs
- Disease modifying antirheumatic drugs (DMARD).

Steroids especially intraarticular injections have an important role.
- *First line of drugs (NSAIDs):* These are aspirin/ ibuprofen/ketoprofen/diclofenac sodium napro-xen/piroxicam, etc. They are the major pharma-ceutical agents for pain relief in rheumatic diseases. Though useful, they have significant side effects. Aspirin is the drug of first choice.
- *Second line of drugs (DMARDs):* Second line of drugs are used only if an adequate trial of first line drugs have failed to relieve symptoms satisfactorily or if there is radiological evidence of progressive disease. Second line drugs are alternatively known as disease modifying antirheumatic drugs (DMARD) and are slow acting drugs. It would seem that they have influence on the underlying disease process, and may take several weeks or months to exert this effect. Commonly prescribed drugs are Injectable gold and oral gold (sodium aurothiomalate), Penicillamine, Sulphasalazine, Antimalarial drugs (e.g. chloro-quine), Dapsone and levamisole.
- *Third line of drugs:* Steroids, Azathioprim, cyclo-phosphamide and chlorambucil can exert a third line effect in patients with rheumatoid arthritis, and are considered when the first two lines of drugs fail to relive symptoms.
- *Role of local corticosteroid* treatment is considered when the rheumatoid arthritis affects one or two joints. It is also indicated in tendinitis, capsular or ligament involvement, carpal tunnel and compression syndromes. It is given weekly in acute cases and three monthly in chronic. If two injections are ineffective, the treatment is discontinued.

Physiotherapy Measures in Rheumatoid Arthritis
- Measures to prevent deformities: Splintages.
- Measures to relieve pain: Heat therapy, tens, etc.
- Measures to mobilize the joints: Active and passive exercises.
- Measures to strengthen the muscles: Various active, resistive, isometric exercises.
- Walking aids.

Surgery: Aim of surgery in rheumatoid arthritis is to:
- Relieve pain.
- Correct the deformity of the joints.
- Reduce joint instability.
- Improve the range of movements of the joints.

Surgical Methods

Synovectomy: It may be indicated in patients with rheumatoid arthritis if joint destruction is minimal and if the main cause of pain and swelling is synovitis, which is resistant to medication and physiotherapy. Synovectomy is usually carried out over the knee, ankle, elbow and wrist.

Osteotomy: This should be considered in patients under the age of 60 with osteoarthritis of the hip or knee due to rheumatoid arthritis. Osteotomy has the advantage of relieving pain without sacrificing the joint surfaces which have only been partially damaged (Fig. 56.8).

At the hip, intertrochanteric osteotomy, which contains the femoral head within the acetabulum, is preferred. At the knee, abduction osteotomy is preferred.

Arthrodesis of the joint gives excellent long-term pain relief. It is reserved for peripheral joints, such as the wrist, ankle, and IP joints of the hands and feet where

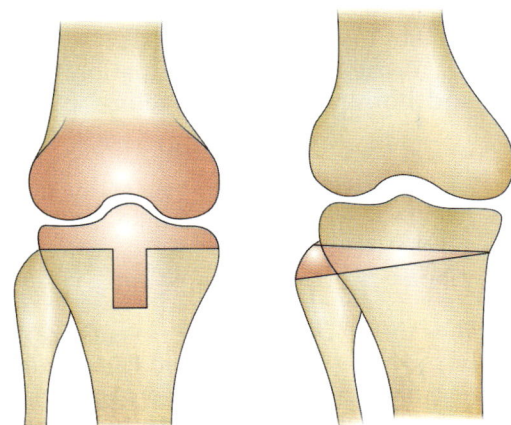

Fig. 56.8: Osteotomy in rheumatoid knee

the functional loss is less disabling and arthroplasty is less reliable.

Arthroplasties of the hip, knee (Figs 56.9 and 56.10), ankle, shoulder, elbow, wrist, and hand is indicated in advanced diseases causing severe pain and incapacitating disability due to stiffness and instability.

Self-management techniques for rheumatoid and other forms of arthritis: This is the most important aspect of the treatment of rheumatoid and other forms of arthritis. People practicing self-management techniques tend to experience less pain and are more active than those who do not practice self-management. In this management, the patient is made aware of the disease and the rationale behind the treatment. They are made to realize that the success of the treatment is their ultimate responsibility (Fig. 56.11).

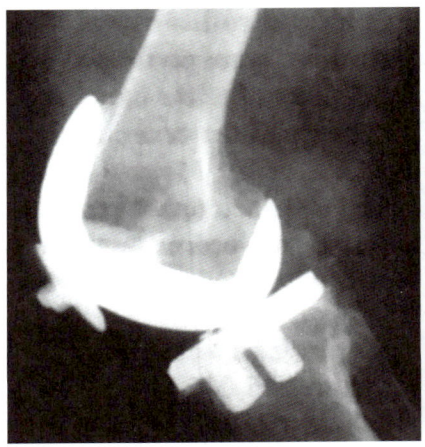
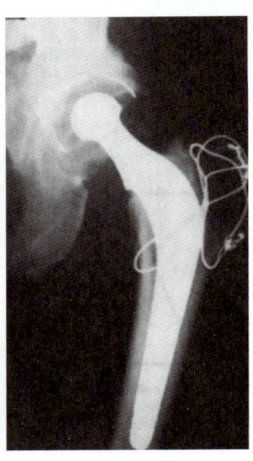

Fig. 56.9: Total knee replacement for RA knee

Fig. 56.10: Total hip replacement for RA hip

56

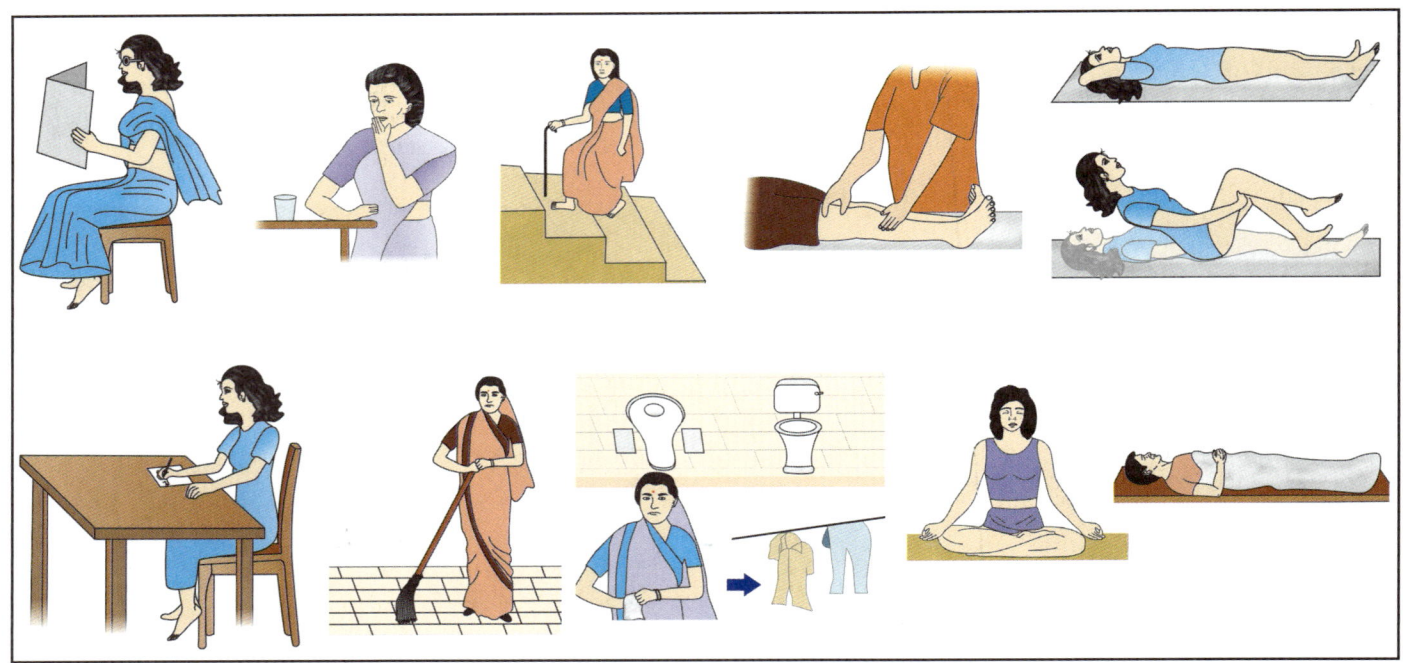

Fig. 56.11: Modifications of activities of daily living

Seronegative Spondyloarthropathies

Ankylosing spondylitis
Crystalline arthropathies
Monosodium urate arthropathy (Gout)
Pseudogout (CPPD)

Seronegative spondyloarthropathies (SSA) group is gradually emerging as a new entity. These disorders are labeled as *seronegative* to indicate that they have in common the *absence of the rheumatoid factor*. The term spondyloarthropathies is used because in many cases there is involvement of the *spine and sacroiliac joints*. Hence, SSA can be defined as an *acute or chronic condition with characteristic involvement of axial joints, absence of RA factor and HLA abnormality.*

The clinical entities, which appear to justify inclusions in the SSA group, are as follows (Table 57.1).
• Ankylosing spondylitis
• Reiter's disease
• Psoriatic arthritis
• Enteropathic arthritis (Ulcerative colitis, Crohn's disease, Whipple's disease)
• Behcet's syndrome.

Note: HLA-B27 shows a strong association with SSA.

ANKYLOSING SPONDYLITIS (MARIE-STRÜMPELL DISEASES)

This is a chronic progressive inflammatory disease of the sacroiliac joints and the axial skeleton.

Causes

Causes are unknown. It is found to be strongly associated with HLA-B27 genetic marker in about 85 percent of the cases.

Age/Sex

Common in young male adults (M: F = 10:1), in the 15–30 age group.

Pathology

The initial inflammation of the joints is followed by synovitis, arthritis and cartilage destruction, fibrous and later bony ankylosis. The joints commonly affected are SI joints, spine, hip, knee and manubrium sterni.

Clinical Features

Patient usually complains of early morning stiffness and pain in the back. The pain is worse at night and during rest and relieved after some activity. On examination patient has a stiff spine. In the later stages the patient may develop a stopped posture and a bent spine that is stiff (Fig. 57.1A).

Cervical spine involvement (Fig. 57.1B) is tested by asking the patient to touch the wall with the back of the head without raising his or her chin (Fleche's test). If the chest expansion is less than 5 cm, involvement of thoracic spine is suspected (Fig. 57.2).

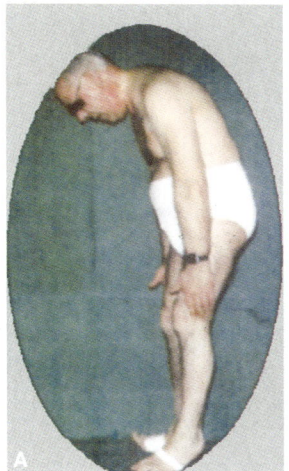 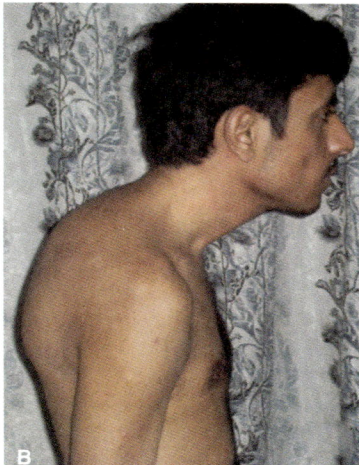

Figs 57.1A and B: (A) Deformity of the back (B) Deformity of the neck

Tests for sacroiliac joint involvement are positive (Figs 57.3 to 57.5).

Extraarticular Manifestations

These include acute iritis (25%), pericarditis, aortic incompetence, subluxation of atlantoaxial joints, apical lobe fibrosis, generalized osteoporosis, etc.

Note: Enthesopathy: This is the condition of calcification at the end of the attachments of the muscles, ligaments, tendons especially of the pelvis, joints, heel, etc.

Table 57.1: Differential Diagnosis SSA

Disease	Sex and age	Onset	Signs and symptoms	Joints involved	Extraarticular lesions	HLA-B27
Ankylosing spondylitis	Predominantly males < 40 years	Insidious	Low back pain, morning stiffness in heart, CNS disturbances, and pain > 3 months	Intervertebral joints	Uveitis, conduction defects pulmonary complications	94%
Psoriatic arthritis	Predominantly females > 50 years	Variable affected joints	Pain and stiffness on IP joints	Distal and proximal urethritis, and skin lesions	Uveitis, conjunctivitis,	100%
Reiter's disease	Predominantly females. 16-35 years	Sudden	Pain and stiffness of affected joints, diarrhea, dysuria, etc.	Weight bearing joints (knee and ankle)	Conjunctivitis, uveitis, buccal erosions, urethritis	83%
Enteropathic arthropathies (Crohn's disease, ulcerative colitis, Whipple's disease)	Predominantly males. Age group is not clear	Variable	Pain and stiffness of the affected joints, weight loss, diarrhea, abdominal pain	Knee, ankle (most common), shoulder wrist, elbow also involved	Aphthous ulcers, uveitis, erythema nodosum	50%
Behcet's syndrome	Predominantly males. 15–40 years	Variable	Pain and stiffness of affected joints.	Knee, hand, ankle and wrist joints are primarily affected. There is involvement of elbow, shoulder and hip joints	Painful oral ulcers, genital ulcers, ocular lesions, skin lesions.	16%

57

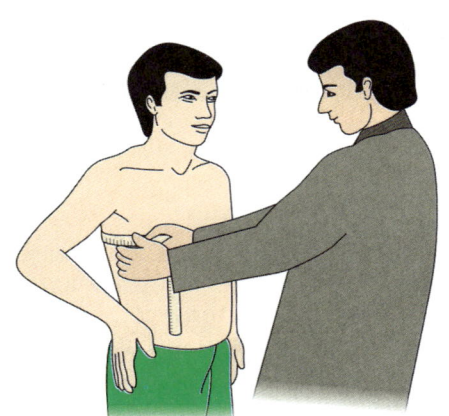

Fig. 57.2: Assessment of chest expansion in ankylosing spondylitis

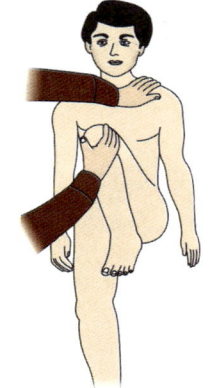

Fig. 57.3: Sacroiliac joint involvement: Pump handle test

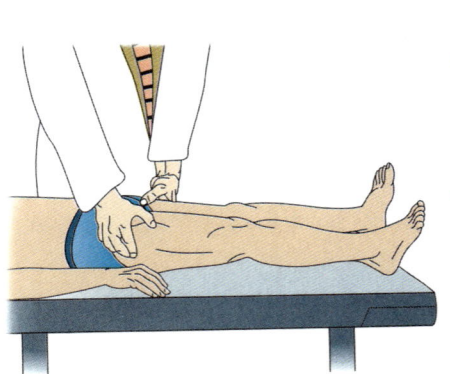

Fig. 57.4: Sacroiliac joint involvement: Pelvic compression test

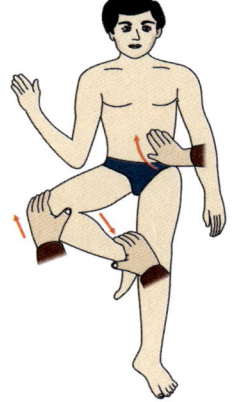

Fig. 57.5: Sacroiliac joint involvement: Fabre test

Investigations

Radiographs of SI joint show haziness, subchondral erosions, sclerosis (Fig. 57.6) widening of SI joint, etc.

Radiographs of spine show squaring of the vertebra, loss of lumbar lordosis, calcification of anterior longitudinal ligament, bridging osteophytes (called Syndesmophytes), bamboo spine (Fig. 57.7), etc.

Treatment

Conservative treatment consists of rest, NSAIDs (indomethacin) physiotherapy, back exercises, etc. Radiotherapy may also help. Surgical treatment consists of spinal osteotomy to correct spine deformity, total hip replacement and total knee replacement for hip and knee joint ankylosis.

CRYSTALLINE ARTHROPATHIES

This group includes two interesting clinical entities:
- Monosodium urate arthropathies (gout)
- Calcium pyrophosphate deposition disease (CPPD).

MONOSODIUM URATE ARTHROPATHY (GOUT)

This is known as *gout* and may manifest itself as *acute* or *chronic*.

57

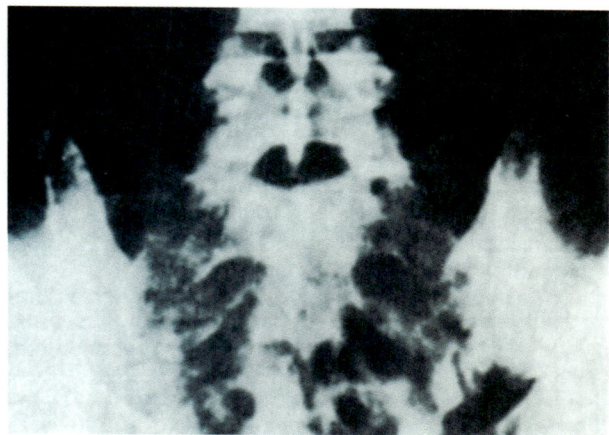

Fig. 57.6: X-ray of the pelvis showing sacroiliac joint sclerosis

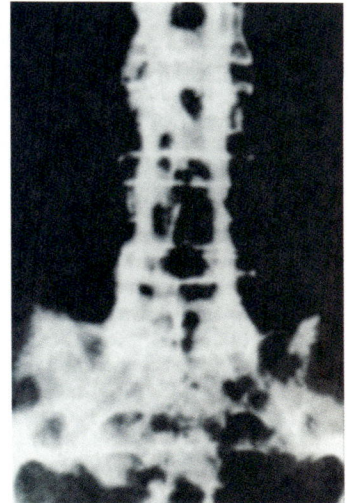

Fig. 57.7: X-ray of the lumbar spine showing bamboo spine in ankylosing spondylitis

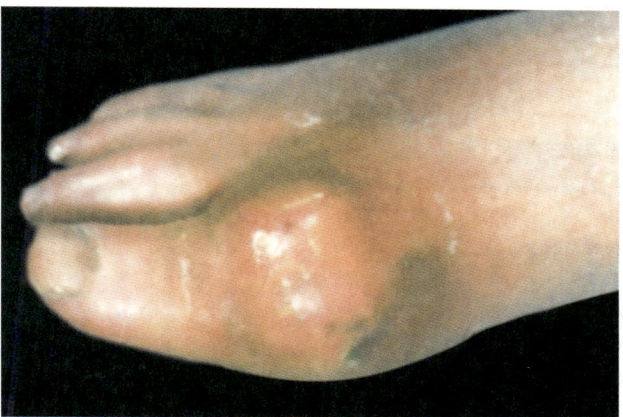

Fig. 57.8: Acute gout

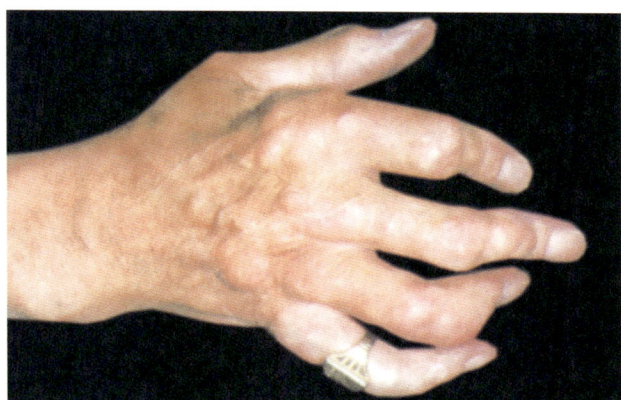

Fig. 57.9: Chronic gout

Investigations

Laboratory tests reveal leucocytosis, ESR is increased. Synovial fluid study is done under polarised microscopy for the presence of monosodium urate crystals. This is the most important diagnostic method (Fig. 57.10).

Sites: It is usually monoarticular and the first metatarso-phalangeal joint is the most common site of involvement (Fig. 57.8). Ankle, knee, wrist, fingers (Fig. 57.9) and elbow are the other joints affected. Distal and lower extremity joints are involved more often.

Role of hyperuricemia: Gout is usually associated with hyperuricemia and may be associated with hypertension, obesity and atherosclerosis.

Clinical Features

It has an abrupt onset. Patient may complain of pain, swelling, tenderness and increased temperature of the first metatarsophalangeal joint. Frequent gouty attacks disturb the sleep. Sometimes the inflammation is so gross that it may resemble cellulitis. Attacks are provoked by surgery, trauma, etc. Mild attacks resolve spontaneously within two days, more severe attacks may last for 7 to 10 days.

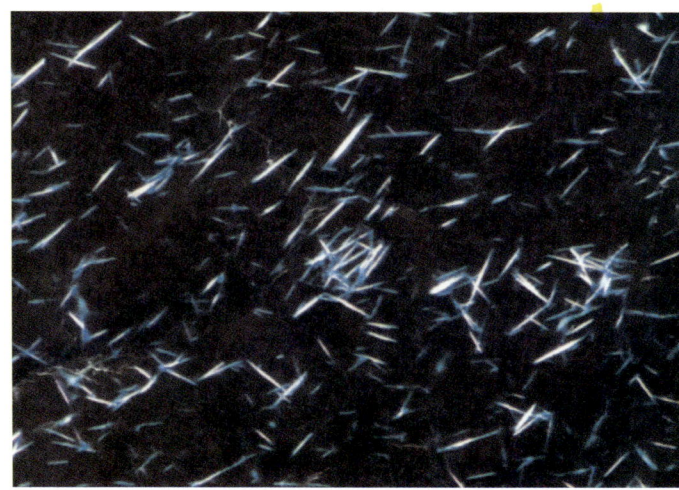

Fig. 57.10: Polarised microscopy picture

Radiology

It is usually normal but may provide a helpful clue to detect chondrocalcinosis.

Treatment

Conservative method is the mainstay of treatment. The following measures are recommended: Indomethacin 75 to 100 mg oral initially. Later it is given as 50 mg every 6 hrs. As the attack subsides the drug may be tapered off. Intra-articular steroid also helps. Recurrent gouty arthritic attacks can be prevented by prophylaxis with Colchicine (0.5 mg BD) or Indomethacin (25 to 50 mg every day). When the above two drugs do not help, Allopurinol is indicated on a long-term basis.

PSEUDOGOUT (CPPD)

Pseudogout is due to deposition of calcium pyrophosphate in the joints. Larger joints are more affected and 50 percent involve the knee joints unlike in gout (Fig.57.11). Other areas commonly involved are elbows, wrists, ankles, shoulder and hip. Synovial fluid study under polarised microscopy reveals CPP crystals. The disease is not as severe as gout and is much rarer.

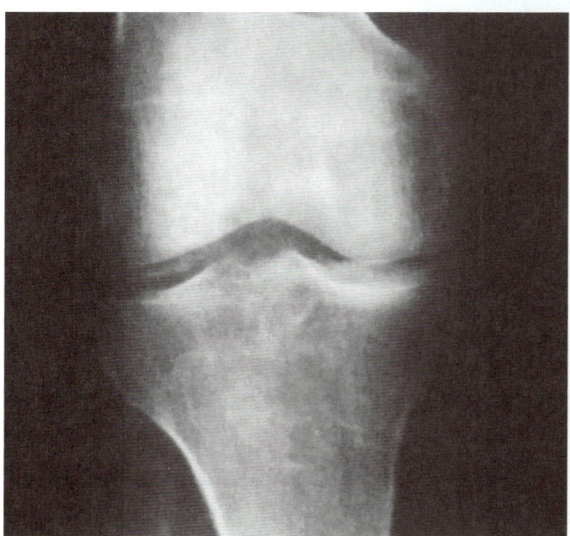

Fig. 57.11: Plain X-ray showing pseudogout

57

Degenerative Arthritis

INTRODUCTION

It is defined as a degenerative, non-inflammatory joint disease characterized by destruction of articular cartilage and formation of new bone at the joint surfaces and margins. There are two varieties, primary and secondary. The former is more common. Knee joint is affected more often than any other joint and is hence discussed first though it can affect any synovial joint in the body (Fig. 58.1).

PRIMARY OSTEOARTHRITIS OF THE KNEE

Etiology: Though exact cause is not known, the following factors are suspected to play an important role in the causation of primary osteoarthritis obesity, genetics and heredity, occupation involving prolonged standing, sports, endocrinal and metabolic disorders.

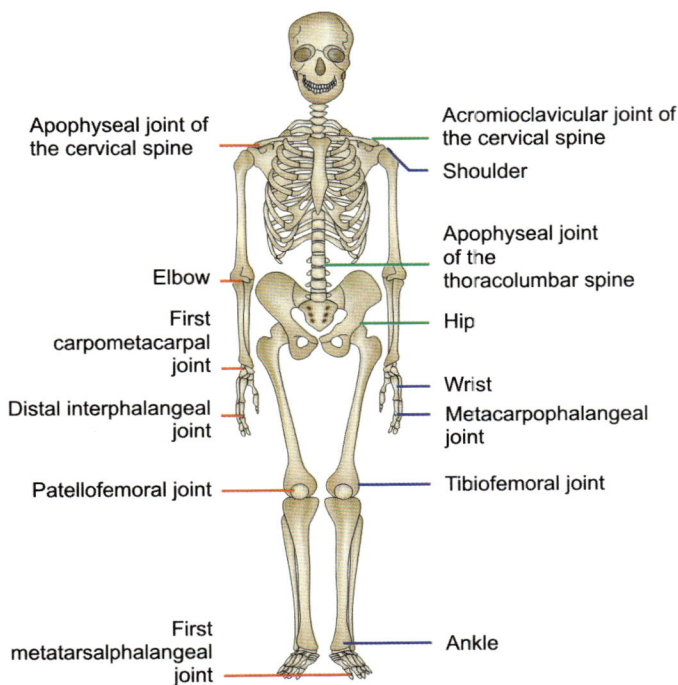

Fig. 58.1: Joints affected in osteoarthritis

Important predisposing factors in the Indians: Use of Indian toilets and squatting cross legged on the ground places the knee joints in extreme flexion and this over the years causes enormous stress on the knees and hastens its degeneration (Fig. 58.2).

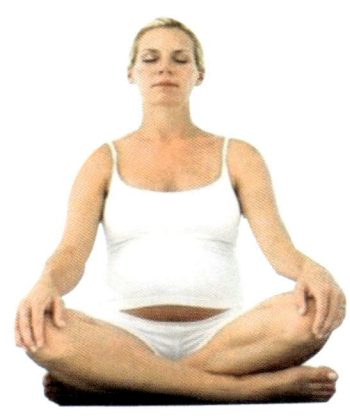

Fig. 58.2: Habit of squatting places abnormal stress on the knee

FEATURES
- It commonly affects the knee joint.
- All races are susceptible.
- Common in older age groups.
- Eighty percent of people are affected by 40 years, but only 40 percent show symptoms.
- It causes varus deformity of the knee in the late stages.

Sequence of pathological events in osteoarthritis: Fibrillation due to loss of fluids of the weight bearing articular cartilage is seen in early stages of the disease followed by complete loss of articular cartilage (Figs 58.3A and B). This puts enormous pressure on the underlying bone which causes sclerosis and later eburnation. Cysts may develop in the subchondral area due to micro fractures that degenerate. New bone formation takes place and results in osteophyte formation. Synovial inflammation and capsular thickening causes effusion and joint stiffness.

Clinical Features

Predominant symptom is pain which increases on walking and is relieved by rest. The pain is poorly localized and is dull aching in nature. Patient has mild swelling of the knee joint and complains of early

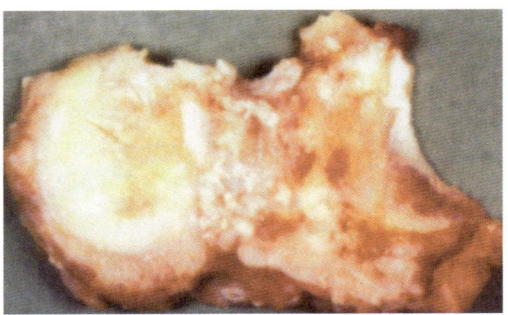

Fig. 58.3A: Pathological specimen of osteoarthritis knee

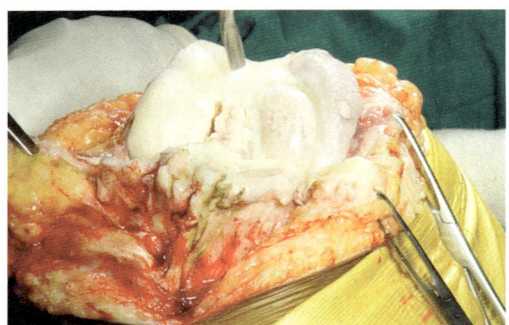

Fig. 58.3B: Arthroscopic view showing damaged cartilage stiffness

morning stiffness. Minimal tenderness and coarse crepitus can be elicited. If there are loose bodies in a joint, patient gives history of locking or giving way. Terminal movements of the knee are restricted (Fig. 58.5). Patient complains of early morning stiffness which subsides over the day after some activity. Genu varum deformity may be seen in very advanced cases (Fig. 58.4). Minimal quadriceps muscle wasting may be seen.

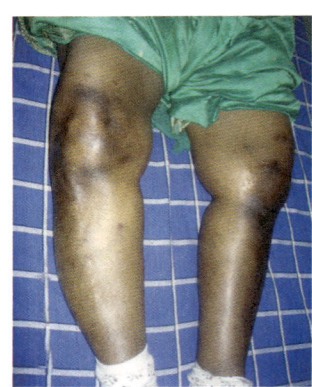

Fig. 58.4: Genu varum deformity in osteoarthritis knee

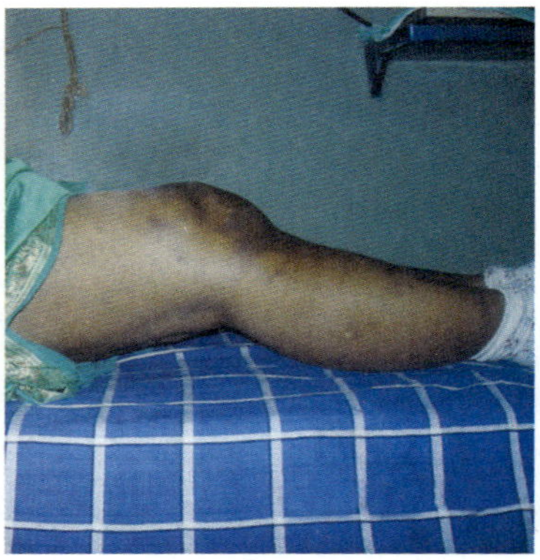

Fig. 58.5: Loss of terminal flexion in osteoarthritis knee

QUICK FACTS: OSTEOARTHRITIS

- *Who is prone to get osteoarthritis?*
  - Middle-aged patients
  - Women have a greater tendency than men
  - One in three people over 60 years are affected and more than three in four persons over the age of seventy show some radiographic evidence of the condition
  - Very rarely it can be seen in younger people
- *What are the typical symptoms of osteoarthritis?*
  - Pain
  - Early morning stiffness
  - Restricted range of joint movements
  - Swelling of the joints
- *What joints are usually affected?*
  - Weight bearing joints like hip, knee, ankle, etc.
  - Spine
  - Fingers
- *What causes osteoarthritis?*
  - Age more than 40 years
  - Female
  - Hereditary conditions
  - Previous joint injuries
  - Obesity
  - Diseases of the joints
  - Poor posture
  - Occupational stress and strain
  - A combination of the above factors
- *How to make a diagnosis?*
  - Physical examination
  - Symptomatology
  - Radiography
  - Blood tests
  - CT scan and MRI

Investigations

Laboratory *investigations* are usually within normal limits. Radiological examination of the knee joint is the most important diagnostic tool. The following are the radiological features seen in osteoarthritis (Fig. 58.6) of the knee.

- Loss of joint space (due to destruction of articular cartilage).
- Sclerosis (due to increase cellularity and bone deposition).

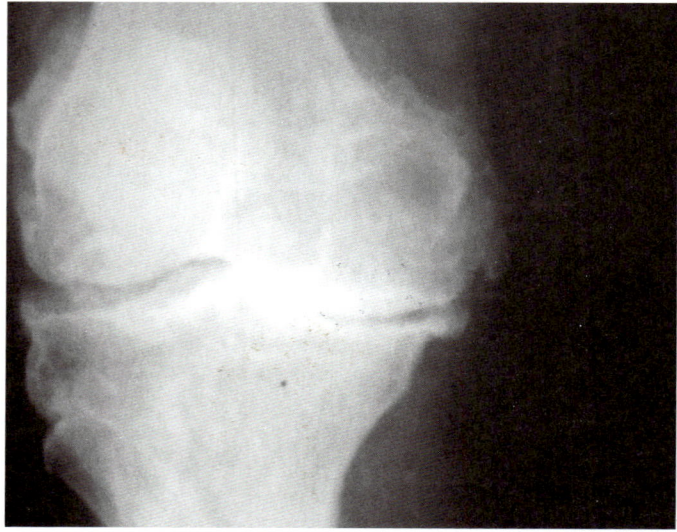

Fig. 58.6: Radiological features in osteoarthritis knee

- Subchondral cysts (due to synovial fluid intrusion into the bone).
- Osteophytes (due to revascularization of remaining cartilage and capsular traction).
- Bony collapse (due to compression of weakened bone).
- Loose bodies (due to fragmentation of osteochondral surface).
- Deformity and malalignment (due to destruction of capsules and ligaments).

Other Investigations

Synovial fluid analysis shows non-inflammatory picture. Bone scan shows increased uptake of technetium-99m, MRI and CT scan also helps to diagnose, subchondral cysts, osteophytes, etc. but are rarely employed. Arthroscopic procedure helps both in diagnosis and therapy.

Treatment

Conservative treatment: This forms the mainstay of management in osteoarthritis of the knee. About 50 percent of patients respond to conservative treatment, which consists of the following measures:

Non-pharmacological Therapy

According to the American College of Rheumatology guidelines, this is the most important part of the treatment and involves the following measures:
- Patient education
- Reduction of weight.
- Isometric quadriceps exercises (Figs 58.7A to C).
- *Physiotherapy:* This consists of heat therapy and is given through ultrasound, short wave diathermy, TENS, etc. This helps to relieve pain and muscle spasm.

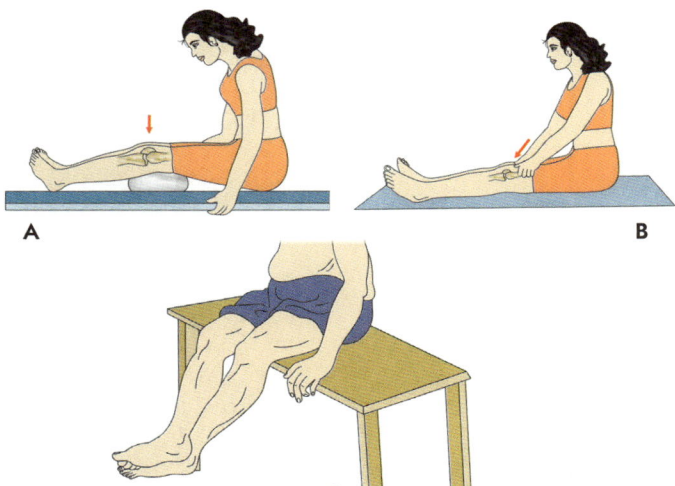

Figs 58.7A to C: Method of quadriceps exercises: (A) pressing the knee against a support, (B) pressing against the patella, (C) self resistance exercises

- *Exercises:* Exercises play a very vital role in improving the joint mobility and strengthening the muscles of the hip, knee and legs (Figs 58.7C).
- *Modifications of daily living activities:* This is the most important aspect of the management of knee joint osteoarthritis.

Pharmacological Therapy

- *Acetaminophen (Paracetamol):* This is an analgesic and is the first line of drug as OA is not an inflammatory condition. It is a least toxic drug and can be given up to 4 gm/day.
- *Non-steroidal anti-inflammatory drugs (NSAIDs):* These are indicated if the patient fails to respond to Paracetamol. It is known for the GI side effects, e.g. rofecoxib, celecoxib.
- *Cartilage protective drugs:* Like glucosamine, chondroitin sulfate are being tried with varied success.
- *Viscosupplementation:* It consists of injecting hyaluronidase drug into the joint. It is known to slow the destruction of the cartilages.
- *Intraarticular injections of steroids:* If the patient fails to respond to the drugs (not more than 3 recommended, local anesthetic is avoided for fear of developing neuropathic joint).
- *Topical application* of pain killer gels and ointments.

Surgery

Indications for Surgery

- Pain that is refractory to conservative measures.
- History of frequent locking episodes.
- Deformity usually genu varum.
- Joint instability.
- Progressive limitation of knee motion.
- Hemarthrosis due to loose bodies or osteochondral fractures.

Surgical Methods

- *Excision* of osteophytes is rarely done alone.
- *Arthroscopic treatment:* Excision of loose bodies, meniscectomy, synovectomy, joint lavage and reconstruction or joint debridement are best done by arthroscopy.
- *Proximal tibial osteotomy (Slocum's):* Indicated for unicompartmental osteoarthritis of knee with pain and also to correct varus (less than 15°) or valgus deformity (less than 12°). Pain is decreased in 80 percent of the cases following surgery as osteotomy changes the line of weight bearing and brings the more normal surface to carry out the function of load transmission (Figs 58.8A and B).
- *Distal femoral osteotomy:* This is indicated when varus or valgus deformity of the knee is more than 12 to 15°.
- *Total knee arthroplasty:* This is indicated when both the compartments of the knee joint are destroyed or

if valgus or varus deformity is more than 15°. It is also indicated in failed conservative treatment (Fig. 58.9).

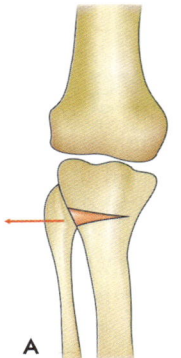 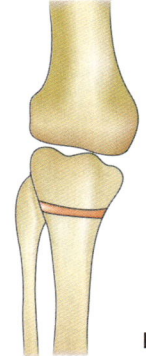 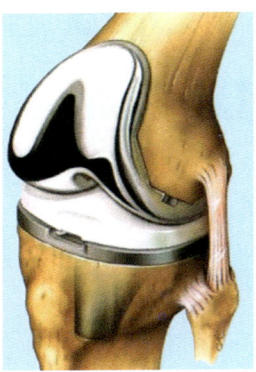

Figs 58.8A and B: High tibial osteotomy in osteoarthritis: (A) before operation, (B) after operation

Figs 58.9: Total knee replacement in OA knee

- *Arthrodesis* is indicated less commonly than arthroplasty. If the patient is young and involved in heavy occupations, arthrodesis is indicated to give him a stable and strong knee. However arthrodesis results in a stiff knee which is a severe disability.
- *Patellectomy:* It is rarely done except as a last resort. Contemplated in osteoarthritis present for several years.

SECONDARY OSTEOARTHRITIS OF THE KNEE

The causes for secondary osteoarthritis of the knee are as follows:
- Obesity, valgus and varus deformities of the knee
- Intraarticular fractures of the knee, etc.
- Rheumatoid arthritis, infection, trauma, TB, etc.
- Hyperparathyroidism
- Hemophilia
- Syringomyelia
- Neurological disease like diabetes
- Overuse of intraarticular steroid therapy.

It is generally observed that secondary osteoarthritis occurs in the younger age groups and is more severe than the primary. Apart from all the features of osteoarthritis, secondary osteoarthritis has the features of the corresponding etiological condition.

Osteoarthritis in Other Regions

Osteoarthritis spine (lumbar spondylosis) it is usually seen in the elderly age group and the patient presents with low backache. Osteophytes may compress the nerve roots at their exit at the intervertebral foramen and may cause neurological disturbances. Plain X-ray of the LS spine shows reduction in joint space, presence of osteophytes, sclerosis, etc. (Fig. 58.10). Conservative treatment usually helps but surgery may be required for prolonged pain and neurological deficits.

Osteoarthritis of the small joints: Osteoarthritis may affect the peripheral joints of the hand and foot. It may cause ankylosis at an increased rate in these joints (Figs 58.11A

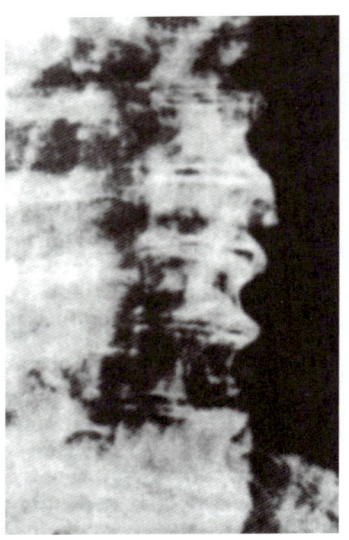

Fig. 58.10: Lumbar spine: Narrowing of disc space and osteophyte formation

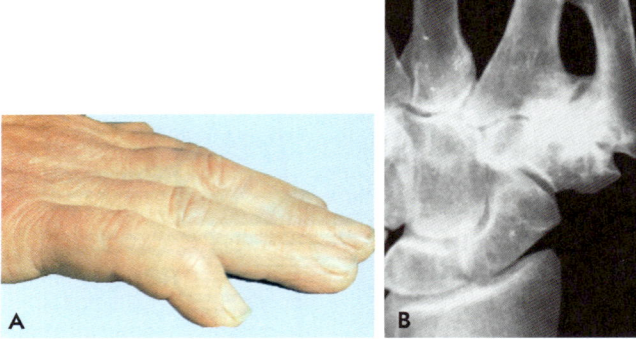

Figs 58.11A and B: Osteoarthritis of the carpometacarpal joint of the thumb: loss of joint space and sclerosis

and B).

Cervical Disc Syndromes

Cervical spondylosis has been discussed at depth in the chapter on regional disorders of the neck.

58

59 Cerebral Palsy, Polio and Other Neuromuscular Disorders

Cerebral palsy
Poliomyelitis
Arthrogryposis multiplex congenita
Leprosy in orthopedics
Myopathy
Muscular dystrophies
Spina bifida

CEREBRAL PALSY (CP)

This is a disorder of movement and posture caused by a non-progressive lesion in the immature brain.

Lesions: In cerebral palsy the lesion could be either in the brain or in the upper cervical cord.
   Incidence is 0.6–5.9/1000 live birth.

Lesions in the brain: In Cerebral Palsy, the lesions in the brain can occur in the following four areas:
1. Cerebral cortex (spastic type)
2. Midbrain (dyskinesia)
3. Cerebellum (ataxic)
4. Widespread brain involvement (rigidity and mixed).

Causes: In Cerebral Palsy, the causes are different in prenatal, natal, postnatal and perinatal period and are listed as in Table 59.1.

Table 59.1: Causes of cerebral palsy			
Prenatal	*Natal*	*Postnatal*	*Perinatal (0–7) days*
• Rubella infection	• Birth trauma	• Trauma	• Most lesions causing CP occur during this period
• Fetal anoxia		• Encephalitis	
• Maternal diabetes	• Anoxia	• Meningitis	
	• Prematurity		

Note: Birth Asphyxia is the commonest cause of CP.

Clinical Features

It could be mild, moderate or severe. This depends on the location of lesions in the brain. Single muscle involvement is rare as in polio and entire portion of the body supplied by that area of brain is involved. Patients show delayed milestones and primitive reflexes are usually preserved.

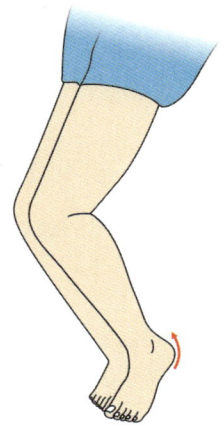

Fig. 59.1: Spastic contractures of the hip, knee and foot in cerebral palsy

Other clinical features depend on the geographic distribution of cerebral palsy and the associated handicapping situations. Involvement of pyramidal tract (65%) causes spasticity, increased reflexes, clonus, etc. This may involve one or more limbs. The most common lower limb deformities are flexion and adduction of the hip, flexion of the knee and equinus of the ankle. Spastic equinovarus are other common deformities of the foot (Fig. 59.1). In the upper limbs, it is flexion of the wrist and fingers, pronation of the forearm and thumb abduction (Fig. 59.3). Variable muscle weakness leads to muscle imbalance and deformities. Sustained pressure helps overcome the spasticity at the joints only to return in toto with vengeance once the pressure is released (Fig. 59.4). Involvement of extrapyramidal tract causes ataxia,

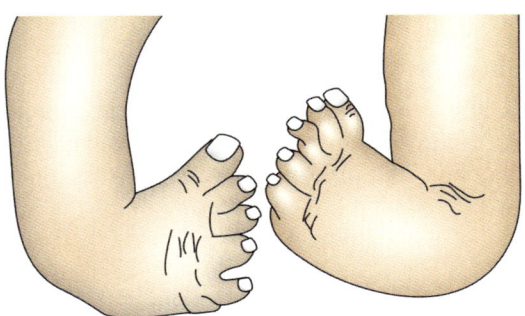

Fig. 59.2: Spastic equinovarus

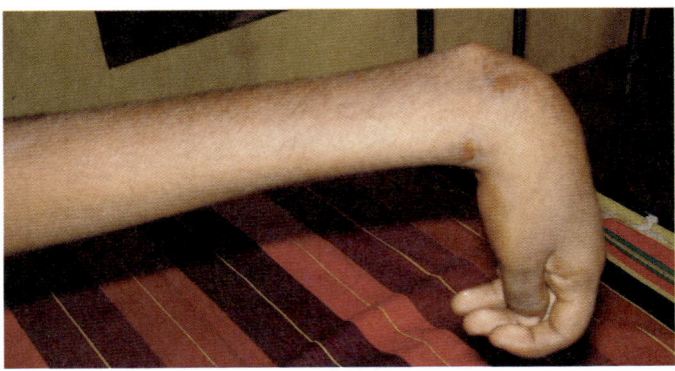

Fig. 59.3: Spastic hand in cerebral palsy

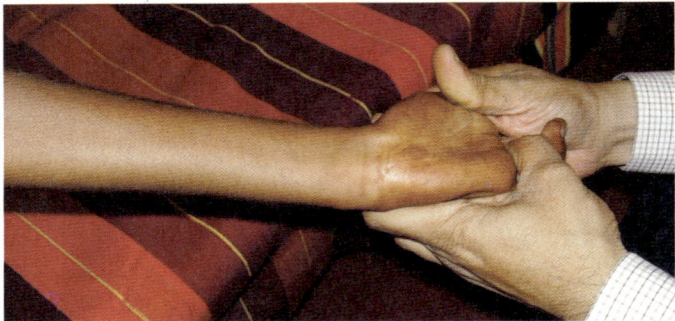

Fig. 59.4: Sustained pressure is required to overcome spasticity

athetosis, dystonia, etc. there could be one or more associated findings.

QUICK FACTS

Common causes of CP and types
- Diplegia—seen in premature infants
- Athetoid—kernicterus
- Hemiplegia—trauma, cerebrovascular accidents, infection, etc.
- Quadriplegia—brain anoxia

Treatment

Unfortunately there is no cure for cerebral palsy. Hence, the aim of treatment is to increase patient's assets as much as possible and minimize his or her defects.

Order of preference to improve the quality of life in cerebral palsy is as follows:
- Education and communication is the first priority.
- Training and assistance in the activities of daily life.
- Mobility
- Ambulation.

The role of orthopedic surgeon starts when the child is 12 months of age and seldom before.

Methods

- *Motor age test.*
- *Physiotherapy,* occupational therapy, speech therapy, etc. are the most important adjunctive treatment measures.

- *Use of braces to:*
  - Improve function.
  - Control unnecessary movements.
  - Prevent and correct deformities.
- *Drug therapy:* The role of drug therapy is disappointing. Muscle relaxants, antiepileptic may have a role.
- *Surgery*
  - Not done till 5 years of age.
  - Indicated to correct deformity in an ambulatory patient and to make him or her socially more acceptable.
  - Commonly indicated in spastic type of CP.

  Aim of surgery in cerebral palsy is
- To correct the deformity.
- To balance the muscle power.
- To stabilize uncontrollable joints.

Choice of Surgery

- *Operation on nervous system:*
  - Sympathectomy, rhizotomy (anterior or posterior).
  - Neurectomy: This helps to control severe muscle spasm which hinders rehabilitation, e.g. obturator neurectomy in hip adduction contractures.
- *Operation on muscles and tendons:*
  - Tenotomy, tendon lengthening and tendon transfers.
  - Myotomy and muscle transposition.
- *Operation on bones and joints:*
  - Bone lengthening or bone shortening to equalize the limb lengths.
  - Osteotomies to correct knock knee and other bone deformities.
  - Arthrodesis of wrist, hip and foot to correct deformity, provide stability and to improve functions.

Prognosis in Cerebral Palsy

- The dictum in brain damage is once damaged, forever damaged, as there is no regeneration. Hence, permanent cure eludes this unfortunate group.
- There is no permanent cure.
- Athetoid child is more intelligent than the spastic child.
- Twenty-five percent go to schools.
- Twenty-five percent are mentally retarded.
- Twenty-five percent are not educable.
- All hemiplegics will walk (by 12 to 16 months).
- Most diplegics will walk (by 4 years).
- Quadriplegics and total body involvement will never walk but can be propped sitters.

POLIOMYELITIS

This is a viral infection of the anterior horn cell of the spinal cord or nerve cells of brainstem, resulting in

59

temporary or permanent paralysis. Common in children, often attacks young adults.

Viruses: The following Picorna group of viruses is known to cause poliomyelitis: Brunhilde (type I), Leon (type II), and ansing (type III).

Pathogenesis: The virus is transmitted and enters the body through the faecooral route, multiplies in the intestines, reaches the regional lymph nodes and enters the blood stream. It enters the nervous tissue and destroys the anterior horn nerve cells because of which the peripheral nerve degenerates resulting in muscle and tendon atrophy. The damage to the anterior horn cells may be mild, moderate or severe (Fig. 59.5). While the first two may cause reversible paralysis, the last causes permanent damage resulting in residual paralysis. The bones become small, the joint capsules and ligaments become lax, as there is no protection by the healthy muscles. All these results in development of various deformities.

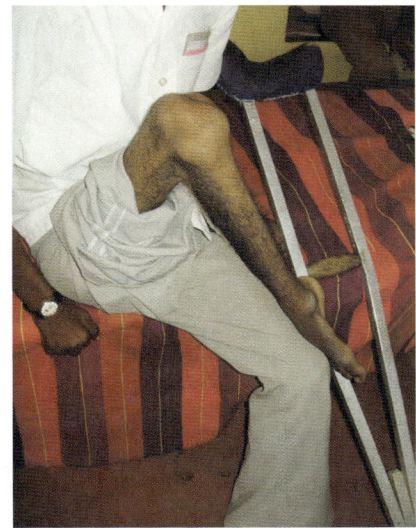

A

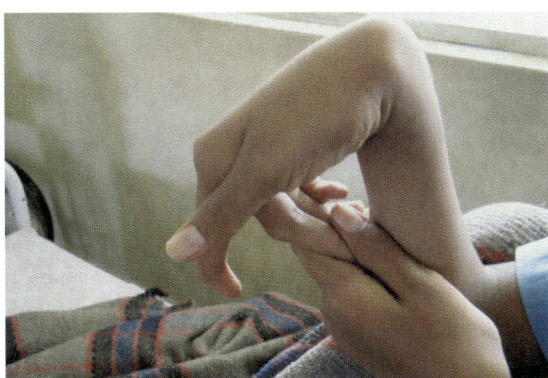

B

Figs 59.6A and B: (A) Showing various lower limb deformities (B) hand deformities in poliomyelitis

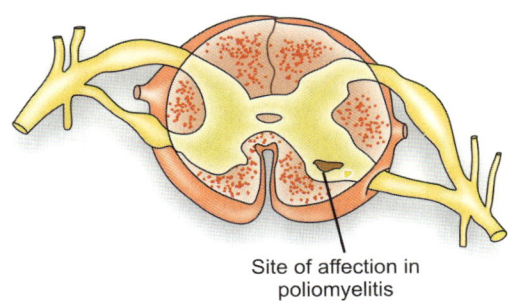

Site of affection in poliomyelitis

Fig. 59.5: Site of affection in polio

QUICK FACTS

In polio, the scene is set by the infection only something needs to pull the trigger to target the anterior horn cells. The trigger is let loose by one of the following events:
- Falls or any other trauma.
- Intramuscular injections.
- Any strenuous physical activity.
- Surgeries like tonsillectomy, adenoidectomy, etc
- Tooth extraction.

Clinical Features

Polio usually affects children less than 12 months. There is a mild episode of fever, headache and diarrhea. On examination, there could be mild neck stiffness and the child may find it difficult to move the affected limb (pre-paralytic). The lower limbs are more commonly affected and the paralysis could be partial or total (paralytic stage) (Figs 59.6A and B).

The paralysis of the muscles whether spinal (75%) or bulbar (25%) usually lasts until two months. Then there may or may not be recovery for a period of two years. Any residual paralysis after two years of affection is permanent with no chance of recovery. Bulbar poliomyelitis is rare and affects the respiratory muscles. It may be fatal.

Orthopedic deformities: Orthopedic deformities encountered in poliomyelitis are listed in the Table 59.2.

Differential Diagnosis

Poliomyelitis has to be differentiated in the acute stages from:
- Pyogenic meningitis
- Guillain-Barré syndrome
- Post-diphtheritic paralysis
- Acute osteomyelitis
- Scurvy, etc.

In the late stages from
- Cerebral palsy
- Spina bifida
- Myopathies
- Muscular dystrophies, etc.

Treatment of poliomyelitis: Supportive treatment during the early stages of the disease.

Table 59.2: Common orthopedic deformities encountered in poliomyelitis

I. **Foot and ankle**	• Claw toes
	• Claw foot
	• Talipes equinus
	• Talipes equinovalgus
	• Flail foot
	• Pes cavus
	• Dorsal bunion
	• Talipes equinovarus
	• Talipes calcaneovalgus
II. **Knee**	• Flexion contracture of the knee
	• Quadriceps paralysis
	• Genu recurvatum
	• Flail knee
III. **Hip**	• Flexion abduction contractures of the hip
	• Paralysis of gluteus medius, maximus
	• Paralytic dislocation of hip
IV. **Iliotibial band contractures** (results in 9 classical deformities)	• Lumbar scoliosis
	• Pelvic obliquity
	• Hip flexed and abducted
	• External rotation of femur
	• Flexion and valgus of knee
	• Posterior and lateral subluxaion of tibia
	• External rotation of tibia
	• Foot in equinus
	• Shortening
V. **Spine**	• Kyphosis
	• Scoliosis
	• Kyphoscoliosis
VI. **Upper limbs**	• Paralysis of shoulder, elbow, forearm

(Fig. 59.7). The commonly prescribed appliances in Table 59.3.

Table 59.3: External appliances in poliomyelitis

1. Spinal brace	To support weak spine
2. Abdominal support	To check abdominal protrusion when abdominal muscles are weak
3. Hip, knee, ankle, foot pelvic support	For deformities of the hip, knee and orthosis with or without ankle
4. Knee caliper	To hold knee extended in quadriceps palsy
5. Below knee brace	To stabilize a flail ankle or foot
6. Single below knee	To control varus or valgus (lateral or medial)
7. Drop foot appliance	For mobile equinus deformity

Quick facts: Conservative treatment

1. Stage of onset	• Bed rest
2. Stage of greatest	• Splints paralysis
	• Artificial respiration, etc.
3. Stage of	• Physiotherapy recovery
	• Walking aid
	• Crutches, etc.
4. Stage of residual	• Can be corrected by provision of suitable paralysis Orthotic appliances or by operation

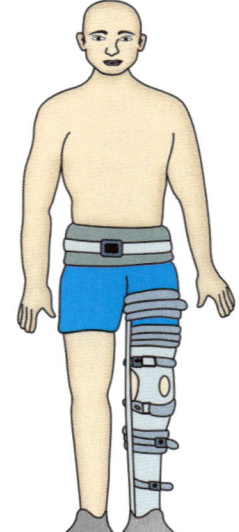

Fig. 59.7: An above knee caliper (KAFO) in a polio patient

• To prevent deformities from developing.
• To assist returning of muscle power by graduated exercises.
• To reduce disability by appropriate appliance or by operations on joints and muscles.

Treatment Methods

Early stages: During the stages of onset, maximum paralysis and the stages of recovery, the child is admitted into the hospital and supportive treatment is given. The child is put on a ventilator support if there is respiratory paralysis due to bulbar polio. Warm and moist packs are given to the joints and all intramuscular injections are avoided during this phase. Plaster splints in functional positions immobilize the affected joints.

Recovery stages: In this stage, the joints are properly splinted through various appliances to prevent or correct the deformities.

Role of Appliances

The purpose of external appliances is to support joints that have lost their normal control. They are more often required for lower limbs rather than upper limbs

Stage of post polio residual paralysis: During this stage the role of orthopedic surgeon is predominant and surgery is the treatment of choice.

Goals of Surgery

• To obtain muscle balance.
• To prevent or correct soft tissue contractures.
• To prevent or correct bony deformities.

Surgical Methods

Soft tissue release for soft tissue contractures, e.g.
- *Soutter's release:* Structures arising from anterior superior iliac spine are released for hip contractures.
- *Ober-Yount's procedure:* It consists of sectioning the iliotibial band (ITB) contractures.
- *Tendo Achilles:* Lengthening for equinus deformity of the foot.
- *Steindler's release:* Plantar fascia for cavus foot
- *Wilson's release:* For knee flexion deformity release.

Tendon transfers: This is indicated when dynamic muscle imbalance produces deformity requiring brace protection.

Aims of tendon transfers: To replace the function of a paralyzed muscle. To remove the deforming force. To provides stability by improving the muscle balance. Tendon transfers are not limited to any age group.

Arthrodesis: This is done to stabilize a flail joint, eliminate the need for brace and to improve function for permanent method of joint stabilization, etc.

Osteotomies: To correct deformities like genu valgum, etc. Ilizarov technique for leg length equalization.

ARTHROGRYPOSIS MULTIPLEX CONGENITA: (Syn: Multiple Congenital Contractures (MCC))

In the year 1841, Otto first described AMC. Swinyard and Beck gave the name MCC. AMC is a non-progressive syndrome characterized by:
- Rigid and deformed joints.
- Muscle absence or atrophy.
- Cylindrical or ellipsoid joints with skin crease loss and subcutaneous atrophy.
- Contractures of capsules and periarticular structures.
- Dislocation of joints like hip and knee.
- Normal mentality and intact sensation.

Causes: Intrauterine immobilization of joints at various stages of development is due to:
- Myopathic cause seen in 10 percent of cases. Autosomal recessive.
- Neurogenic cause is due to reduced number or improper organization of anterior horn cells, peripheral nerves and motor end plates, weakness of muscles, etc.
- Mechanical causes like breech, twins, oligohydramnios amniotic bands, etc. which reduce the intrauterine space.

Classification (Sharrard, Brown and Robson)

Eight types: Two upper limb and six lower limb deformities are encountered. Common variety is quadriplegic type (Fig. 59.8). Scoliosis is associated in 20 percent of the cases of AMC; webbing of the knees is seen in some.

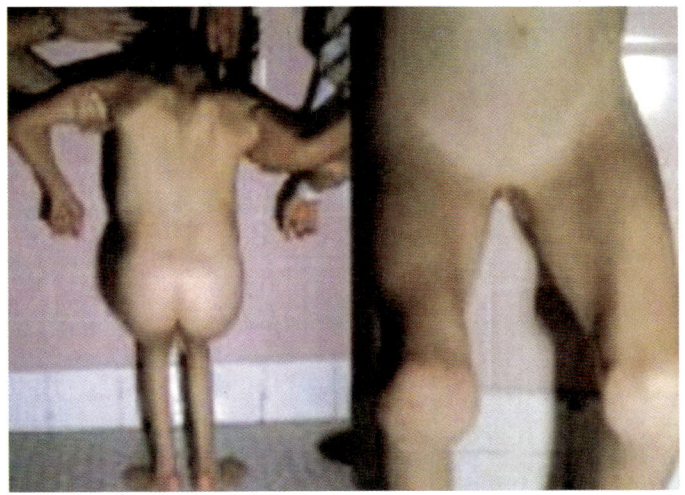

Fig. 59.8: Quadriplegic type is the most common variety of arthrogryposis multiplex congenita (AMC)

COMMON ORTHOPEDIC DEFORMITIES IN AMC
a. *Foot:* Planovalgus and equinovarus.
b. *Knee:* Flexion contracture and fixed in extension.
c. *Hip:* Extension, abduction, external rotation.
d. *Shoulder:* Medial rotation of shoulder.
e. *Elbow and wrist:* Flexed.

Investigations: Muscle biopsy, electromyography, nerve conduction studies, radiograph for scoliosis, dislocation, chromosomal studies are helpful.

Treatment: The treatment consists of passive stretching exercises, serial splinting of the limbs and surgical correction of the contractures and deformities.

LEPROSY IN ORTHOPEDICS

Leprosy is a chronic infectious disease caused by *Mycobacterium leprae*. It affects mainly the peripheral nerves and affects the skin, muscles, bones, testes and internal organs. Clinically it is characterized in early stages by hypopigmented patches, rashes (Fig. 59.9) loss of cutaneous sensation, thickened nerves, and presence of acid-fast bacilli in the skin or nasal smears. In late *stages* trophic *ulcers, foot-drop; claw toes claw hand, nasal bridge* collapse, loss of *fingers or toes.*

QUICK FACTS
Peripheral nerve involvement in leprosy
- Facial nerve—face
- Ulnar nerve—elbow
- Median nerve—wrist
- Common peroneal nerve—fibular head

Pathogenesis of the deformities: Peripheral nerve involvement affects all its three components namely sensory, motor and autonomous. Loss of sensation in

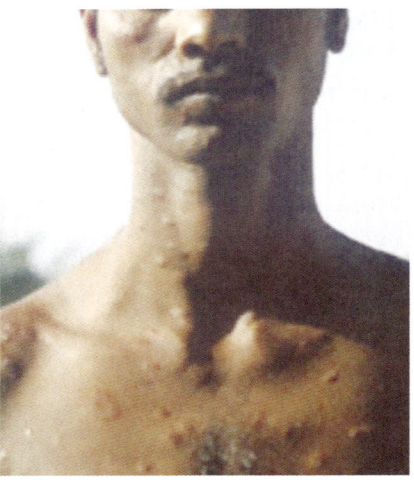

Fig. 59.9: Rashes over the body in leprosy

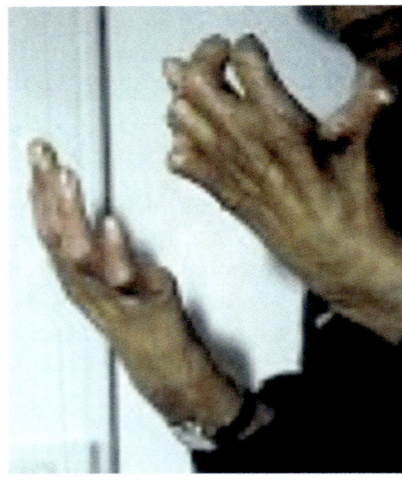

Fig. 59.10: Clinical photograph of bilateral clawing

hands and feet leads to injury, ulcers and scarring. Loss of autonomic function causes dryness of the skin, which in turn causes fissures, ulceration and scarring. Motor loss leads to paralysis and contractures. The ultimate result of this scarring and contractures are various deformities and mutilation, so commonly associated with leprosy.

Classification

Three classifications proposed are Indian, Madrid, Ridley and Jopling types

Investigations

Bacteriological examination of material obtained from the skin or nasal smears, footpad culture of mice is 10 times more sensitive than the skin slit smears. Histamine test biopsy, immunological tests are some of the other important tests.

Tests for detecting CMI Lepromin test, Lymphocyte transformation test, etc.

Tests for detecting humoral antibodies ELISA test, etc.

Treatment

Primary prevention by vaccine is not possible, so leprosy control is based on effective chemotherapy.

Multibacillary	Paucibacillary
Ripampicin 600 mg/month	R-cin 600 mg/month for 6 months
Dapsone 100 mg/day	+
Clofazimine 300 mg/month	Dapsone 100 mg/day for 6 months

If Clofazimine is not acceptable, Ethionamide—250-375 mg/day. *Duration of treatment* is at least for 2 years until smear is negative. *BCG vaccine* showed a high degree of protection in 80 percent and 30 percent in some cases.

Preventive Measures

To prevent deformities and ulcerations, proper splinting of the joints, care of the skin by practicing proper antisepsis and protective foot wears are advocated.

Surgical Measures

Ulcer debridement, tendon transfers and bony surgeries, etc. are indicated in appropriate situations for correction or prevention of various deformities.

Orthopedic Affections in Leprosy

Affections of the Hand in Leprosy

The following are the common hand deformities encountered in leprosy.
- *Ulnar claw hand* is due to affection of ulnar nerve at the elbow.
- *Total claw hand* is due to affection of ulnar nerve at elbow and median nerve at the wrist.
- *Triple nerve palsy* the following nerves are affected: ulnar nerve at the elbow, median nerve at the wrist and radial nerve at the spiral groove.

Surgery for hand: Brands many tailed tendon transfer operation (EF4T) Developed by Paul Brand at the Christian Medical College, Vellore, India is the most common surgical procedure.

Extensor carpi radialis longus is released from its insertion and brought into the flexor aspect of the forearm. Free graft from palmaris longus tendon is taken and is split into four strips, which are then attached to the extensor expansion of the respective fingers (EF4T).

Ankle and Foot

Every kind of deformity is seen in the foot. Deformity is gross, because patient continues to use the foot due to loss of sensations. Ankle is rarely affected in this

59

disease. In leprosy due to loss of sensation, there is absence of warning pain because of which, there is injury. Secondary infection following the injury is common.

Foot Drop

This is one of the very common complications encountered in leprosy (Fig. 31.22). It is seen in 2 percent of the cases. Common peroneal nerve is more commonly involved. Usually it is completely damaged, sometimes only deep peroneal or superficial branch is involved and occasionally only external hallucis longus muscle is involved.

Treatment

For recent or incomplete drop foot: toe raising spring, physiotherapy, short wave diathermy, ultrasound, local steroids, etc. are the recommended forms of treatment. If more than one year after affection or if the lesion is complete surgical correction is needed.

Surgical Methods for Foot Drop

- When there is no contracture and if the foot is mobile, tibialis posterior transfer is indicated.
- Triple arthrodesis of Lambrunidi for fixed equino-varus deformity of the foot.

Plantar Ulcers

This is the other important foot complication in leprosy. It is also known as trophic ulcers due to neurological deficit. It has a spontaneous onset, it is painless, persists, and recurs. Healing process is not defective. Recurrent ulceration causes progressive destruction of the skeleton.

Sites

Plantar ulcers are commonly seen over the ball of feet especially first metatarsal, and heel (Fig. 59.11) and tips of the fingers.

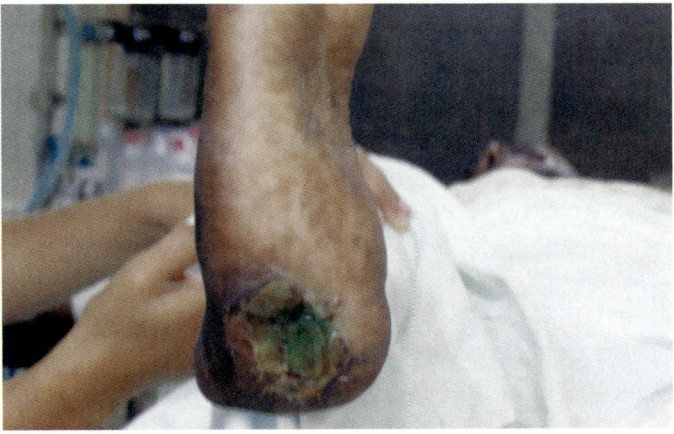

Fig. 59.11: Plantar heel ulcer in leprosy

Treatment of Plantar Ulcers

Aim is to get the ulcer healed by various measures and to prevent its recurrence by various non-surgical and surgical measures.

Methods: The treatment methods consist of rest, antibiotics, regular washing with eusol solution, protective footwear, braces, excision, arthritis, etc. Surgery consists of debridement, curettage, plastic surgery to cover the defect, excision and amputation in recalcitrant cases.

MYOPATHY

This refers to muscle disorders per se due to somatic motor dysfunctions. CNS, lower motor neuron, neuromuscular junction are all-normal. Myopathies may be inherited or acquired and may sometimes even affect other organs in the body apart from the skeletal muscles.

Muscular dystrophies are 'inherited' variety of myopathies in which the major offending cause is an abnormal structural protein (other noted errors in inherited myopathies are abnormal cellular enzymes or both). Acquired myopathies may be due to certain infections, toxic drugs, etc.

Muscular dystrophies show the following interesting characteristic features:
- Strong family history.
- Frequently bilateral.
- Muscular weakness and wasting.
- No specific laboratory and histological findings.
- Relentless progression over the years.
- Atypical forms cause diagnostic dilemmas.

Can one distinguish individual muscular dystrophies: Though confusing, with proper systemic approach dystrophies can be identified by keeping in mind the following criteria:
- Age of onset
- Sex
- Inheritance types whether autosomal or sex linked.
- Arrangement and distribution of physical features.
- Presence of any other genetic abnormality.
- Maintaining a profile on the progression of the disease.

MUSCULAR DYSTROPHIES

These are difficult problems to treat and the cause is usually not known. A few important muscular dystrophies in each variety is described below

Duchenne muscular dystrophy this is the most common type of muscular dystrophy encountered.

Clinical Features (Figs 59.12A and B)

Duchene's dystrophy is more common in boys. This consists of delayed walking, abnormal gait and multiple

falls (in less than 3 years child does). Gower's sign is positive, hypertrophy of calf muscles, waddling gait, increased lumbar lordosis and weakness of shoulder muscles. Serrati, pectorals, deltoid, latissimus dorsi, biceps, triceps and brachialis muscles are weak. In lower limbs weakness of hip flexors, evertors of feet, tibialis anterior are seen, ocular, pharyngeal and masticatory muscles are never involved. Knee jerk is absent earlier than ankle jerk. Tendo Achilles contractures appear first, later hamstrings, hip flexors and elbow follow. Intellectual impairment is present. Death below 16 years is due to respiratory infection or cardiac failure.

Investigations

Serum glutamic oxaloacetic transminase (SGOT), serum glutamate pyruvate transaminase (SGPT), lactate dehydrogenase$_5$ (LDH$_5$) aldolase and creatinine phosphokinate (CPK) levels are raised, muscle biopsy and electromyography (EMG) helps, electrocardiogram (ECG) shows biventricular hypertrophy.

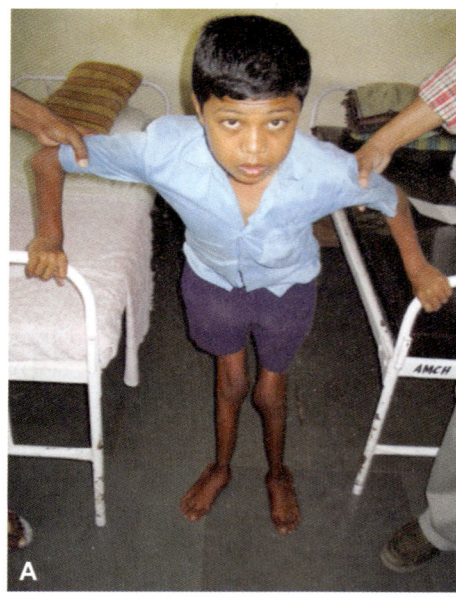

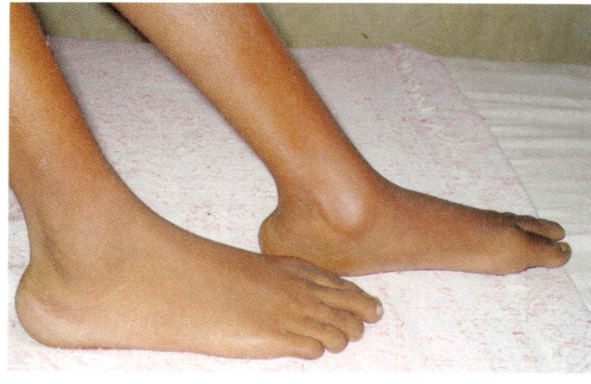

Figs 59.12A and B: Posture and foot deformities in muscular dystrophies

FASCIOSCAPULOHUMERAL MUSCULAR DYSTROPHY

It is seen in second decade of life and the fascial musculature is involved early. Patient complains of inability to close the eyes, slurred speech, etc. Elevation of the scapula on abduction is characteristic. In the upper limbs, deltoid and wrist flexors are spared. In the lower limbs, anterior tibial muscle is involved earlier. Majority of the patient suffering from this dystrophy have a normal lifespan.

LIMB GIRDLE MUSCULAR DYSTROPHY

It is seen in second or third decade. Lower limb girdle weakness appears first followed by upper limb. Muscular hypertrophy is rare. Winging of the scapula is seen. There is no involvement of cardia.

Treatment for Muscular Dystrophies

An attempt is made to treat underlying cause. *Supportive therapy* consists of physiotherapy, mental and physical support, speech therapy, and mechanical aids like splints, walking aids, etc. Care of the anesthetic skin, proper splint age to prevent deformities is the other recommended forms of treatment.

SPINA BIFIDA

Embryo logically the mesoderm around the notochord develops into vertebral body. The vertebral arch is formed by two projections from the vertebral body which grow backward enclosing in between them the neural canal and fuse in the center. The fusion starts at the thoracic region and extends up and down. When these vertebral arches err in fusion, spina bifida results. The failure of fusion could be limited, only to the spinous process resulting in spina bifida occulta, the most common variety or the entire vertebral arch including the neural elements may fail to fuse giving rise to the rare variety of spina bifida aperta. Figures 59.13A to D show different varieties of spina bifida.

Spina Bifida Occulta

This is the most common variety and is generally mild. Lumbosacral spine and the first sacral vertebra are commonly affected. The overlying skin may be normal or there may be presence of a tuft of hair, pigmentation, lipoma, dimple, etc. There may be muscle imbalance in the lower limbs resulting in equinovarus or cavus deformity of the foot due to tethering of the cord by a membrane either to the skin or filum terminale. Rarely there could be a bifid cord. Plain X-ray of the spine reveals the bifid spine (Fig. 59.14).

Treatment

Asymptomatic cases require no treatment except physiotherapy and back exercises. Surgical correction of foot deformities is as discussed in earlier chapters.

59

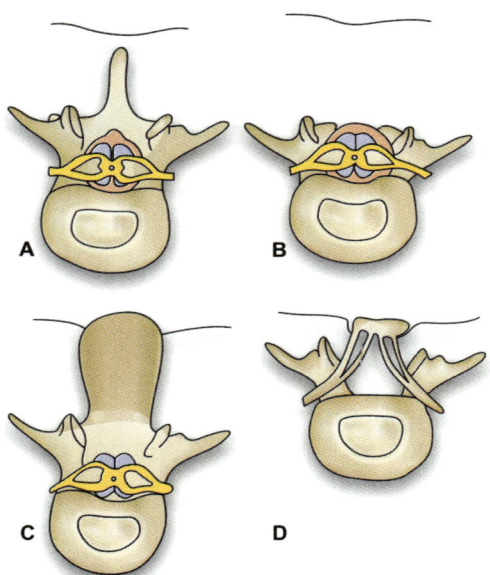

Figs 59.13A to D: Different types of spina bifida: (A) spina bifida occulta, (B) spina bifida aperta (meningocele), (C) myelomeningocele, (D) myelocele

Spina Bifida Aperta

Here the defect involves the vertebral arches, skin, meninges and cord. The following varieties are described.

Meningocele in which there is protrusion of the meninges.

Myelomeningocele in which there is protrusion of meninges and cord (Fig. 59.15).

Syringomyelocele in which central canal of the cord is dilated and the cord is protruded.

Myelocele in which the central cord remains unfused and exposed.

Next to spind bifida occulta, myelocele is the next common variety. Most of the cases of spina bifida aperta are either stillborn or die within few days of birth. The surviving children may suffer from severe orthopedic deformities, bladder and bowel incontinence and foot deformities.

Treatment is aimed to correct the spina bifida, foot deformities and other orthopedic deformities. Bladder incontinence may require urological treatment.

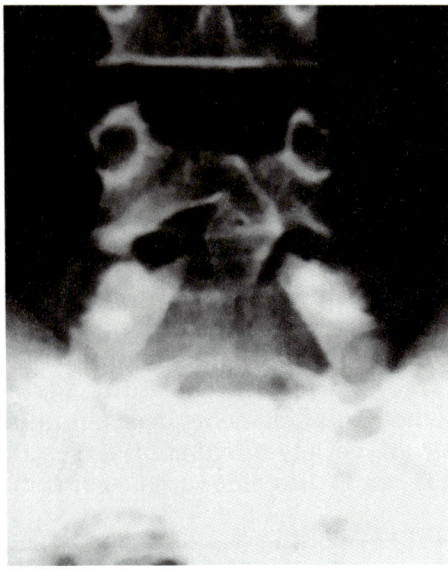

Fig. 59.14: Plain X-ray showing spina bifida occulta

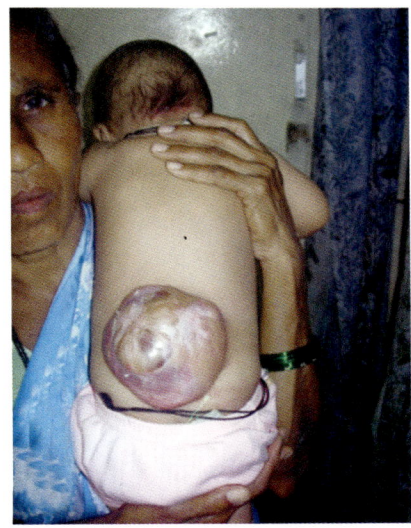

Fig. 59.15: Clinical photograph of myelomeningocele

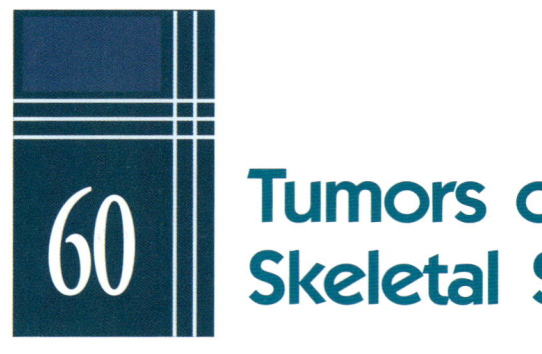

60 Tumors of the Skeletal System

INTRODUCTION

Like other systems in the body, musculoskeletal system may also develop tumors, either as a **primary** from this system itself or as a **secondary** from a distant primary location. The *latter appears to be more common*. Some of the tumors are benign and others are malignant. The accurate diagnosis of a neoplasm is a must before planning the treatment strategy. Diagnosis is best established by history, a proper physical examination and investigations like histopathological examination, biochemical assays, X-ray, CT scan, MRI, bone scans, arteriography, ultrasound, biopsy (both frozen section and permanent paraffin section), etc.

Primary bone tumors may be benign or malignant. Tumors spreading secondarily to the bone are generally primary carcinomas of breast, kidney, thyroid and lung. These tumors are called *metastatic carcinomas* because the tissue of origin is ectoderm. Secondaries of the bone are always malignant .

Classification of Bone Tumors

Various classifications have been proposed for bone tumors like Dahlia's classification, Mercer's classification, Turek's classification, etc. The ABC classification of *Bristol bone tumor registry* proposed by *Charles price* is by far the easiest to understand and remember (Table 60.1).

BONE TUMORS OF CARTILAGINOUS ORIGIN

OSTEOCHONDROMA

This is the most common benign bone tumor. It is an offshoot from the spongy bone tissue covered with a cartilaginous cap (size of the cap may vary from 1 to 40 cm).

Age: It is common during the growth period and ceases to grow once the growth plate fuses. Hence it is not a true tumor.

Sex: It has a male preponderance.

Area: Location favors the sites of *tendinous attachments, which* are usually around the metaphysis of long bones in the region of knee, ankle, hip, shoulder and elbow.

Clinical Features

Symptoms: Usually it is symptomless but patient may complain of pain, swelling, etc. once complications like bursitis, fracture, malignant change, etc. have developed (Fig. 60.1A).

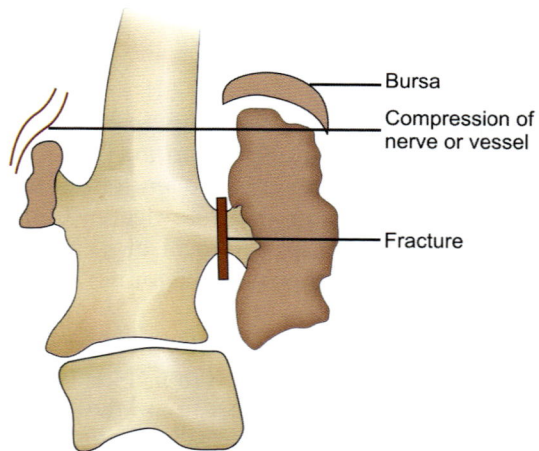

Fig. 60.1A: Osteochondroma and some of its complications

60

Table 60.1: Classification of bone tumors

Section	Benign	Malignant
Section A Angioid tumors	• Angioma • Aneurysmal bone cyst • Glomus tumor	• Angiosarcoma
Section B Bone forming tumor	• Osteoma • Osteoblastoma • Osteoid osteoma osteosarcoma	• Osteosarcoma • Parosteal • Chondroma
Section C Cartilage forming tissue	• Chondrosarcoma • Osteochondroma • Chondroblastoma	
Section D Dental and allied structure	• Odontogenic cyst • Amelloblastoma odontoma	• Malignant
Section E Embryonic vestigeal tissue		• Chordoma
Section F Fibroblastic	• Fibroma	• Fibrosarcoma
Section H Heterotrophic tissue of long bones	• Dermoid	• Adamantinoma
Section N Nonosseus connective tissue	• Lipoma • Neurofibromatosis • Neurilemmoma sarcoma	• Liposarcoma • Reticulum cell • Myeloma • Leukemia • Hodgkin's • Ewing's • Leiomyosarcoma
Section S Synovial tissue	• Synovioma • Chondroma	• Synovial sarcoma
Section U Undifferentiated osteoclastoma connective tissue	• Osteoclastoma	• Malignant
Section X	• Undiagnosed primary bone tumors	• Undiagnosed primary bone tumors

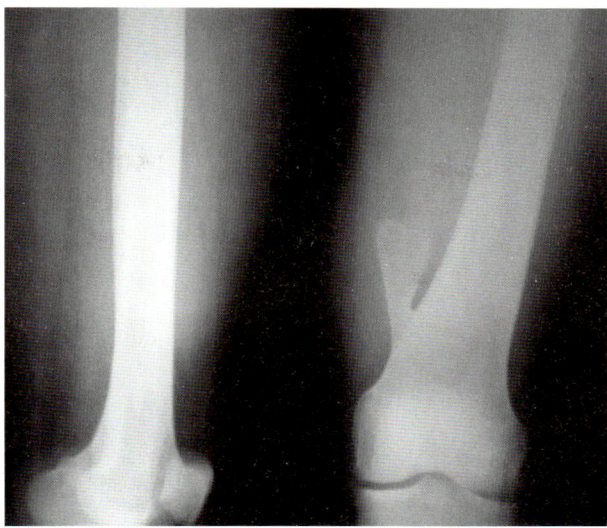

Fig. 60.1B: Plain X-ray showing osteochondroma

Signs: A firm non-tender swelling fixed to the bone around the joints is the most common clinical finding. A bursa if inflamed will give rise to tenderness and local warmth. Joint movements may be decreased because of the tumor causing a mechanical block rather than the extension of the tumor into the joint.

Radiographic Features

This consists of an outgrowth of bone at the metaphysis. This attachment is sessile or pedunculated. The tumor is composed of cortical and medullary portions, which are continuous with the main bone. The cartilage and capsules are not seen unless it calcifies (Fig. 60.1B).

Treatment

Usually it requires no treatment but complete surgical excision is indicated in the following situations.
- *Joint interference* if the tumor is large and obstructing the joint movements, it needs excision of the tumor along with its periosteal cover to prevent recurrence of the tumor.
- *Painful bursitis* a bursa usually develops because of the constant friction between the tumor and the surrounding soft tissues. If inflammation develops within this bursa, it gives rise to pain necessitating its excision.
- *Fracture* of the bony stalk may occur due to trauma.
- *Malignant change* (1–2%) Local irradiation may convert this benign tumor into malignant. It grows rapidly and has to be excised.
- *Pressure on the neighboring vessels* and nerves may give rise to neurovascular complications.

CHONDROMA (Enchondroma, Chondromyxoma)

This is a benign cartilaginous tumor centrally located when it occurs in phalanges and humerus. It causes destruction of the cancellous bone and has a potential for undergoing malignant change, especially when it is situated in the long bones.

Age: 10 to 50 years.

Site: Metaphysis is usually involved. It is common in the phalanges of hand (little finger common) and feet. Innominate and long bones may also be involved.

Clinical Features

Symptoms are practically none. There may be slight pain and the phalanx may be enlarged. The course of the tumor is very slow.

Radiology

The tumor appears cystic (loculated or non-loculated), cortex is thin and expanded, it may be perforated and at the center fibrous septa may be seen interspersing the central cavity. Stippling or calcification may be present. There is no reactive bone formation (Fig. 60.2).

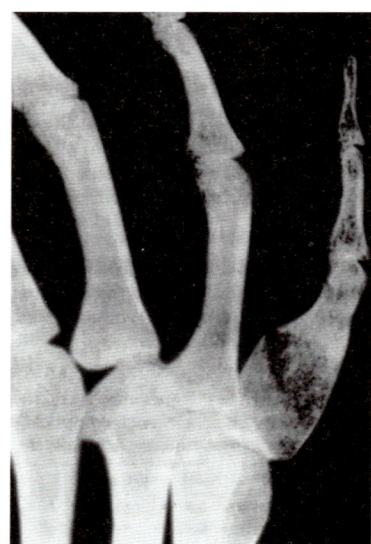

Fig. 60.2: Radiograph showing enchondroma with pathological fracture

Treatment

Curettage is done and the wall is cauterized if the tumor is small. The surgery done in cases of large tumors is excision and removal of the capsule to prevent recurrence. Radical resection is done for tumors of long bones and pelvis. Recurrence is common with chondromas of the long bones.

Prognosis

The incidence of malignant change is 25 percent especially in the pelvis.

CHONDROBLASTOMA

This is a highly cellular, vascular, and cartilaginous benign bone tumor of the cancellous bone. Here the cancellous bone is destroyed and multiple calcium deposits are usually found within the tumor.

Age: 10 to 20 years.

Sex: Male preponderance.

Sites: Epiphyseal ends of long bones are commonly affected.

Clinical Features

The patient may present with pain, swelling, joint effusion, etc.

Radiology

Radiographic features of the tumor are areas of rarefaction at epiphysis, eccentric position of the tumor, thin cortex and mottled areas of calcification.

Treatment

This consists of curettage and bone grafting if the lesion is small, excision in bigger tumors. If it is accidentally irradiated it may turn malignant. Recurrence rate after excision is 25 percent.

CHONDROSARCOMA

This is *second* in frequency to osteosarcoma. It arises from the cartilage cells. It is a malignant but *slow* growing tumor. It has a long history and a better prognosis. Unlike osteogenic sarcoma, there is *no neoplastic osteoid formation and alkaline phosphatase is usually not raised.* It ranges from being locally aggressive to high-grade malignancy.

Classification

Primary/secondary: Secondary tumors develop when benign cartilaginous tumors are irradiated.

Peripheral/central/juxtacortical: Depending on the situation of the tumor within the bone.

Low, medium and high-grade malignancy: Depending on the cellularity.

Location: It is common at the sites of proximal femur, humerus, ribs, and scapula, innominate bones, rare in hands and feet except in calcaneus, and occur in pelvis or upper femora.

Sex: Males are more commonly affected than females.

Age: Twenty to sixty years, rare below twenty years, peak in the sixth decade.

Clinical Features

The duration of symptoms are usually less than 2 years in 75 percent of the cases and less than 5 years in the remaining 25 percent. Pain is usually not a prominent feature unlike osteogenic sarcoma. The central tumor remains entirely asymptomatic until it has eroded and penetrated the cortex or caused a pathological fracture. A palpable firm mass attached to the bone is the common physical sign. The tumor may assume large proportion (Fig. 60.3A).

Radiology

Central lytic lesion with calcification gives a fluffy, cotton wool, popcorn or breadcrumb appearance (Fig. 60.3B). Metaphysis or diaphysis of the long tubular bone is usually affected. Greater degree of calcification is observed in slow growing tumors.

60

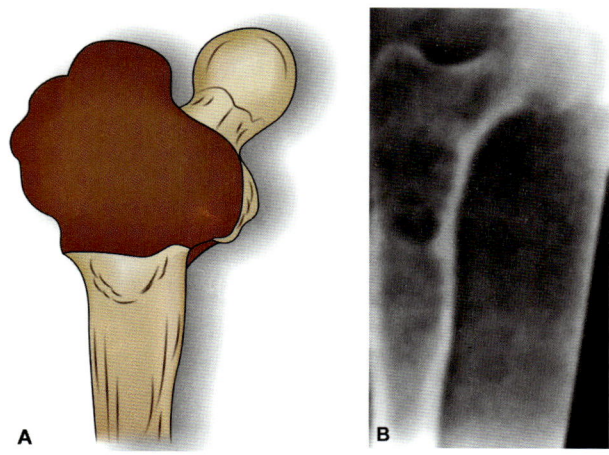

A **B**

Figs 60.3A and B: (A) Chondrosarcoma affecting the upper end of the femur (B) Radiograph showing chondrosarcoma upper end of femur

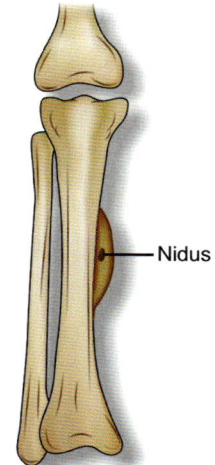

— Nidus

Fig. 60.4A: Osteoid osteoma in tibia

60

Treatment

Surgery is the treatment of choice.

Low and medium grade lesions: Require wide excision, e.g. Forequarter amputation (Thikor-Linberg) for the shoulder girdle; hindquarter amputation for the pelvic girdle.

High-grade lesions: Require radical marginal excision Role of systemic chemotherapy in chondrosarcoma is controversial.

Palliative radiotherapy: It is indicated when the tumor cannot be resected because of its enormous size or if the tumor is present in an accessible region.

QUICK FACTS IN CHONDROSARCOMA
- Second in frequency to osteosarcoma
- No neoplastic osteoid
- Long history
- Pain is not a prominent feature
- X-ray—popcorn appearance
- Wide excision is the treatment of choice
- Better survival rate.

OSSEOUS ORIGIN BONE TUMORS

OSTEOMA

It is a benign bone tumor, occurs in membranous bones of skull and face. Usually there are very few complaints, the history is long and the finding is a diffuse bony hard tumor. It rarely requires treatment.

OSTEOID OSTEOMA

This is a benign osteoblastic tumor with a well-demarcated nidus of less than 1 cm surrounded by a distinct reactive bone (Fig. 60.4A). This tumor presents very interesting clinical features. It is a tumor of young adults, benign in nature and occurs in enchondral bones.

Age: It is common in young adults between 10 and 25 years of age

Sex: Male preponderance (M: F = 2:1)

Sites: The diaphysis of long bones usually tibia, femur are more commonly affected. The posterior vertebral elements are the other favorable sites.

Clinical Features

Patient complains of vague and intermittent pain, which is more at night. The pain dramatically decreases after giving aspirin so much so that this is called the 'Therapeutic test'. Patient also complains of limp due to pain. There is a mild swelling, the local area may be tender, temperature is not raised, and the skin is not stretched, shiny or warm. When the lesion occurs in the spine, patient presents with acute low backache.

Radiology

It usually shows small-rarefied lesion <2 cm in diameter found in either the cortex, subcortical or subperiosteal regions. It is surrounded by a thick sclerotic bone. A small dense center of ossification seen in the center as the nidus (Fig. 60.4B). Five percent of the cases of sciatica are due to osteoid osteoma. CT scan and MRI also help in diagnosing this tumor.

Treatment

Conservative line of treatment consists of rest to the part and analgesics. If the tumor is too troublesome, complete excision of the cortex, containing the nidus is sufficient.

Note: Osteoid osteoma is the commonest 'true' bone tumor.

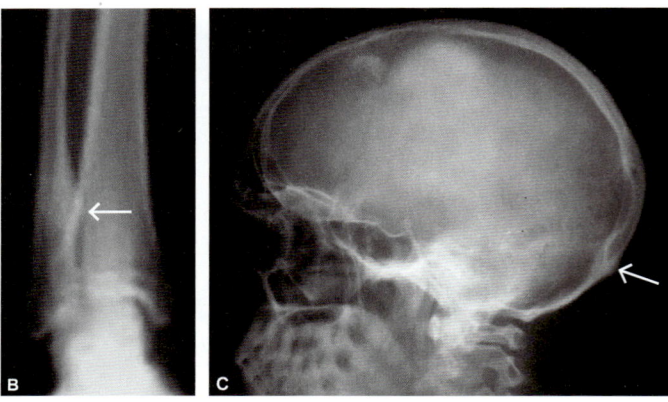

Figs 60.4B and C: Radiograph showing osteoid osteoma of tibia and skull

OSTEOGENIC SARCOMA

Osteogenic sarcoma is a highly malignant primary bone tumor. Here tumor cells invariably form a neoplastic osteoid, bone, or both. It arises from a common multifactorial mesenchymal tissue and hence the tumor could be either *fibroblastic, osteoblastic* or *chondroblastic*. This is the most frequent primary bone tumor next only to multiple myeloma.

Age: It is common in the second decade, rare below 10 years of age, 75 percent of the cases are seen below the age of 25.

Sex: Male preponderance, when found in females it starts at an early age.

Incidence is 1/75,000 population.

Site: Ninety percent of the tumor occurs in the metaphysial region of the ends of long bones. It has a predilection around the knee and upper humerus. It may affect the jaws in the aged.

Location (in the decreasing order of frequency)
- Fifty-two percent of the cases occur in the femur (9% in greater trochanter).
- Twenty percent of cases are seen in the tibia (90% in upper medial aspect).
- Nine percent are seen in the humerus. It is common in the upper end but rare below the deltoid tubercle.

Exciting Factors

The predisposing factors of this tumor are:

Virus
- *DNA virus:* Polyoma and SV 40 virus.
- *RNA virus:* Harvey and Moloney mouse sarcoma virus. These are known to produce tumors in experimental animals but not known in humans.

Radiation: If a dose of more than 2000 rads is given to osteoprogenitor cells situated in areas of active growth at the metaphysis malignancy sets in.

Chemicals: Twenty methyl cholanthrene, beryllium compounds are known to induce malignancy changes.

Pathology

The tumor could be either osteoblastic, chondroblastic or fibroblastic. Consequently the tumor may be osteosclerotic or osteolytic. Most common tumor is both a combination of osteosclerotic and osteolytic variety.

Gross: The tumor is more commonly situated in metaphysis of a long bone. It is a large tumor with areas of destruction (Fig. 60.5A) gives an appearance of leg of mutton. The consistency ranges from stony hard to soft. At the areas of rapid growth, there are necrotic foci, cavitations and hemorrhage.

Histology: Small spindle cells with hyper chromatic nuclei are seen. Cells are pleomorphic in nature. Large spindle-shaped cells are rare. Giant cells are often present. Matrix may be myxomatous, cartilaginous or osseous. Areas of hemorrhage may be present.

Classification

1. Primary and secondary
2. *Dahlin's (prognostic)* classification:
   a. *Osteoblastic:* Poor five-year survival rate.
   b. *Chondroblastic*: Five-year survival rate is three-times more than that of osteoblastic variety.
   c. *Fibroblastic*: Five-year survival rate is two-times more of osteoblastic variety.
3. *Geschickter and Copeland* classification:
   a. Sclerosing type
   b. Osteolytic type
   c. Mixed type of both osteoblastic and osteolytic verities.
   d. Telangiectatic type.
   Secondary osteosarcoma: This is less malignant than the primary, develops in bones affected with Paget's disease, diaphyseal aclasia, enchondromas, irradiation, etc. It is more common is older age groups and is treated on the same lines as the primary.
   Lichtenstein's criteria to identify osteogenic sarcoma include the presence of the following:
   a. Sarcomatous stroma
   b. Spindle cells
   c. Direct formation of neoplastic osteoid and bone.

Clinical Features

The patient usually presents with pain as the first symptom. It precedes the tumor, is seen first at night and is intermittent in nature. History of mild trauma is a common feature. Patient complains of tired feeling and limp. General condition is good till the late stages. Pyrexia is seen with increased WBCs. Patient is usually anemic than cachectic. Swelling develops later and the skin over the tumor is stretched, shiny and mobile (Figs 60.5A and B). Local temperature is raised,

60

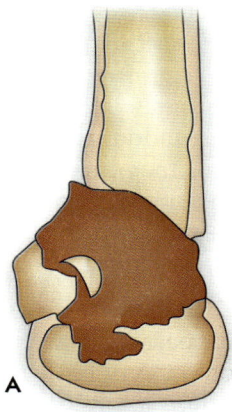 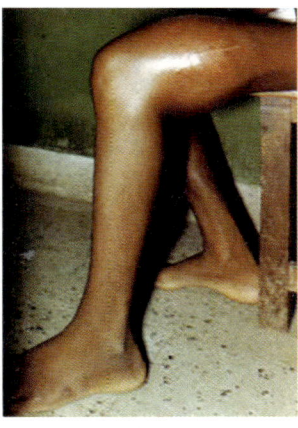

Figs 60.5A and B: (A) Areas of destruction (B) osteosarcoma lower end of femur

consistency of the tumor is variable, dilated veins are present (and is evident at an early stage). Pathological fracture is not typical of osteogenic sarcoma since the swelling and pain keeps the patient off his or her feet. The nearest joint may show pain and effusion. Joint movements may be unimpaired but there could be a mechanical block caused by the tumor bulk. Neurovascular structures could be compressed.

Spread

- It is mainly by blood spread, lungs are involved in 80 percent of the cases.
- Lymphatic spread to regional lymph nodes is seen in 30 percent of the cases.

Investigations

Laboratory tests reveal Hb percentage decreased, alkaline phosphate (Alk PO_4) increased, ESR increased, WBCs increased, etc.

Radiology

Four types are usually described. Sclerotic type, Osteolytic type, Mixed type, Radiating, Spicule type. The typical radiograph features are (Fig. 60.6):

Sunray appearance: It is seen in the subperiosteal space and it is due to deposition of tumor osteoid along the vessels.

Codman's triangle: This is a reactive bone formation parallel to the bone and is triangular, it is not specific to osteosarcoma as it is also seen in Ewing's sarcoma and chronic osteomyelitis.

Pathological fracture: If the bone tumor grows fast, new bone formation is weak and pathological fracture may occur. It is commonly not seen.

Other Investigations

- *Tomograms* of the entire bone are done to define the extent of the tumor.

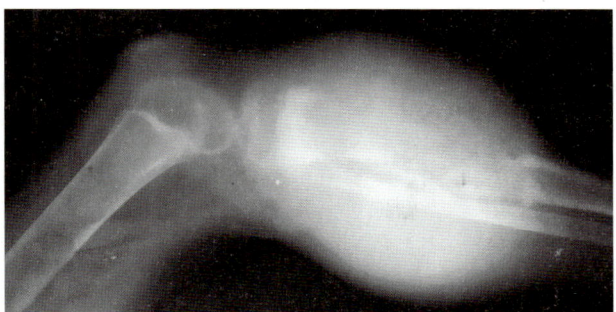

Fig. 60.6: Osteosarcoma upper end of tibia

- *Complete skeletal survey* is done using radioactive isotopes to determine the metastatic lesions elsewhere.
- *Chest X-ray* helps to determine the lung metastasis.
- *CT scan* helps to study the cross-section of the tumor and enables to detect the chest metastasis as small as 2 mm.
- *MRI* helps to define the medullary spread and soft tissue involvement.
- *Biopsy* of the tumor is very useful in arriving at a definitive diagnosis. Fine-needle aspiration cytology (FNAC) is preferred as incision may further provoke the spread.

Treatment

General principles
- Early radical amputation is done to remove the primary tumor.
- An attempt is made to prevent metastasis or control it if it has already formed by preoperative irradiation, chemotherapy, or both.
- Resection of large pulmonary metastasis is carried out.

Surgery

Early and radical ablation is the surgical procedure of choice. Having first established the diagnosis by biopsy, the level of amputation is determined after carrying out the various investigations mentioned above. Surgery is done at the earliest possible time.

QUICK FACTS

Osteosarcoma: Levels of amputation
  a. Upper end of humerus: Forequarter amputation.
  b. Upper end of tibia: Midthigh amputation.
  c. Upper end of femur: Hindquarter amputation and hip disarticulation.
  d. Lower end of femur: Midthigh amputation and hip disarticulation.

Megavoltage Radiotherapy

Megavoltage irradiation is given preoperatively before amputation to decrease the viability of the cells that may be disseminated into bloodstream by surgical trauma. It is a useful adjunct in the treatment of

resectable tumors. Its efficacy is doubtful in the non-resectable tumors, e.g. vertebra. Irradiation destroys tumor cells with minimal effect on the uninvolved parts.

Chemotherapy (CT)

Earlier osteogenic sarcoma was refractory to chemo-therapy. Nevertheless, it has now been found that high doses of methotrexate, citrovorum factor rescue (CFR) and Adriamycin are effective. By using the above drugs in short cyclical courses, toxic effects can be held to a minimum. Addition of an alkylating agent like cyclo-phosphamide has increased the interval between the administrations of individual drugs. This has marke-dly reduced the toxicity of the drugs. The treatment triads in order of sequence are shown in Fig. 60.7.

Surgery

In summary, after having established the diagnosis of osteogenic sarcoma with certainty, patient is initially put on chemotherapy. Local irradiation of the tumor is done next. Early radical surgical ablation is then carried out at the appropriate time. This limb saving surgery is followed up with fitting of a custom made prosthesis.

Prognosis of osteogenic sarcoma has dramatically improved by the combined approach of ablation, mega-voltage irradiation and chemotherapy. In untreated cases, survival time after pulmonary metastasis has developed is around 2.9 percent. With the combined approach of chemotherapy, radiotherapy and pulmonary resection, the five-year survival rate has increased by 60 percent.

Remember

Characteristic facts of osteogenic sarcoma
- Highly malignant bone tumor.
- Arises from multipotent cells.
- Most frequent primary bone tumor next only to multiple myeloma.
- Seventy-five percent are below 25 years of age.
- Ninety percent occur in the metaphysis.
- Neoplastic osteoid is always present.
- Both osteosclerotic and osteolytic variety is the most common.
- Leg of mutton appearance.
- Spindle cells.
- No giant cells.
- Pain is the first symptom.
- Skin is stretched shiny, dilated veins are present.
- Pathological fractures are not common.
- Eighty percent has blood spread.
- Sunray appearance and Codman's triangle are special X-ray features.
- Multipronged approach gives better survival rate.

RESORPTIVE BONE TUMORS

These are not true tumors but tumor like conditions (hamartoma). These are benign and may cause patho-logical fractures.

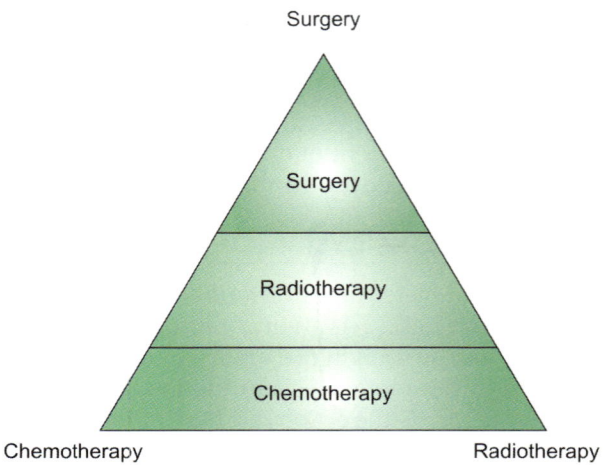

Fig. 60.7: Triad of treatment in osteogenic sarcoma

ANEURYSMAL BONE CYST

60

Aneurysmal bone cyst is a benign lesion eccentrically situated in the metaphyseal ends of the long bones. It grows outwards and is located subperiosteally.

Age: 10 to 30 years.

Sex: Males are more commonly affected than females.

Clinical Features

Patient usually gives history of mild trauma. Pain and swelling are the main complaints. Joint movements may be decreased.

Radiology

Radiographic features of the tumor consists of radio-lucent area situated at the metaphysis. It extends outwards eccentrically, periosteal new bone formation is seen, and pathological fractures may be present (Fig. 60.8).

Pathology

It is a thin shell of bone enclosing cystic blood filled spaces. Partially organized clots remains in the center

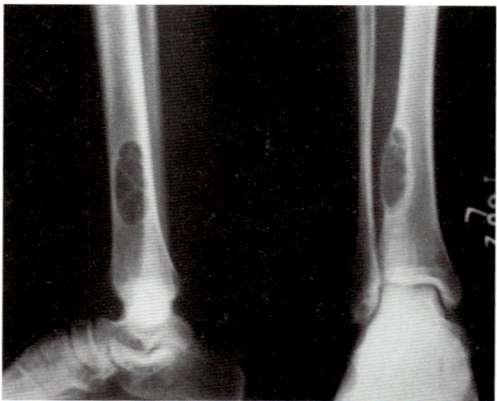

Fig. 60.8: Aneurysmal bone cyst lower end of tibia (Eccentric situation)

of the tumor. Microscopy show blood filled spaces. Giant cells are seen.

Treatment

Surgery is the treatment of choice. Curettage and bone grafting is the procedure commonly followed.

UNICAMERAL BONE CYST

Jaffe and Lichtenstein first described unicameral bone cyst in the year 1942. It is an uncommon, non-neoplastic lesion commonly seen in the first two decades of life. It is situated in the metaphysis of the long bones and its proximity towards the epiphysis may affect the growth plate. Pathological fracture is a common entity. The cyst will not disappear on its own and remains so unless obliterated by surgery.

Age: Fifty percent lesions are seen in less than 10 years of age, 40 percent between 10 and 20 years.

Sex: The male to female ratio is 2:1.

Location: Upper end of humerus in 55 percent, upper end of femur in 26 percent.

Pathology

Gross: It is a fusiform swelling, occupying the metaphyseal region of the bone. The underlying bone is thin with areas of hemorrhage present.

Microscopy: The cells are flat and vascular tissue is present. It has characteristic *giant cells*.

Clinical Features

The tumor is asymptomatic until fracture occurs through the cyst wall, which causes pain and draws the attention of the patient towards the problem. In most cases the cyst is juxtaepiphyseal. Due to its proximity to the growth plate the cysts may cause shortening, lengthening, coxa vara or coxa valga deformities. The tumor weakens the bone and the patient is susceptible to pathological fractures. Spontaneous obliteration of the cyst is seen in 15 percent of the cases and in 30 percent of the cases, cyst is displaced down the shaft due to continuous bone growth.

Radiology

Radiographic examination of the tumor shows lytic lesion in the juxtaepiphyseal portion of the metaphysis, the lesion is expansive, the regional cortex is attenuated and pathological fractures may be seen (Figs 60.9A and B).

Complications

Since the tumor is situated in the juxtaepiphyseal region, complications like shortening, coxa vara, coxa valga and bone overgrowth may develop.

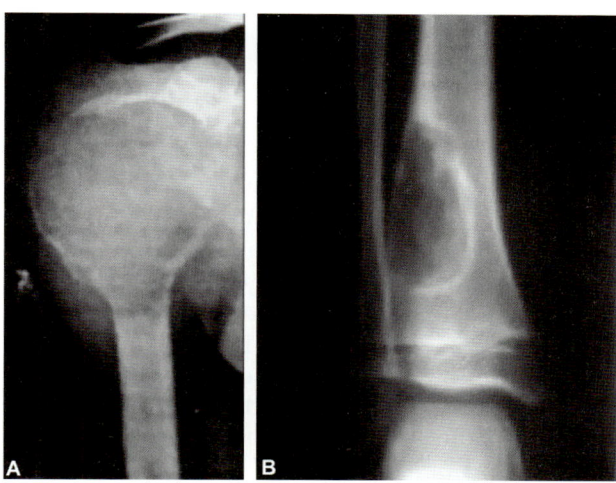

Figs 60.9A and B: Unicameral bone cyst of upper end of humerus and lower end of tibia

Treatment

Surgical excision is the treatment of choice.

BENIGN GIANT CELL TUMOR (GCT) (Syn: Osteoclastoma)

Benign giant cell tumor is an osteolytic tumor arising from the *epiphysis* and is common in young adults. Though it is benign, it is *locally* malignant. The presence of *tumor giant cells* is the hallmark of this tumor.

Sex: The male: female ratio is 1.5:1.

Age: It is common between 15 and 35 years. 80% occur in more than 20 years of age and the average age group is 35 years.

Areas affected are asymmetric portions of the epiphysis of long bones. About 75 percent of GCT occurs in lower end of femur, upper end of tibia, fibula and the distal end of radius.

Pathology

Gross: The tumor consists of ragged, friable, bleeding tissue filled with old or fresh blood clots with various sized cysts and cavities. Color varies from red to brown. Epiphyseal end of the bone is distorted. Tumor extension into the joint cavity is usually not seen and there is no evidence of periosteal reaction.

Microscopy: The tumor is encompassed by a fibrous capsule at the periphery. Presence of abundant tumor giant cells is quite characteristic. These cells are characterized by their larger size, multiple nuclei more than 150 in number, which are distributed throughout the cell. Appearance of spindle cells indicates *malignant* potential.

Clinical Features

The course of the tumor is chronic. Unlike osteogenic sarcoma, pain is not the presenting feature but trauma

is, the patient complains of swelling which is situated on one side of the bone. Skin over the tumor is stretched but there are no dilated veins (Fig. 60.11A). Tenderness is moderate or absent, egg shell crackling sensation may be present or absent. Limitation of joint movements is not seen till the late stages. There is no increase in joint fluid and the joint is rarely invaded. Pathological fracture is a late feature.

Radiology

Plain X-ray of the affected bone shows:
- An eccentrically situated swelling
- An osteolytic area is seen near the epiphysis
- The cortex is expanded and thin
- There is no periosteal new bone formation
- Thin septa of bone traverse the interior and produce a *soap-bubble appearance* (Figs 60.10A to C)
- The cortex may be disrupted in late stages
- Joint extension is rare.
- There is no calcification within the tumor.

Malignant GCT

Primary: This develops as a frank sarcomatous lesion.

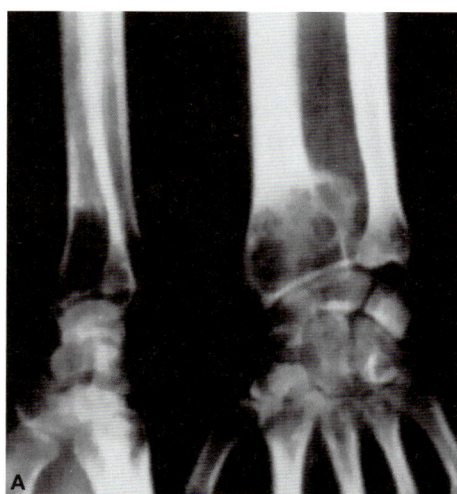

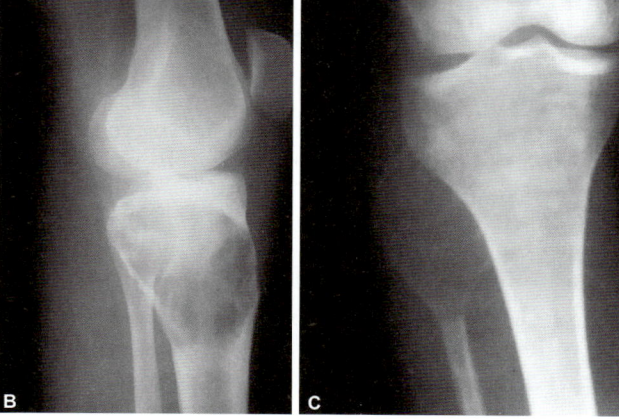

Figs 60.10A to C: (A) Giant cell tumor of the lower end of radius (B and C) upper end of tibia and fibula

Secondary: This develops at the site of previously treated GCT. Figure 60.11B shows gross destruction of the affected bone in malignant GCT.

QUICK FACTS

GCT is it benign or malignant? A confusing question:
- 1/3 cases are benign.
- 1/3 cases are locally malignant.
- 1/3 cases are malignant.

Treatment of GCT

Principles of tumor treatment
- The tumor is invasive and aggressive.
- It commonly recurs, may become malignant after unsuccessful removal.
- Recurrence is treated with *en bloc* excision.
- *En bloc* excision is also indicated if the tumor has eroded the cortex and extended into the soft tissues.

Surgical Methods

Approach that is more aggressive is adopted for lesions that are more aggressive and the surgical methods described are:

Curettage and bone grafting: It is a simple technique but is associated with high recurrence rate (about 30%).

En bloc excision: This is the initial procedure of choice and here 2 cm of normal tissue is also excised. Defects are filled with cancellous bone grafts, freeze-dried allograft or prosthesis. This technique has low recurrence rate.

Curettage and acrylic bone cementation: This has a low rate of recurrence and the heat of polymerization destroys residual stromal and giant cells (0.5 cm).

Curettage and cryosurgery: This destroys the residual tumor at its margin of curettage by repetitive freezing and thawing by liquid nitrogen. Malignancy change rate decreases from 15 to 1.9 percent.

60

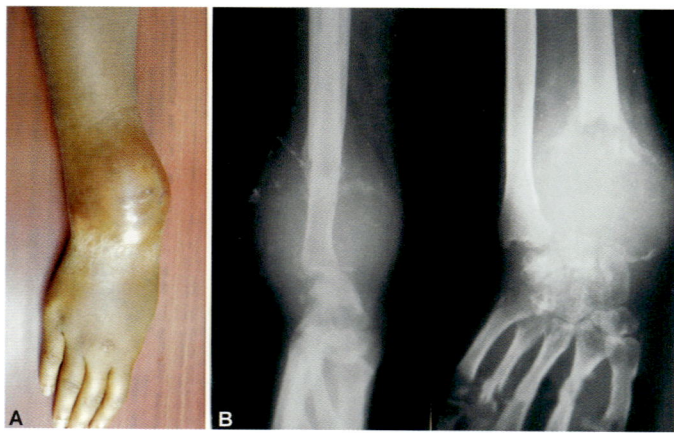

Figs 60.11A and B: (A) Clinical photograph of GCT lower end of radius, (B) radiograph showing malignant GCT

Excision and reconstruction: This procedure can be followed for GCT affecting the lower end of femur or upper end of tibia. After *en bloc* excision, reconstruction can't be done:

Turn-O-plasty technique: Here after excision of the tumor in the lower end of femur, the required length of the proximal tibia is chosen, split into two halves and one-half of it is turned upside down and fixed with the left over stump of the femur. If the lesion is in the tibia the procedure is done by taking half of the femur.

Arthrodesis: This is done by using the fibula from both the sides to bridge the excised gap.

Arthroplasty: After tumor excision, arthroplasty is done either by using an autograft, allograft or prosthesis.

Irradiation therapy: Induces malignant change if it is given to the benign lesion. Megavoltage therapy is permissible only for inaccessible lesions located in the spine, sacrum, pelvis, etc. The recommended dosage is 1500 to 5000 rads for 5 to 6 weeks.

Other Methods

Marginal resection with curettage: This is done using power burrs with copious irrigation of 5 percent phenol and 70 percent alcohol.

Resection of distal radius and using ipsilateral proximal fibula to reconstruct the wrist joint.

Amputation: This is done for widespread aggressive tumor as a last resort.

Treatment facts of GCT

Sites	Surgical options
I. Upper limb	
a. Lower end of ulna	Excision
b. Lower end of radius	Excision with reconstruction by ipsilateral fibula
II. Lower limbs	
a. Lower end of femur	Excision with Turn-O-graft
b. Upper end of tibia	Excision with Turn-O-graft

Quick facts of GCT
- Locally malignant
- Affects young adults
- Arises from the epiphysis
- Giant cells are characteristic
- Egg shell crackling may be present
- Soap-bubble appearance is characteristic
- *En bloc* excision and reconstruction is the surgical method of choice
- One-third is benign, one-third is locally malignant and one-third is malignant.

TUMORS OF NON-OSSEOUS ORIGIN

EWING'S SARCOMA

It was first described by Ewing in the year 1928. This is a rare primary malignant bone tumor (10–14% of all malignant bone tumors) affecting children. It is a lethal tumor with a poor 5-year survival rate.

Features

Age: Persons commonly affected are four to twenty-five age group (about 80%).

Sex: More common in males.

Site: Long bones affected are femur, tibia, fibula and humerus in that order. About 20 percent of tumors are seen in flat bones.

Location: Diaphysis of the long bones is commonly affected.

Pathology

Gross: It is a grayish white tumor encapsulated by fibrous tissue. It may contain hemorrhagic foci and areas of cystic formation. From the medulla, it reaches to the surface through the haversian canals.

Histology: The tumor is very *cellular.* The cells may be small, round or polyhedral in shape and may be arranged as cords or sheets. Intercellular substance is minimal. Necrosis is common. Cells are arranged round the vessels justifying the term *perithelioma.* Many tumors show *Rosette* formation with central fibril. *Pseudo rosettes* are more common (no central fibril). Giant cells are not found and there is no new bone formation.

Clinical Features

Patient presents with pain, which is intermittent in nature. The pain is worse at night. The tumor is fixed to the bone, swelling is tense, skin is red, dilated veins may be present (Fig. 60.12). Some times the tumor may present with constitutional symptoms like fever, sweating, chills, leucocytes, and anemia. This may create confusion as it mimics acute osteomyelitis.

Course

- Exacerbation and remission is characteristic.
- Blood and lymphatic spread is common.
- Metastasis to other bones like skull, vertebrae, ribs, lungs, etc. may occur.

Investigations: Radiographic Features

- The lesion could be lytic, sclerotic or mixed.
- Diaphysial lesion with irregular destruction (moth-eaten appearance or cracked ice appearance).
- Periosteal new bone formation is in layers giving an *onion peel* appearance (Fig. 60.13).
- It has a permeative margin.

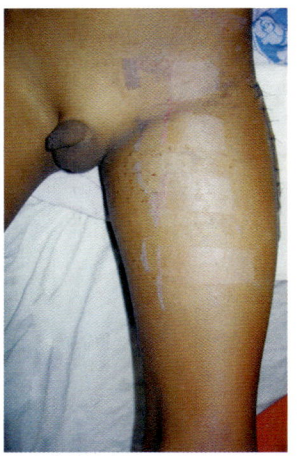

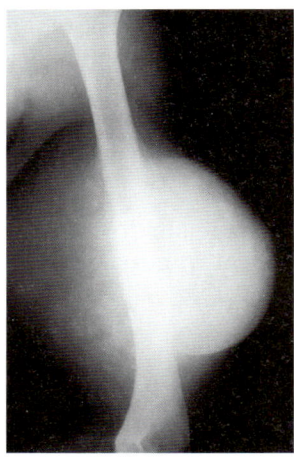

Fig 60.12: Clinical photograph of Ewing's sarcoma of the femur

Fig 60.13: Plain x-ray showing Ewing's sarcoma of the femur

Biopsy

It is necessary for diagnosis

Other Tests

- *Urine* for vanillylmandelic acid (VMA).
- *Tissue* for glycogen stain.
- Immunohistochemical markers.
- *Electron microscopy study.*

N.B. Onion peel appearance is also seen in:
- Osteomyelitis
- Osteosarcoma
- Malignant lymphoma

Recommended Treatment

This tumor is highly radiosensitive, disappears with radiation only to recur (melts like snow). Hence a combination of local radiotherapy with systemic chemotherapy brings down the recurrence rate dramatically. However, even this treatment has a recurrence rate of 20 to 30 percent and because of the possibility of radiation-induced sarcomas; surgical resection for the control of the primary lesion is being used. The surgery planned is conservative in nature and aims at limb preservation.

Effective chemotherapy is given using newer chemotherapeutic drugs like ifosfamide, cisplatinum, epipodophyllin toxin for a short period of time.

Radiation is the mainstay of local treatment especially in axial skeleton. Dose required is high 4000 rads for the entire limb and 1000 rads as boost to the tumor.

Surgery: Conservative surgery like debulking of the tumors or limb preservation surgery has a role.

Primary irradiation followed by amputation has a two-year survival rate of 15 percent. A combination of chemotherapy, radiotherapy with surgery improves the survival rate to 50 to 75 percent for 3 to 5 years.

Unfavorable prognostic features
- Male patients
- Humerus if involved
- Pelvic bones if involved
- Distant metastasis.

Ewing's sarcoma
- Rare primary malignant tumor.
- Common between 5 and 15 years.
- Tumor of the diaphysis.
- Clinically may mimic acute osteomyelitis.
- X-ray shows moth-eaten appearance and onion peel appearance.
- Tumor is highly cellular.
- Highly radiosensitive (melts like snow).
- High rate of recurrence.
- Combination of radiotherapy, chemotherapy and surgery has improved 2-year survival rate.

MULTIPLE MYELOMA (PLASMACYTOMA)

60

This is the most common bone tumor in adults. It accounts for 50 percent of all bone tumors. Here plasma cells replace the bone. It affects elderly persons between 40 and 60 years of age.

Sex: Males and females are equally affected.

Clinical Features

Typical Radiological Lesions

- Osteolytic lesion penetrates the cortex, but there is no periosteal reaction.
- Rarefaction of vertebrae may be extensive *(disappearing vertebrae),* vertebral pedicle involvement is more common, when involved it is called as the "pedicle sign" (common in secondaries).

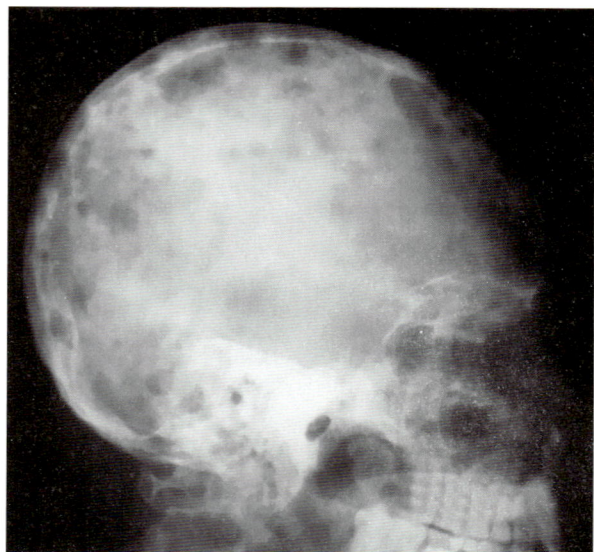

Fig. 60.14: Punched out skull appearance

- Skull X-ray may show the typical punched out lesion (Fig. 60.14).

Treatment

When the tumor is widespread it is usually fatal and then the treatment is only palliative. The tumor is radio-sensitive.

Chemotherapy: Agents like steroids, cyclophosphamide, urethane and melphalan (SCUM) are found to be effective.

Surgery

- Laminectomy is done when there is evidence of compression of spinal nerves.
- Intramedullary fixation is done for pathological fractures of long bones. (Also, see section on the treatment of pathological fractures.)

Complications

- Pathological fracture of the ribs.
- Spinal cord or nerve root compression.
- Anemia, leucopenia, thrombocytopenia.
- Renal failure.
- Severe infection.
- Amyloidosis.

Prognosis

- The disease is widespread and fatal.
- Death occurs within three years in majority of cases and in all by five years.

INCLUSION TUMORS SYNOVIOMA (SYNOVIAL SARCOMA)

Synovioma is a slowly growing malignant tumor occurring in juxtaposition to and attached to the synovial tissue but almost invariably lies outside the joint. It commonly occurs in and around the knee joints.

Pathology

Gross: It is difficult to find the synovial attachment of the tumor. The tumor may be circumscribed, rounded, lobulated, and may be surrounded by a pseudo capsule. The tumor lies closely to the tendons, bursae and joint capsules.

Microscopy: Three basic patterns indicate synovial origin (i) formation of tissue spaces, (ii) formation of cell tufts, and (iii) the presence of epithelial cell tufts.
Evidence of malignancy is seen in fibrosarcomatous stroma.

Clinical Features

This is a tumor of young adults, rare in people more than 40 years of age, common in the lower extremity, around the knee. Soft tissue outside the joint is involved, painful swelling, slowly increasing in size, firm or soft and tender. Restriction of joint movements may be seen.

Course: The course is very slow, metastasizes eventually to the lungs.

Radiology

Soft tissue shadows are seen. Stippling is observed if the tumor contains small areas of calcification (Fig. 60.15).

Treatment

Synovioma is a slow growing tumor. It metastasizes late. Surgery is the treatment of choice and includes local excision. Radical amputation is preferred if the tumor has a widespread involvement.

METASTATIC TUMORS OF BONES

These are cancerous tumors originating in other organs and involving the skeletal structures of the body. Bones may be involved by

- Direct invasion.
- Blood borne metastasis (most common route).
- Very rarely through the lymphatic.

Blood borne metastases to the bone greatly outnumber the primary bone tumors.

Incidence is twenty-seven to seventy percent.

QUICK FACTS: TENDENCY PERCENTAGEWISE	
Ca Breast	73%
Ca Lungs	32%
Ca Kidneys	24%
Ca Rectum	13%
Ca Stomach	11%

Sites: The secondary bone tumors commonly involve vertebrae (Fig. 60.15), ribs, pelvis, sternum, skull and proximal ends of femur and humerus. It is unusual for metastasis neoplasm is to involve bones distal to the elbows or knees.

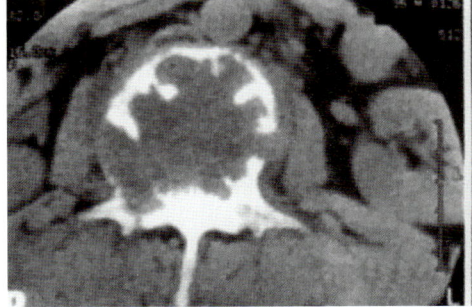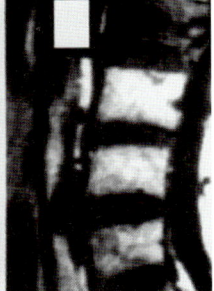

Fig. 60.15: Metastasis in a vertebral body

Clinical Features

Patient is usually an adult, in the middle or late life, and may present with pain, pathological fracture or anemia. Patient complains of headache if the skull is involved. Spine involvement causes girdle pains, spastic paralysis, etc. Pathological fractures are frequent in femur. Collapse of vertebrae may be present. In few cases, patient may present with complaints peculiar to the primary malignancy.

Laboratory Diagnosis

- Blood picture may be normal or bizarre showing features of anemia, thrombocytopenia or thrombocytosis, leucocytes or leucopenia, eosinophilia, etc.
- Sometimes anemia is associated with leucoerythroblastic reaction.
- Sometimes a syndrome of hemolytic anemia, thrombocytopenia, and fibrinogenopenia can be seen with cancer of stomach and pancreas, etc.
- Alkaline phosphatase is increased normally, but acid phosphatase increases in cancer of prostate.
- High ESR and increased serum calcium.

Radiology

Radiographs fail to detect secondaries in the bone in 20 to 25 percent of the cases. Two types are recognized
- Osteolytic variety is frequent.
- Osteoblastic variety shows increased density (cancer prostate).
  Periosteal reaction and mottled or marble appearance are the other radiographic features.

Bone Scan

This is the most sensitive method of investigation.

Fine needle biopsy is accurate in over 90 percent of the cases.

CT scan and MRI

These are the other very useful investigative procedures.

Treatment

The following are the various modalities of treatment.

Radiotherapy is by ^{60}Co 3000 to 4000 rads for 3 to 4 weeks.

Surgery: If the patient has developed pathological fracture, internal fixation with acrylic cement is done. Decompressive laminectomy is done for secondaries in the spine. Endocrine surgery for cancer breast, cancer prostate, etc.

Hormone therapy
- For prostatic cancer, estrogen.
- For breast cancer, diethylstilbestrol.
- For thyroid cancer, T3 and ^{131}I.

Radioisotope therapy is by using
- Radioactive phosphorus
- Radioactive ^{131}I

Chemotherapy is by using drugs like alkylating agents, antimetabolites, etc.

Treatment of hypocalcemia is by using cortisone, mithramycin, etc.

Amputation is indicated for intractable pain and as a last resort.

Prophylactic nailing is considered for those cases with more than 50 percent destruction of the cortex.

60

QUICK FACTS
Silent primary: Here there are no features of primary but present with features of secondary for the first time:
- Ca thyroid
- Renal cell sarcoma
- Ca bladder, etc.

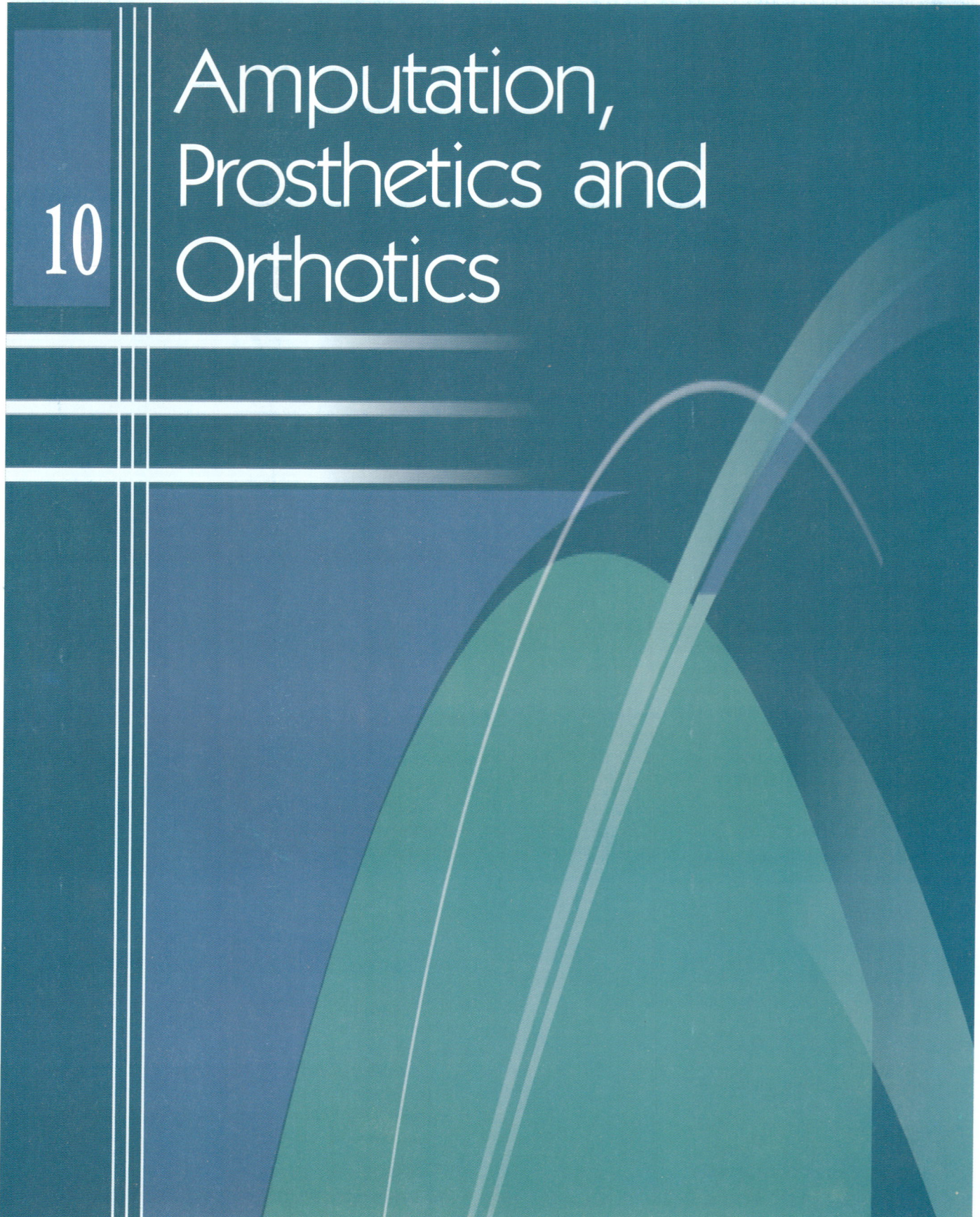

10

Amputation, Prosthetics and Orthotics

61 Amputations

GENERAL PRINCIPLES

Amputation is defined as removal of the limb through a part of a bone. Disarticulation is the removal of the limb through a joint.

Incidences

Age: Common in 50 to 75 age group.

Sex: 75% men, 25% women

Indications: Eighty-five percent is through the lower limbs, 15 percent is through the upper limbs. Injuries leading to amputations are the ones which are severe and leave the limbs badly mutilated. High speed RTAs, major falls, and crushing injuries due to industrial or agricultural accidents spell unmitigated disaster to the limbs making amputation a logical solution. However, in children, congenital anomalies and in the elderly, peripheral vascular disease is the common cause of amputation.

Other indications:
- Malignant bone tumours like osteogenic sarcoma, Ewing's sarcoma, etc.
- Gross bony deformities
- TAO, frostbite, etc.

Remember
The only real absolute indication for amputation is irreparable loss of blood supply of a diseased or injured limb.

QUICK FACTS
Common Indications for amputations vs age
- Children—Congenital anomalies
- Young adults—Injuries
- Elderly patients—Peripheral vascular disease

Amputation: Types and Levels

Upper limbs: Various levels of amputation at the upper limbs (Fig. 61.1)

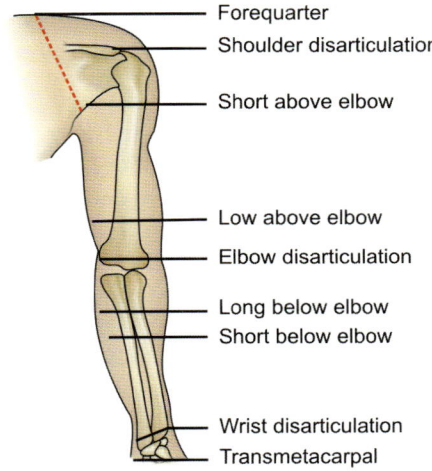

Fig. 61.1: Levels of upper limb amputations

- Shoulder disarticulation
- Standard above elbow
- Very short below elbow
- Long below elbow
- Short above elbow
- Elbow disarticulation
- Medium below elbow
- Krukenberg's amputation

Lower limbs: Levels of amputations at the lower limbs are (Fig. 61.2):
- Hip disarticulation
- Short above knee
- Long above knee
- Knee disarticulation
- Short and below knee.
- Very short above knee
- Medium above knee
- Very long above knee
- Very short below knee

Ankle Amputation

- *Syme's amputation:* Here the level of bone section is 0.6 cm proximal to the ankle joint. The weight bearing function is retained due to the retention of the heel pad.
- *Sarmiento's amputation:* Here the level is 1.3 cm proximal to the joint.
- *Wagner's:* This is two-stage Syme's amputation.
- *Boyd's:* This consists of talectomy and calcaneotibial arthrodesis.
- *Pirogoff's amputation:* In this only anterior part of the calcaneum is removed.

Foot Amputation

- *Ray amputation:* Amputation of great toes and other toes.

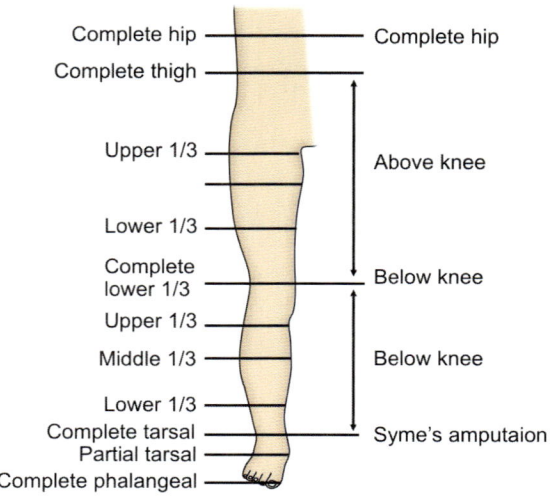

Fig. 61.2: Levels of lower limb amputations

- *Gille's operations:* Amputation through the metatarsal bones.
- *Lisfranc's operation:* Amputation is at the level of the the tarsometatarsal joints.
- *Chopart's operation:* Amputation is through the mid-tarsal joints.

Closed Amputation

This is done most of the times as an elective procedure and may be above knee or below knee, above elbow and below elbow, etc. In this, the skin is closed primarily after amputation (Fig. 61.3).

- *Tourniquets:* These are desirable except in ischemic limbs.

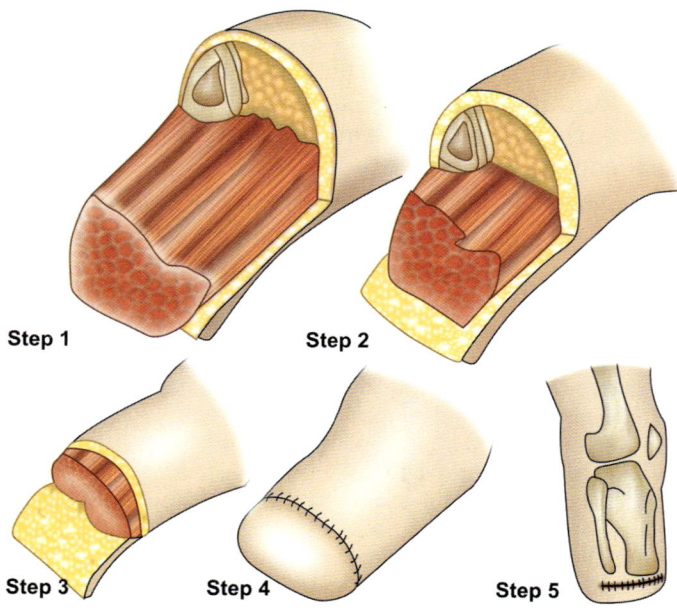

Fig. 61.3: Steps of below knee closed amputation

- *Level of amputation:* As in the past the level of amputation is no longer important, thanks to the modern and sophisticated present-day prosthesis.

THE CARDINAL RULE

Amputate through the tissues that will heal satisfactorily and preserve all possible lengths consistent with good surgical judgment.

- *Skin flaps:* Good skin coverage for the amputation site is of vital importance. The skin should be mobile and sensitive. Location of the scar is not important.
- *Muscles:* The muscle is divided at least 5 cm distal to the level of intended bone section and sutured.

TWO METHODS OF MUSCLE SUTURE

- *Myodesis:* Here muscle is sutured to the ends of the bone stump.
- *Myoplasty:* Here muscles are sutured to the opposite muscle group under appropriate tension.

Note: These are unpreferred methods in peripheral vascular disease.

61

These two techniques of *myodesis and myoplasty* help improve the function of the muscles and circulation in the stump and thereby helps to prevent phantom pain.

- *Nerves:* The nerves are pulled down and cut proximally and allowed to retract. Larger nerves like the sciatic nerve needs to be ligated before cutting.
- *Blood vessels:* These are doubly ligated with non-absorbable sutures and cut.
- *Bone:* The bone is sectioned above the level of muscle section. Ragged irregular bone edges need to be smoothened before closure.
- *Drains:* These are removed after 48 to 72 hours to prevent stump edema.

Open Amputation (Guillotine Operation)

In this type of amputation the skin is not closed primarily and later it is followed by any one of the closure methods like secondary closure, reamputation, revision amputation or plastic repair depending upon the prevailing local situations.

Indications: Severe infections, severe crush injuries, etc.

Types
1. *Open amputation:* With inverted skin flaps is the method of choice.
2. *Circular open amputation:* Here the wound is kept open and closed secondarily either by secondary suture after a few days, split thickness skin graft, revision of the stump or by re-amputation.

After treatment:
Following amputations: Two concepts are widely accepted.

Rigid dressing concept: Here plaster of Paris cast is applied to the stump over the dressing after surgery. This presents the following advantages:
- Prevents edema.
- Enhances wound healing.
- Decreases postoperative pain.
- Encourages early upright posture, which has both physiologic and psychological benefits.
- Reduces hospital stay.
- Helps in early temporary prosthetic fitting.

Soft dressing concept: This is the conventional method wherein the stump is dressed with a sterile dressing and elastocrepe bandages are applied over it (Figs 61.4 and 61.5). The bed is elevated to facilitate venous drainage and prevent stump edema. The sutures are removed after 10 to 14 days and the muscle exercises are commenced. Prosthetic fitting is taken up as the last step.
- Stump elevation prevents edema and prevents healing.
- Stump exercises enable the muscles to regain its strength and joints its mobility.
- Prosthetic fitting and gait training follows next.
  Figure 61.6 shows a below knee stump and Fig. 61.7 shows an above elbow stump.

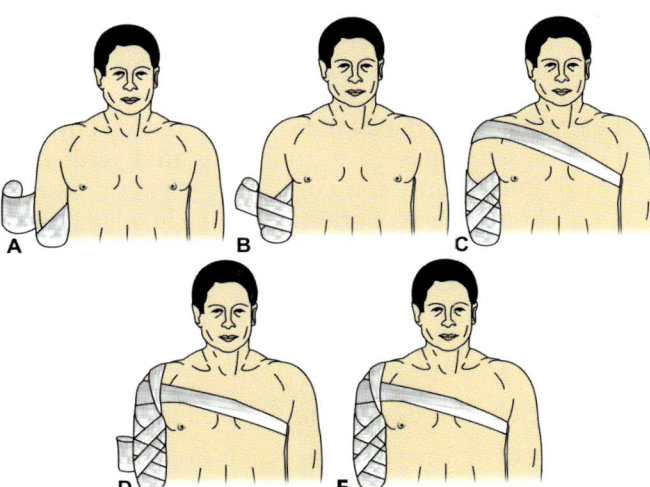

Fig. 61.4: Bandaging of the above elbow stump

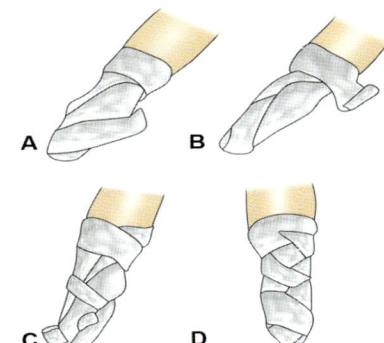

Fig. 61.5: Bandaging techniques of below knee stump

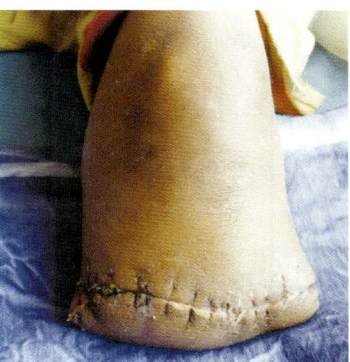

Fig. 61.6: Below knee stump

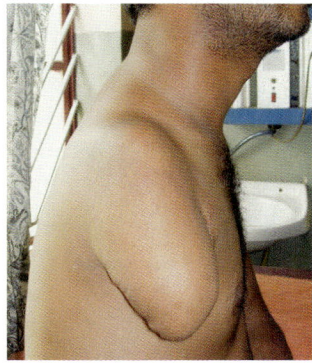

Fig. 61.7: Above elbow stump

Complications of Amputations

Hematomas: These are due to slipping of ligatures, inadequate hemostasis, etc. This delays the wound healing and acts as a culture media for the growth of the organisms. The treatment consists of aspiration and pressure bandaging.

Infection: This is more common in peripheral vascular disease and diabetics. Appropriate antibiotics needs to be given.

Necrosis of the skin flaps are usually due to insufficient circulation and requires revision amputation or redesigning of the skin flaps.

Contractures: This is largely preventable by positioning the stump properly. Physiotherapy and severe ones by surgery can correct mild contractures.

Neuromas form always on the end of a cutaneous nerve and any pain from a neuroma is usually caused by traction on a nerve when it is embedded within the scar tissue.

Phantom sensation: This is a pseudo feeling of the presence of the amputated limb. It could be of a painless or a painful variety. This is predominantly felt during the early stages of amputation. Treatment is challenging.

Causalgia: It is due to division of the peripheral nerves. Even local stimulus stimulates pain.

Remember
- Eighty-five percent amputations are through the lower limbs.
- Severe injury forms the most common indication in adults PVD is elderly and congenital in children.
- Level of amputation is no longer important as in the past due to efficient prosthesis.
- The latest concept is to preserve as much stump length as possible.
- Guillotine amputations are salvage procedures for life-threatening infections.
- Stump care is very vital to prevent post-amputation problems.

62 Prosthetics

INTRODUCTION

Prosthesis in Greek means "in addition". Thus, prosthesis is *defined as a replacement or substitution of a missing or a diseased part.* Prosthetics is the theory and practice of the prescription, fitting, design, assessment and production of prosthesis.

Classification

End prostheses: These are implants internally used in orthopedic surgery to replace joints, e.g. Austin Moore prosthesis.

Exoprostheses: These are for external replacement for the lost part of a limb. They are more extensively used in the lower limbs.

Types

- *Temporary prosthesis (e.g. Pylon):* These are used following an amputation till the patient is fitted with permanent prosthesis (Fig. 62.1).
- *Permanent prosthesis:* PTB prosthesis, Syme's prosthesis, SACH foot, Jaipur foot are some of the examples of permanent prosthesis.

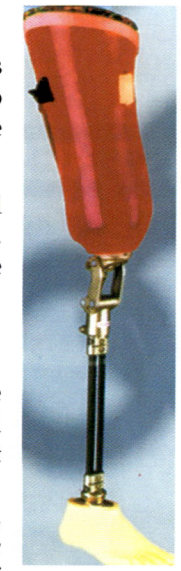

Fig. 62.1: A temporary prosthesis

PARTS OF PROSTHESIS (LOWER LIMBS)

Prosthesis has three components, the proximal, middle and distal parts.

Proximal Part

This consists of two components namely, socket and suspension. Socket is the lodging space for the stump and is usually double walled. The sockets are usually designed according to the shape of the stump, first by taking a plaster of Paris mold and finally the plastic mold. The final fit should be comfortable. If the weight bearing is through the end of the stump, it is called "End bearing stump" and if it is through the entire stump area, it is called the "Total Contact Socket". The other important component of the proximal part is the suspension which holds the socket to the stump.

Middle Part

This is the link between the proximal and distal parts and consists of joints and an extension, which is a link between the middle and distal parts.

Distal Part

This belongs to the prosthetic foot. Traditionally it is the SACH foot, with a wooden core and peripheral rubber components. SACH foot is designed to look like a normal foot and make walking on uneven surfaces easier. Indian modification to the SACH foot is the 'Jaipur Foot' (Fig. 62.2). Modifications are done keeping the Indian interest of 'barefoot walking' in mind. We all should be proud of our very own Dr PC Sethi of Jaipur whose pioneering work in devising Jaipur foot has come as a boon to our fellow citizens.

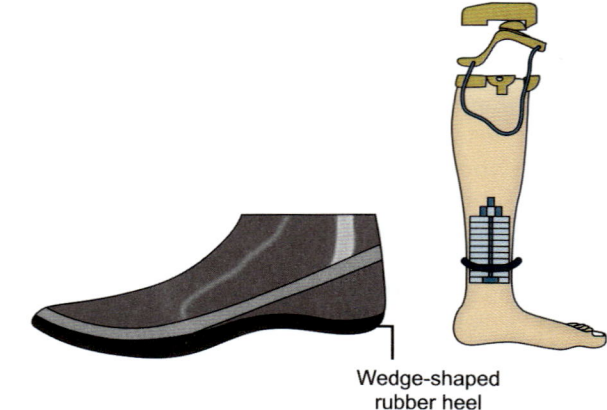

Wedge-shaped rubber heel

Fig. 62.2: SACH foot and Jaipur foot

Recent trends: Use of computers in designing lightweight materials, battery and electronically operated devices, etc. has revolutionized prosthetic designing and wear.

PROSTHESIS FOR THE LOWER LIMBS

Prosthesis for the lower limbs is required in the following situations:

1. For disarticulation of hip and hemipelvectomy (Fig. 62.3).
2. Following transfemoral amputations: Two types of prostheses are recommended.
   a. *Suction-socketed limb:* This is useful in young adults and is best suited for cylindrial tumps. It snugly fits and has a two-way valve mechanism to maintain negative pressure (Fig. 62.4).
   b. *Non-suction-socketted limb:* Here no negative pressure is employed to hold the prosthesis, but pelvic bands or harness are made use of for holding.

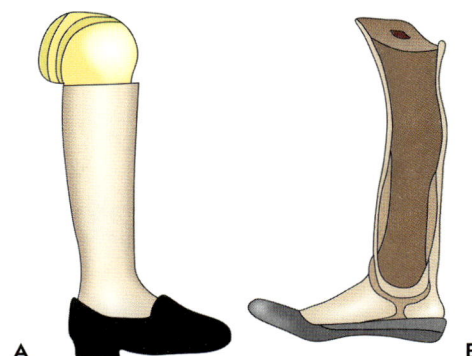

Figs 62.5A and B: Below knee prosthesis (A) PTB prosthesis and (B) Syme's prosthesis

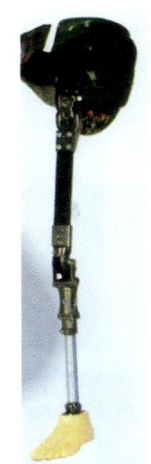
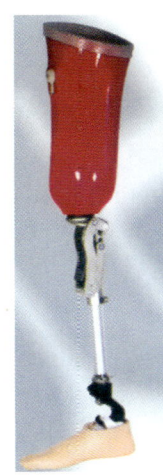

Fig. 62.3: Prosthesis for hemipelvectomy and hip disarticulation

Fig. 62.4: Prosthesis for above knee amputation

3. Prosthesis for through knee amputation.
4. Prosthesis for below knee amputation two varieties are described:
   - *Patellar tendon bearing (PTB) prosthesis:* In this, the socket is made in such a way that it fits exactly over the patellar tendon and the sides of the tibial condyles (Fig. 62.5A).
   - *Conventional type prosthesis:* This consists of the thigh corset, the side steels, the knee joint, shin piece, ankle joint unit and the foot piece.
5. *Prosthesis for Syme's amputation:* This is a below knee. Prosthesis used after Syme's amputation (Fig. 62.5B). These prostheses may have closed sockets or open sockets and may be full weight bearing or modified end bearing.

QUICK FACTS
- Quadrilateral socket prosthesis for above knee amputation.
- PTB prosthesis for below knee amputation.
- Syme's prosthesis for Syme's amputation.
- Shoe fillers for partial foot amputation.

Aims of prosthetic fitting
- To substitute for a lost part.
- To restore a lost function.
- In lower limbs it must provide a comfortable ambulation with minimal expenditure of energy.

Prosthesis for the Upper Limb Amputation

Forequarter amputations: Here the prosthesis merely serves a cosmetic purpose. A sleeve fitter prosthesis with a plastozoate cap-padded inside with foam and retaining straps is used.

Shoulder Disarticulation

- *Shoulder piece:* Extended cap to hold the prosthesis.
- *Elbow piece:* It can be flexed by pulling on the flexion cord with the protractors of the shoulder.
- *Hand piece:* Either cosmetic or splint hook type.

Above elbow amputation: Same as above except that the elbow flexion is stronger due to the action of the arm muscles along with the protractors of the shoulder.

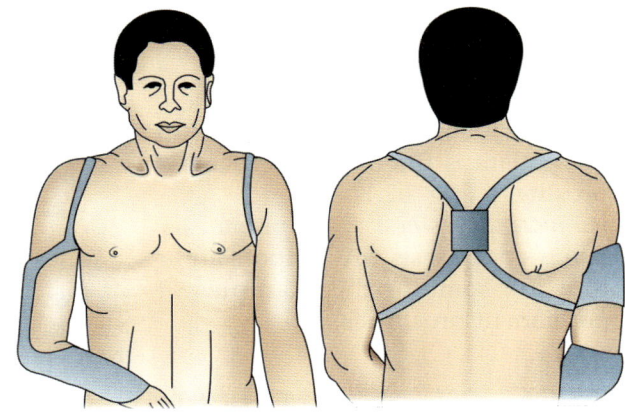

Fig. 62.6: Below elbow prosthesis

Below elbow amputation: Here there is a cup socket attached to the terminal device through an operational cord. The terminal device can be activated through a loop harness (Fig. 62.6).

For wrist disarticulation: In this, a split socket forearm and a wrist rotation device is provided. A device can be provided to lock for supination and pronation.

62

63 Orthotics

Orthotics is an appliance, which is *added* to the patient to enable better use of that part of the body to which it is fitted. In cataracts, prosthesis replaces a missing part of the body. An orthotist is a person qualified to measure and fit all types of orthoses.

LOWER LIMB ORTHOSIS

Caliper is an orthosis for the lower limb, which may be used permanently or for a very short time only.

Hip-knee-ankle-foot Orthosis (HKAFO) and Lumbosacral Hip-knee-ankle-foot Orthosis (LSHKAFO)

A pelvic band may be attached to the KAFO with or without a hip joint to convert it to an HKAFO. In addition, if this is extended upwards, a lumbosacral support is obtained converting it to an LSHKAFO (Fig. 63.1A). The purpose of the pelvic band at the hip joint is to:
• Prevent development of a flexion deformity in polio, cerebral palsy
• To increase the stability of spine.

Knee-ankle-foot Orthosis (KAFO)

These are either weight relieving or non-weight relieving calipers (Fig. 63.1B). It consists of the following parts, an upper end that may be made up of ring, cuff or bucket top. It has two sidebars or upright, the knee joint, the ankle joint, a shoe, thigh, knee and calf bands.

Ankle-foot Orthosis (AFO)

This is a below-knee orthosis in which the ankle joint can be controlled by mechanical ankle joints or by heel straps (Fig. 63.2).

All the above lower limb orthoses so far mentioned are useful either to prevent or correct deformities due to polio, cerebral palsy, spina bifida, etc. They can be used either temporarily or permanently.

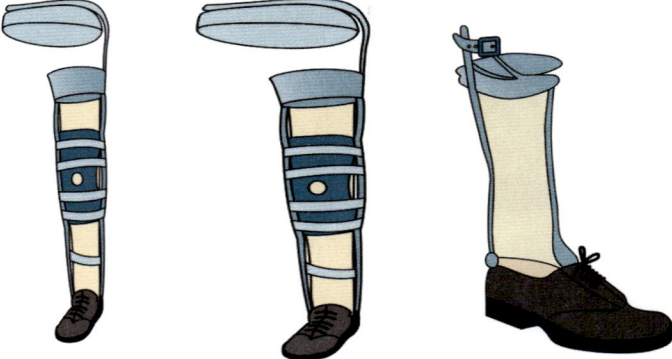

Fig. 63.1A: Hip-knee-ankle-foot orthosis (HKAFO) **Fig. 63.1B:** Knee-ankle-foot orthosis (KAFO) **Fig. 63.2:** Ankle-foot orthosis AFO (Plastic)

> **Remember**
>
> The functions of calipers
> • It provides stability
> • It relieves weight bearing
> • It relieves pain
> • It controls deformity
> • It restricts movements
> • It assists movements
> • A combination of the above functions

FOOT ORTHOSIS

The following are some of the modifications of surgical footwear useful in the clinical situations mentioned below:
a. *Rocker bar* for hallux rigidus.
b. *Outside heel float* for lateral ligament injuries of the ankle.
c. *Heel pad* for heel pain.
d. *Medial longitudinal arch support* to relieve pain the following supports are used.
   • Valgus insole
   • Thomas heel (extension of medial aspect of the heel)
   • Filling of the medial half of the shank of the shoes (medial shank filler).
e. *Metatarsal arch* is supported by the doom-shaped metatarsal bars (Fig. 63.3).

347

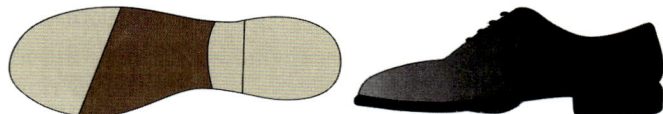

Fig. 63.3: Metatarsal bars under the sole of the footwear

f. *More roomy footwear:* To accommodate deformed toes.
g. *CTEV shoes:* To maintain the corrections obtained (Fig. 63.4) after manipulation of the clubfoot.

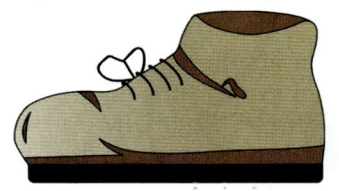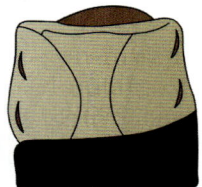

Fig. 63.4: CTEV shoes

63

QUICK FACTS: SURGICAL FOOTWEAR

Footwear with	Indications
a. Thomas heel	Flat foot
b. Arch support	Flat foot
c. CTEV shoes	For CTEV
d. Heel pad	Calcaneal spur and plantar fasciitis
e. Metatarsal pad	For corns
f. Metatarsal bar	Metatarsalgia
g. Medial raise	Genu valgum
h. Lateral raise	Genu varum
i. Universal	For short leg

ORTHOTIC FACTS

Nomenclature for orthosis now used has the first letter of the name of each joint which the orthosis crosses in power sequence, and the letter 'O' for orthosis is attached at the end. Accordingly, we have the following types of orthoses:
a. CO—Cervical orthosis
b. CTLSO—Cervico-thoraco-lumbar-sacral orthosis
c. WHO—Wrist hand orthoses
d. HKAFO—Hip-knee-ankle-foot orthoses
e. KAFO—Knee-ankle-foot orthoses
f. KO—Knee orthoses
g. AFO—Ankle foot orthoses
h. FO—Foot orthoses

SPINAL ORTHOSES

These fall into two categories: Supportive and corrective.

Supportive Spinal Orthosis

Belts and corsets: These are most commonly used for the treatment of low backache. It mainly provides support and rest to the painful back (Fig. 63.5).

Corrective Spinal Orthosis

Milwaukee brace is an active corrective spinal orthosis used almost exclusively in the ambulant treatment of structural scoliosis. The main aim of Milwaukee brace is to postpone, temporarily or permanently, the need for operation (Fig. 63.6).

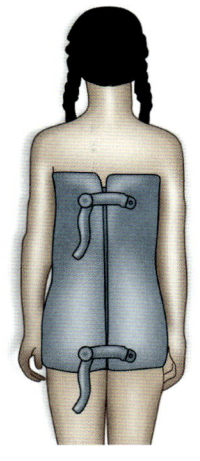

Fig. 63.5: Lumbosacral belt   **Fig. 63.6:** Milwaukee brace

ORTHOSIS FOR CERVICAL SPINE

Cervical collar (Fig. 63.7) SOMI (sterno-occipit mandibular immobilization) brace, four post-cervical brace (Fig. 63.8), Halo body orthosis (Fig. 63.9), Minerva jacket are some of the important cervical orthoses.

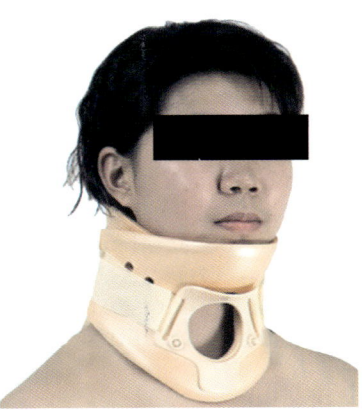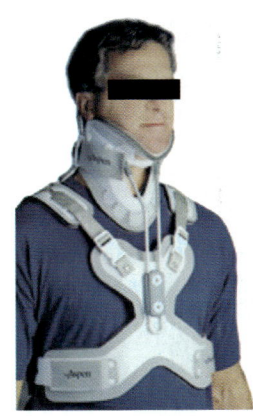

Fig. 63.7: Cervical collar   **Fig. 63.8:** Four post-cervical brace

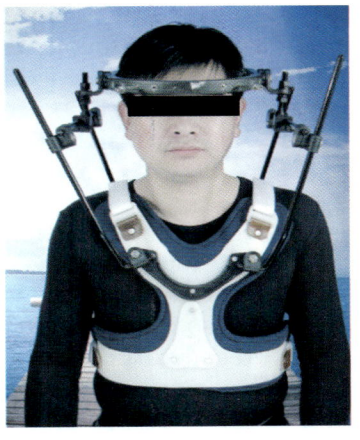

Fig. 63.9: Halo body orthosis

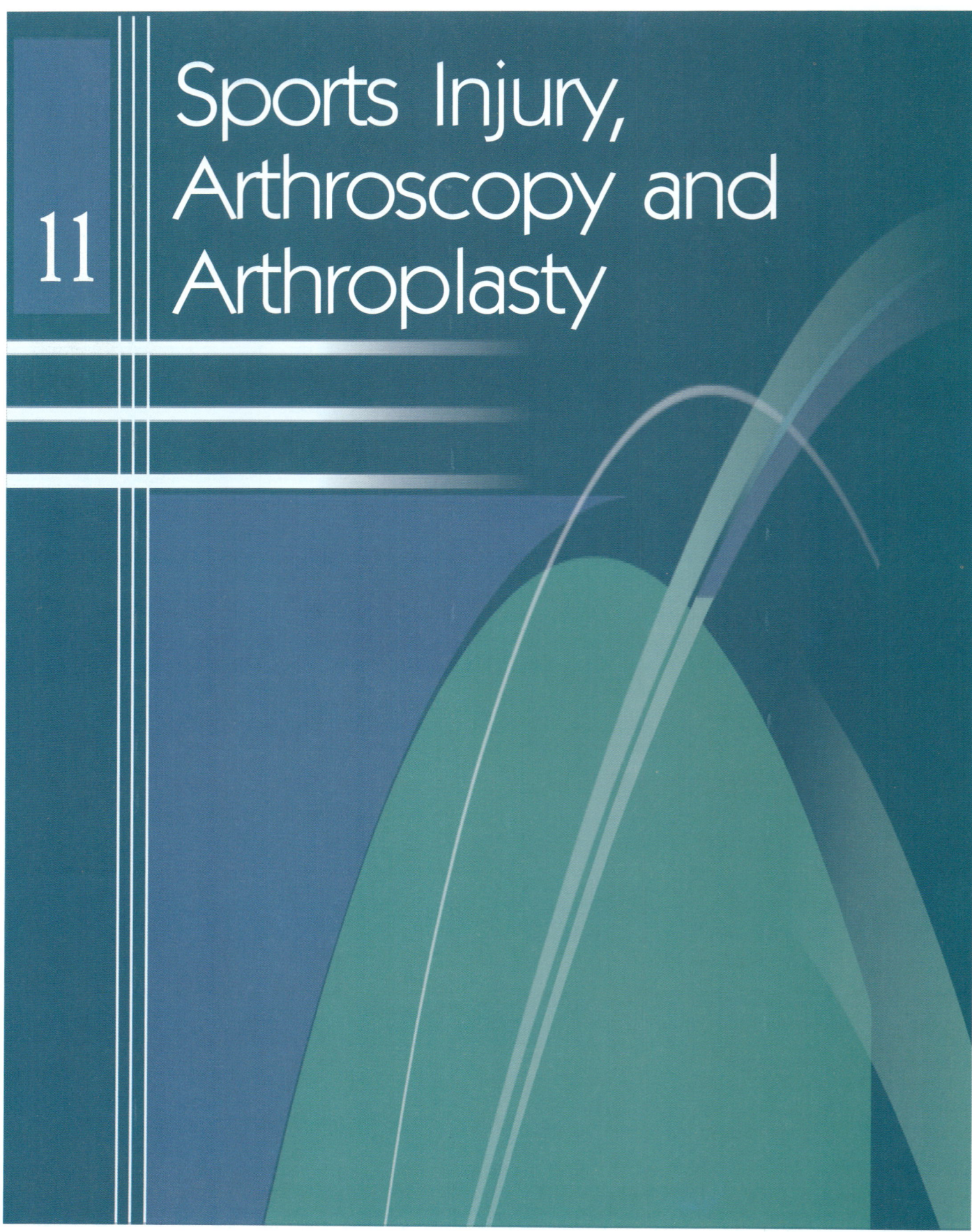

11

Sports Injury, Arthroscopy and Arthroplasty

64 Sports Injuries

Introduction
Common sports injuries
Investigations
Treatment

Sports medicine usually deals with minor orthopedic problems like soft tissue trauma (Fig. 64.1). Very rarely, there may be serious fractures, head injuries or on the field deaths. There is nothing unusual about these injuries except that a sportsperson demands a 100 percent cure and recovery while an ordinary person is satisfied and happy with a 60 to 80 percent recovery. The difference is because of the desire of the sportsperson to get back to the sport again, which requires total fitness.

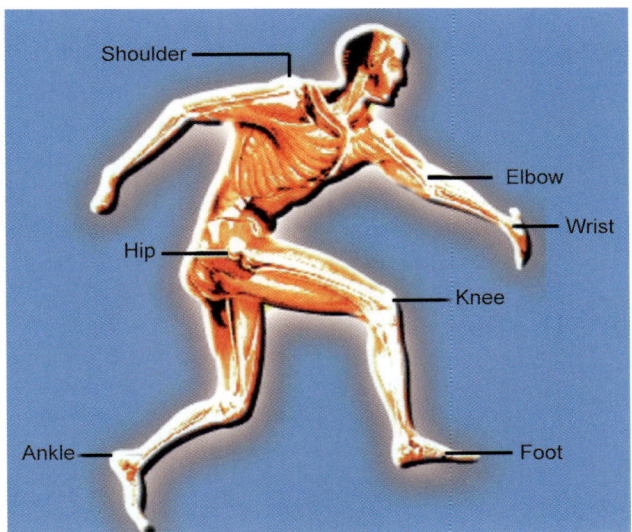

Fig. 64.1: Sites of common soft tissue injuries in sports injuries

Note: The incidence of sports injuries among all orthopedic injuries is 5 to 10 percent.

COMMON SPORTS INJURIES

The following are some of the most common sports-related injuries one encounters in clinical practice.

Upper Limbs

1. *Shoulder complex*
   a. Rotator cuff injuries

   b. Shoulder dislocations
   c. Fracture clavicle
   d. Acromioclavicular injuries
   e. Bicipital tendinitis or rupture.

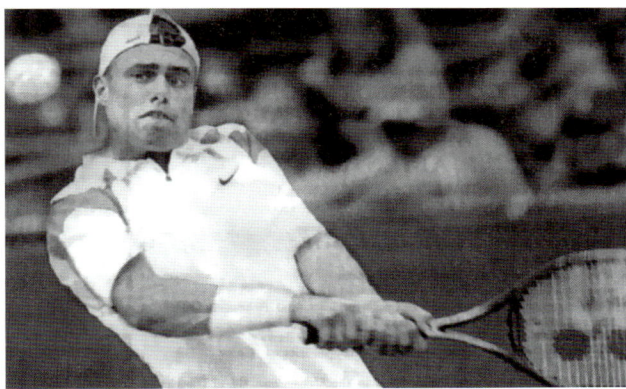

Fig. 64.2: Tennis elbow is a very common sport injury

2. *Elbow*
   a. Tennis elbow (Fig. 64.2)
   b. Golfer's elbow
   c. Dislocation of elbow.
3. *Wrist*
   a. Wrist pain
   b. Carpal tunnel syndrome.

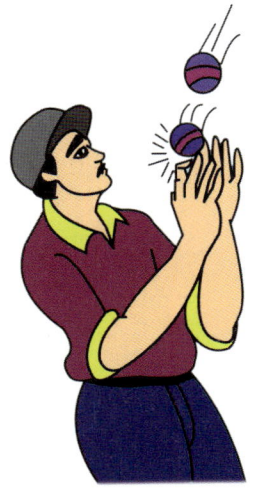

Fig. 64.3: Mechanism of mallet injury

4. *Hand*
   a. Mallet injury (Fig. 64.3)
   b. Baseball finger
   c. Jersey thumb
   d. Injuries to the finger joints.

Lower Limbs

1. *Hip*
   a. Iliotibial or tract syndrome
   b. Quadriceps strain
   c. Hip pain
   d. Groin pain due to adductor strain.
2. *Knee joint*
   a. Jumpers knee
   b. Chondromalacia
   c. Fracture patella
   d. Knee ligament injuries
   e. Meniscal injuries.
3. *Legs*
   a. Calf muscle strain
   b. Hamstring sprain
   c. Stress fracture tibia
   d. Compartmental syndrome of the leg.
4. *Ankle injuries*
   a. Ankle sprain
   b. Injuries to tendo-Achilles
   c. Tenosynovitis.
5. *Foot*
   a. March fracture
   b. Jones fracture
   c. Forefoot injuries
   d. Injuries of sesamoid bone of the great toe.
6. *Head, Neck, Trunk and Spine* (Fig. 59.4)
   a. Head injuries
   b. Whiplash injuries
   c. Rib fractures
   d. Trunk muscle strains
   e. Abdomen muscle strain
   f. Low backache.

Serious injuries like fractures, dislocations, head injuries, chest injuries and rarely even death can happen in high contact sports injuries like football, hockey (Fig. 64.4).

All these injuries have been discussed in relevant sections.

Investigations

These are the same as for any orthopedic-related disorders and consists of plain X-ray, CT scan, bone scan, MRI, arthroscopy, arthrography, stress X-rays, etc.

TREATMENT OF SPORTS INJURY

This is discussed under three headings: prevention, treatment proper and training.

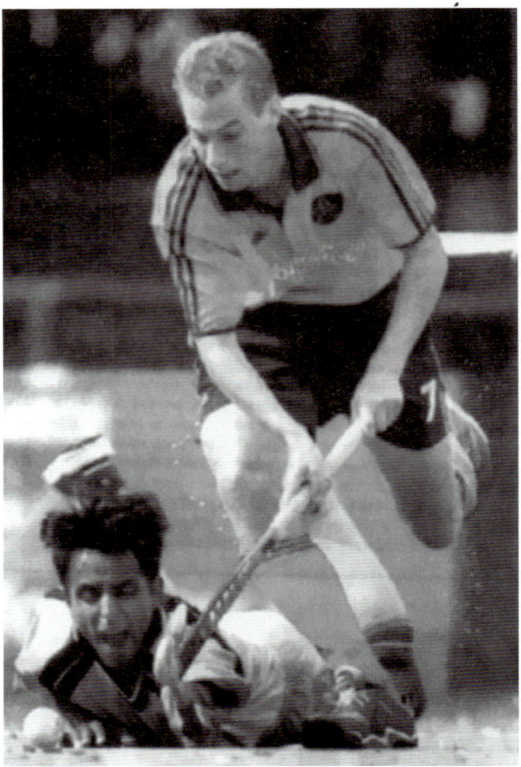

Fig. 64.4: High contact sports can cause serious injury

Preventive Measures

The best way to treat a sport injury is to prevent it from happening. Nothing is better than preventing the injury.

QUICK FACTS: PREVENTIVE MEASURES
a. Proper clinical examination to identify any bodily defects.
b. Fitness training
c. Correcting the wrong body mechanics and posture
d. Conditioning exercises to overcome particular deficiencies
e. Cardiopulmonary conditioning exercises to develop endurance
f. Proper warm up exercises and relaxation techniques before and after the sports
g. Wearing proper footwear's and other protective devices like helmet, gloves, etc.
h. To prevent overuse syndrome, taking adequate breaks in between the vigorous sports is advised
i. Avoiding sports in very high or low temperature climates
j. Not allowing aggravating minor problems like contusion, sprain, etc. by taking adequate rest and treatment.

Treatment

Treatment of individual sports-related disorders is discussed under suitable sections. However, a mention is made here of the general principles of treatment which is applicable to all sports injuries.

64

General Principles

1. *Concept of* **RICEMM**: This sums up the early treatment methodology of sports-related soft tissue injuries and consists of:

   R Rest to the injured limb
   I Ice therapy
   C Compression bandaging
   E Elevation of the injured part
   M Medicines like painkillers, etc.
   M Modalities like heat, straps, supports, etc.

2. After immobilization and rest, early vigorous exercises should be commenced at the earliest to prevent muscle weakness and atrophy.

3. To prevent joint stiffness, early mobilization has to be done first by passive movements and later by active movements. To improve the strength, resistive exercises are added.

4. Unlike the conventional once-a-day treatment, a sportsperson needs to be seen at least 2 to 3 times a day.

5. As mentioned earlier, allow resumption of sporting activity only after the sportsperson assumes 100 percent fitness.

6. Mind training is as important as physical training. By repeated counseling, improve the psychological status of the patient to avoid depression, anxiety and negative attitudes, which may develop during the injury.

7. Orthopedic and surgical treatment to be undertaken at appropriate situations.

Training

The physiotherapist has to train a sportsperson in various exercises to enable him to keep his fitness level very high. After conducting a fitness testing, (mentioned earlier), the therapist has to subject an athlete to various forms of exercises to increase the endurance, strength, running, weight-bearing, etc. The following are the various forms of exercises.

Exercises to Increase the Cardiopulmonary Capacity

These exercises are done to increase the endurance level of an athlete or sportsperson.

Exercises to Increase the Muscle Strength

By carefully planned, graded, progressive resistive exercises (PRE), the therapist aims at improving the strength of the muscles of the upper limbs, lower limbs, trunk and spine.

> **QUICK FACTS: PRE (PROGRESSIVE RESISTIVE EXERCISES)**
> - For upper limb muscles—bench press
> - For lower limb muscles—squatting exercises
> - For trunk and muscles of the limbs—power clean.

Exercises for Free Weight Training

Strength training with machines has a disadvantage in training only the prime movers. This anomaly is converted by free weight training, which helps to strengthen not only the prime movers but also the synergistic and stabilizing groups of muscles (e.g. exercises with dumb bells). They are also known to increase the tensile strength of the muscles, ligaments and tendons.

Measures to Improve the Agility

The measures to improve the agility levels of sportsperson are two-leg hops, one-leg hop, cross over-run turning, bending and backward running. These exercises help to improve balance, coordination and movements at a faster rate.

Measures to Improve the Speed-Polymetrics

In this, the neuromuscular system is trained to such an extent that it can react very quickly to sudden increase of speed and power, which is so often required in sporting activities.

Measures of Relaxation

After the vigorous work out mentioned above, the sportspersons are taught methods of relaxation and body stretches.

> **QUICK FACTS: ABOUT POLYMETRICS**
> - Hops
> - Speed jumps
> - Running drills
> - These above exercises must be done very fast with sudden burst of energy.
> - The speed strength of a sportsperson depends on how fast the muscle action changes from eccentric to concentric ones.
> - This is then followed with graded resistance exercises.

Before an athlete or a sportsperson resumes his sporting activities, a fitness testing is carried out and only then, he is allowed to take to the sports provided he is 100 percent fit.

65 Arthroscopy

INTRODUCTION

Thousands of years ago, star gazing to unravel the secrets of the skies was a favorite pass time of the yesteryear Greek scientists. The human eye could not match this enthusiasm and belied all their interests. Then came Galileo with his phenomenal invention of a telescope which opened up the secrets of astronomy and lo and behold the beautiful galaxy was now suddenly seen in all its splendor and glory.

Something similar happened in the field of surgery. The morbidity and mortality associated with long incision, wide surgical approaches was getting increasingly alienated. The patients and the surgeons yearned for something small and less morbid. They realized that they had to open less, see more, and do more. How could that be possible they wondered. Again that wonder tool called the telescope made this a reality. Peeping inside a joint through a telescope suddenly exposed the joint in all its grandeur. That joint which had a myriad of fascinating structures within it could be accessed for diagnosis and thereafter treatment by a telescopic like instrument that was christened as Arthroscopy. Like telescope, arthroscope revolutionized the way we look and treat joint conditions. Great deeds could now be performed through small nicks courtesy arthroscopy. Joints now heaved a sigh of relief that no longer they need to be subjected to mutilating knives of a marauding surgeon.

What is an Arthroscopy?

It is a 4-mm telescope like optical instrument (range 1.7 mm to 7 mm) used to visualize the inside of a joint, detect pathology if any and then treat it. The angle of inclination of the scope at the tip varies from 25 to 90 degrees. The former is commonly used and the latter helps to see corners of the joints. Thus the equipment for arthroscopy consists of the following:
- An arthroscope
- A fiberoptic light source to adequately and effectively light up the interior of the joints.
- A video camera to catch the glimpses and visualize the joint interiors
- A TV monitor to see the interiors of the joints in all its grandeur on the screen.

If after introduction and inspection of the joint, a pathology is seen and needs to be tackled by an operation following instruments are required:
- *A Probe:* This is the most vital instrument which is known to extend the surgeons fingers inside the joint to palpate its structures. This also helps in the all important triangulation techniques.
- *Scissors:* Obviously have to be small (3–4 mm) to cut, trim and remove the damaged and frayed joint structures. The jaws of the scissors could be straight or hooked.
- *Punch or basket forceps:* This enables to remove or punch the damaged structures and flush it out with saline later. It makes pulling the forceps out to deliver the debris out unnecessary.
- *Grasping forceps:* Obviously are used to grasp the loose bodies, meniscus, synovial folds, ligaments, etc. while operating.
- *Blade knives:* Inserted through a cannula to prevent damage to surrounding structures and minimize the chances of breakage, blades could be straight, curved, hooked, retrograde, undercut, etc.
- *Motorized shavers:* These are used to shave the damaged joint structures. To do this there is a hollow rotating cannula with compounding windows within a sheath.
- *Electrocautery:* This is an underwater cutting cautery and is used for cutting and hemostasis purposes.
- *Laser:* It can be used for cutting purposes that is precise and causes minimal thermal damage. But it has its own disadvantages like bone and joint damage and is yet to be used widely.
- *Implants:* Include suture anchors, materials for cartilage repair, tendon and ligament fixation, etc. and can be both metallic and biodegradable with the latter being slightly better.
- *Sheaths and trocars:* To pass and hold arthroscopic instruments.
- *Irrigation systems:* This consists of a 6 to 6.2 mm sheath to allow Ringer lactate or Normal saline to flow inside a joint for continuous joint irrigation.
- *Tourniquet:* To obtain a bloodless field for surgery.
- *Leg holder:* To position the legs properly for the procedure.

INDICATIONS FOR ARTHROSCOPY

Cartilage conditions
- Excision of damaged cartilage
- Mosaicplasty

Synovium conditions
- Excision of the plicas
- Trimming of the plicas
- Synovial biopsy
- Synovectomy

Meniscal pathology
- Repair
- Resect

Ligament structures
- Repair
- Reinforce
- Reconstruct

Loose bodes
- Crushing
- Removal

Patellar problems
- Lateral release
- To correct maltracking

Joints pathology
- Arthrolysis
- Debridement
- Shaving
- Stabilization as in recurrent dislocation of shoulder
- Excision of the joints, e.g. ACM joint
- Fusion of the joints
- To detect and reconstruct tibial plateau fractures

Procedure: A step by step account of the surgical steps is given here to make it easy for the students to understand

- Patient is under spinal or general anesthesia
- Tourniquet is applied
- Legs are positioned properly
- Painting of the limb is done
- Draping is done next
- Through an Anterolateral portal the scope is introduced (Fig. 65.1)
- The joint is distended with running RL or Saline
- Through an Anteromedial portal the instruments are introduced

- The joint structures are now visualized on a TV monitor
- Thorough inspection of the joint structures is done
- Achieve triangulation by bringing the scope and the instruments in front of the telescope
- Joint is continuously irrigated
- The required procedure is carried out
- Thorough joint lavage is done
- Compression bandage applied
- Mobilize the patient the same day or the next day
- Thorough skill is required to carry out the arthroscopy procedures.

Advantages

- Less morbid
- Faster return to activity
- Less bleeding
- Less damage to structures
- Smaller incision and hence smaller scar
- Live joint assessment and thus helps to detect the pathology (Fig. 65.2).
- Dynamic joint assessment possible
- Better diagnostic potential
- Faster rehabilitation.

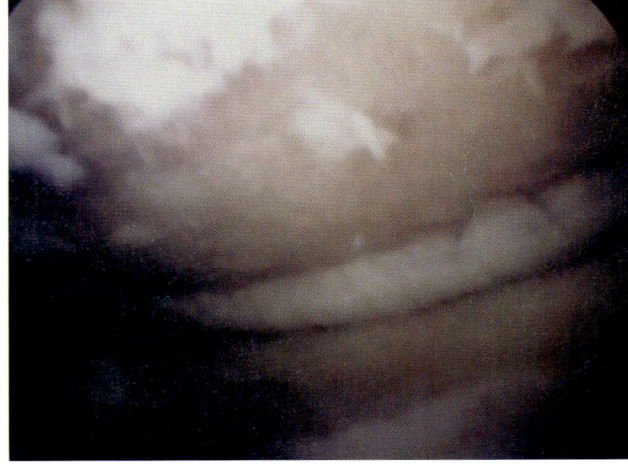

Fig. 65.2: An internal arthroscopic view showing cartilage destruction in OA knee

Limitations

- Steep learning curve
- Great surgical skill required
- Sophisticated instrumentation
- Good infrastructure needed
- Instruments are costly and expensive
- Not useful in conditions like infection, bleeding diathesis, nueropathic conditions, etc.
- Not useful in Recurrent dislocations as in shoulder and patella.

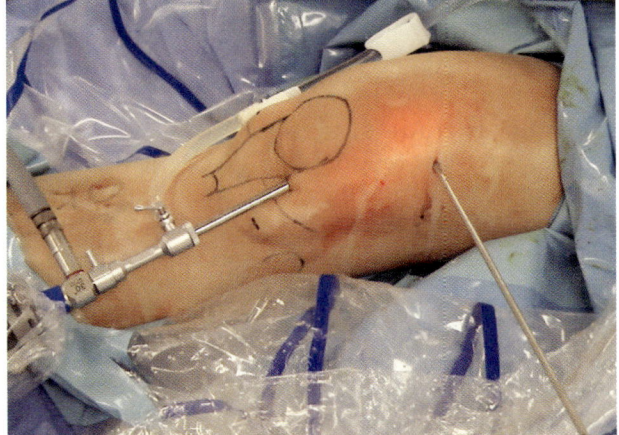

Fig. 65.1: Operative photograph showing instruments of the arthroscope through anterolateral approach

65

66 Arthroplasty

INTRODUCTION

Total knee and hip arthroplasty has become the definitive treatment for rheumatoid arthritis and end-stage osteoarthritis. They have proved to be reliable and successful allowing patients to resume their normal activities. Hip arthroplasty can be performed using cement or biologic fixation.

HISTORY

- In 1960, Sir John Charnley first replaced a hip with a metallic femoral stem and a polyethylene acetabular cup.
- In 1968, Frank Gunston performed the first knee replacement surgery
- In 1972, John Insall designed the modern knee designs

TOTAL HIP REPLACEMENT

Total hip replacement has stood the test of time and today commands its own place as an effective option for end-stage arthritis of the hip

In cement fixation there is mechanical interlock of methylmethacrylate to the interstices of bone. Biological fixation can be either a porous-coated metallic surface that provides bone ingrowths fixation or by a grit-blasted metallic surface that provides bone ongrowth fixation.

The choice of method of fixation remains controversial. In hip arthroplasty the tendency is towards the use of uncemented prosthesis in younger active patients because cemented prosthesis have reported a higher loosening rate in long-term follow up. In total knee arthroplasty the cemented prosthesis have reported good results in long-term follow up and is more widely used than the cementless ones.

Aseptic loosening is the most common indication for revision surgery. In cemented hip the most common reason for revision is failure of the cemented acetabular component, while in the uncemented ones the most common cause for failure of the femoral component. In knee arthroplasty aseptic failure can be caused by many factors as component loosening, polyethylene wear, ligament instability and patellofemoral maltracking.

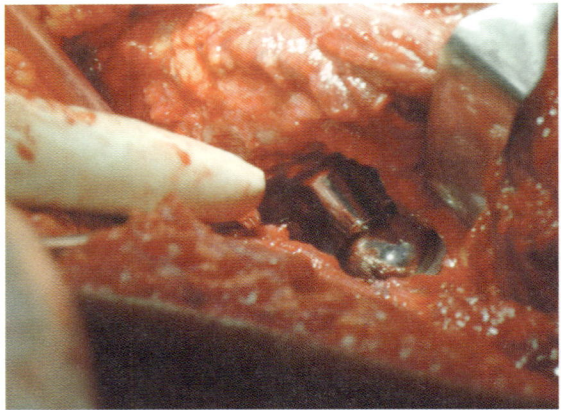

Fig. 66.1A: Total hip replacement

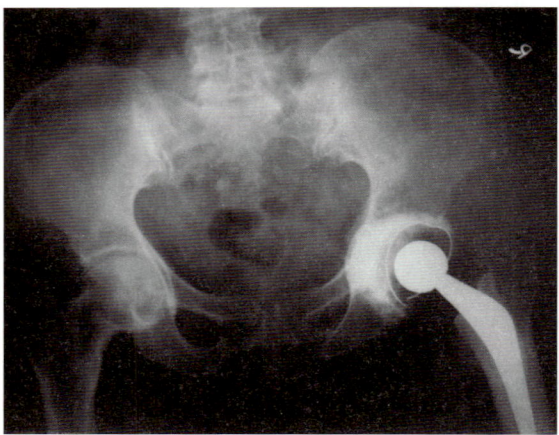

Fig. 66.1B: Plain X-ray

Articular bearing in hip arthroplasty is mainly on "hard on soft couple" which include metallic heads coupled with polyethylene cup. The other hard on soft couple is ceramic head with polyethylene cup. Titanium alloy head should be avoided because it is liable to scratching which will cause rapid wear of the polyethylene surface. In knee arthroplasty the majority of articular bearing components are metallic femoral surface (cobalt, chromium) coupled with polyethylene tibial surface.

In 1997 *Birmingham hip resurfacing* was introduced using metal on metal prosthesis. It is a bone conserving operation with minsimal or virtually no dislocation which makes it ideal for young active people (Fig. 66.2).

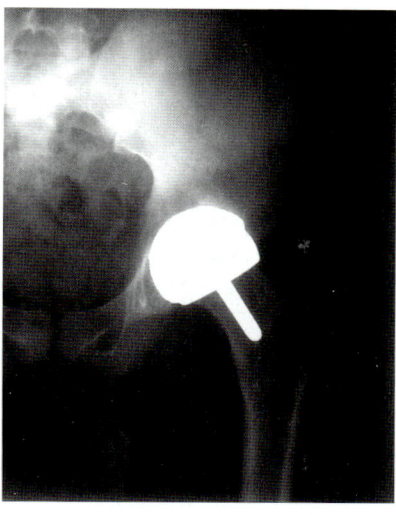

Fig. 66.2: Birmingham hip resurfacing

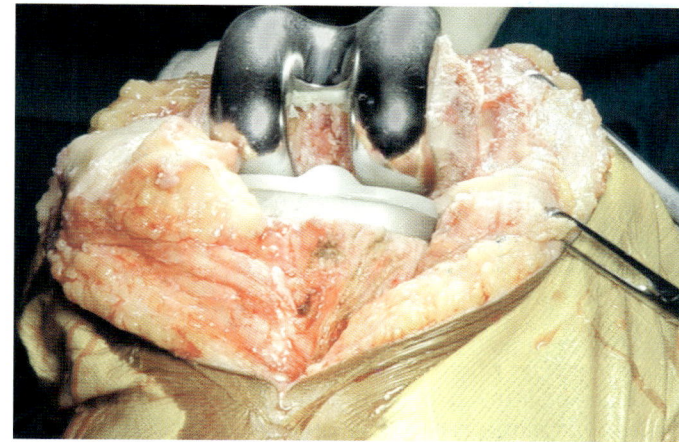

Fig. 66.4: Surgical photograph of TKR

Indications

- Osteoarthritis
- Secondary osteoarthritis
- Failed Hemi replacement arthroplasty
- Rheumatoid arthritis
- Avascular necrosis of the head of femur
- Ankylosed hip
- Tuberculosis hip.

Contraindications

- Infection is an absolute contraindication
- Obesity
- Poor medical risk
- Poor anesthetic risk
- Neuropathic joints.

Complications

- DVT
- Infection
- Loosening of implants
- Periprosthetic fractures
- Heterotrophic ossification
- Fat embolism
- Breakages of implants
- Osteolysis
- Dislocation
- Vascular and nerve injuries.

Types

- Uni-condylar replacement
- Total knee replacement: This could be cemented or uncemented, PCL sacrificing or sparing or rotating platform (Fig. 66.5)
- Minimally invasive TKR.

Total shoulder, total elbow, total ankle are the other prosthetic replacement surgeries graining importance worldwide.

Components

- A metallic femoral component
- Tibial base plate
- A plastic component
- A patellar component

Indications, contraindications and complications more or less remain the same as for THR.

TOTAL KNEE REPLACEMENT

This is increasingly gaining popularity thanks to the high incidences of osteoarthritis of the knee joints world-wide. Though not as popular or as successful as Total hip replacement, TKR nevertheless is catching the attention of both orthopedic surgeons and patients alike and is being commonly performed across the country (Figs 66.3 and 66.4).

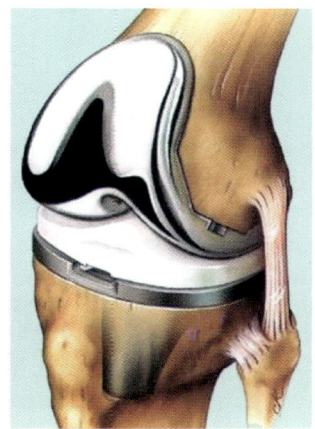

Fig. 66.3: TKR

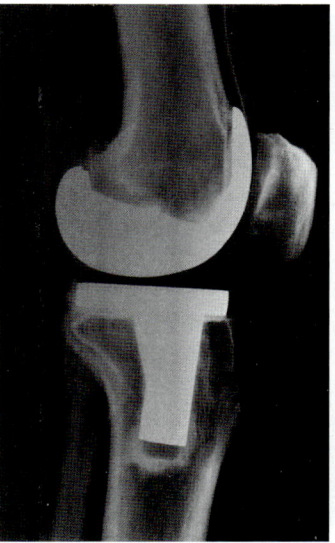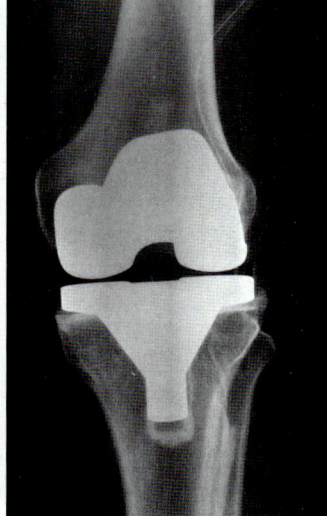

Fig. 66.5: X-ray of TKR

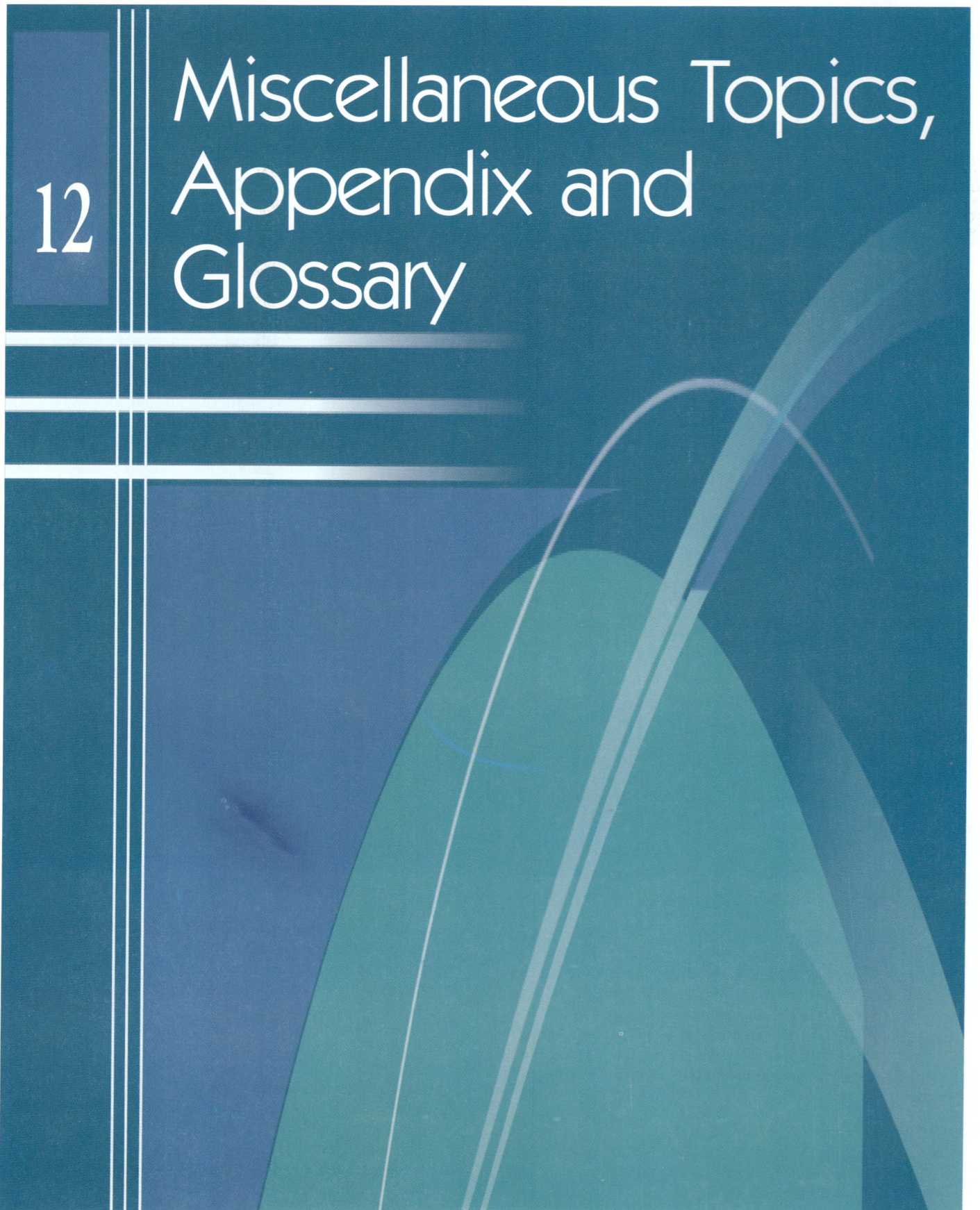

12

Miscellaneous Topics, Appendix and Glossary

Clinical Examinations in Orthopedics

I

EXAMINATION OF A BONY SWELLING

A lesion in the bone could be congenital, developmental, metabolic, infective, inflammatory, neoplastic or traumatic. To diagnose a bony lesion, a proper history and an accurate examination is necessary.

HISTORY

Age of Onset

Ewing's sarcoma is seen in children less than 10 years. Osteogenic sarcoma in the second decade, multiple myeloma in the fourth decade, etc.

Thus, the age of onset of a bony lesion has a special reference to the diagnosis.

Sex

Osteoid osteoma, osteomyelitis, osteogenic sarcoma are more common in males.

Role of Trauma

Trauma could be a contributory factor (e.g. fracture and its problems like malunion, non-union) or could be a precipitating factor or aggravating factor (e.g. osteogenic sarcoma, Perthes' disease, tuberculosis).

Pain

This is the most common complaint given by the patient with a bony lesion.

Duration

This will be short in acute osteomyelitis, osteogenic sarcoma, etc. but long in cases of chronic osteomyelitis, benign bone tumors, etc.

Deformity

Deformities may develop due to the effects of a bony lesion near the growth plate in children (e.g. genu varum or valgum). Malunion or nonunion of fractures can also cause deformities. In congenital problems like congenital talipes equinovarus (CTEV) or developmental disorders like osteogenesis imperfecta, the patient can present with deformity as the main complaint.

Other Complaints

There may be complaints of restriction of movements, discharging sinuses, limp, etc. Constitutional symptoms are present in tuberculosis, malignancy, etc.

PHYSICAL EXAMINATION OF A BONY LESION

Inspection

It is important to make the patient as comfortable as possible and the examining part should be adequately exposed and examined in broad daylight. Look for the following points during inspection.

1. *Site of the lesion:* An accurate diagnosis of the bony lesion can be made depending upon the site of involvement. Hence, determine first whether the lesion is epiphyseal (e.g. giant cell tumor—GCT), metaphyseal (e.g. osteomyelitis) or diaphyseal (e.g. Ewing's sarcoma) (Fig. I.1).

2. *Extent of involvement:* After having established the site of lesion, it is now important to determine the extent of bone involvement. In GCT, one aspect of the bone is involved while in osteogenic sarcoma, the entire circumference of the bone may be involved.

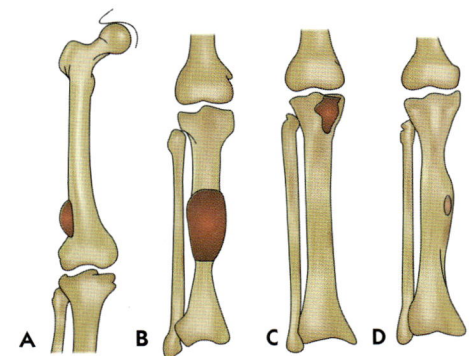

A   B   C   D

Fig I.1: Different sites of bony lesions

3. *Color and texture of the overlying skin:* The skin will be stretched and shiny with dilated veins in osteogenic sarcoma and will appear redder. In GCT, the skin may be just stretched and shiny.

4. *Presence of any scars or sinuses:* These indicate the presence of chronic osteomyelitis or old infections.

5. *Deformities:* Like cubitus varus, valgus, genu valgus or varus, flexion deformities, etc. should be looked for.

6. *Length of the bone:* Due to the effects of a bony lesion, there could be alteration in the length of the bone like shortening (common) or lengthening (rare).

7. *Shape of the lesion:* Find out whether the lesion is globular, oval, etc. by a 3-dimensional examination.

8. *Size of the lesion:* Huge swelling is commonly seen in osteogenic sarcoma, chondrosarcoma, etc. Medium-to-small sized swellings are common in bone cysts, GCT, etc.

9. *Surface:* In benign bone tumors, the surface is smooth and regular; while in chronic osteomyelitis, malignant bone tumor the surface may be irregular.
10. *Edge of the swelling:* Determine whether the edge of the swelling is indistinct or clearly defined.
11. *Pressure effects:* Edema of the limb distal to the swelling indicates the pressure effect.
12. *Gait:* Find out whether the patient has limp, antalgic gait, short-limbed gait, etc.
13. Look for muscle wasting proximal and distal to the swelling.

Palpation

In this step, effort is made to confirm most of the findings observed during inspection.

1. *Local rise of temperature:* This is elicited by examining the bony lesion with the dorsum of the hand since it helps detect even minor changes in the temperature, as this is the most sensitive part. Increased warmth indicates increased inflammatory activity of the bony lesion. Compare this with the opposite side.
2. *Tenderness:* It has to be elicited and graded carefully as described previously (Fig. I.2).
3. *Size and shape:* The size and shape of the swelling is measured and expressed in centimeters.

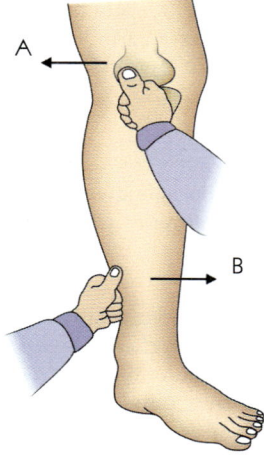

Fig. I.2: Method of eliciting joint line: (A) tenderness, and (B) bone tenderness

4. *Consistency:* The whole swelling is gently palpated and the consistency is graded as follows:
   Grade I—very soft (like jelly)
   Grade II—soft (as a relaxed muscle)
   Grade III—firm (as a contracted muscle)
   Grade IV—hard (as a contracted biceps)
   Grade V—stony or bone hard.
   Bony lesions are usually hard, but there can be variable consistency as in osteogenic sarcoma or eggshell crackle like consistency as in GCT.
5. *Situation of the bony lesion:* By careful palpation, determine:
   a. Whether the swelling is epiphyseal (e.g. GCT)
   b. Whether near the epiphyseal line (e.g. exostosis)
   c. Whether the swelling envelopes the whole circumference or is eccentric (e.g. GCT)

d. Whether swelling is metaphyseal (e.g. osteomyelitis)
   e. Whether swelling is diaphyseal (e.g. Ewing's sarcoma).
6. Palpate the surface and find out whether it is regular or irregular.
7. *Edge:* In soft tissue tumors like lipoma, the edge of the swelling slips under the examining finger.
8. *Fluctuation:* This can be elicited in a cystic swelling.
9. *Translucency:* This can be demonstrated in a cystic swelling.
10. *Fixity of the swelling:* A bony lesion is usually fixed to the underlying bone and cannot be moved independent of it.
11. *Plane of the swelling:* It is important to determine the anatomical plane of the swelling. By putting the muscle over the swelling into contraction, the plane of the swelling can be determined:
    • If it is situated on the bone beneath the muscle—the swelling reduces in size.
    • If in the muscle—gets fixed and slightly reduces in size.
    • Above the muscle—no change in the size of the swelling.
12. *Scars and sinuses:* The presence of scars and sinuses near a bony lesion indicates an old infection and chronic osteomyelitis (see Fig. 51.7). Find out whether the sinuses are old and healed or contains sprouting granulation tissue. If present, it indicates a nonhealing sinus and could be due to:
    • Anaerobic infection
    • Sequestrum
    • Foreign bodies
    • Epithelialization of the sinus tract
    • Diabetes
    • Steroid treatment
    • Secondary infection
    • Neoplasm
    • Anemia and debility.
13. *Neurovascular status:* It is important to determine the effects of the swelling due to compression of the nerves and vessels.

Due to the compression over the vessels, there could be distal limb edema, discoloration of skin and weak or absent peripheral pulses.

Compression over the nerves causes impairment of the neurological status of the limb distal to the lesion. Examination of the sensory system, motor system and reflexes has to be carried out.

Movements of the neighboring joints near the bony lesion could be restricted due to:
1. The mechanical block created by the swelling near the vicinity of a joint.
2. Soft tissue and muscle contractures.
3. Intraarticular extension of the swelling (e.g. osteogenic sarcoma).
4. Neurovascular compression.

Measurements

The limb is measured for shortening, lengthening and wasting of the muscles. This is compared with the normal side.

OTHER EXAMINATIONS

A complete systemic examination is carried out to find out if the bony lesion is a local manifestation of a generalized disorder.

Examination of a bony lesion
- Age of onset
- Trauma
- Sex
- Duration of symptoms
- Where is the swelling—epiphyseal, metaphyseal or diaphyseal?
- How much bone circumference is affected—half/entire?
- Plane of the swelling—bone/muscle/above the muscle.
- Scars and sinuses—indicate chronic infections.
- Size, shape, surface and edges
- Consistency—hard/variable/egg shell crackles.
- Fixity
- Pressure effects.
- Movements of the neighboring joints.
- Measurements done to know the length of the limb and extent of muscle wasting.
- Neurovascular status.
- Constitutional symptoms.

EXAMINATION OF THE HIP JOINT

History

How Does the Patient with Hip Disorders Present?

Interestingly, a patient with a hip problem can present with either symptoms (e.g. pain, commonest symptom) or signs (e.g. limp, commonest sign) or both. The following are the common modes of presentations in order of importance.

Pain due to the hip proper is experienced in the groin or in front of the thigh or rarely in the knee.

Limp: This is the second commonest complaint. It could be painful as in acute hip condition (e.g. arthritis) or painless as in congenital dislocation of hip (CDH). *Limp is usually noticed and told by the relatives than by the patient himself.*

IMPORTANT PRESENTING SIGNS

Gait disorders: Alteration in the normal gait pattern varies according to the cause.

Problems with hip joint activities: Inability or difficulty in sitting, squatting or walking. The reasons could be painful muscle spasms, joint adhesions or arthritis.

Movements: There could be restriction of all movements (e.g. arthritis) or a few movements (e.g. decreased abduction as in CDH).

Deformity: The patient can present with flexion, abduction, adduction or rotational deformities of the hip.

OTHER RELEVANT POINTS

Age

TB hip is common in children and young adults.

Sex

Perthes' disease and tuberculosis are more commonly seen in males, while slipped capital femoral epiphysis, rheumatoid arthritis, etc. are common in females.

Trauma

This could be the cause (e.g. neck femur) or a precipitating or aggravating factor (e.g. Perthes' disease, tuberculosis).

Duration

Longer duration of symptoms and signs are noticeable in chronic disorders like tuberculosis, rheumatoid arthritis.

Constitutional Symptoms

These are commonly seen in problems like tuberculosis, rheumatoid arthritis.

Clinical Examination

Ideally, the hip joint should be examined in four positions namely walking, standing, lying and sitting in that order. The examination methods include inspection, palpation, measurement and movement.

Preparation for the Examination

The best way to examine the hip joint is that the patients have no clothing on the body. However, this is ideally possible only in children and is impractical in adults especially women, for obvious practical reasons. Hence, a man is allowed to keep his shirts on and cover the genitalia. For females, adequate cover should be provided to cover the private parts and the presence of a *female attendant* or *nurse* cannot be less emphasized in females and it is in them that the hip joint examination provides the greatest difficulty.

Examination in Walking (Gait)

A proper inspection of the gait gives an insight into the hip problem, which the patient might have been affected with.

Method of Examination

The legs of the examining patient should be adequately exposed and the feet should be bare. There should be no constricting clothing like gown. The patient should walk away from the examiner first, then turn around at a given point and come towards him again.

Points to be Noted

During the examination of gait, the following points should be noted; Can the patient walk? Does he or she walk in a straight line? Does he fall? Does he or she walk with a limp? If so, does he or she lurch towards the affected side (e.g. coxa vara, CDH) or does he or she lean towards the sound side (e.g. arthritis) or does he or she waddle or lurch on both sides? Is the patient carrying a walking stick and holding it in the same hand or opposite hand?

EXAMINATION IN STANDING POSITION

Spine

This is best seen from the sides. Increase in the lumbar lordosis of the spine suggests a compensatory mechanism to conceal a fixed flexion deformity (FFD) of the hip.

The level of **anterior superior iliac spine (ASIS) normally**, both the ASISs should be in the same horizontal line and should be at 90° to the vertical line or spine. In this position, pelvis is said to be "square" (Fig. I.3).

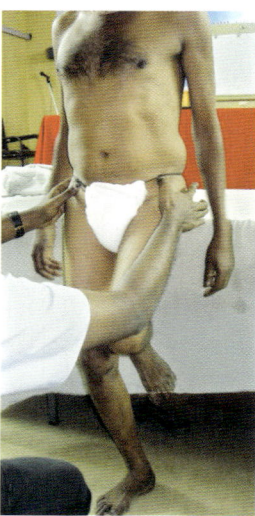

Fig. I.3

The ASIS will be at a higher level in fixed adduction deformity, and lower in fixed abduction deformity (Fig. I.4) *Swellings:* Look for any swellings in and around the hip joint indicate the following:

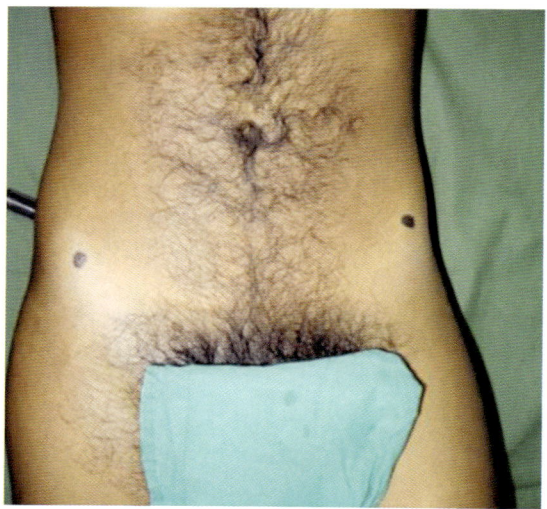

Figs I.4: Fixed adduction deformity

Old Healed Scars and Sinuses

The presence of these indicates chronic hip disorders like tuberculosis, osteomyelitis.

Wasting of muscles

This is particularly noted in the glutei, thigh and hamstring muscles and indicates chronic disorders of the hip.
Asymmetry of glutei folds: It indicates posterior dislocation of hip, CDH, etc.

Stance

A patient with pain in the hip due to arthritis tends to bear most of the weight on the *normal* leg to lessen the weight bearing.

Shortening of the Lower Limb

The limb may be really short (no pelvic tilt) or apparently short (pelvic tilt present).

Level of Patella

The level and position of patella gives valuable clinical "clues" for diagnosis of hip disorders.

Level of Popliteal Fossa

Alteration of the level of popliteal folds when viewed from the back indicates discrepancies in the length of the legs.

EXAMINATION IN THE LYING DOWN POSITION

STEP I (ROUTINE EXAMINATION)

a. Feel for the rise in local temperature
b. Elicit and grade tenderness
c. Feel and palpate for a mass (e.g. head of femur) in the glutei region or in the femoral triangle.
d. The greater trochanter could be tender (fractured or inflamed bursa), thickened (malunited trochanteric fracture or growth), shifted up (fracture neck femur or dislocation), or not easily palpable (due to rotation as in femoral ante version).
e. Look for increased lumbar lordosis (called swayback deformity)
f. Palpate both the ASIS on both the sides simultaneously and find out their levels.
g. Feel for the femoral artery pulsation. Normally, it should be just felt.
h. Test for the mobility of the scars and sinuses.
i. Feel and examine the enlarged group of inguinal lymph nodes.

STEP II (DEFORMITY ESTIMATION)

Fixed Flexion Deformity

If a patient has fixed flexion deformity, there is increased lumbar lordosis and the clinician can easily pass the hand between the back and the table.

Methods to Unveil the Deformity

Thomas test (Figs I.5A and B)
Method:

The patient lies supine. With the palm of the hand facing upwards, the clinician passes the hand beneath the spine. Now flex the "Normal" hip until the thigh touches the abdomen.

The affected hip now shows flexion and the concealed deformity stands revealed. The angle formed between the back of the thigh and the table is the angle of fixed flexion deformity. *Limitations of the test:* This test is not useful in bilateral fixed flexion deformity.

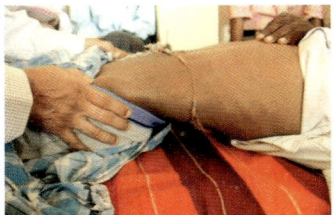 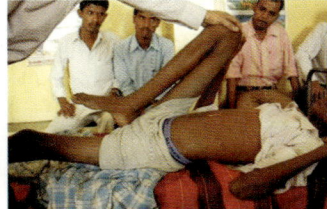

Figs I.5A and B: Method of performing the Thomas test (A) Thomas test: Exaggerated lordosis (B) Obliteration of the ordosis

Fixed Adduction Deformity

Attitude: The patient lies with the pelvis tilted up on the affected side (Fig. I.4).

Methods to Measure the Deformity

Decompensation method: This method aims at revealing the "concealed" deformity. Here the affected limb is adducted till both the ASIS come to lie in the same horizontal line and at right angles to the midline of the body, the angle between the long axis of the limb and the straight line is the angle of fixed "adduction."

Fixed Abduction Deformity

Attitude: The patient lies with the pelvis tilted down (See Fig. 54.3B).

Estimations of the Angle of Fixed Abduction

Method of Decompensation

Here the "concealed" deformity is "revealed". The affected limb is abducted until the interspinous line becomes horizontal and is at right angles to the body. The angle between the long axis of the limb and the straight line is the angle of fixed abduction deformity.

Fixed Medial or Lateral Rotational Deformities

Attitude

The patient lies with the limb in either internal (medial) or external rotation (lateral).

Methods of Estimation

Note the direction of the patella. Normally, the anterior surface of the patella is 5 to 10° externally rotated. In the lateral rotational deformity, the angle will be more and in medial rotational deformity, the patella looks towards the ceiling or inwards.

STEP III

Apparent length of the whole limb: due to the bone or joint diseases, the limbs may appear of different lengths. Technique of measuring (Fig. I.6) the apparent length (in supine position)

Step I: Place the limbs parallel to one another and in line with the trunk.

Step II: Measurement is made bilaterally from any fixed point in the midline of the trunk (e.g. umbilicus) to the apex of each medial malleoli.

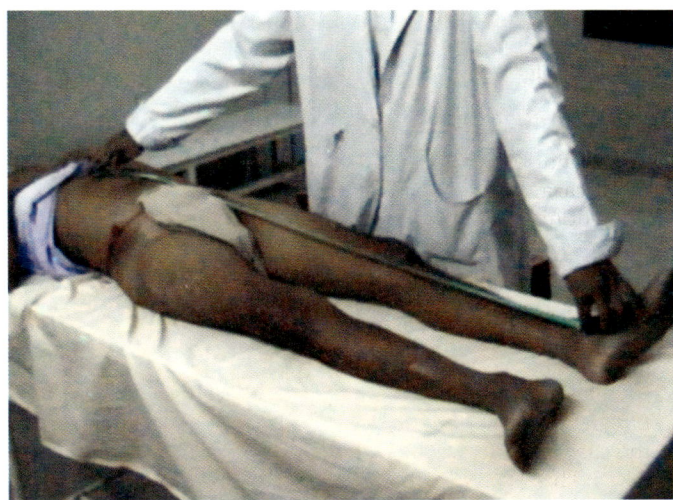

Fig. I.6: Measurement of apparent lengthening

Step III: Determine the true length of the limb (discussed next).

Note: It is noted that apparent lengthening is seen in abduction deformity of the hip and apparent shortening in adduction deformity.

Actual, real, or true length of a limb: This is the combined length of the bones and joints not altered by the position of the spine, pelvis or hip joints. The real length of the limb has to be measured between the ASIS and the tip of the medial malleolus with the joints being in the "identical" positions (Fig. I.7).

Technique to Measure the Actual Leg Length

Step I: The patient is supine. First, bring the two limbs to the same identical position by squaring the pelvis.

Step II: Fix the tape measure to the ASIS with a flat metal end.

Step III: At the medial malleolus, the tip of the index finger is placed immediately distal to the medial malleolus and pushed up against it. After recording the actual length of the limb, if

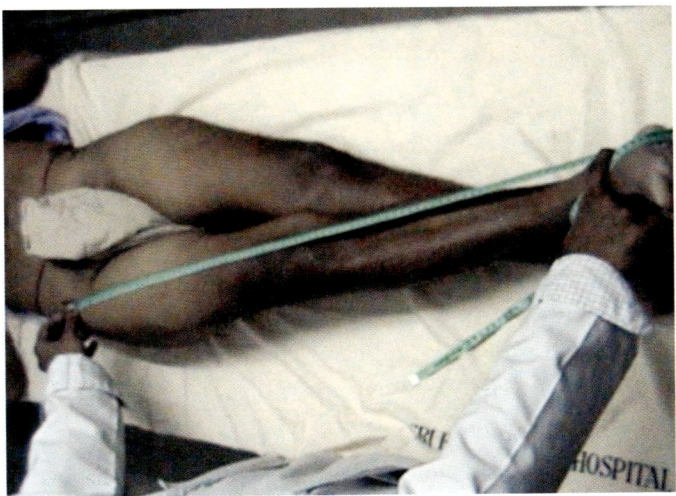

Fig. I.7: Measurement of true shortening

there is 'real' shortening, it is now imperative to find out the source of the shortening whether it is 'supratrochanteric' or 'infratrochanteric'.

Supratrochanteric Shortening

Here the shortening is above the trochanter and could be due to Coxa cara, CDH, fracture neck femur, dislocation of hip, arthritis of hip TB or rheumatoid.

Methods of Measurement

1. *Bryant's triangle* (Fig. I.8)
   This triangle is constructed on both sides as follows:
   Line 1: This is drawn between the ASIS and the greater trochanter.
   Line 2: This is an imaginary line dropped perpendicular to the examination table from the ASIS.
   Line 3: This is a vertical line drawn from the greater trochanter to line two above.

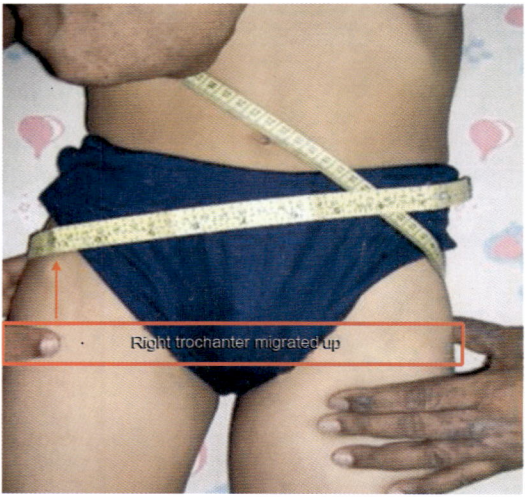

Figs I.9: Schoemaker's line

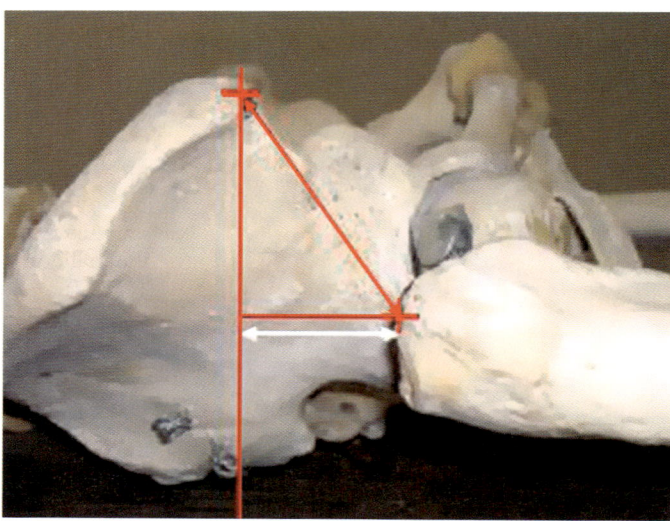

Fig. I.8: Bryant's triangle

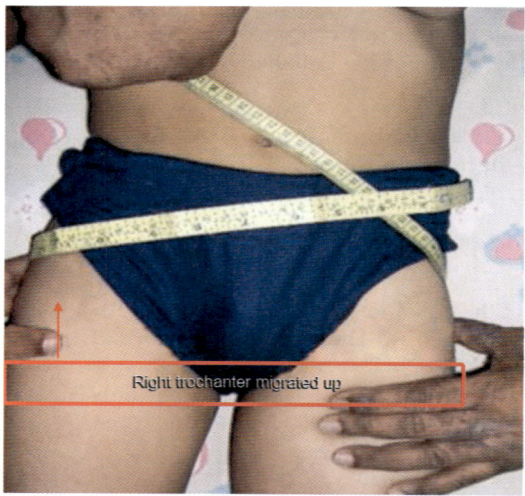

Figs I.10: Chiene's lines

2. *Schoemaker's line:* The lines joining the greater trochanter and the ASIS when extended up from both sides (Fig. I.9):
   • May cross above the umbilicus in the midline—normal.
   • May cross above the umbilicus away from the midline—supratrochanteric shortening on one side.
   • May cross in the midline below the umbilicus—bilateral supratrochanteric shortening.
3. *Chiene's lines:* The lines joining the two ASIS and the two greater trochanter are normally parallel to each other. This is disturbed if the trochanter is shifted up (Fig. I.10).
4. *Nelaton's line:* The patient lies on the side. A line is drawn from the ischial tuberosity to the ASIS. Normally, the greater trochanter just touches this line. If it lies above this line, supratrochanteric shortening is confirmed (Fig. I.11).
5. *Morris Bitrochateric line:* This is the line that measures the distance between the greater trochanter and the pubic symphysis on both the sides (Fig I.12)

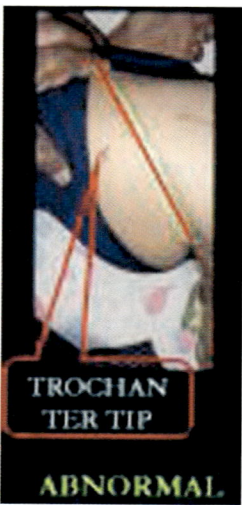

Fig. I.11: Nelaton's line

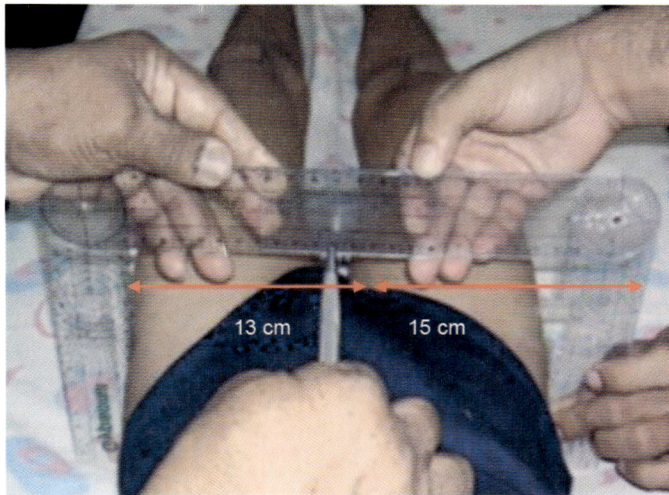

Fig. I.12: Morris Bitrochanteric lines

Advantage: In this test, upward displacement of the greater trochanter can be demonstrated without having to compare it with the opposite side unlike in the Bryant's triangle.

If shortening is below the trochanter: If Bryant's triangle, Nelaton's line, etc. are normal, the cause of the real shortening could be below the trochanter and could be due to old mal-united fracture femur, old fracture tibia, growth disturbances, etc.

Method of Estimation

1. *Galleazi's or Allen's test:* The patient is supine. Slightly flex both the hips and knees, square the heels together by placing a hand behind the heels and record the observations (Fig. I.13).
   a. *In femoral shortening* Here both the thighs are level but the knee is lower than the normal one. The leg is also slightly "behind" the normal leg.

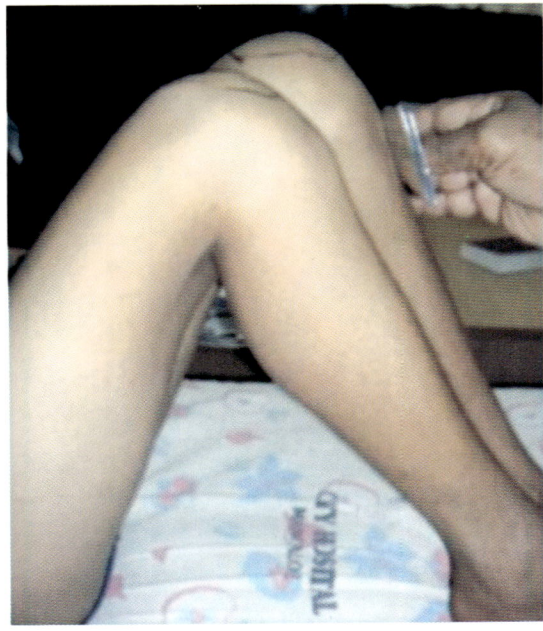

Fig. I.13: Galeazzi or Allis Test

b. *In tibial shortening* here both the legs are level, but the thighs are not level and the knee appears pushed forwards.

2. *Direct measurement:* Tibial shortening is now confirmed by taking direct measurement from the medial joint line to the medial malleolus.

Step IV (examination of the movements of the hip joint) hip joint is a multiaxial ball and socket joint with flexion, extension, adduction, abduction, internal or medial rotation, external or lateral rotation and circumduction.

Flexion: Normal range with the thigh flexed, it is 0 to 120°. With the thigh extended, it is 0 to 75 to 90° (due to tight hamstrings).

Methods of examination:
Supine method: If the patient does not have fixed flexion deformity, flexion of the hip is tested with both the knees flexed and extended. If there is FFD, Thomas test is done first and the angle is recorded. Further, flexion is then done and measured (Fig. I.14).

Extension: Normal range 0 to 15°
Method: The patient is in prone position. The examiner passively lifts the thigh from the bed to record the extension (Fig. I.15).

Adduction: Normal range is 30°

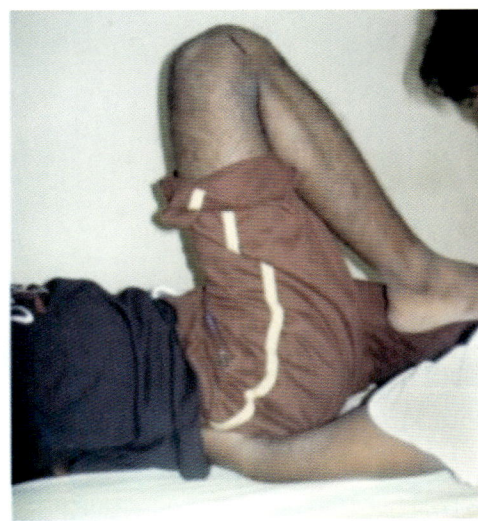

Fig. I.14: Measurement of flexion

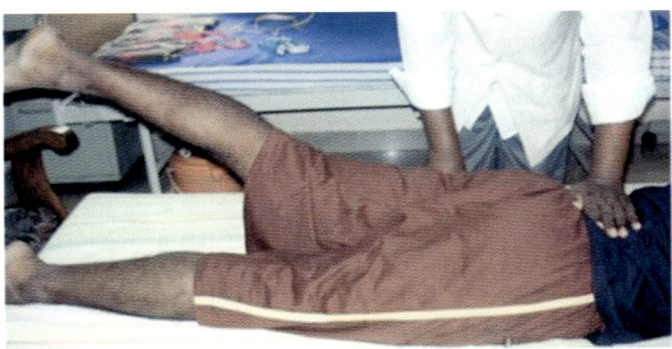

Fig. I.15: Measurement of extension

Method: The patient is supine. The examiner fixes the pelvis by holding the ASIS and the limb is adducted. Note at what level the limb crosses the opposite thigh (Fig. I.16):

a. In the middle 1/3—Normal
b. In the upper 1/3—Adduction is increased.
c. In the lower 1/3 or less—Adduction is decreased.

If there is fixed adduction deformity, square the pelvis and then test for further adduction.

Abduction: Normal range is 45°

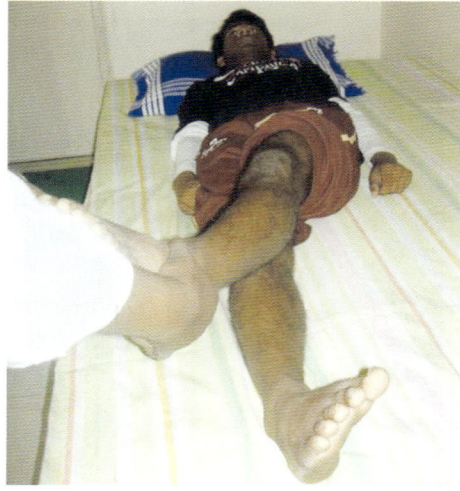

Fig. I.16: Measurement of adduction

Method: The patient is in supine position. Steady the pelvis by fixing the ASIS and the limb is slowly abducted and the angle is measured. In fixed abduction deformity, first square the pelvis and then test for further "free" abduction and compare with the normal limb (Fig. I.17).

Rotations: Normal range is 35 to 40°. External Rotation Normal range is 45° (Fig. I.18)
Methods of Examination: In supine position

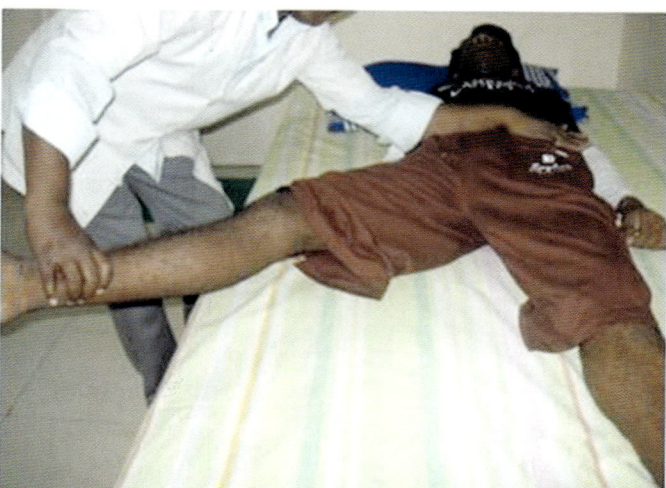

Fig. I.17: Measurement of abduction

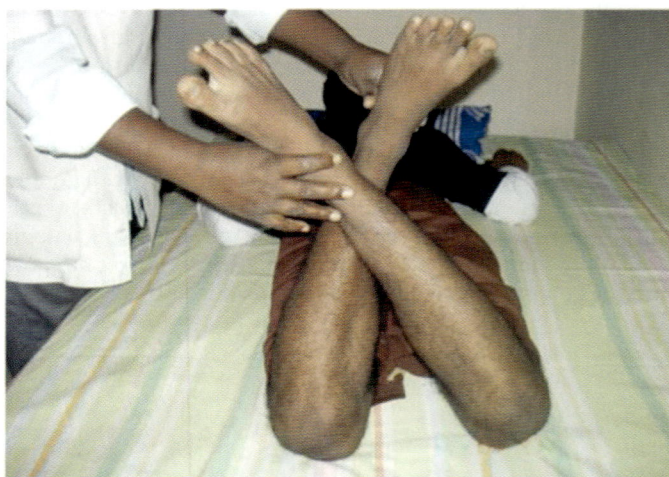

Fig. I.18: Measurement of external rotation

a. By rolling the limb gently sideways in the supine position, internal and external rotations can be determined by looking at the direction of the toes and patella.
b. By flexing the hip and knee to 90°, both the legs are simultaneously rotated internally or externally and the range is recorded.

In the prone position: Hip is extended and the knee is flexed to 90°. The patient is asked to internally and externally rotate and the range is recorded (Fig. I.19).

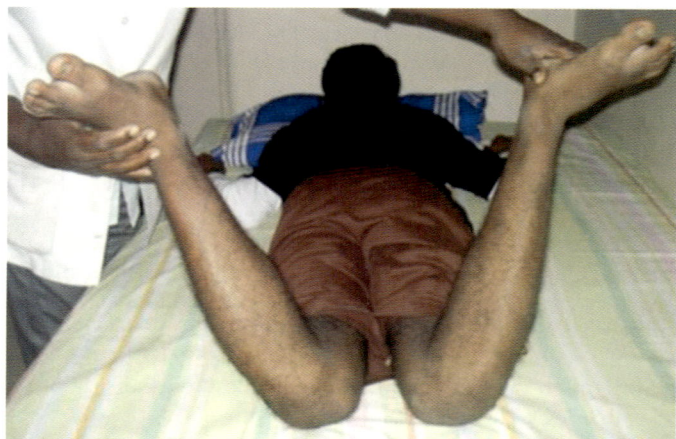

Fig. I.19: Measurement of internal rotation

Tests for Hip Stability

A normal stable hip is required for locomotion, walking, etc. the stability of the hip is dependent upon a good abductor mechanism of the hip. The following tests enable to determine the stability of the hip.

IN STANDING POSITION

Trendelenburg test: This is a test for the abductor mechanism of the hip. The abductor mechanism of the hip consists of the head of the femur (fulcrum), the neck of the femur (lever) and the abductor mechanism (power).

In the normal posture, the weight of the body is distributed equally on both the lower limbs and the center of gravity falls between the two limbs. If, for example, left limb is lifted, the weight of the body and the weight of the left lower limb now falls on the right lower limb. Consequently, the center of gravity automatically shifts to the left to maintain balance. This tends to pull the opposite pelvis down. To counter this pelvic tilt, on the left side, the right abductor muscles of the hip contract and pull the (left) side of the pelvis up and prevent it from sinking. If there is a failure of the abductor mechanism, this no longer happens and the pelvis on the opposite side sinks (Figs I.20A and B).

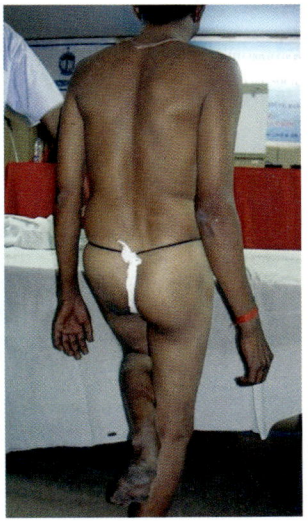 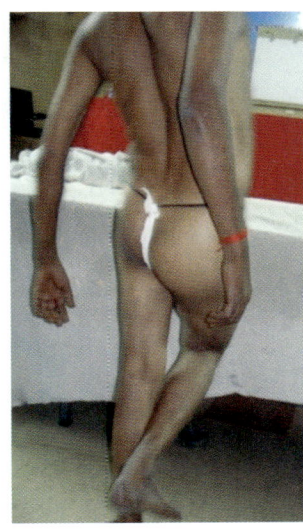

Fig. I.20A: Patient stands on the affected limb, pelvis drops on the opposite side

Fig. I.20B: Trendelenburg test—Patient stands on the normal limb

Test: The patient is first asked to stand on the normal limb. The pelvis on the opposite side rises (or alternatively the iliac crest will be low on the standing side and high on the side of the elevated leg) due to the intact abductor mechanism of the hip on the normal side. The patient is now made to stand on the affected limb. Due to the faulty abductor mechanism, the opposite side of the pelvis sinks (or alternatively the iliac crest will be high on the standing side and low on the side of the elevated leg). The test is said to be positive.

Causes

1. *Failure in power:* Gluteus medius weakness or paralysis due to polio, etc.
2. *Failure in lever:* Fracture neck femur, trochanteric fracture, etc.
3. *Failure in fulcrum:* Arthritis due to TB and rheumatoid, dislocation of hip, etc.
   Sometimes two or more factors operate: In upward dislocation of the hip, there is a failure in the fulcrum and slack abductor muscles due to upward shift of the greater trochanter.

IN LYING DOWN POSITION

Telescopy Test

Principle this is a test for hip stability.

Procedure

The patient is in supine position, the patient's knee and hip are flexed to 90°. One hand is placed beneath the greater trochanter to feel for it. The femur is now pushed down into the examination table. The femur and leg are then lifted up. In a normal hip, little movement occurs during the action. In a dislocated hip, there will be a lot of relative movement felt by the hand. This excessive movement is called the telescoping of the hip (Fig. I.21).

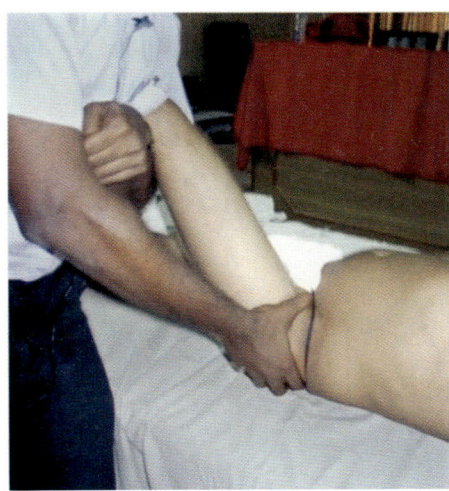

Fig. I.21: Telescopy test

Other Tests

Measurement of muscle wasting: The thigh and the leg muscles are measured for muscle wasting as follows. Marks are made at a convenient distance from the ASIS from the patella (say about 18 cm up) on both the sides and the measurement is taken. The difference between the circumference of the two thighs or legs is the amount of wasting (Figs I.22A and B).

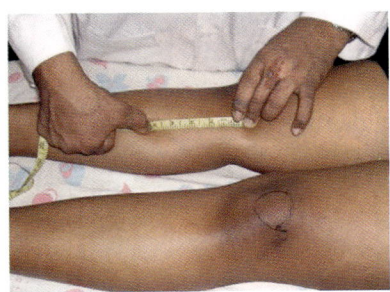

Fig. I.22A: Measurement of the leg girth

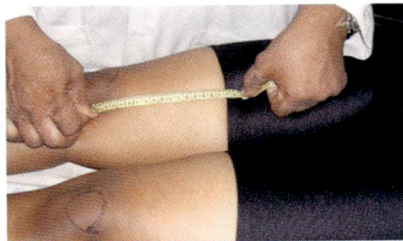

Fig. I.22B: Measurement of the thigh girth

EXAMINATION OF THE KNEE JOINT

Clinical Examination

This consists of history, observation and physical examination.

History

A patient with knee problems usually presents with the following complaints.

Pain

This may be acute or chronic and there may be a history of trauma. History of night cries if present suggests TB arthritis.

Swelling

This could be due to effusion or synovial membrane thickening. The duration of the swelling following trauma gives a clue to the probable diagnosis—if a swelling develops within 2 hours of the injury, it suggests hemarthrosis and if it develops after 2 to 24 hours, it suggests traumatic synovitis. Approximately 75 percent of the cases of hemarthrosis are due to anterior cruciate ligament (ACL) tears. Localized swellings could be due to bursal enlargement.

Limp: This may be due to pain, muscle spasm, stiffness or arthritis.

Restriction of Movements

Locking: It could be due to menisci tear or loose bodies. In locking, the patient complains of inability to complete the last few degrees of extension.

Deformity: In genu valgum, varum and recurvatum, the patient usually presents with the deformity.

PHYSICAL EXAMINATION OF THE KNEE

As in the other parts of the body, examination of knee joint consists of inspection, palpation, measurements, movements and stability tests peculiar to the knee.

Preparation

The whole limb to be examined is exposed with the patient wearing short trousers. Examination of the knee is carried out from the front, sides and back.

Inspection

Inspection is carried out in the following order:
- First look at the height and weight of the patient.
- Look for standing alignment of the knee, which should be 3 to 7° valgus.
- Look for the abnormality of the feet like flat feet, etc. which may contribute to the knee problems.
- *Gait:* The patient could walk with a limp (e.g. arthritis), circumduction (stiff knee), etc.
- Wasting of the thigh and leg muscles are to be noted.
- *Swelling:* This could be due to intraarticular or extraarticular causes. If all the natural depressions above, below and by the sides of the patella are obliterated, the cause could be intraarticular. In extraarticular causes, not all the natural fossae will be obliterated and the swelling usually extends over the patella.

PALPATION

Temperature: Feel for the local rise of temperature with the dorsum of the hand.

Tenderness: Elicit the tenderness and grade it as described earlier.

Test for the extensor mechanism: The extensor mechanism of the knee consists of the quadriceps muscle, patella, patellar ligament and the tibial tubercle. Palpate these for tenderness, wasting, loss of continuity, etc.

Swelling: Swelling of the joint is usually due to effusion within the joint, which indicates damage to the joint and the presence of a major cause must always be ruled out. Synovial membrane thickness is the other common cause.

CONTENTS OF KNEE EFFUSION
- Synovial fluid (common)
- Blood
- Pus

Types of Swelling

a. *Small:* In these cases, there will be bulging of the sides of the patellar ligament and obliteration of the hollows of the medial and lateral edges of patella.
b. *Medium*
c. *Large:* All the findings noted in the small and medium effusions and distension of suprapatellar pouch.
d. *Localized:* Due to osteophytes, exostosis, bursa, cysts, etc.

Swelling due to Synovial Membrane Thickness

Swelling due to synovial membrane thickness is usually due to chronic inflammatory disorders. The features of the swelling due to the synovial membrane thickness are:
a. Most prominent usually above the patella near the suprapatellar pouch.
b. Boggy to feel.
c. Local raise of temperature.

Tests: The following tests help to evaluate the swellings of the knee:

a. Patellar tap test
b. Fluid displacement test
c. Fluctuation test.

Patellar tap test: This test (Fig. I.23) is carried out as follows:

Step 1: In the horizontal position, a considerable amount of excessive synovial fluid gravitates into the suprapatellar pouch. From 6" above the patella, excess fluid in the suprapatellar pouch is driven back into the joint by sliding down firmly with index finger and the thumb.

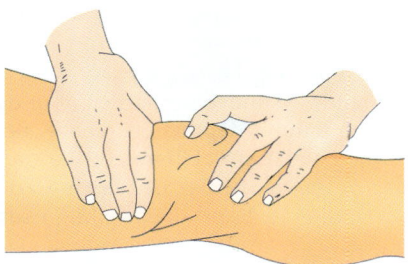

Fig. I.23: Method of eliciting patellar tap

Step 2: The tips of the three fingers and the thumb of the free hand is placed over the anterior surface of the patella and a quick "jerk" is given downwards. If the fluid is present, a "click" is heard as the patella can be felt to strike on the femoral condyle and "bounces" back.

Fluid Displacement Tests

These tests help to detect small effusions. Two methods are described below:

Fluctuation test: This test is particularly useful in large knee joint effusions (Fig. I.24). The method is as follows:

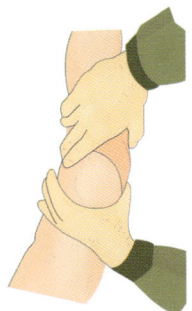

Fig. I.24: Method of eliciting fluctuation test to detect gross knee effusion

Step 1: The patient is in the supine position. Excessive fluid in the suprapatellar pouch is squeezed with the index finger and thumb of the left hand and held in that position.

Step 2: With the thumb and index finger of the (right) hand on either side of the ligamentum patellae, pressure is applied and the (left) hand feels this transmission of force.

Limitations: This test is negative in small effusions.

Localized Swelling of the Knee

These are due to enlarged bursae and cysts, which are present all round the knee, and has been discussed earlier.

Patella: It is very important to carry out a systematic examination of the patella.

   Q-angle (quadriceps angle) is defined as the angle between the quadriceps tendon (primarily the rectus femoris) and the patellar tendon.

Joint line tenderness (Fig. I.2): It is important to elicit joint line tenderness in arthritis, menisci injury or collateral ligament injuries.

Method: The patient is supine. To mark the joint line, flex and extend the knee slowly and feel for the gap between the femoral and tibial condyles. Mark this with a skin pencil on both sides. Now palpate systematically for tenderness from front to back and at the points of attachments of the collateral ligaments.

TESTS PECULIAR TO KNEE

As mentioned earlier, the stability of the knee depends on the soft tissues, the capsule, the meniscus, the quadriceps, the cruciates and the collateral ligaments. To detect the integrity of the above structures, stability tests are carried out.

Tests for collaterals: Abduction or valgus stress test (Fig. I.25A): This test is done to detect the medial collateral ligament injury.

Adduction stress or varus stress test: This test is to detect the lateral collateral ligament injury (Fig. I.25B).

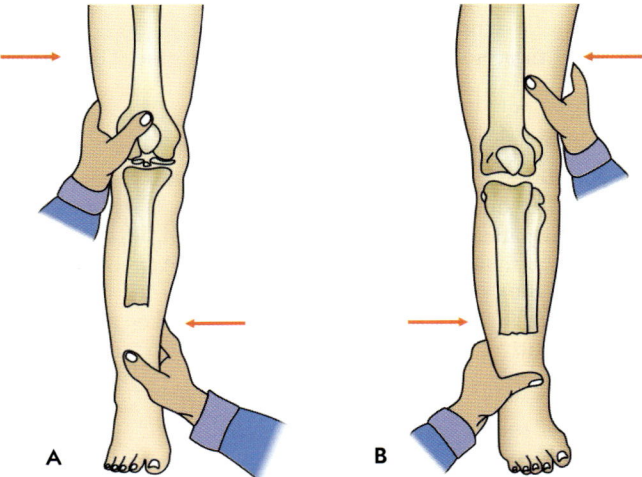

Figs I.25A and B: Stress tests for collateral ligament injuries: (A) Valgus or abduction stress test, (B) Varus or adduction stress test

Tests for cruciates anterior drawer test: This is a one-plane test for anterior instability as it tests the anterior cruciate ligament (ACL) (Fig. I.26).

Tests for menisci: Mcmurray's sign (see Fig. 24.12) the presence of this sign indicates injury to the menisci.

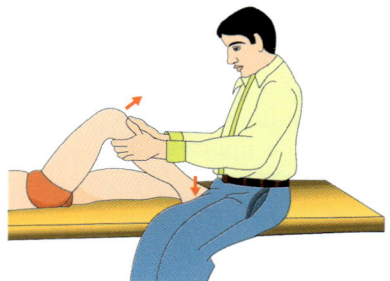

Fig. I.26: Anterior drawer test

Apleys' compression and distraction tests:

The former helps to determine the menisci injury and the latter helps to test the collateral ligaments.

Lachman Test

This test indicates injury to the anterior cruciate ligament. This is a test especially for the poster lateral band, one plane, and anterior instability (Fig. I.27).

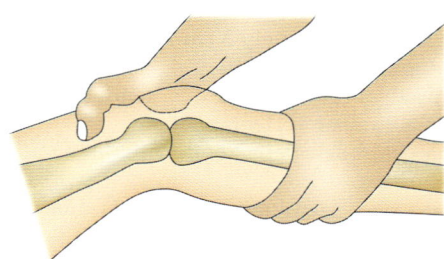

Fig. I.27: Lachman's test

EXAMINATION OF MOVEMENTS

The important movements taking place at the knee joint are flexion and extension. In a semi-flexed position, slight side-to-side and rocking movements are possible.

Flexion: The normal range of knee flexion is 130 to 150°. *Muscle Testing* The patient is prone. The examiner places one hand over the pelvis to stabilize, it while he offers graded resistance with the other hand at the ankle as the patient attempts to flex the knee. If knee flexion is tested with the ankle externally rotated, biceps femoris is tested and if the ankle is rotated medially, semimembranosus and semitendinosus are tested.

Procedure to Record Flexion

1. In the prone position, the patient is asked to flex both the knees simultaneously and the distance between the heels to buttock is noted.
2. In supine position, the patient is asked to flex the knee and the heel to buttock distance is measured by a tape.
3. In sitting position, the patient is asked to flex and extend the knee holding the edge of the table.

Rule of Thumb: For every 1 cm distance restriction, there is 1.5° loss of flexion.

Extension: Normal range the knee should normally extend to a straight line (0°) and occasionally can hyperextend to 15° in some women.

Measurement: The degree of extension is determined by measuring the angle between the thigh and the leg.

Measurements

1. *Measurement of the length of the thigh*: Length of the thigh is recorded by taking a measurement between the ASIS and the medial joint line of the knee.
2. *Measurement of the length of the leg*: This is done by recording the length between the medial joint line and the medial malleolus.
3. Breadth of the lower end of femur and upper end of tibia is recorded by using a caliper.
4. Distance between the tibial tubercle and the head of the fibula is recorded.
5. To measure the muscle wasting, circumference of the thigh and muscles are recorded from fixed points on both sides (e.g. about 6" to 7" above the joint line) (see Fig. 33.6).

EXAMINATION OF THE POPLITEAL FOSSA

Examination of the popliteal fossae is done in standing and prone positions. The following are the important lesions in the popliteal fossa:

- *Baker's cyst:* It is prominently seen and felt during extension of the knee and disappears or becomes less prominent during flexion (see Fig. 40.12).
- *Aneurysm of the popliteal artery*: A pulsatile swelling is in the center of the popliteal fossa.
- *Enlarged popliteal lymph node*: This is enlarged in the early stages of TB arthritis.

OTHER EXAMINATIONS

1. *Systemic examination:* Useful in TB knee, rheumatoid arthritis, Charcot's joint (syphilis), etc.
2. *Examination of other joints*: Especially hip joint as the pain in the knee may be a referred pain from the hip.
3. *Examination of inguinal lymph nodes*: These are enlarged in later stages of TB arthritis.

QUICK FACTS: ORDER OF EXAMINATION OF KNEE
- History
- Inspection
- Palpation
- Tests for stability
- Movements
- Measurements
- Examination of popliteal fossa
- Systemic examination
- Examination of hip and other joints
- Examination of inguinal and popliteal lymph nodes.

EXAMINATION OF SPINE

Systematic examination of the spine will go a long way in making a good and proper diagnosis. The following protocol is helpful. General examination should be done before examining the spine to detect the role of systemic disease in the pathogenesis of back pain.

Inspection: This is first carried out in standing position after the back is adequately exposed. Inspect the skin for cafe-au-lait spots (neurofibromatosis), lipoma and tuft of hair (meningocele), etc.

Posture: Does the patient have a normal posture or whether posture is altered due to deformities? The well-known postural deformities of spine.

Kyphosis: This usually refers to the increased normal posterior convexity of the thoracic spine.

Lordosis: It is increase in the anterior convexity of the lumbar spine (see Fig. 42.13). Lordosis of the spine is best inspected from the sides.

Scoliosis: It is a lateral curvature of the spine.

Spondylolisthesis: The following clinical signs help to detect this deformity (see Fig. 42.12)
- A "step" at the upper angle of the sacrum.
- Increased lumbar lordosis.
- A transverse furrow encircles the body between the coastal margins and the iliac crest.

Other Examinations

Examination of gait, evidence of swelling due to cold abscess. In spina bifida, it could be due to meningocele or myelo-meningocele. In spina bifida occulta, there is no swelling but only a dimple, or dilated vessels or a tuft of hair.

RANGE OF MOVEMENT

Flexion: Normal range is 105° (45° at the thoracic spine; 60° at the lumbar spine).

Method: Ask the patient to bend forward and note the distance between the fingers and the ground. Normally, the patient can touch the ground or reach within 7 cm off the ground. This test indicates the overall movements of the thoracic and lumbar segments ignoring the hip (see Figs 45.12 and 45.13).

Extension: In the standing position, the patient is asked to arch his back while the examiner steadies the pelvis and a pull is exerted on the shoulder (see Fig. 45.15). The angle between the long axis of the spine when erect and bent back is the angle of extension.

Normal range is 30° (thoracic—25°, lumbar—35°).

Lateral flexion: Normal range is 30° (thoracic and lumbar segments are equal).

Methods: Lateral flexion is best examined in standing position (see Fig. 45.14).
a. The patient is asked to slide down the hands on each side of the leg. The distance from the floor in cm or the position that the fingers reach in the legs is measured.
b. The angle formed between the vertical and the line joining T1 and S1 on lateral flexion is measured.

Rotations:
- *Normal range* is 40 to 45° (thoracic—40°, lumbar—5°).
- *Method*: This is best examined in the sitting position. The patient sits at the edge of the table and holds it firmly to fix the pelvis. The patient is then asked to rotate on either side.

The rotation is then measured between the plane of the shoulder and the pelvis (see Fig. 45.11).

Palpation: Palpation is carried out with the patient in standing, sitting or prone positions (Fig. I.15). First, palpate both the groups of paraspinous muscles simultaneously for tenderness and firmness. Next, palpate the bony structures as follows for tenderness.

Percussion: In the standing position, ask the patient to bend forwards. From the root of the neck to the sacrum, the spine is lightly percussed in an orderly fashion. The patient complains of marked pain in TB, infections, etc.

Rotation method: This is the most accurate method. Here an attempt to rotate the vertebra by firmly pushing at the spinous process from the side elicits pain.

Rough method: Gentle blows are given on either side of the spine. It is not advisable.

Anvil method: Application of sudden jerk over the head. This is dangerous and is best avoided.

Other Sites

a. *Facet joints*: Approximately 3 cm lateral to the midline facet joint tenderness can be elicited.
b. In prolapsed intervertebral discs, tenderness is elicited in between the lumbar vertebrae.
c. In mechanical back pain, tenderness is elicited over the lumbar muscles.
d. Tenderness over sacroiliac (SI) joints is due to mechanical back pain or SI joint infection.

Tests to Detect Low Disc Prolapse (L4–L5)

Straight leg raising test (SLRT): It is a delicate accurate test to assess the presence or absence of nerve root irritation. Pain duplicating sciatica that is elicited by this test indicates a space-occupying lesion (SOL) such as lumbar disc herniation at the nerve root level.

Procedure: It is a passive test (see Fig. 45.16) and each leg is tested individually. The patient is supine with the legs extended. With one hand under the heel and the other over the knee, the examiner passively lifts the leg of the patient until the patient complains of pain or tightness. The test is positive if pain extends from the back, down the leg along the sciatic nerve distribution.

Femoral nerve traction test (see Fig. 45.18): The patient lies on the side on the unaffected side with hip slightly flexed. Grasp the affected leg of the patient and gently extend the hip by 15°. This stretches the femoral nerve. Now slowly flex the knee of the affected leg. This further stretches the femoral nerve. If pain radiates to the anterior thigh, it indicates a radiculopathy involving L1, L2, L3 and L4 nerve roots.

Neurological signs: After having ascertained the nerve root compression due to disc prolapse, neurological examination of the lower limbs must be carried out to assess the damage caused to the neuromuscular system.

Motor testing: Test the muscle strength of the following group of muscles and compare it with the normal side:
a. The quadriceps group—test for the L2, L3 and L4 roots (Fig. 45.7).
b. Extensor hallucis longus—test for L5 root (see Fig. 45.8).

c. The gastrocnemius—test for S1 and S2 (see Fig. 45.9).
d. The peroneus longus and brevis—test for S1.

Sensation

There is a considerable variation and overlap of the dermatomal patterns and hence it is difficult to chart the dermatomes precisely. In mapping out a sensory dermatome, it is advisable to go from zone of numbness to normal sensitivity.

General Guidelines

- *L4 dermatome affected:* Medial aspect of foot and leg.
- *L5 dermatome affected:* Dorsum of the foot and great toe.
- *S1 dermatome affected:* Lateral border of the foot.
- *L2, L3, L4 dermatome affected:* Anterior aspect of thigh.
- *S1, S2, S3, S4 dermatome affected:* Perineum, and rectal tone.

Reflexes

a. *Knee reflex:* To test the L4 nerve root.
b. *Ankle reflex:* To test the S1 nerve root.
   No reliable reflex test is available for L5 nerve roots.

Back pain due to spinal pathology: In this group, ankylosing spondylitis is the common cause. Two important clinical tests help to diagnose this condition.

Chest expansion: This is measured with the patient's arm held straight up over the head. In men, measurement is carried out at the level of fourth intercostals space and in women just below the breasts. Measurement is carried out in both inspiration and expiration. Normal expansion is more than 3 cm. It is decreased in ankylosing spondylitis.

QUICK RECAP: EXAMINATION OF SPINE
- General examination
- Inspection
- Palpation
- Range of movements.
- Evaluation of the causes of low back pain.
- Tests for IVDP both high and low.
- Neurological examination.
- Tests to detect malingering.
- Tests for back pain, due to spinal pathology and mechanical back pain.
- Other examinations—for cold abscess, SI joint, systemic examination. Examination of hip joint, etc.

EXAMINATION OF SHOULDER JOINT

History: A patient with shoulder joint problems presents with the following complaints.

Swelling: The swelling could be due to injury or arthritis.

Deformity: In anterior dislocation of the shoulder there will be anterior prominence and the arm will be held in internal rotation.

Loss of contour: This may be due to shoulder dislocation or due to wasting of deltoid muscle in tuberculosis (TB), rheumatoid arthritis, etc.

Restriction and loss of movements: This is particularly seen in frozen shoulder, arthritis, etc.

Physical Examination

Inspection: The patient is stripped down to the waist and is examined in a sitting position. Inspection is carried out from the front, sides, behind and above.

From the front: First note, whether there is any prominence of the sternoclavicular joint. If present, it indicates sternoclavicular joint subluxation or dislocation. Next, look for any deformity along the clavicle. If seen, it could be due to malunion or nonunion of a fracture clavicle. Any prominence near the area of acromioclavicular joint indicates subluxation or dislocation (see Fig. 15.8A). Lastly, look for any wasting of the deltoid muscle. If present, it could be due to axillary nerve palsy or a chronic disease like TB, rheumatoid arthritis.

From behind: Here, the structure to be noted most is the scapula. Look whether the scapula is placed high or low, normal or small in size and if there is any winging of the scapula (due to paralysis of serratus anterior).

From above: Look for asymmetry of the supraclavicular fossae on both the sides. Swelling of the shoulder and any deformity of the clavicle are the other points to be looked for.

From the sides: Note whether there is any swelling of the joint, flattening of the shoulder (anterior dislocation) or rounded fullness of the shoulder (due to effusion).

Palpation

1. *Local temperature:* Feel for the local rise of temperature.
2. *Tenderness:* Try to elicit the tenderness.

Movements

As already mentioned, shoulder joint is highly mobile and consists of (Fig. I.28):

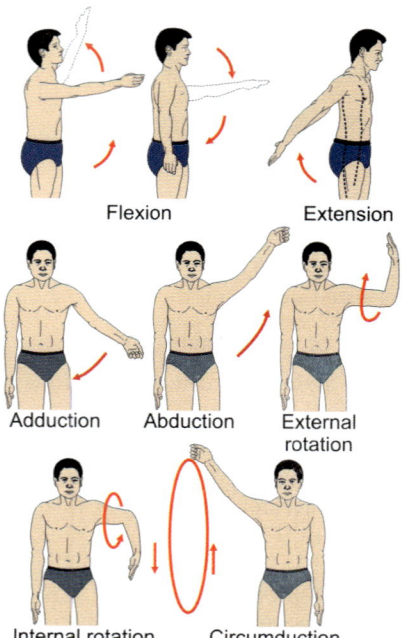

Fig. I.28: Movements of the shoulder joint

Flexion (Normal Range is 180°): Flexion is best tested with the patient seated. Both active and passive movements are tested.

Extension (Normal Range is 45°): Best tested in the seated position.

Abduction (Normal Range is 180°): Best tested in the standing position and both the shoulders are tested simultaneously for comparison.

Other Important Tests

Apprehension test: There is a look of apprehension or the patient resists any attempt made to dislocate the shoulder joint.
Bryant's sign: Lowering of the axillary folds suggests dislocation.
Callaway's test: Girth of the affected shoulder is increased in dislocation.
Duga's test: The patient is seated and places the hand of the affected shoulder on the opposite shoulder. The patient is instructed to touch the chest with the elbow. Inability to do so indicates shoulder subluxation or dislocation.
Hamilton's test: Normally it is not possible to touch the acromion and lateral epicondyle by placing a ruler by the side of the arm due to the rounded contour of the shoulder. In dislocation, this becomes possible.
Painful Arc test (See for Subacromial Bursitis) for description.

Other Examination

1. Examine the cervical spine.
2. Examine the acromioclavicular and sternoclavicular joints.
3. Neurovascular examination of the upper limbs.
4. Systemic examination for tuberculosis, rheumatoid arthritis, etc.

> **RECAP ORDER OF SHOULDER EXAMINATION**
> - History
> - Inspection
> - Palpation
> - Movements
> - Special tests
> - Examination of cervical spine
> - Neurovascular examination of the upper limbs
> - Systemic examination for TB, RA, etc.

EXAMINATION OF THE ELBOW JOINT

History

Patients with elbow disorders usually complain of pain, stiffness and deformity.
Pain in the elbow could be due to disorders of the elbow joint or could be a referred pain from the neck or shoulder.

Stiffness and Loss of Movements

Elbow joint is notorious to develop stiffness and loss of movements early.

Deformity: Patients with elbow deformity usually give a history of childhood injury mismanaged or treated by an osteopath (e.g. cubitus varus deformity in supracondylar fracture humerus).

Inspection

The physical examination of the elbow joint begins with a systematic inspection of the joint and extremity. The entire arm including the elbow, forearm and hand should be exposed. The following points should be noted during inspection:

a. *Carrying angle:* Like the knee joint a true elbow joint is never straight. The carrying angle is determined by measuring the angle between the longitudinal axis of the arm and forearm when the elbow is fully extended and the forearm supinated. Normally, this angle is about 10° in males and 15 to 20° in females (due to wider pelvis). Carrying angle is reduced in cubitus varus deformity (see Fig. 17.3).
b. *Deformities* of the elbow are very much revealed and consist of the following:
   - *Flexion deformity:* Fixed flexion deformity is the commonest elbow deformity since flexion is the position of ease.
   - *Cubitus varus deformity*—(see Fig. 17.3) (gunstock deformity): This is usually due to malunited supracondylar fracture in children.
   - *Cubitus valgus deformity* (see Fig. 17.3): This is commonly due to malunited lateral condyle fractures of humerus and rarely due to supracondylar fractures.
c. *Swelling:* Around the elbow joint could be due to effusion, synovial thickening, periarticular soft tissue inflammation, soft tissue mass, bony enlargement or deformity. The swelling could be generalized or localized. If generalized, it is usually due to effusion in the joint. The features are:
   - Swelling all around the joint.
   - Normal hollows on either side of the olecranon process are obliterated.
   - Fullness in the cubital fossae.
   If localized:
   - Swelling over the olecranon process—olecranon bursitis.
   - Swelling over front of the joint—bicipitoradial bursitis.
d. Inspect the soft tissues and skin about the anterior, posterior, medial and lateral surfaces of the joint. The presence and location of scars, sinuses, discoloration, etc. should be noted.
e. *Muscle wasting:* Look for wasting of the arm and forearm muscles.

PALPATION

1. *Local temperature:* This will be raised in arthritis and bursitis.
2. *Tenderness:* The site of tenderness can give clue to the diagnosis.
3. *Bony relations* (see Figs 17.2A and B): With the elbow flexed to 90°, the lines connecting the lateral and medial epicondyles and the olecranon process form a near isosceles triangle when viewed from behind. When the elbow is extended, these three structures come to lie in a straight line.
   Anteriorly, palpate the margins of the cubital fossae and its contents.
4. *Swelling:* Due to effusion can easily be palpated in the region bordered by the lateral epicondyle, radial head and the lateral margin of the olecranon.
5. Palpate the lower end of the humerus, upper end of the radius and ulna for any bony thickening.
6. Palpate the supratrochlear and axillary lymph nodes (supratrochlear lymph node is situated on the anterior aspect of the medial intermuscular septum one cm above the medial epicondyle. It can be best felt in the flexed position of the elbow. If enlarged on both sides, it indicates syphilis).

Movements: It should be recorded and measured after completion of inspection and palpation. Elbow movements are flexion, extension, and rotations (supination and pronation).

Flexion:

Range: Elbow flexion is measured from the fully extended position (0°) to about 140° to 150° and this is recorded as (0° to 140°). In some patients, the elbow can be extended beyond 0° to say 15° to 20°. This is called hyperextension (HE) and is recorded as 20° HE to 140° flexion. In an individual, where there is a fixed flexion deformity (FFD) of say 40°, the movement is recorded as 40° FFD-140° flexion (Fig. I.30)

Extension Normal is Neutral or 0°

Supination/pronation:

Method: The patient is seated, the side places arm firmly, the elbow is held at 90° flexion and the thumb is straight up. Rotation of the forearm with palm facing down is pronation and is normally 45 to 80° and the opposite movement is supination and is about 85° (Fig. I.31)

Measurements

Limb Length Measurements

The length of the entire upper limb should be measured and compared to the normal side (see Fig. 33.4).

Method: Arm length has to be measured between the angle of the acromion and the lateral epicondyle, while the forearm length has to be recorded between the lateral epicondyle and the radial styloid process (Fig. I.29).

Wasting of Muscles

Mark the identical points on the upper arms and forearms on both sides and measure the girth of the muscles.

SPECIAL TESTS

Cozen's test (for lateral epicondylitis): Affected elbow is slightly flexed and pronated. The patient is instructed to make a fist and actively dorsiflex the hand and wrist against full resistance. If this produces pain at or near the lateral epicondyle, it is suggestive of tennis elbow.

Golfer's elbow test (Reverse Cozen's test): The elbow is in slight flexion. The hand and wrist of the patient is in supination. Steady pressure is applied to the supinated hand in an attempt to extend the elbow. The patient resists this movement with active flexion. If pain is elicited at the medial epicondyle, it suggests golfer's elbow.

Other Examinations

Examine the shoulder joint, the neck and the wrist joints. Systemic examination is required in TB and rheumatoid arthritis.

ORDER OF EXAMINATION
- History
- Inspection
- Palpation
- Measurements
- Special tests
- Examination of neck, shoulder and wrist joints
- Systemic examination in tuberculosis and rheumatoid arthritis

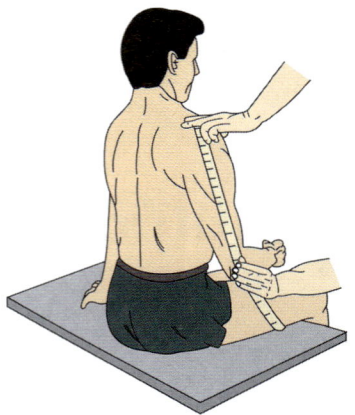

Fig. I.29: Measurement of the upper arm

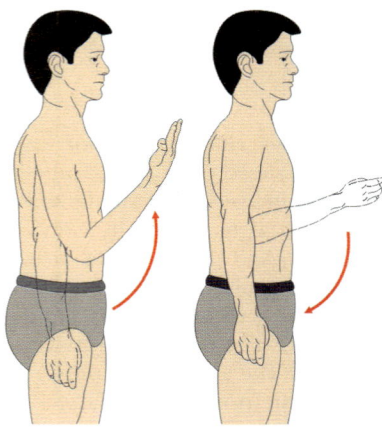

Fig. I.30: Movements of flexion and extension of the elbow

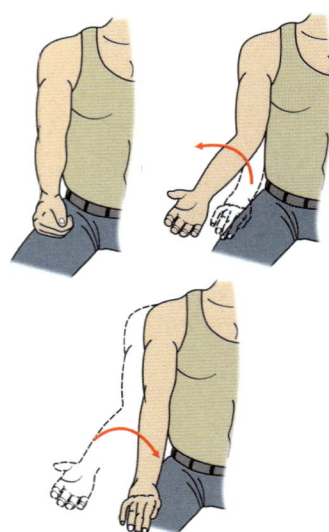

Fig. I.31: Supination and pronation of the forearm

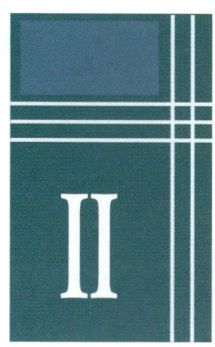

Human Gait

INTRODUCTION

What is Gait?

It is a term used to describe the style of walking. Through evolution, man has changed from a quadruped gait to a biped gait. The gait in the animals is more stable, since it walks on all the four limbs and the center of gravity is in between the fore limbs and hind limbs. And the 'speed' is also more in animal gait, since the trunk musculature helps the limbs in locomotion. This stability and speed is compromised in human gait because of the two legged gait. The center of gravity keeps changing and is above the base. The gait in each person is different and has a characteristic pattern which helps in the identification of that person.

Study of human gait is a fascinating subject. Even a subtle variation in the gait has a story to tell and only a discerning and knowledgeable eye will be able to detect the cause for such a change.

GAIT CYCLE

Definition

It can be defined as all the activities that occur from heel contact of one foot to the next heel contact of the same foot (alternatively it can be from toe off of one foot to the next toe off of the same foot). (Fig. II.1).

Phases of the Gait Cycle

There are two phases:
1. The stance phase
2. The swing phase.

Fig. II.1: Human gait

Stance phase: This comprises 60 percent of the normal adult gait cycle. It begins with the initial heel contact and ends with the toes coming off the ground.

Swing phase: This forms 40 percent of the gait cycle in adults. It begins when the concerned foot lifts off the ground and ends when the same foot comes in contact with the ground.

Terminology of the Gait Cycle

Two gait terminologies are described:
1. Traditional terms.
2. Rancho Los Amigos (RLA) terms.

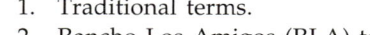

QUICK FACTS: TRADITIONAL TERMS vs RLA TERMS	
Traditional	*RLA*
1. Heel strike	Initial contact
2. Foot flat	Loading response
3. Midstance	Midstance
4. Heel off	Terminal stance
5. Toe off	Preswing
6. Acceleration	Initial swing
7. Midswing	Midswing
8. Deceleration	Terminal swing

Stance phase (Figs II.2A and B)
This consists of the first five phases.
- Heel strike—here, the heel strikes the ground.
- Foot flat—here, the foot is flat on the ground.
- Midstance.
- Heel off—here, the heel is off the ground.
- Toe off—here, the toes are off the ground.

Swing phase (Fig. II.3)
- Acceleration—here the leg is in front of the body.
- Midswing—here the leg continues to swing forward.
- Deceleration—here the swing slows down and the heel is ready for the strike.

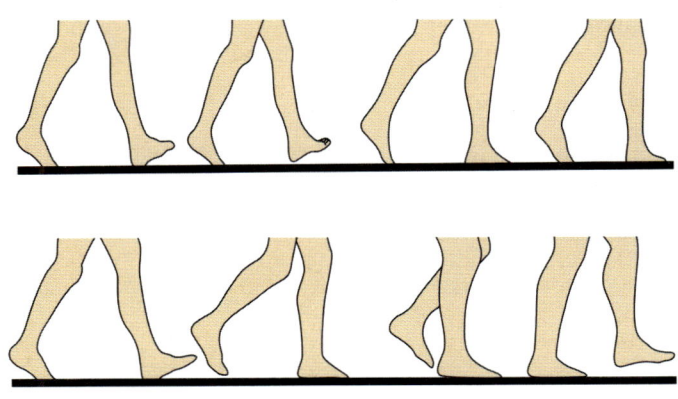

Figs II.2A and B: Stance phase

In a normal gait, each leg alternatively goes through a stance phase and a swing phase. Thus, the body is carried forward in normal walking by these rhythmic cycles.

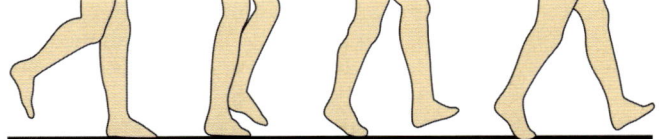

Fig. II.3: Swing phase

What is the percentage of each phase in the gait cycle?

I. **Stance phase (60%)**
a. Heel strike	0–2%
b. Foot flat	0–10%
c. Midstance	10–30%
d. Heel off	30–50%
e. Toe off	50–60%

II. **Swing phase (40%)**
a. Acceleration	60–73%
b. Midswing	73–85%
c. Deceleration	85–100%

Note
- *The swing stance ratio is 0.66.*
- *Double limb support* Here both the limbs are on the ground for a brief period of time. This constitutes 20 percent of the gait cycle.

Q<small>UICK</small> FACTS: I<small>NTERESTING</small> 'GAIT' FACTS
- *The passenger unit* (This represents 70 percent of the body weight). According to Perry 1992. It is the head, neck, arms and trunk.
  According to Elthman (1954) It is head, arms and trunk (denoted by the acronym—HAT).
  This is so called, because they do not directly contribute to the act of walking but 'go along for the ride,'
- *The locomotor unit* This is the functioning system which is comprised of the pelvis and both the lower limbs.

Note
The locomotor unit consists of 19 joints:
• Lumbosacral	• Both hips
• Both knees	• Both ankles
• Both subtalars	• Both MTP joints

Q<small>UICK</small> FACTS: V<small>ITAL</small> FACTS
1. **Single limb support** here only one foot is in contact with the ground. Forms 80% of the gait cycle.
2. **Double limb support** both limbs are on the ground. Forms the remaining 20% of the gait cycle.

3. **Stride length** it is the distance the 'body' has traveled in one gait cycle (Fig. 20.4A).
   Men 4.8 feet
   Women 4.2 feet. Overall average is 4.6 feet.
4. **Step length** it is the distance one foot has traveled during a gait cycle (Fig. 20.4B).
   Men 2.4 feet
   Women 2.1 feet, both (average)—2.3 feet.
5. **Cadence** number of steps taken in a specified time.
   Men 111 steps/min, Women: 117 steps/min.
   Both 113 steps/min (average).
6. **Walking velocity** the speed of walking on a smooth snail surface.
   Men 276 ft/min
   Women 250 ft/min
   Both 262 ft/min (average).

KINETICS AND KINEMATICS OF GAIT

Stance phase: The following table gives an insight into the kinetics and kinematics of gait (see Table 20.2) during the stance phase.

Thus during
- *Heel strike:* The hip is in flexion of 25–30°, the knee is in 50° flexion and the ankle is at 0° plantar flexion. The GRFV is anterior to the hip and knee joints, posterior to the ankle joints.
- *Foot flat:* The hip is still in 25–30° flexion, the knee in flexion and the ankle in plantar flexion. However, the GRFV is anterior to the hip but posterior to the knee and ankle joints.
- *Midstance:* The hip is in extension the knee is also in extension and the ankle is in dorsiflexion. The GRFV is passing anterior to posterior in the hip region, posterior to anterior in the knee region and anterior to the ankle joint.
- *Heel off:* During heel off the hip is in extension, the knee is passing slowly from extension to flexion and the ankle from dorsiflexion to plantar flexion.
- The GRFV passes posterior to the hip, anterior to posterior in the knee and anterior at the ankle joints.
- *Toe off during* toe off, the hip is in flexion, the knee is also in flexion and the ankle joint is in plantar flexion. The GRFV is posterior to hip and knee and anterior in the ankle joints.

Swing phase
- During acceleration phase, the hip joint is in flexion, the knee joint is also in flexion and the ankle joint is in dorsiflexion.
- During midswing, the hip is in flexion, the knee is in extension and the ankle joint is in dorsiflexion.
- During deceleration phase, the hip joint progresses from flexion to extension, the knee joint from extension to flexion and the ankle joint continues to be in dorsiflexion.

PATHOLOGICAL GAIT

To diagnose a pathological gait, a sound knowledge of the normal ambulation, locomotion, etc. is a must.

Instead of labeling the abnormal gaits as antalgic, circumduction, etc. which is wholly inadequate, it is better if by careful analysis, a gait in question is described, how it differs from the normal ambulation. The following are some of the pathological gaits.

Hip Abnormalities

1. Lateral trunk bending	Here the patient leans towards the affected side on bearing weight on that side
2. Hip pain	Patient leans towards the affected side
3. Hip abductor weakness	Here the pelvis drops on the unaffected side when patient bears weight on the affected leg (Trendelenburg or glutes medius, dip gait)
4. Hip/knee flexion contracture	Swing phase is shortened, the trunk bends backwards with circumduction, trunk dips sideward and the hip is elevated on the affected side
5. Hip extensor weakness (Gluteus maximus gait)	Backward thrust of the trunk, affected hip is protruded, lumbar lordosis is increased.
6. Hip hiking (seen in hip flexor weakness, extensor spasticity, dorsiflexor weakness, etc.)	By the action of quadratus lumborum and lateral abdominalis, patient elevates The pelvis on the affected side and advances the affected limb by increased pendulum action.
7. Circumduction	To clear the ground, the limb goes around a laterally curved path. Seen in spastic limb.
8. Internal rotation of the hip:	Seen in biceps femoris weakness, fixed inversion of the heel, spastic cerebral palsy, etc.
9. External rotation of the hip	Seen in hamstring weakness, fixed eversion of the heel, weakness of tibialis anterior, posterior and plantar flexors muscles.

Knee Abnormalities

1. Quadriceps paralysis	In this condition the patient cannot stabilizes the knee in early stance phase and the knee bends backwards.
2. Knee instability	In this condition the knee flexes abruptly after midstance causing the patient to buckle.
3. Hyperextended knee	Here the knee bends backwards during the stance phase. The trunk is bent forwards, pushing back with forceful contractions of the gluteus maximus helps to overcome this problem
4. Arthritic knee	A patient with rheumatoid and OA knee walk with a limp which increases with speed.

The knee is flexed and there is lateral trunk bending

Foot Abnormalities

1. High step	Here patient walks with a high stepping gait to clear the ground as in the case of foot drop
2. Push off	Weight is borne mainly on the heel and the entire foot leaves the flour simultaneously instead of the roll from heel to toes. Seen in tendo-Achilles rupture
3. Pes calcaneus	Here the patient uses the entire sole for push off. Seen in hammer toes, metatarsalgia, etc.

Trunk Abnormalities

1. Lordosis	During weight-bearing on the affected side, the lumbar curvature is increased and the upper trunk is displaced posteriorly. Seen in hip extensor, abdominal muscle weakness or both.
2. Anterior trunk bending	Here the patient bends the trunk forwards while walking. Seen in quadriceps weakness combined with weakness of gluteus, maximus, gastrocnemius or both.
3. Posterior trunk	Here the patient extends the upper trunk bending backwards while walking. Seen in hip extension and weakness of both the hips.

CNS Abnormalities

1. Rhythmic disturbances	In this condition the patient takes a quick short steps with the affected limb and a corresponding long slow step with the normal leg, e.g. Parkinsonism, ataxia.
2. Cerebellar gait (Drunken or reeling gait)	Here the gait is wide-based unsteady and irregular, seen in cerebellar dysfunction.
3. Gait in sensory ataxia	The leg is wide based, lifts the legs high and stamps the foot firmly on the ground. Seen in Friedreich's ataxia, etc.
4. Hemiplegic gait	Circumduction gait (see page 330)
5. Paraplegia gait	In spastic paraplegia, there may be crossing of the legs in front, e.g. scissors gait
6. Festinant gait (Parkinsonism)	Short steps, trunk bent forwards, arms flexed leg stiff and flexed at hip and knee.
7. Hysterical gait	The patient does not lift the leg, but drags it like a useless member of the body. Maybe monoplegic or paraplegic

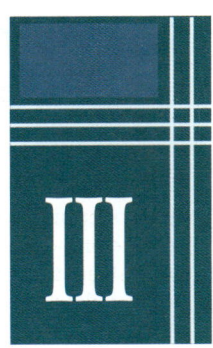

Appendix: Instruments and Implants in Orthopedics

For convenience and easy understanding, instruments used in orthopedic surgery can be categorized into three groups:
1. General surgical instruments
2. Regular orthopedic instruments
3. Instruments used in special orthopedic situations.
   Now let us try to analyse each one in detail.

GENERAL SURGICAL INSTRUMENTS

a. Surgical knife and blade is used to incise the skin and soft tissues.
b. Artery forceps is used to catch the bleeding vessels.
c. Allis forceps is used to catch the soft tissues.
d. Retractors are used to retract the soft tissues.
e. Scissors are used to cut the soft tissues.
f. Tissue holding forceps, needles, etc.
   The general surgical instruments help in the initial stage of surgery, for exposure, to deal with the soft tissue structures, to expose the bones, etc.

REGULAR ORTHOPEDIC INSTRUMENTS

After reaching the bone, general orthopedic instruments help to deal with the bone to place implants, etc. The following are the general orthopedic instruments mentioned in order of priority.

BONE HOLDING, PLATE HOLDING AND ROD HOLDING INSTRUMENTS

Instruments

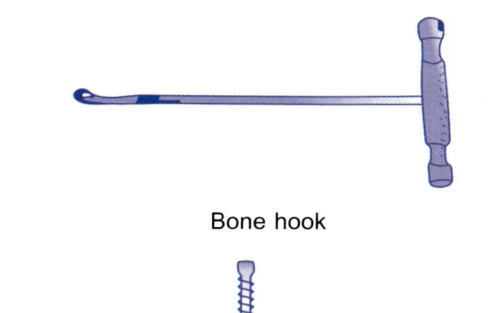

Bone hook

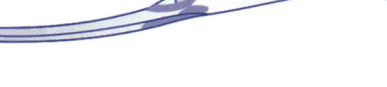

AO forceps

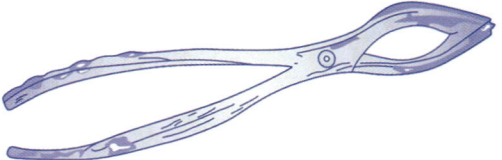

Fergusson's lion-toothed bone holding forceps

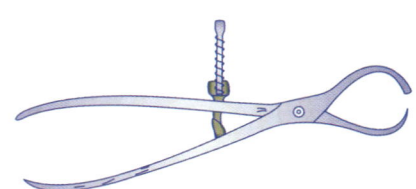

Patella forceps

INSTRUMENTS USED TO CUT, NIBBLE, CURETTE AND MAKE HOLES IN THE BONES

Instruments

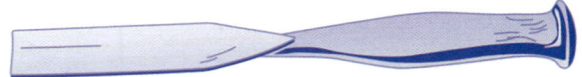

Smith-Peterson osteotome—straight

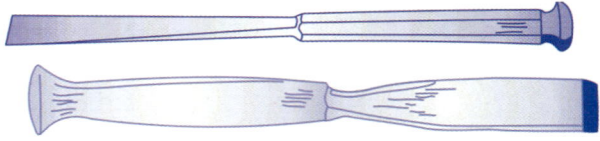

Stille type chisel—straight 7"
(sizes 5 to 30 mm with 5 mm variation)

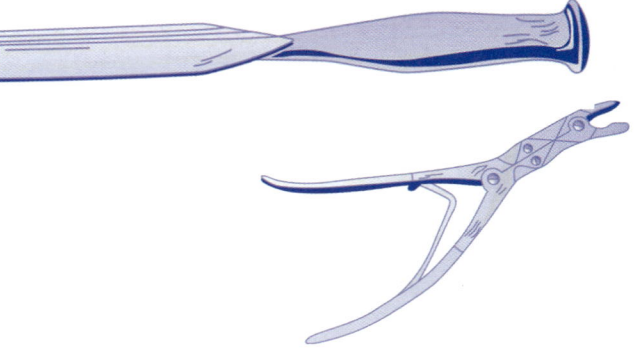

Leksell's rongeur (double action)

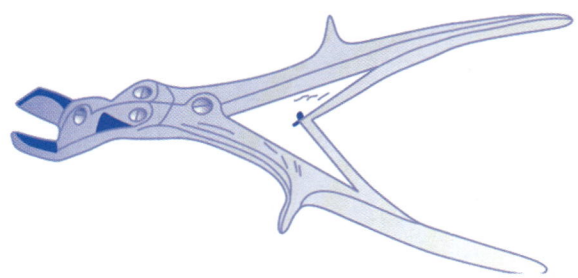

Stille-Horsley bone cutting forceps (10" length)

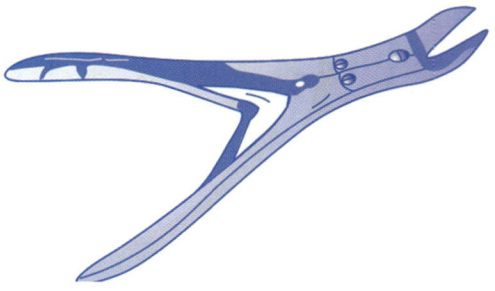

Ruskin bone cutting forceps (double action) 7½"

Cup curette (sizes 3 to 10 mm)

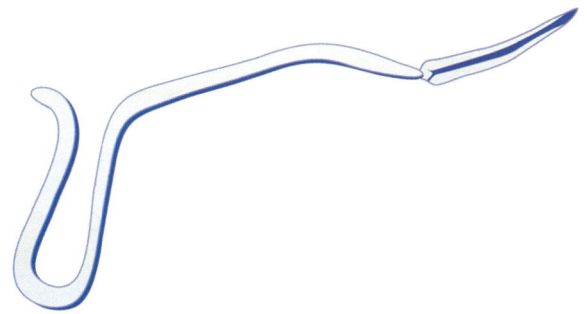

Kuntscher's diamond pointed AWL

MISCELLANEOUS ORTHOPEDIC INSTRUMENTS

Instruments

I. Periosteal Elevators

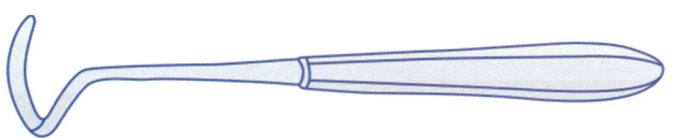

Doyan's periosteal elevator Adult—right/left

II. Bone Levers

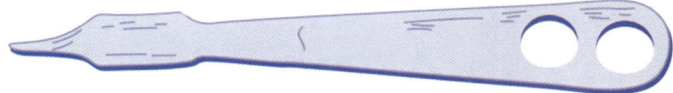

Retractor long narrow tip (for hip surgery)—width 18 mm

III. Fracture Reduction Forceps

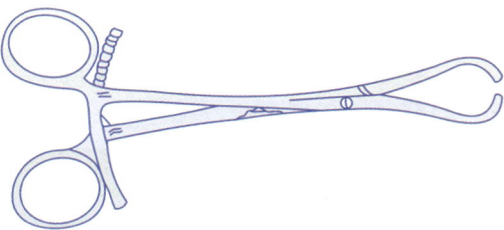

1. Ratchet lock

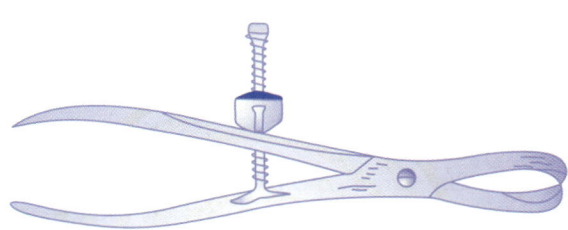

2. Speed lock

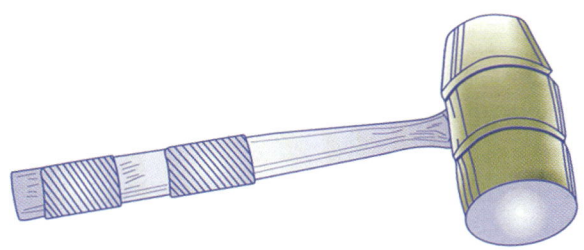

3. Mallet

INSTRUMENTS USED FOR INSERTION OF PLATE AND SCREWS

Instruments

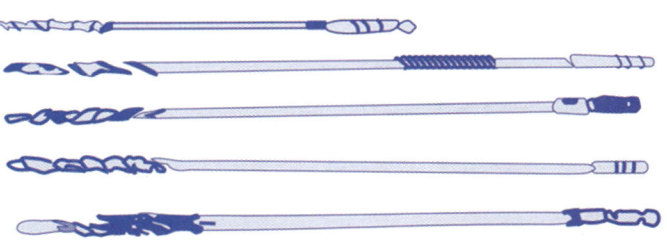

Drill bits

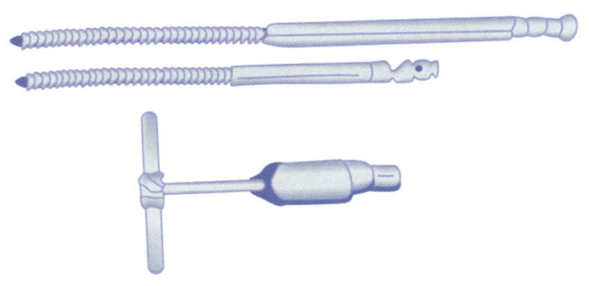

Tap and T-handle

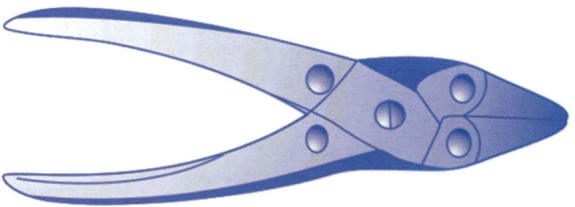

Cutting pliers

Depth gauge

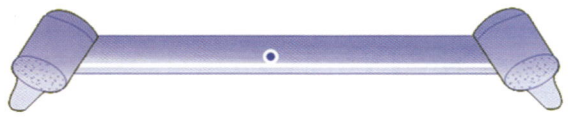

DCP drill guide position

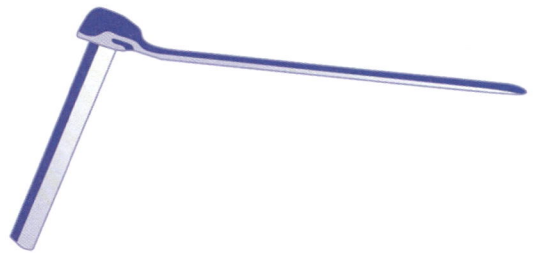

Protection sleeve

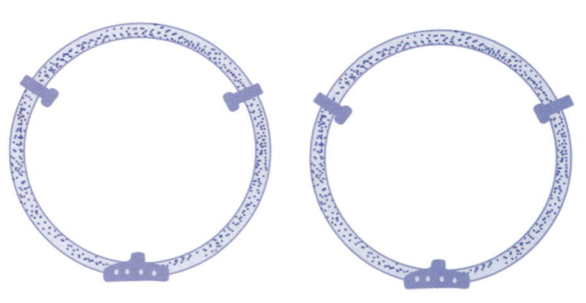

Circlage wire

IMPLANTS IN ORTHOPEDICS

Different types of Plates used in Orthopedics

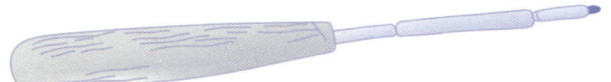

Hexagonal screwdriver

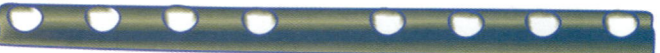

1. Semitubular plate

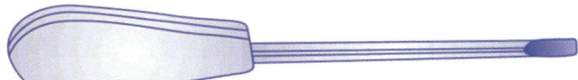

Ordinary screwdriver

2. Narrow DCP 4.5

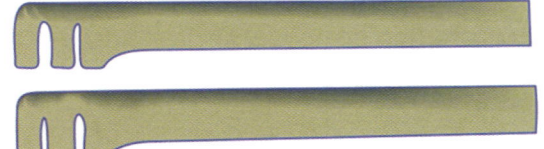

Plate benders

3. Narrow LC-DCP 4.5

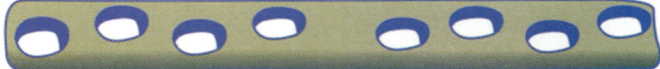

4. Broad DCP 4.5

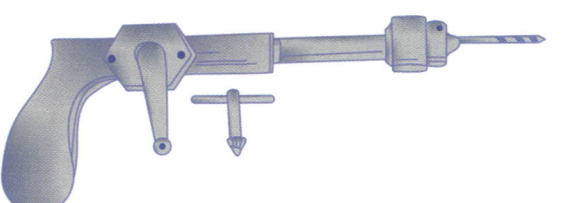

Hand operated drill and chuck

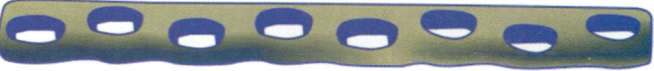

5. Broad LC-DCP 4.5

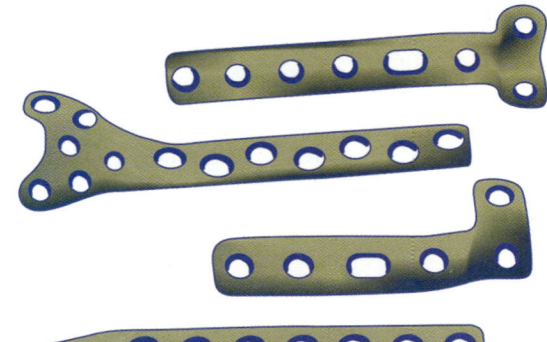

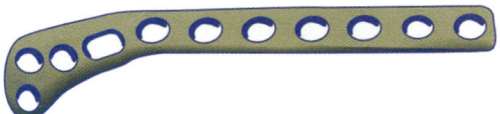

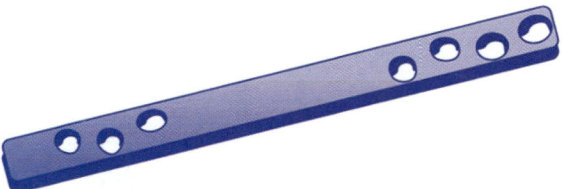

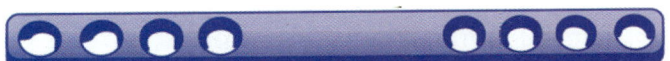

6. Form plates

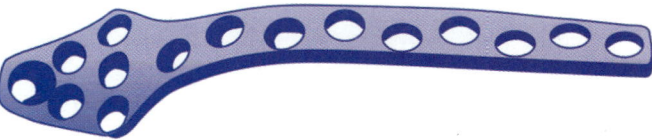

7. Broad lengthening plate

8. Narrow lengthening plate

9. Cobra head plate

Semitubular plate is used for fracture of subcutaneous bones like ulna

Note
Narrow DCP—is used for tibia and is not intended for femur
Broad DCP—is used for femur and humerus and is not intended for tibia
LC-DCP—is a limited contact dynamic compression plate.

Different Sets of Screws

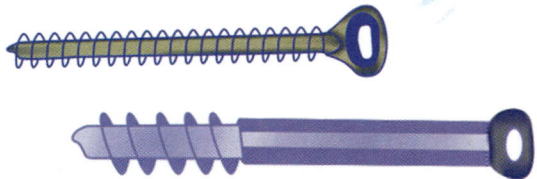

4.5 mm malleolar screw

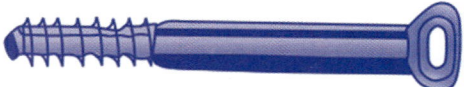

cortex screw
4.5 shaft screw

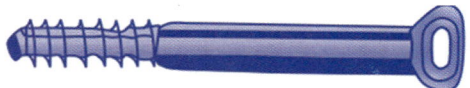

6.5 mm cancellous bone screw/fully threaded

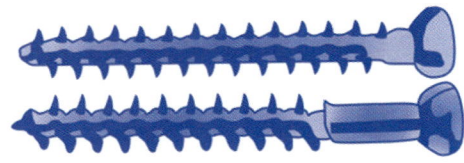

6.5 mm cancellous bone screw/32 mm

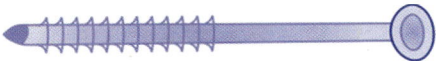

6.5 mm cancellous bone screw/16 mm

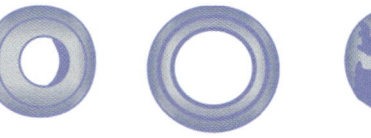

Nuts and washers

Different Conventional Intramedullary Nails

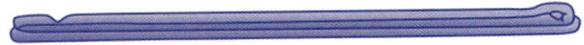

Küntscher's cloverleaf medullary
nail with two slots for femur (K-nail)

INSTRUMENTS USED FOR K-NAIL INSERTION FOR FEMUR

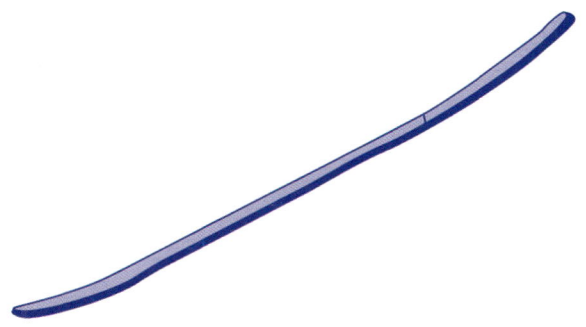

Nail set

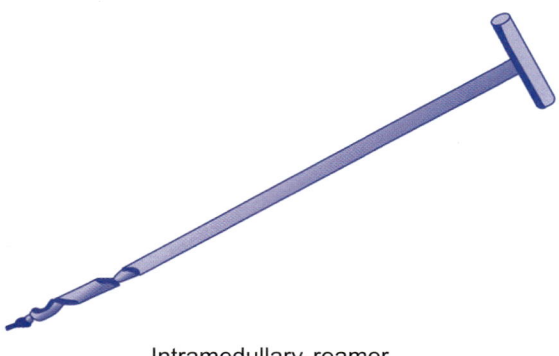

Intramedullary reamer
(Sizes 6 to 15 mm with 1 mm variation)

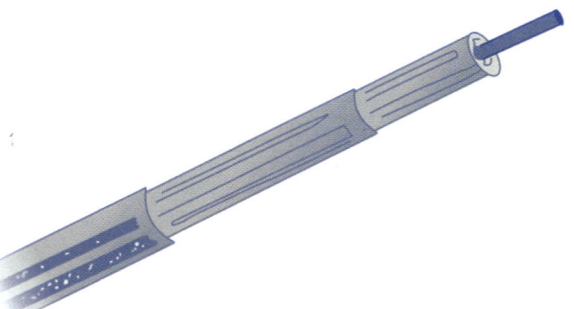

Küntscher's nail driver

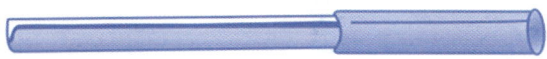

Küntscher's nail punch for final tapping

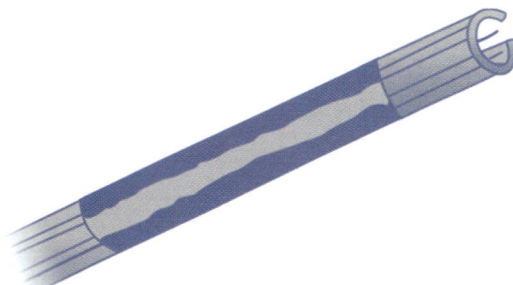

K-nail impactor

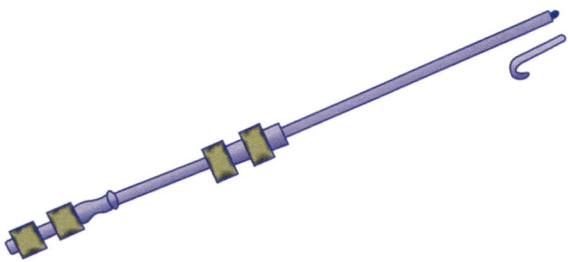

K-nail extractor with two hooks

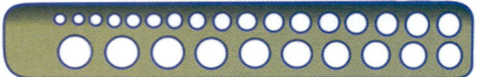

Diameter measuring gauge

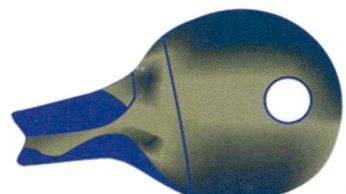

Tissue protector

PROSTHESIS OF THE HIP

Prostheses are used for replacement of head of femur following nonunion and avascular necrosis due to fracture neck of femur.

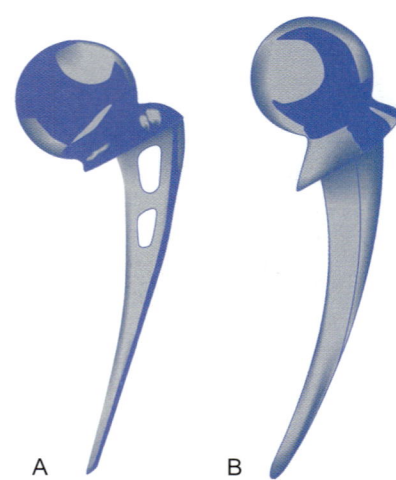

A   B

Figs III.1A and B: (A) Austin Moore and (B) Thompson's prosthesis

DIFFERENT HIP IMPLANTS

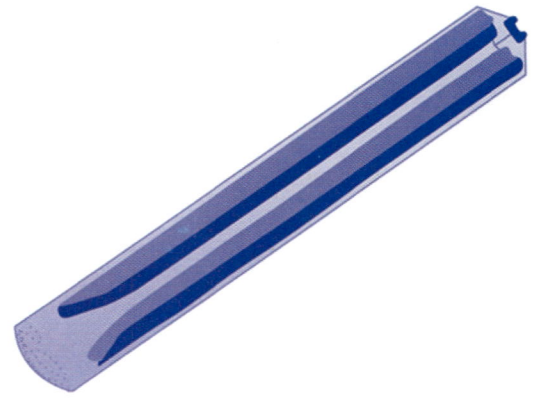

1. Fixed angles nails and plates (sizes 2.5" to 7" with 0.25")
   a. Smith-Peterson nail

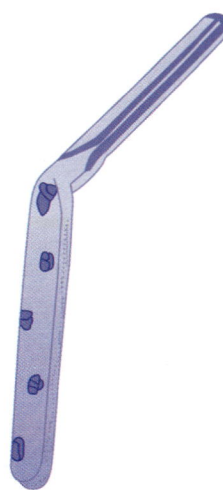

Rasp for intramedullary canal
reaming for AM prosthesis

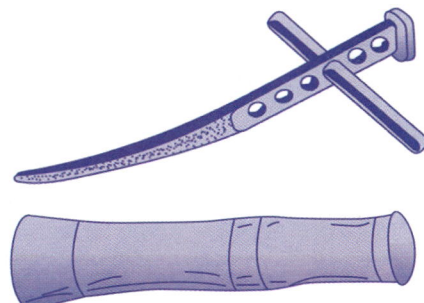

Alluminium impactor for AM prosthesis

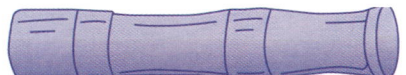

Alluminium impactor with tufnol
head for AM prosthesis

b. Jewett nail 120 DEG, pin length 2.5" to 4"
   with 0.25" variation (Plate sizes 3 to 6 holes)

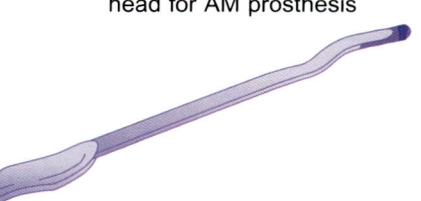

Murphy skid

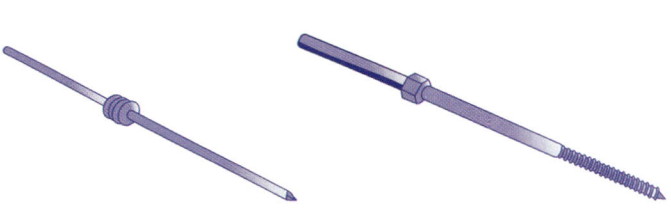

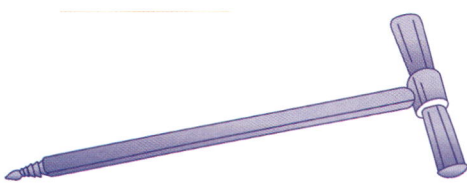

2. Hip fixation pins
   a. Moore pin with two nuts
      Sizes 2.5" to 5" with 0.25" variation
   b. Knowles pin 4 mm diameter
      Sizes 2.5" to 5" with 0.25" variation

Head extractor—Judet extractor

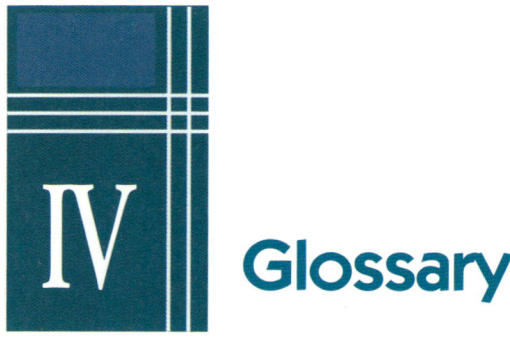

Glossary

IMPORTANT CLASSIFICATIONS IN ORTHOPEDICS

Spine

- Allen's—for cervical spine injuries.
- Anderson and D'olonzo's—for odontoid process fractures.
- McAffee's—for thoracolumbar fractures.

Upper Limbs

- Neer's—for proximal humeral fractures
- Gartland's—for supracondylar fractu: of the humerus (extension type).
- Bado's—for Monteggia's fractures in adults.
- John Weins—for Monteggia's fractures in children.
- Stimson's—for posterior dislocation of the elbow joint.
- Shorbe's—for side swipe injuries of the elbow.
- Colton's—for olecranon fractures.
- Frykmann's—for Colles' and Smith's fractures
- Mason's—for radial head fractures.

Pelvis Fractures

- Key and Conwell's.
- Tile's.

Lower Limbs

Hip Joint

- Garden's—for fracture neck of femur (intracapsular).
- Pauwell—for intracapsular fracture neck of femur.
- Perlington—for intracapsular fracture neck of femur.
- Delbet's—for fracture neck of femur in children.
- Seinsheimer's—for subtrochanteric fracture of femur.
- Thompson Epstein—for fracture dislocation of the hip.
- Fielding's—for subtrochanteric fracture of the femur.
- Judet—for central dislocation of the hip.
- Neer—for supracondylar fracture of the femur.

Knee and Proximal Tibia

- Smillie's—for meniscal injury.
- Hohl and Moore's—for fracture of the proximal tibia.
- Elli's—for fracture of shaft of tibia and fibula.

Ankle

- Lauge Hansen—for ankle injuries.
- Dennis Weber—for ankle injuries.

Foot

- Essex-Lopresti—for calcaneal fractures.
- HAWKINS—for talar neck fracture

Peripheral Nerve Injuries

- Sunderland.
- Seddon.

Epiphyseal Injuries

- Salter and Harris.

Miscellaneous

- Gustilo and Anderson's—for open or compound fractures.

IMPORTANT RADIOLOGICAL APPEARANCES

Hip Joint

- Trethovan' sign—seen in slipped capital femoral epiphysis.
- Risser's sign—seen in iliac bone epiphysis.
- Shenton's line—for hip dislocations and displaced hip fractures.
- Hilgenreiner's line—for CDH.
- Perkin's line—for CDH.
- Sagging rope sign—for Perthes' disease.
- Tear drop sign—for Perthes' disease.
- Garden's criteria—for fracture neck of femur.
- Salter extrusion angle—Perthes' disease.

Knee Joint

- Insaal and Blumensaat's lines—for patella alta.

Ankle Joint

- Hawkin's sign—avascular necrosis talus.
- Bohler's angle—for calcaneum.
- Crucial angle of Gissane—for calcaneum.

Shoulder

- Goldie's sign—for periarthritis or frozen shoulder.
- Maloney's line—for shoulder joint, similar to the Shenton's line.

Elbow Joint

- Crescent sign—absence of the normal radiolucent gap of the elbow on the lateral view.
- Tear drop sign—seen in the lateral view of the elbow.
- Anterior humeral line—a line drawn along the anterior border of the distal humeral shaft.
- Fish tail sign—the sharp anterior border of the proximal fragment in supracondylar fracture of the humerus.
- Coronoid line—a line directed proximally along the anterior border of the coronoid process of the ulna.
- Bauman's angle—angle between the horizontal line of the elbow and the line drawn through the lateral epiphysis and the long axis of the forearm.
- Maclaughlin's line—a straight line drawn along the center of the shaft of the radius cuts the capitulum in the center irrespective of the position of the elbow.

Hand

- Kaplan's lesion—presence of a sesamoid bone within the metacarpophalangeal joint of the finger (commonly index).
- Scapholunate angle—for carpal injuries.

Spine

- Aneurysmal sign—Pott's spine (anterior type).
- Scottish terrier sign—for spondylolysis due to fracture in pars.

Infection

- Sequestrum—seen in chronic osteomyelitis.
- Cloacae and involucrum—chronic osteomyelitis.
- Spina ventosa—tubercular dactylitis.
- Protrusio acetabuli, Mortal Pestle appearance—TB hip.
- Concertina collapse—TB spine.

Metabolic Disorders

- Champagne glass appearance—rickets.
- Moth-eaten appearance—renal rickets.
- Looser's or Milkman's line—osteomalacia.
- Pin head stippling—primary hyperthyroidism.
- Ground glass and biconcave vertebrae—osteoporosis.
- White line of Frankel—scurvy.
- Scurvy line—scurvy.
- Wimberger's line—scurvy.
- Pelkan spur—scurvy.

Developmental Disorders

- Shepherd's crook deformity—fibrous dysplasia.
- Ribbon ribs—von Recklinghausen's disease.
- Marble bone—osteopetrosis.
- Quadrilateral ilium—achondroplasia.

Congenital Disorders

- Von Rosen line—CDH.
- Kite's index—CTEV.
- Hourglass tibia—congenital pseudoarthrosis of tibia.

Bone Tumours

- Soab-bubble appearance—seen in giant cell tumour.
- Onion peel—seen in Ewing's sarcoma.
- Sunrise sign—seen in osteogenic sarcoma.
- Codman's triangle—seen in osteogenic sarcoma.
- Nidus—osteoid osteoma.
- Fluffy, cotton wool, bread crumb or popcorn—chondrosarcoma.
- Pedicle sign—multiple myeloma.

IMPORTANT FRACTURES WITH EPONYMS

Spine

- Hangman's fracture—fracture pedicle lamina of C2 vertebra.
- Jefferson fracture—fracture of C1 vertebra.
- Whiplash injury—ligament injury of the neck.
- Chance fracture—horizontal avulsion fracture of lumbar spine.

Upper Limbs

- Essex-Lopresti fracture—fracture head of the radius with dislocation of the inferior radioulnar joint.
- Nightstick fracture—fracture of the shaft of the ulna.

- Galeazzi fracture—fracture distal radius with subluxation or dislocation of the inferior radioulnar joint.
- Fracture of necessity—other name for Galeazzi.
- Reverse Monteggia's fracture—other name for Galeazzi.
- Colles' fracture—fracture distal end of radius.
- Smith's fracture—fracture distal end of radius with palmar displacement.
- Chauffeurs fracture—fracture of the radial styloid process.
- Bennett's fracture—intra-articular fracture of the base of the first metacarpal bone.
- Rolando's fracture—extra-articular fracture of the base of the first metacarpal bone.
- Jersey finger rupture of ulnar collateral ligament of the thumb.
- Baseball thumb avulsion of femur digitarum profundus from its insulin or distal phalanx (opposite of mallet finger).
- Mallet finger or baseball finger—avulsion of the extensor tendon from base of the distal phalanx.
- Barton's fracture—rim fracture of the distal end of the radius.

Pelvis

- Malgaigne's fracture—disruption of the pelvic ring with injury to the pubic symphysis and sacroiliac joint on the same side.

Lower Limbs

- Dash board fracture—fracture patella.
- Bumper's fracture—comminuted lateral condyle fracture tibia.
- Pott's fracture—bimalleolar fracture.
- Cotton's fracture—trimalleolar fracture.
- Aviator's fracture—fracture neck of the talus.
- Jones fracture—fracture base of the fifth metatarsal bone.
- March fracture—stress fracture of the second metatarsal bone.

IMPORTANT CLINICAL TESTS IN ORTHOPEDICS

Neck

- Adson's test—for thoracic outlet syndrome.

Shoulder Joint

Tests for anterior dislocation of shoulder:
- Bryant's test.
- Callaway's test.
- Dugas test.
- Hamilton ruler test.
- Regiment badge test—for axillary nerve injury.

Elbow Joint

- Cozen's test—for tennis elbow.
- Gunstock deformity—malunited supracondylar fracture humerus.
- S-shaped deformity—seen in supracondylar fracture humerus.

Forearm

- Volkmann's test—for Volkmann's ischemia of the forearm.

Wrist Joint

- Wrist drop—for radial nerve injury.
- Thumb and finger drops—for radial nerve injury.
- Finkelstein's test—for de Quervain's disease.

Hand

- Police tip deformity—for Erb's palsy.
- Claw hand—for ulnar nerve injury.
- Benediction test—for median nerve injury.
- Ape thumb deformity—for median nerve injury.
- Pointing index—for median nerve injury.
- Kanaval sign—for ulnar nerve bursitis.
- Froment's sign—for ulnar nerve injury.
- Tinel's sign—for peripheral nerve injury recovery.

Spine

- Anvil test—percussion by fist thumping to elicit spine tenderness.
- Straight leg raising test (SLRT)—passive straight leg raising test in disc prolapse.
- Fazerstazan test—SLRT with dorsiflexion of the foot.
- Lasegue test—hip flexed, knee flexed and the leg is slowly straightened.
- Buckling sign—after doing SLRT knee is suddenly flexed.
- Sicard test—after doing SLRT great toe is dorsiflexed.
- Well leg raise test—SLRT of the normal leg.
- Bilateral SLRT—SLRT of both the legs.
- Femoral nerve stretch test—reverse SLRT for high disc prolapse.
- Coin test—for TB spine.

Sacroiliac Joint

- Pump handle test.
- Gaenslon test.

Hip Joint

- Barlow test—test for CDH in the newborn.
- Ortolani's test—test for CDH in infant between 3 and 9 months.
- Galeazzi's test—knee flexion test for CDH.
- Thomas test—for fixed flexion deformity of the hip.
- Trendelenburg's test—test for abductor mechanism of the hip.
- Ober's test—test for iliotibial band contracture as in polio.

Pelvis

- Destot's sign—pelvic fracture.
- Roux's sign—pelvic fracture.
- Earle's sign—pelvic fracture.

Knee Joint

- Lachman's test—anterior drawer test at 30 degrees knee flexion in acute injuries.
- Drawer's test—for anterior cruciate ligament (ACL) tear.
- McMurray's test—test for meniscal injuries.
- Ludloff's test—for avulsion of the lesser trochanter.
- Apley's compression test—for meniscal injuries.
- Apley's distraction test—for knee collateral ligament injuries.
- O'Donoghue's triad—injury to the medial meniscus, medial collateral and anterior cruciate ligaments.
- Pivot shift test—for ACL tear.

IMPORTANT ORTHOPEDIC SURGERIES BY NAMES

Upper Limbs

Shoulder Joint

- Putti-Platt's—Overlapping and tightening of subscapularis tendon for recurrent dislocation of shoulder.

- Bankart's—detached anterior structures attached to glenoid rim by sutures.
- Bristow's—transplantation of coracoid process to anterior rim of the glenoid cavity in recurrent dislocation of shoulder.
- Staple capsulorrhaphy of Destot's and Roux—same as Bankart's but staples used instead of sutures.
- Magnusan and Stack—lateral advancement of subscapularis tendon.
- Eden Hybinette—anterior bone graft over glenoid and scapular neck.
- Maclaughlin—for posterior dislocation of the shoulder.

Elbow Joint

- French osteotomy—lateral closed wedge osteotomy for cubitus varus.
- King's osteotomy—medial open wedge osteotomy for cubitus varus.
- Max page—releasing of structures from medial epicondyle of humerus for VIC.

Wrist Joint

- Fernandez—dorsal wedge osteotomy for Colles.
- Campbell—lateral wedge osteotomy for Colles.

Lower Limbs

Hip Joint

- Souter—release of structures arising from anterior superior iliac spine (ASIS) for polio.
- Yount—sectioning of iliotibial band.
- Meyer—muscle pedicle (quadratus femoris) graft for posterior wall comminution in fracture neck of femur.
- Girdlestone—surgical excision of the hip joint.

Knee Joint

- Wilson—for flexion deformity of the knee.
- Hauser—for recurrent dislocation of the patella.
- Campbell—for recurrent dislocation of patella.

Foot

- Triple arthrodesis—fusion of the calcaneousboid, subtalar and talonavicular joints.
- Lambrinudi—for severe equinus deformity of the foot.
- Dwyer—lateral closed osteotomy for varus foot deformity.
- Evan—resection of calcaneocuboid joint for CTEV.
- Garceau—transfer of tibialis anterior to middle cuneiform for CTEV.
- Turco—one-stage release of posteromedial structures in mild CTEV.
- Mackay—one-stage release of posteromedial and posterolateral structures in severe CTEV.
- Grice-Green—subtalar fusion.
- Jones'—surgical correction of foot deformity.
- Keller's—surgical correction of halux valgus deformity.
- Steindler's—release of plantar fascia in cavus foot deformity.

TERMINOLOGIES ASSOCIATED WITH FRACTURES

- Fracture—a break in the continuity of the bone.
- Simple fracture—fracture that does not have an open wound in the skin.
- Compound or open—fracture in which there is an open wound at the skin or soft parts that leads into the fracture.

IV

- Comminuted fracture with multiple fragments.
- Avulsion fracture—small fracture near a joint that usually has a ligament or tendon attached to it.
- Impacted fracture—fracture whose ends are driven into each other.
- Displaced fracture—fracture whose ends are separated.
- Undisplaced fracture—fracture whose ends are not separated.
- Greenstick fracture—incomplete fracture due to break in one cortex of the bone in children.
- Pathologic fracture—fracture that occurs due to bone weakness due to a local or generalised bone disorder.
- Intra-articular fracture—fracture that involves a joint surface of a bone.
- Fatigue or stress fracture—fracture due to repeated minor stresses.
- Torus or buckle fracture—fracture caused by compression of the cortex most commonly in the distal region.
- Epiphyseal fracture—fracture of the growth plate usually in the long bones.
- Occult or hidden fracture—as clinical condition that suggests a fracture. Radiographs 2 to 3 weeks later may show the fracture line or a new bone formation.
- Nonunion—complete failure of fracture union.
- Malunion—union or fractured bone in a position other than anatomical.
- Cross-union—side to side union of fracture.

IMPORTANT ORTHOPEDIC TERMINOLOGIES

Joint

- Ankylosis—restriction of joint motion.
- Arthrodesis—surgical fusion of a joint.
- Arthroplasty—surgery to restore motion and function to a joint.
- Arthrotomy—opening of a joint.
- Effusion—escape of fluid into a joint cavity.
- Dislocation—complete disruption in the continuity of a joint.
- Subluxation—partial disruption in the continuity of the joint.
- Fracture dislocation—dislocation that occurs in conjuncton with a fracture of the bone if incomplete it is called fracture subluxation.
- Osteoarthritis—degeneration of a joint.
- Osteophytes—new bone growth due to degeneration of the joint.
- Arthrocentesis—joint aspiration.
- Arthroscopy—inspection of a joint through an arthroscope.
- Strain—muscle tear.
- Sprain—ligament tear.
- Genu—pertains to knee.
- Cubitus—pertains to the elbow.

Movements

- Flexion—forward bending of the joint.
- Extension—backward bending of a joint.
- Abduction—movement away from the midline.
- Adduction—movement towards the midline.
- Pronation—to rotate the forearm in such a way that the palm looks downwards when the arm is in the anatomical position.
- Supination—to rotate the forearm in such a way that the palm looks forward when the arm is in the anatomical position.
- Eversion—turning outward in the foot.
- Inversion—turning inward in the foot.

Spine

- Spondylitis—inflammatory condition of the spine.
- Spondylosis—degenerative condition of the spine.
- Spondylolysis—defect in the parts portion of the spine.
- Spondylolisthesis—slipping of one vertebra over the other.
- Kyphosis—curvature of the spine with posterior convexity.
- Lordosis—curvature of spine with anterior convexity.
- Scoliosis—abnormal lateral curvature of the spine.
- Radicular pain—shooting pain due to a spinal nerve involvement.
- Sciatica—shooting pain along the course of sciatic nerve.
- Laminotomy—opening made in the lamina.
- Hemilaminectomy—partial removal of the lamina.
- Laminectomy—complete removal of the lamina.
- Fenestration—opening made in ligamentum flavum between two laminae.

Foot and Ankle

- Equinus—plantar flexion of the foot.
- Calcaneus—dorsiflexion of the foot.
- Planus—flat foot.
- Cavus—hollow foot.
- Talipes—talus (ankle) + pes (foot).
- Pes—foot.
- Hallux—great toe.

Tendons and Nerves

- Tenotomy—cutting a tendon.
- Tenodesis—attaching a tendon to another tendon or bone.
- Tenolysis—freeing a tendon from adhesions.
- Tendon transfer—transferring a tendon from one site to the other.
- Neurolysis—freeing a nerve from adhesions.
- Neurorrhaphy—repairing a sectioned nerve.
- Neurectomy—sectioning a nerve.

IMPORTANT OSTEOTOMIES IN ORTHOPEDICS

Upper Limbs

- French—for cubitus varus deformity.
- King's—for cubitus varus deformity.

Hip Joint

- Mc Murray—for nonunion fracture neck femur.
- Shanz—for nonunion fracture neck femur.
- Pauwel—for nonunion fracture neck femur.
- Salter—for CDH.
- Pemberton—for CDH.
- Steel—for CDH.
- Chiari—for CDH.
- Derotation osteotomy—for CDH.
- Innominate osteotomy—for Perthes' disease.

Knee

- High tibial—for genu varus deformity in osteoarthritis.

Spine

- Spinal osteotomy—for ankylosing spondylitis.

Foot

- Dwyer's—for varus deformity of the heel.

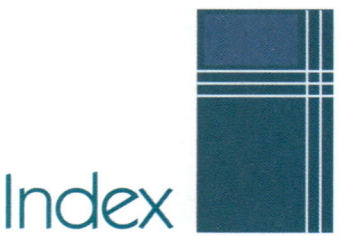

Index

Science of
Dental Materials
with Clinical Applications

Third Edition